F I R S T

PDR®

Drug Guide for Mental Health Professionals™

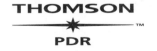

THOMSON
™
PDR

Contents

Foreword v

Section 1 1
Psychotropic Drug Profiles
In-depth descriptions of 72 medications used in the treatment of
emotional and psychological disorders.

Section 2 245
Interactions with Psychotropic Drugs
Details potential interactions with the psychotropic medications
described in Section 1, including ratings of onset, severity, and
evidence of the interaction.

Section 3 377
Common Prescription Drugs
Brief descriptions of the most frequently used prescription medications
and their uses. Includes over 1,100 entries.

Section 4 633
Mental and Emotional Side Effects
Part 1: Psychological Side Effects and Drugs That Can Cause Them, 633
Part 2: Common Drugs and Their Psychological Effects, 701

Section 5 783
Psychotropic Herbs and Supplements
Overviews of 35 herbs and nutritional supplements currently advocated
for relief of mental and emotional problems.

Appendix 845
Prescription Drugs with Potential for Abuse
Lists over 500 prescription drug products with high, medium, or low
potential for abuse.

Indices 853
Psychotropic Drugs Indexed by Brand and Generic Name, 853
Psychotropic Drugs Indexed by Indication, 855
Psychotropic Drugs Indexed by Category, 859
Psychotropic Herbs and Supplements Indexed by Indication, 861

iv

PDR® Drug Guide
for Mental Health Professionals™

FIRST EDITION

Foreword by Ronald J. Comer, Ph.D.
Director of Clinical Psychology Studies
Department of Psychology, Princeton University

Editor: David W. Sifton
Associate Editors: Edward P. Connor, Lori Murray
Assistant Editor: Gwynned L. Kelly
Project Manager: Catherine Accardi
Production Design Supervisor: Adeline Rich
Electronic Publishing Designers: Bryan Dix, Rosalia Sberna, Livio Udina

PHYSICIANS' DESK REFERENCE

Executive Vice President, Directory Services: Paul Walsh
Vice President, Clinical Communications and Strategic Initiatives: Mukesh Mehta, RPh
Vice President, Sales and Marketing: Dikran N. Barsamian
Director of Product Management: Valerie Berger
Senior Product Manager: Jeffrey D. Dubin
Senior Director, Publishing Sales and Marketing: Michael Bennett
Director of Trade Sales: Bill Gaffney
Direct Mail Managers: Jennifer M. Fronzaglia, Lorraine M. Loening
Promotion Manager: Linda Levine
Senior Director, Operations: Brian Holland
Manager of Production Operations: Thomas Westburgh
Senior Data Manager: Jeffrey D. Schaefer
Director of Client Services: Stephanie Struble
Fulfillment Manager: Louis J. Bolcik

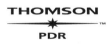

Officers of Thomson Healthcare: *President and Chief Executive Officer:* Richard Noble; *Chief Financial Officer and Executive Vice President, Finance:* Paul Hilger; *Executive Vice President, Directory Services:* Paul Walsh; *Senior Vice President, Planning and Business Development:* William Gole; *Vice President, Human Resources:* Pamela M. Bilash

ISBN: 1-56363-457-0

Foreword

The mental health field has changed enormously during the past half-century. Today fewer than one of every ten clinicians is a psychiatrist. In contrast to the 35,000 physicians currently in psychiatric practice in the United States, there are 70,000 psychologists, nearly 200,000 social workers, and 50,000 marriage and family therapists. It is for all these other clinicians that the *PDR Drug Guide for Mental Health Professionals* has been designed. Although they do not actually prescribe medications, these professionals often play a key collaborative role in medication decisions, and an increasing percentage of their psychotropic drugs. Clearly an effective drug guide is a necessity for today's mental health practitioner—and this book does an outstanding job of addressing this long-overlooked need.

In the past, the mental health field was dominated by narrow schools of thought and heated conflicts. Clients were forced to choose—between psychotherapy and medications, between psychologists and psychiatrists, between outpatient resources and inpatient care. Today, although the field is still marked by wide differences of opinion, approach, and professional training, there is a growing movement toward collaboration and integration. Practitioners have been pushed in this direction—sometimes kicking and screaming—by the results of clinical research.

Studies have revealed, for example, that psychotherapy and medication are each of great help to people suffering from depression. About two-thirds of such individuals are able to overcome their disorder when they receive cognitive, interpersonal, or certain other types of psychotherapy; a similar percentage are helped by antidepressant drug therapy; and, according to some research, an even higher percentage may be helped by a combination of the two approaches. A parallel story has unfolded in the treatments of panic, obsessive-compulsive, and several other disorders. Even treatments for schizophrenia and bipolar disorder—where medication typically plays a dominant role—are, according to research, greatly enhanced by the addition of psychotherapy, community interventions, and/or case management.

Just as medications and psychotherapy are often used together in the clinical field today, it is now common for psychiatrists and other mental health professionals to work side by side. In mental hospitals, clinics, and counseling centers, patients often work with a team of professionals, receiving medication from one, therapy from another, and, in some cases, case management from a third. Similarly, in private practice, clients' psychotherapy sessions with psychologists, social workers, or other professionals are often supplemented by visits to psychiatrists (also referred to as "psychopharmacologists" in this context) who focus exclusively on their medication needs. In all such instances, mental health professionals play a key role in drug therapy—whether by referring the client to the best psychopharmacologist, by discussing the case and the impact of medication with the psychopharmacologist, or by watching for the effects of medication—both wanted and unwanted—over the course of psychotherapy. It is also worth noting that this role may soon become even more prominent, since some state legislatures are now deciding whether to license psychologists to prescribe drugs.

All these changes in the clinical field point in the same direction: mental health professionals today must be as knowledgeable as possible about psychotropic drugs. A key resource in the acquisition and application of this knowledge is an effective drug reference, and, as I noted earlier, the *PDR Drug Guide for Mental Health Professionals* addresses this need extraordinarily well. There are a number of very useful features in this book. Let me cite several that I find particularly valuable.

First, the book is structured specifically to meet the needs of clinicians in practice. It readily provides complete profiles of each psychotropic drug, including such information as when and when not to use the drug, undesired effects, interactions with foods and other drugs, and other special precautions. One section of the book is even organized by side effect rather than drug name, to help clinicians determine whether a symptom is drug-related or not.

Second, the book reaches beyond psychotropic drugs to include information on psychotropic herbs and supplements, which have become such an important force in our society. Similarly it includes descriptions of the many other common prescription drugs that a patient may be taking along with psychotropic medication.

Third, the book is written without medical jargon in a manner that is clear, yet detailed and informative. This is not a cut-and-paste version of the *PDR*. It was obviously written especially for mental health professionals—taking into consideration their background as well as their clinical needs.

Whenever I am asked to write a foreword, my initial reaction is one of extreme caution and even reluctance. A foreword is, after all, perceived by some as an implicit endorsement, and is not something to be undertaken lightly. Obviously, I have been impressed by this book and by the importance of such a reference work given the current climate in the field of mental health care. In addition to the features that I have already mentioned, two other aspects of this book finally won me over and convinced me to write the foreword. One, the book emphasizes the *limitations* of each drug every bit as much as its potential strengths. It is not a "pro-drug" book. Instead, it simply seeks to inform professionals, even-handedly and authoritatively. Two, the book maintains a good feel for the importance of psychotherapy. For example, in the discussion of a drug for attention deficit hyperactivity disorder, the book states, "It is important to remember that the drug is only part of the overall management of ADHD, and that the doctor should also recommend counseling or other therapy." That is my kind of guide book—balanced, evidence-based, and genuinely informative.

Ronald J. Comer, P.h. D.
Director of Clinical Psychology Studies
Department of Psychology, Princeton University

Section 1

Psychotropic Drug Profiles

In this section you'll find detailed overviews of 72 medications commonly used in the treatment of mental and emotional disorders. The drugs are organized alphabetically by brand name and cross-referenced by generic name. The information is drawn from the drug's government-approved product labeling as submitted for publication in *Physicians' Desk Reference*®. Included are the drug's potential side effects and interactions, reasons the drug should *not* be prescribed, necessary precautions, typical dosage regimens, and signs of overdose. A more detailed review of each drug's possible interactions with other medications can be found in Section 2.

Brand name:

Adderall

Pronounced: ADD-ur-all
Generic ingredients: Amphetamines

Why is this drug prescribed?

Adderall is prescribed in the treatment of Attention Deficit Hyperactivity Disorder (ADHD). It is used as part of a broader treatment plan that includes psychological, educational, and social measures.

Adderall is also prescribed for narcolepsy.

Most important fact about this drug

Adderall, like all amphetamines, has a high potential for abuse. If used in large doses over long periods of time, it can cause dependence and addiction. It's important for patients to use Adderall only as prescribed.

How should this medication be taken?

Patients should use no more than the prescribed amount of Adderall. It should not be taken for a longer time or for any other purpose than prescribed.

The first dose should be taken upon awakening. If additional doses are prescribed, they should be taken at intervals of 4 to 6 hours. Patients should avoid late evening doses, which can interfere with sleep.

■ *Missed dose...*
If the patient is taking 1 dose a day, and at least 6 hours remain before bedtime, the dose should be taken as soon as remembered. If it's not remembered until the next day, the patient should skip the dose and go back to the regular schedule.

If the patient is taking more than 1 dose a day, and remembers within an hour or so of the scheduled time, the missed dose should be taken immediately. Otherwise, the patient should skip the dose and go back to the regular schedule.

Patients should never take 2 doses at once.

■ *Storage instructions...*
Adderall should be stored at room temperature in a tight, light-resistant container.

What side effects may occur?

Side effects cannot be predicted. If any develop or change in intensity, patients should inform their doctor as soon as possible.

■ *Side effects may include:*
Changes in sex drive, constipation, depression, diarrhea, dizziness, dry mouth, exaggerated feelings of well-being, headache, high blood pressure, hives, impotence, insomnia, loss of appetite, mental distur-

bances, overstimulation, rapid or pounding heartbeat, restlessness, stomach and intestinal disturbances, tremor, twitches, unpleasant taste, weakened heart, weight loss, worsening of tics (including Tourette's syndrome)

Why should this drug not be prescribed?

Adderall should never be prescribed for patients with any of the following conditions:

Heart disease
Hardening of the arteries
High blood pressure
High pressure in the eye (glaucoma)
Overactive thyroid gland

Patients should avoid using Adderall within 14 days of taking a drug classified as an MAO inhibitor, such as the antidepressants Nardil and Parnate. A potentially life-threatening spike in blood pressure could result.

Adderall should not be prescribed for patients who have ever had a reaction to similar stimulant drugs. Adderall is also contraindicated for patients who appear agitated or are prone to substance abuse.

Special warnings about this medication

Adderall should be used with caution if the patient has even a mild case of high blood pressure. Patients should be careful, too, about driving or operating machinery until they know how this drug affects them. It may impair judgment and coordination.

Adderall can make tics and twitches worse. If the patient or a family member has this problem (or the condition called Tourette's syndrome), the doctor should be made aware of it.

If the problem is attention-deficit disorder, the doctor should do a complete history and evaluation before prescribing Adderall, taking particular account of the severity of the symptoms and the age of the child. If the problem is a temporary reaction to a stressful situation, Adderall is probably not called for.

There are no data on long-term Adderall therapy in children. However, other amphetamine-based medications have been known to stunt growth, so the child should be watched carefully.

Possible food and drug interactions when taking this medication

If Adderall is taken with certain other drugs, the effects of either could be increased, decreased, or altered. Here is an overview of the drugs that may cause a problem:

Acetazolamide (Diamox)
Antihistamines such as Benadryl and Chlor-Trimeton

Antipsychotic drugs such as Haldol and Thorazine

Drugs classified as MAO inhibitors, including the antidepressants Nardil and Parnate

Drugs that make the urine more acid, such as Uroquid-Acid No. 2

Fruit juices and vitamin C

Glutamic acid (an amino acid related to MSG)

High blood pressure medications such as Calan, HydroDIURIL, Hytrin, Procardia, and Serpasil

Lithium (Eskalith)

Meperidine (Demerol)

Methenamine (Urised)

Norepinephrine (Levophed)

Propoxyphene (Darvon)

Seizure medications such as Dilantin, phenobarbital, and Zarontin

Tricyclic antidepressants such as Norpramin, Tofranil, and Vivactil

Special information about pregnancy and breastfeeding

Heavy use of amphetamines during pregnancy can lead to premature birth or low birth weight. Pregnant women should avoid taking Adderall unless absolutely necessary.

Amphetamines do find their way into breast milk, so patients should not take Adderall while breastfeeding.

Recommended dosage

Whether the problem is attention-deficit disorder or narcolepsy, the dosage should be kept as low as possible.

ATTENTION DEFICIT HYPERACTIVITY DISORDER

Children 3 to 5 Years of Age

The usual starting dose is 2.5 milligrams daily. Each week, the daily dosage may be increased by 2.5 milligrams until the condition is under control.

Children 6 Years of Age and Older

The usual starting dose is 5 milligrams once or twice a day. Each week, the daily dosage may be increased by 5 milligrams. Only in rare cases will a child need more than 40 milligrams per day.

Therapy may be interrupted occasionally to see if the drug is still needed.

NARCOLEPSY

Adults

The usual total daily dose ranges from 5 to 60 milligrams, taken as 2 or more smaller doses.

Children under 12 Years of Age
The usual starting dose is 5 milligrams daily. Each week, the daily dose may be raised by 5 milligrams until the condition is under control.

Children 12 Years of Age and Older
The usual starting dose is 10 milligrams daily, with weekly increases of 10 milligrams daily until the drug takes effect.

Overdosage
A large overdose of Adderall can be fatal. Warning signs of a massive overdose include convulsions and coma.

■ *Symptoms of Adderall overdose may include:*
Abdominal cramps, assaultiveness, changes in blood pressure, confusion, diarrhea, hallucinations, heightened reflexes, high fever, irregular heartbeat, nausea, panic, rapid breathing, restlessness, tremor, vomiting

If an overdose is suspected, seek emergency treatment immediately.

Generic name:
Alprazolam

See Xanax, page 230

Brand name:
Ambien

Pronounced: AM-bee-en
Generic name: Zolpidem tartrate

Why is this drug prescribed?
Ambien is used for short-term treatment of insomnia. A relatively new drug, it is chemically different from other common sleep medications such as Halcion and Dalmane.

Most important fact about this drug
Sleep problems are usually temporary and require medication for a week or two at most. Insomnia that lasts longer could be a sign of another medical problem. Patients should check with their doctor if they find that they need this medicine for more than 7 to 10 days.

How should this medication be taken?
Ambien works very quickly. Patients should take it just before going to bed, and should take no more than the prescribed dose.

■ *Missed dose...*
Ambien should be taken only as needed. Patients should never double the dose.

■ *Storage instructions...*
May be stored at room temperature. Protect from extreme heat.

What side effects may occur?
Side effects cannot be predicted. If any develop or change in intensity, patients should inform their doctor as soon as possible.

■ *More common side effects may include:*
Allergy, daytime drowsiness, dizziness, drugged feeling, headache, indigestion, nausea

■ *Less common side effects may include:*
Abdominal pain, abnormal dreams, abnormal vision, agitation, amnesia, anxiety, arthritis, back pain, bronchitis, burning sensation, chest pain, confusion, constipation, coughing, daytime sleeping, decreased mental alertness, depression, diarrhea, difficulty breathing, difficulty concentrating, difficulty swallowing, diminished sensitivity to touch, dizziness on standing, double vision, dry mouth, emotional instability, exaggerated feeling of well-being, eye irritation, falling, fatigue, fever, flu-like symptoms, gas, general discomfort, hallucination, hiccups, high blood pressure, high blood sugar, increased sweating, infection, insomnia, itching, joint pain, lack of bladder control, lack of coordination, lethargy, light-headedness, loss of appetite, menstrual disorder, migraine, muscle pain, nasal inflammation, nervousness, numbness, paleness, prickling or tingling sensation, rapid heartbeat, rash, ringing in the ears, sinus inflammation, sleep disorder, speech difficulties, swelling due to fluid retention, taste abnormalities, throat inflammation, throbbing heartbeat, tremor, unconsciousness, upper respiratory infection, urinary tract infection, vertigo, vomiting, weakness

■ *Rare side effects may include:*
Abnormal tears or tearing, abscess, acne, aggravation of allergies, aggravation of high blood pressure, aggression, allergic reaction, altered production of saliva, anemia, belching, blisters, blood clot in lung, boils, breast pain, breast problems, breast tumors, bruising, chills with high temperature followed by heat and perspiration, decreased sex drive, delusion, difficulty urinating, excessive urine production, eye pain, facial swelling due to fluid retention, fainting, false perceptions, feeling intoxicated, feeling strange, flushing, frequent urination, glaucoma, gout, heart attack, hemorrhoids, herpes infection, high cholesterol, hives, hot flashes, impotence, inability to urinate, increased appetite, increased tolerance to the drug, intestinal

blockage, irregular heartbeat, joint degeneration, kidney failure, kidney pain, laryngitis, leg cramps, loss of reality, low blood pressure, mental deterioration, muscle spasms in arms and legs, muscle weakness, nosebleed, pain, painful urination, panic attacks, paralysis, pneumonia, poor circulation, rectal bleeding, rigidity, sciatica (lower back pain), sensation of seeing flashes of lights or sparks, sensitivity to light, sleepwalking, speech difficulties, swelling of the eye, thinking abnormalities, thirst, tooth decay, uncontrolled leg movements, urge to go to the bathroom, varicose veins, weight loss, yawning

Why should this drug not be prescribed?

There are no known situations in which Ambien cannot be used.

Special warnings about this medication

When sleep medications are used every night for more than a few weeks, some may lose their effectiveness. People can also become dependent on sleep medications if they are used for a long time or at high doses. Anyone who has had previous problems with addiction to alcohol or drugs should make sure the doctor knows about it.

Some people using Ambien—especially those taking serotonin-boosting antidepressants—have experienced unusual changes in their thinking and/or behavior. Patients should alert the doctor if they notice a change.

Ambien and other sleep medicines can cause a special type of memory loss. It should not be taken on an overnight airplane flight of less than 7 to 8 hours, since "traveler's amnesia" may occur.

Until patients know whether the medication will have any "carry over" effect the next day, they should use extreme care while doing anything that requires complete alertness, such as driving a car or operating machinery. Older adults, in particular, should be aware that they may be more apt to fall.

Patients with liver problems should use Ambien with caution. It will take longer for its effects to wear off.

Patients should consult with their doctor before stopping Ambien if they've taken it for more than 1 or 2 weeks. Sudden discontinuation of a sleep medicine can bring on withdrawal symptoms ranging from unpleasant feelings to vomiting and cramps.

When taking Ambien, patients should not drink alcohol. It can increase the drug's side effects.

Patients with breathing problems may find that the condition worsens while they use Ambien.

Possible food and drug interactions when taking this medication

If Ambien is used with certain other drugs, the effects of either drug could be increased, decreased, or altered. Here is an overview of drugs that can cause a problem:

The antipsychotic agent, chlorpromazine (Thorazine)
The antidepressant drug, imipramine (Tofranil)
Serotonin-boosting antidepressants such as Paxil, Prozac, and Zoloft
Drugs that depress the central nervous system, including Valium, Percocet, and Benadryl

Special information about pregnancy and breastfeeding

Patients should inform their doctor immediately if they are pregnant or plan to become pregnant. Babies whose mothers take some sedative/hypnotic drugs may have withdrawal symptoms after birth and may seem limp and flaccid. Ambien is not recommended for use by nursing mothers.

Recommended dosage

ADULTS

The recommended dosage for adults is 10 milligrams right before bedtime. The doctor will prescribe a smaller dose if the patient is likely to be sensitive to the drug or has a liver problem. No one should ever take more than 10 milligrams of Ambien per day.

CHILDREN

Safety and effectiveness have not been established in children below the age of 18.

OLDER ADULTS

Because older people and those in a weakened condition may be more sensitive to Ambien's effects, the recommended starting dosage is 5 milligrams just before bedtime.

Overdosage

People who take too much Ambien may become excessively sleepy or even go into a light coma. The symptoms of overdose are more severe if the person is also taking other drugs that depress the central nervous system. Some cases of multiple overdose have been fatal. If an overdose is suspected, seek medical attention immediately.

Generic name:

Amitriptyline

See Elavil, page 66

Generic name:

Amitriptyline with Chlordiazepoxide

See Limbitrol, page 97

Generic name:

Amitriptyline with Perphenazine

See Triavil, page 212

Generic name:

Amoxapine

Pronounced: a-MOCKS-a-peen

Why is this drug prescribed?

Amoxapine relieves the symptoms of depression. It is believed to work by readjusting the balance of certain natural chemicals in the brain.

Most important fact about this drug

Serious, sometimes fatal, reactions can occur when drugs such as amoxapine are taken with the type of antidepressant classified as an MAO inhibitor. Drugs in this category include Nardil and Parnate. Amoxapine should be avoided within two weeks of taking one of these drugs.

How should this medication be taken?

It's not unusual to feel no immediate effect from this medication. However, relief of symptoms usually begins within 2 weeks, and sometimes in as few as 4 to 7 days.

Amoxapine can cause dry mouth. Sucking hard candy or chewing gum can help this problem.

■ *Missed dose...*

Patients who take amoxapine once a day at bedtime and don't remember until morning should skip the missed dose. If they take several doses per day, the forgotten dose should be taken as soon as it's remembered. If it is almost time for the next dose, they should skip the one they missed and return to their regular schedule. Doses should never be doubled.

■ *Storage instructions...*

Amoxapine can be stored at room temperature. It should be protected from excessive heat.

What side effects may occur?

Side effects cannot be predicted. If any develop or change in intensity, patients should inform their doctor as soon as possible.

■ *More common side effects may include:*

Anxiety, blurred vision, confusion, constipation, difficulty sleeping, dizziness, drowsiness, dry mouth, excessive appetite, excitement, fatigue, fluid retention, headache, increased perspiration, lack of muscle coordination, nausea, nervousness, nightmares, fluttery heartbeat, restlessness, skin rash, tremors, weakness

■ *Less common side effects may include:*

Abdominal pain, blood disorders, breast enlargement and excessive or spontaneous flow of milk in women, diarrhea, difficulty urinating, dilation of the pupils of the eye, disorientation, disturbed concentration, extremely high body temperature, fainting, fever, gas, hepatitis, high blood pressure, hives, impotence, incoordination, increased or decreased sex drive, itching, low blood pressure, menstrual irregularity, numbness, painful ejaculation, peculiar taste, rapid heartbeat, ringing in the ears, seizures, sensitivity to light, stuffy nose, teary eyes, tingling or pins and needles in arms and legs, upset stomach, vomiting, weight gain or loss

Why should this drug not be prescribed?

Amoxapine must be avoided by anyone taking an MAO inhibitor. (See "Most important fact about this drug.") Patients should also avoid this medication if recovering from a heart attack, or if they have ever had an allergic reaction to amoxapine or dibenzoxazepine medications.

Special warnings about this medication

Amoxapine may cause the facial and body twitching known as tardive dyskinesia.

Neuroleptic malignant syndrome (NMS) has also occurred in people using amoxapine. NMS is characterized by extremely high body temperature, rigid muscles, excessive perspiration, altered mental state, and irregular pulse, blood pressure, and heartbeat. If any of these symptoms develop, they should be reported to the doctor immediately.

Amoxapine should be used with care in patients who have difficulty urinating, and in those who suffer from increased pressure within the eye (glaucoma). It should also be used cautiously by anyone who has a seizure disorder or has had one in the past.

The antidepressant drug Prozac can increase the effects of amoxapine. If the patient is switching from Prozac to amoxapine, the doctor may wait 5 weeks or more before starting the new drug.

Patients with a heart condition should use amoxapine with caution. There have been reports of heart attack and stroke in patients taking this type of antidepressant.

Antidepressants can cause allergic reactions such as skin rashes or fever in some people. This usually occurs during the first few days of treatment. Patients should stop taking the medication and consult their doctor if these symptoms develop.

Amoxapine may cause drowsiness. Caution is warranted when driving, operating machinery or appliances, or doing any activity that requires full mental alertness until it's known how the patients reacts on amoxapine.

Possible food and drug interactions when taking this medication

Amoxapine may increase the effects of alcohol. Patients should not drink alcohol while taking this medication.

If amoxapine is taken with certain other drugs, the effects of either could be increased, decreased, or altered. Here is an overview of drugs that can cause a problem:

Antipsychotic drugs such as Mellaril and Thorazine
Barbiturates/sedatives such as phenobarbital and Seconal
Cimetidine (Tagamet)
Flecainide (Tambocor)
Fluoxetine (Prozac)
MAO inhibitors such as the antidepressant drugs Nardil and Parnate
Other central nervous system depressants such as Percocet and Halcion
Paroxetine (Paxil)
Propafenone (Rythmol)
Quinidine (Quinaglute)
Sertraline (Zoloft)

Special information about pregnancy and breastfeeding

Although the effects of amoxapine during pregnancy have not been adequately studied, stillbirths and decreased birth weight have appeared in animal studies. Amoxapine should be used only if the potential benefits outweigh the potential risks. Patients should inform their doctors immediately if they are pregnant or plan to become pregnant.

Amoxapine appears in breast milk and could affect a nursing infant. If this medication is essential to the patient's health, her doctor may advise her to stop breastfeeding until her treatment is finished.

Recommended dosage

Effective dosages of amoxapine may vary from one person to another.

ADULTS

The usual starting dosage is 50 milligrams 2 or 3 times daily. If the patient tolerates the drug well, the doctor may increase the dosage to 100 milligrams 2 or 3 times daily by the end of the first week. If that dose is not effective after 2 weeks, the doctor may increase the dose even further.

When the effective dosage has been established, the doctor may prescribe a single dose (not to exceed 300 milligrams) at bedtime.

CHILDREN

Safety and effectiveness have not been established in children under the age of 16.

OLDER ADULTS

In general, lower dosages are recommended for older people. The recommended starting dosage of amoxapine is 25 milligrams 2 or 3 times daily. If this is well tolerated, the doctor may increase the dosage by the end of the first week to 50 milligrams 2 or 3 times daily. A daily dosage of 100 to 150 milligrams may be enough for many older people, but some may need up to 300 milligrams.

Overdosage

Any medication taken in excess can have serious consequences. If an overdose is suspected, seek medical treatment immediately.

■ *Symptoms of amoxapine overdose may include:*
Coma, convulsions, kidney failure, severe, protracted epileptic seizures

Generic name:

Amphetamines

See Adderall, page 1

Brand name:

Anafranil

Pronounced: an-AF-ran-il
Generic name: Clomipramine hydrochloride

Why is this drug prescribed?

Anafranil, a chemical cousin of tricyclic antidepressant medications such as Tofranil and Elavil, is used in the treatment of obsessive-compulsive disorder.

Most important fact about this drug

Serious, even fatal, reactions have been known to occur when drugs such as Anafranil are taken along with drugs classified as MAO inhibitors.

Drugs in this category include the antidepressants Nardil and Parnate. Anafranil must never be combined with one of these drugs.

How should this medication be taken?

Anafranil should be taken with meals at first, to avoid stomach upset. After a regular dosage has been established, patients can take 1 dose at bedtime to avoid sleepiness during the day.

This medicine may cause dry mouth. Hard candy, chewing gum, or bits of ice may relieve this problem.

■ *Missed dose...*

Patients who take 1 dose at bedtime should consult their doctor if they miss a dose. The missed dose should not be taken in the morning. Patients who take 2 or more doses a day can take the missed dose as soon as they remember. If it is almost time for their next dose, they should skip the one they missed and go back to their regular schedule. Doses should never be doubled.

■ *Storage instructions...*

Anafranil should be stored at room temperature in a tightly closed container, away from moisture.

What side effects may occur?

Side effects cannot be predicted. If any develop or change in intensity, patients should inform their doctor as soon as possible.

The most significant risk is that of seizures. Headache, fatigue, and nausea can be problems. Men are likely to experience problems with sexual function. Unwanted weight gain is a potential problem for many people who take Anafranil, although a small number actually lose weight.

■ *More common side effects may include:*

Abdominal pain, abnormal dreaming, abnormal tearing, abnormal milk secretion, agitation, allergy, anxiety, appetite loss, back pain, chest pain, confusion, constipation, coughing, depression, diarrhea, dizziness, dry mouth, extreme sleepiness, failure to ejaculate, fast heartbeat, fatigue, fever, flushing, fluttery heartbeat, frequent urination, gas, headache, hot flushes, impotence, inability to concentrate, increased appetite, increased sweating, indigestion, inflamed lining of nose or sinuses, itching, joint pain, light-headedness on standing up, memory problems, menstrual pain and disorders, middle ear infection (children), migraine, muscle pain or tension, nausea, nervousness, pain, rash, red or purple areas on the skin, ringing in the ears, sex-drive changes, sleeplessness, sleep disturbances, sore throat, speech disturbances, taste changes, tingling or pins and needles, tooth disorder, tremor, twitching, urinary problems, urinary tract infection, vision problems, vomiting, weight gain, weight loss (children), yawning

■ *Less common side effects may include:*

Abnormal skin odor (children), acne, aggression (children), eye allergy (children), anemia (children), bad breath (children), belching (children), breast enlargement, breast pain, chills, conjunctivitis (pinkeye), difficult or labored breathing (children), difficulty swallowing, difficulty or pain in urinating, dilated pupils, dry skin, emotional instability, eye twitching (children), fainting (children), hearing disorder (children), hives, irritability, lack of menstruation, loss of sense of identity, mouth inflammation (children), muscle weakness, nosebleed, panic, paralysis (children), skin inflammation, sore throat (children), stomach and intestinal problems, swelling due to fluid retention, thirst, unequal size of pupils of the eye (children), vaginal inflammation, weakness (children), wheezing, white or yellow vaginal discharge

Why should this drug not be prescribed?

This medication cannot be used by patients who are sensitive to or have ever had an allergic reaction to a tricyclic antidepressant such as Tofranil, Elavil, or Tegretol.

Anafranil must be avoided if the patient is taking, or has taken within the past 14 days, an MAO inhibitor such as the antidepressants Parnate or Nardil. Combining Anafranil with one of these medications could lead to fever, seizures, coma, and even death.

Patients who have recently had a heart attack should not take Anafranil.

Special warnings about this medication

If the patient has narrow-angle glaucoma (increased pressure in the eye) or is having difficulty urinating, Anafranil could make these conditions worse. Anafranil should also be used with caution in patients with limited kidney function.

If the patient has a tumor of the adrenal gland, this medication could cause blood pressure to rise suddenly and dangerously.

Because Anafranil poses a possible risk of seizures, and because it may impair mental or physical ability to perform complicated tasks, patients should take special precautions if they need to drive a car, operate complicated machinery, or take part in activities such as swimming or climbing in which suddenly losing consciousness could be dangerous. Note that the risk of seizures is increased if the patient:

Has ever had a seizure
Has a history of brain damage or alcoholism
Is taking another medication that increases the risk of seizures

As with Tofranil, Elavil, and other tricyclic antidepressants, an overdose of Anafranil can be fatal. To minimize the risk of overdose, the doctor may prescribe only a small quantity of Anafranil at a time.

Anafranil may cause the skin to become more sensitive to sunlight. Prolonged exposure to sunlight should be avoided.

Before any kind of surgery involving the use of general anesthesia, the doctor or dentist should be informed that the patient is taking Anafranil. The drug may have to be temporarily discontinued.

When it is time to stop taking Anafranil, patients should not quit abruptly. Their doctor will have them taper off gradually to avoid withdrawal symptoms such as dizziness, fever, general feeling of illness, headache, high fever, irritability or worsening of emotional or mental problems, nausea, sleep problems, and vomiting.

Possible food and drug interactions when taking this medication

Patients should avoid alcoholic beverages while taking Anafranil.

If Anafranil is taken with certain other drugs, the effects of either could be increased, decreased, or altered. Here is an overview of the drugs that may cause a problem.

Barbiturates such as phenobarbital
Certain blood pressure drugs such as Ismelin and Catapres-TTS
Cimetidine (Tagamet)
Digoxin (Lanoxin)
Drugs that ease spasms, such as Donnatal, Cogentin, and Bentyl
Flecainide (Tambocor)
Methylphenidate (Ritalin)
Major tranquilizers such as Haldol and Thorazine
MAO inhibitors such as Nardil and Parnate
Phenytoin (Dilantin)
Propafenone (Rythmol)
Quinidine (Quinidex)
Serotonin-boosting drugs such as the antidepressants Luvox, Paxil, Prozac, and Zoloft
Thyroid medications such as Synthroid
Tranquilizers such as Xanax and Valium
Warfarin (Coumadin)

Special information about pregnancy and breastfeeding

The doctor should be informed immediately if the patient is pregnant or plans to become pregnant. Some babies born to women who took Anafranil have had withdrawal symptoms such as jitteriness, tremors, and seizures. Anafranil should be used during pregnancy only if absolutely necessary.

Anafranil appears in breast milk. Patients should not breastfeed while taking this medication.

Recommended dosage

ADULTS

The usual recommended initial dose is 25 milligrams daily. The doctor may gradually increase this dosage to 100 milligrams during the first 2 weeks. During this period the patient should take this drug, divided into smaller doses, with meals. The maximum daily dosage is 250 milligrams. After the ideal dose has been determined, the doctor may switch the patient to a single dose at bedtime, to avoid sleepiness during the day.

CHILDREN

The usual recommended initial dose is 25 milligrams daily, divided into smaller doses and taken with meals. Within 2 weeks, the doctor may gradually increase the dose to 100 milligrams or 3 milligrams per 2.2 pounds of body weight per day, whichever is smaller. The maximum dose is 200 milligrams or 3 milligrams per 2.2 pounds of body weight, whichever is smaller. Once the dose has been determined, the child can take it in a single dose at bedtime.

Overdosage

An overdose of Anafranil can be fatal. If an overdose is suspected, seek medical attention immediately.

■ *Critical signs and symptoms of Anafranil overdose may include:*
Impaired brain activity (including coma), irregular heartbeat, seizures, severely low blood pressure

■ *Other signs and symptoms of overdosage may include:*
Agitation, bluish skin color, breathing difficulty, delirium, dilated pupils, drowsiness, high fever, incoordination, little or no urine output, muscle rigidity, overactive reflexes, rapid heartbeat, restlessness, severe perspiration, shock, stupor, twitching or twisting movements, vomiting

There is a danger of heart malfunction and even, in rare cases, cardiac arrest.

Brand name:

Aricept

Pronounced: AIR-ih-sept
Generic name: Donepezil hydrochloride

Why is this drug prescribed?

Aricept is one of the few drugs that can provide some relief from the symptoms of early Alzheimer's disease. (Cognex, Exelon, and Reminyl are others.) Alzheimer's disease causes physical changes in the brain that disrupt the flow of information and interfere with memory, thinking, and behavior. Aricept can temporarily improve brain function in some Alzheimer's sufferers, although it does not halt the progress of the underlying disease.

Most important fact about this drug

To maintain any improvement, Aricept must be taken regularly. If the drug is stopped, its benefits will soon be lost. Patience is in order when starting the drug. It can take up to 3 weeks for any positive effects to appear.

How should this medication be taken?

Aricept should be taken once a day just before bedtime. Caregivers should make sure it's taken every day. If Aricept is not taken regularly, it won't work. It can be taken with or without food.

■ *Missed dose...*
It should be made up as soon as it's remembered. If it is almost time for the next dose, caregivers should skip the one that was missed and go back to the regular schedule. Doses should never be doubled.

■ *Storage instructions...*
Aricept may be stored at room temperature.

What side effects may occur?

Side effects cannot be predicted. If any develop or change in intensity, the doctor should be informed as soon as possible.

Side effects are more likely with higher doses. The most common are diarrhea, fatigue, insomnia, loss of appetite, muscle cramps, nausea, and vomiting. When one of these effects occurs, it is usually mild and gets better as treatment continues.

■ *Other side effects may include:*
Abnormal dreams, arthritis, bruising, depression, dizziness, fainting, frequent urination, headache, pain, sleepiness, weight loss

Why should this drug not be prescribed?

There are two reasons to avoid Aricept: an allergic reaction to the drug itself, or an allergy to the group of antihistamines that includes Claritin, Allegra, Atarax, Periactin, and Optimine.

Special warnings about this medication

Aricept can aggravate asthma and other breathing problems, and can increase the risk of seizures. It can also slow the heartbeat, cause heart-beat irregularities, and lead to fainting episodes. The doctor should be contacted if any of these problems occur.

In patients who have had stomach ulcers, and those who take a non-steroidal anti-inflammatory drug such as Advil, Nuprin, or Aleve,

Aricept can make stomach side effects worse. Aricept should be used with caution in such patients, and all side effects should be reported to the doctor.

Possible food and drug interactions when taking this medication

Aricept will increase the effects of certain anesthetics. The doctor should be made aware of Aricept therapy prior to any surgery.

If Aricept is taken with certain other drugs, the effects of either could be increased, decreased, or altered. Here is an overview of the drugs that may cause a problem:

Drugs that quell spasms, including Bentyl, Cogentin, and Donnatal
Bethanechol chloride (Urecholine)
Carbamazepine (Tegretol)
Dexamethasone (Decadron)
Ketoconazole (Nizoral)
Phenobarbital
Phenytoin (Dilantin)
Quinidine (Quinidex)
Rifampin (Rifadin, Rifamate)

Special information about pregnancy and breastfeeding

Since it is not intended for women of child-bearing age, Aricept's effects during pregnancy have not been studied, and it is not known whether it appears in breast milk.

Recommended dosage

ADULTS

The usual starting dose is 5 milligrams once a day at bedtime for at least 4 to 6 weeks. The dose should not be increased during this period unless directed. The doctor may then change the dosage to 10 milligrams once a day if response to the drug warrants it.

CHILDREN

The safety and effectiveness of Aricept have not been established in children.

Overdosage

Any medication taken in excess can have serious consequences. If an overdose is suspected, seek medical attention immediately.

■ *Symptoms of Aricept overdose include:*
Collapse, convulsions, extreme muscle weakness (possibly ending in death if breathing muscles are affected), low blood pressure, nausea, salivation, slowed heart rate, sweating, vomiting

Brand name:

Atarax

Pronounced: AT-a-raks
Generic name: Hydroxyzine hydrochloride
Other brand name: Vistaril

Why is this drug prescribed?

Atarax is an antihistamine used to relieve the symptoms of common anxiety and tension and, in combination with other medications, to treat anxiety that results from physical illness. It also relieves itching from allergic reactions and can be used as a sedative before and after general anesthesia. Antihistamines work by decreasing the effects of histamine, a chemical the body releases that narrows air passages in the lungs and contributes to inflammation. Antihistamines reduce itching and swelling and dry up secretions from the nose, eyes, and throat.

Most important fact about this drug

Atarax is not intended for long-term use (more than 4 months). The doctor should reevaluate the prescription periodically.

How should this medication be taken?

This medication should be taken exactly as prescribed.

■ *Missed dose...*

Generally, the dose should be taken as soon as remembered. However, if it is almost time for the next dose, the patient should skip the missed dose and go back to the regular schedule. Doses should never be doubled.

■ *Storage instructions...*

Tablets and syrup should be stored away from heat, light, and moisture. Syrup should be kept from freezing.

What side effects may occur?

Side effects cannot be predicted. If any develop or change in intensity, patients should inform their doctor as soon as possible.

Drowsiness, the most common side effect of Atarax, is usually temporary and may disappear in a few days or when dosage is reduced. Other side effects include dry mouth, twitches, tremors, and convulsions. The last two usually occur with higher-than-recommended doses of Atarax.

Why should this drug not be prescribed?

Atarax should not be taken in early pregnancy. It should be avoided by anyone who is sensitive to or has ever had an allergic reaction to it.

Special warnings about this medication

Atarax increases the effects of drugs that depress the activity of the central nervous system. If the patient is taking narcotics, non-narcotic analgesics, or barbiturates in combination with Atarax, the dosage should be reduced.

This medication can cause drowsiness. Driving or operating danger-ous machinery or participating in any hazardous activity that requires full mental alertness is not recommended until patients know how they react to Atarax.

Possible food and drug interactions when taking this medication

Atarax may increase the effects of alcohol. Patients should avoid alcohol while taking this medication.

If Atarax is taken with certain other drugs, the effects of either could be increased, decreased, or altered. Here is an overview of the drugs that may cause a problem:

Barbiturates such as Seconal and phenobarbital
Narcotics such as Demerol and Percocet
Non-narcotic analgesics such as Motrin and Tylenol

Special information about pregnancy and breastfeeding

Although the effects of Atarax during pregnancy have not been ade-quately studied in humans, birth defects have appeared in animal studies with this medication. Patients should avoid Atarax in early pregnancy, and inform their doctor immediately if they are pregnant or plan to become pregnant.

Atarax may appear in breast milk and could affect a nursing infant. If this medication is essential to the patient's health, the doctor may advise her to discontinue breastfeeding until her treatment is finished.

Recommended dosage

When treatment begins with injections, it can be continued in tablet form. The doctor will adjust dosage based on the patient's response to the drug.

FOR ANXIETY AND TENSION

Adults
The usual dose is 50 to 100 milligrams 4 times per day.

Children under Age 6
The total dose is 50 milligrams daily, divided into several smaller doses.

Children over Age 6
The total dose is 50 to 100 milligrams daily, divided into several smaller doses.

FOR ITCHING DUE TO ALLERGIC CONDITIONS

Adults
The usual dose is 25 milligrams 3 or 4 times a day.

Children under Age 6
The total dose is 50 milligrams daily, divided into several smaller doses.

Children over Age 6
The total dose is 50 to 100 milligrams daily, divided into several smaller doses.

BEFORE AND AFTER GENERAL ANESTHESIA

Adults
The usual dose is 50 to 100 milligrams.

Children
The usual dose is 0.6 milligram per 2.2 pounds of body weight.

Overdosage
Any medication taken in excess can have serious consequences. If an overdose of Atarax is suspected, seek medical attention immediately.

The most common symptom of Atarax overdose is excessive calm; blood pressure may drop, although it is not likely.

Brand name:
Ativan

Pronounced: AT-i-van
Generic name: Lorazepam

Why is this drug prescribed?
Ativan is used in the treatment of anxiety disorders, and for short-term (up to 4 months) relief of the symptoms of anxiety. It belongs to a class of drugs known as benzodiazepines.

Most important fact about this drug
Tolerance and dependence can develop with the use of Ativan. Patients may experience withdrawal symptoms if they stop using it abruptly. A change in dose or discontinuation of the drug should be done only under the supervision of a doctor.

How should this medication be taken?
This medication should be taken exactly as prescribed.

■ *Missed dose...*
If it is within an hour or so of the scheduled time, the forgotten dose should be taken as soon as remembered. Otherwise, it should be skipped and the patient should go back to the regular schedule. Doses should never be doubled.

■ *Storage instructions...*
Ativan should be stored at room temperature in a tightly closed container, away from light.

What side effects may occur?
Side effects cannot be predicted. If any develop or change in intensity, patients should inform their doctor as soon as possible.
If any side effects develop, they will usually surface at the beginning of treatment. They will probably disappear as the patient continues to take the drug, or if the dosage is reduced.

■ *More common side effects may include:*
Dizziness, sedation, unsteadiness, weakness

■ *Less common or rare side effects may include:*
Agitation, change in appetite, depression, eye function disorders, headache, memory impairment, mental disorientation, nausea, skin problems, sleep disturbance, stomach and intestinal disorders

■ *Side effects due to rapid decrease or abrupt withdrawal of Ativan:*
Abdominal and muscle cramps, convulsions, depressed mood, inability to fall or stay asleep, sweating, tremors, vomiting

Why should this drug not be prescribed?
Patients who are sensitive to or have ever had an allergic reaction to Ativan or similar drugs such as Valium should not take this medication.

Ativan should also be avoided if the patient has acute narrow-angle glaucoma (a type of high pressure in the eyes).

Anxiety or tension related to everyday stress usually does not require treatment with Ativan. Symptoms should be thoroughly evaluated prior to treatment.

Special warnings about this medication
Ativan may cause patients to become drowsy or less alert. Therefore, driving or operating dangerous machinery or participating in any hazardous activity that requires full mental alertness is not recommended.

This drug should be used with caution in patients who are severely depressed or have suffered from severe depression. A risk of suicide exists.

Ativan should also be used cautiously in patients with decreased kidney or liver function.

Older patients and those who have been using Ativan for a prolonged period of time should be closely watched for stomach and upper intestinal problems.

Possible food and drug interactions when taking this medication

Ativan may intensify the effects of alcohol. Patients should avoid alcohol while taking this medication.

If Ativan is taken with certain other drugs, the effects of either could be increased, decreased, or altered. It is especially important for patients to check with their doctor before combining Ativan with barbiturates (phenobarbital, Seconal, Amytal) or sedative-type medications such as Valium and Halcion.

Special information about pregnancy and breastfeeding

The patient should avoid Ativan if she is pregnant or planning to become pregnant. There is an increased risk of birth defects.

It is not known whether Ativan appears in breast milk like other drugs in this class. However, breastfeeding is not recommended.

Recommended dosage

ADULTS

The usual dosage is a total of 2 to 6 milligrams per day divided into smaller doses. The largest dose should be taken at bedtime. The daily dose may vary from 1 to 10 milligrams.

Anxiety

The usual starting dose is a total of 2 to 3 milligrams per day taken in 2 or 3 smaller doses.

Insomnia Due to Anxiety

A single daily dose of 2 to 4 milligrams may be taken, usually at bedtime.

CHILDREN

The safety and effectiveness of Ativan have not been established in children under 12 years of age.

OLDER ADULTS

To avoid oversedation, the usual starting dosage for older adults and those in a weakened condition should not exceed a total of 1 to 2 milligrams per day, divided into smaller doses. This dose can be adjusted by the doctor as needed.

Overdosage

Any medication taken in excess can have serious consequences. An overdose of Ativan can be fatal, though this is rare. If an overdose is suspected, seek medical attention immediately.

■ *The symptoms of Ativan overdose may include:*
Coma, confusion, drowsiness, hypnotic state, lack of coordination, low blood pressure, sluggishness

Brand name:

Aventyl

See Pamelor, page 132

Generic name:

Bupropion

See Wellbutrin, page 226

Brand name:

BuSpar

Pronounced: BYOO-spar
Generic name: Buspirone hydrochloride

Why is this drug prescribed?
BuSpar is used in the treatment of anxiety disorders and for short-term relief of the symptoms of anxiety.

Most important fact about this drug
BuSpar should not be used with drugs classified as monoamine oxidase (MAO) inhibitors, such as the antidepressants Nardil and Parnate.

How should this medication be taken?
Patients should not be discouraged if they feel no immediate effect. The full benefit of this drug may not be seen for 1 to 2 weeks.

■ *Missed dose...*
Patients should take a forgotten dose as soon as they remember, unless it is almost time for the next dose. If that's the case, they should skip the one they missed and go back to their regular schedule. Doses should never be doubled.

■ *Storage instructions...*
BuSpar should be stored at room temperature in a tightly closed container, away from light.

What side effects may occur?
Side effects cannot be predicted. If any develop or change in intensity, patients should inform their doctor as soon as possible.

■ *More common side effects may include:*
Dizziness, dry mouth, fatigue, headache, light-headedness, nausea, nervousness, unusual excitement

■ *Less common or rare side effects may include:*
Anger/hostility, blurred vision, bone aches/pain, confusion, constipa-

tion, decreased concentration, depression, diarrhea, fast, fluttery heartbeat, incoordination, muscle pain/aches, numbness, pain or weakness in hands or feet, rapid heartbeat, rash, restlessness, stomach and abdominal upset, sweating/clamminess, tingling or pins and needles, tremor, urinary incontinence, vomiting, weakness

Why should this drug not be prescribed?

This drug should be avoided by patients who are sensitive to or have ever had an allergic reaction to BuSpar or similar mood-altering drugs. BuSpar is also inappropriate for people with severe kidney or liver damage.

Anxiety or tension related to everyday stress usually does not require treatment with BuSpar. Symptoms should be thoroughly assessed prior to treatment.

Special warnings about this medication

The effects of BuSpar on the central nervous system are unpredictable. Patients should avoid driving, operating dangerous machinery, or participating in any hazardous activity while they are taking BuSpar.

Possible food and drug interactions when taking this medication

Although BuSpar does not intensify the effects of alcohol, it is best to avoid alcohol while taking this medication.

If BuSpar is taken with certain other drugs, the effects of either can be increased, decreased, or altered. Here is an overview of the drugs that may cause a problem:

The blood-thinning drug Coumadin
Haloperidol (Haldol)
MAO inhibitors such as the antidepressants Nardil and Parnate
Trazodone (Desyrel)

Special information about pregnancy and breastfeeding

The effects of BuSpar during pregnancy have not been adequately studied. Patients should inform their doctor immediately if they are pregnant or plan to become pregnant.

It is not known whether BuSpar appears in breast milk. If this medication is essential to the patient's health, the doctor may advise her to discontinue breastfeeding until her treatment is finished.

Recommended dosage

ADULTS

The recommended starting dose is a total of 15 milligrams per day divided into smaller doses, usually 5 milligrams 3 times a day. Every 2 to 3 days, the doctor may increase the dosage 5 milligrams per day as needed. The daily dose should not exceed 60 milligrams.

CHILDREN

The safety and effectiveness of BuSpar have not been established in children under 18 years of age.

Overdosage

Any medication taken in excess can have serious consequences. If an overdose of BuSpar is suspected, seek medical attention immediately.

■ *The symptoms of BuSpar overdose may include:*
Dizziness, drowsiness, nausea or vomiting, severe stomach upset, unusually small pupils.

Generic name:

Buspirone

See BuSpar, page 23

Brand name:

Celexa

Pronounced: sell-EX-ah
Generic name: Citalopram hydrobromide

Why is this drug prescribed?

Celexa is used to treat major depression. Like the antidepressant medications Paxil, Prozac, and Zoloft, Celexa is thought to work by boosting serotonin levels in the brain. Serotonin, one of the nervous system's primary chemical messengers, is known to elevate mood.

Most important fact about this drug

Celexa must not be taken for 2 weeks before or after using an antidepressant known as an MAO inhibitor. Drugs in this category include Nardil and Parnate. Combining Celexa with one of these medications could lead to a serious—even fatal—reaction.

How should this medication be taken?

Celexa is taken once a day, in the morning or evening, with or without food. It's important to take Celexa regularly, even when feeling better. Depression typically begins to lift in 1 to 4 weeks, but it takes several months for the medication to yield its full benefits.

■ *Missed dose...*
Generally, the forgotten dose should be taken as soon as remembered. However, if it is almost time for the next dose, patients should skip the one they missed and go back to their regular schedule. Doses should never be doubled.

■ *Storage instructions...*
Celexa may be stored at room temperature.

What side effects may occur?
Side effects cannot be predicted. If any develop or change in intensity, patients should inform their doctor as soon as possible.

■ *More common side effects may include:*
Abdominal pain, agitation, anxiety, diarrhea, drowsiness, dry mouth, ejaculation disorders, fatigue, impotence, indigestion, insomnia, loss of appetite, nausea, painful menstruation, respiratory tract infection, sinus or nasal inflammation, sweating, tremor, vomiting

■ *Less common side effects may include:*
Amnesia, attempted suicide, confusion, coughing, decreased sexual drive, depression, excessive urination, fever, gas, impaired concentration, increased appetite, increased salivation, itching, joint pain, lack of emotion, loss of menstruation, low blood pressure, migraine, muscle pain, rapid heartbeat, rash, skin tingling, taste disturbances, visual disturbances, weight gain, weight loss, yawning

■ *Rare side effects may include:*
Abnormal dreams, acne, aggressive behavior, alcohol intolerance, angina (chest pain), arthritis, belching, bone pain, breast enlargement, breast pain, bronchitis, bruising, chills, conjunctivitis (pinkeye), decreased muscle movements, delusions, dermatitis, difficulty breathing, difficulty swallowing, dizziness, drug dependence, dry eyes, dry skin, eczema, emotional instability, excessive milk flow, excessive muscle tone, eye pain, fainting, feeling of well-being, flu-like symptoms, flushing, frequent urination, gum inflammation, hair loss, hallucinations, heart attack, heart failure, hemorrhoids, high blood pressure, hives, hot flashes, inability to hold urine, inability to urinate completely, increased sex drive, increased urination, involuntary muscle movements, leg cramps, mouth sores, muscle weakness, nosebleeds, numbness, painful erection, painful urination, panic, paranoia, pneumonia, psoriasis, psychosis, ringing in the ears, sensitivity to light, skin discoloration, slow heartbeat, stomach and intestinal inflammation, stroke, swelling, teeth grinding, thirst, uncontrollable muscle movements, unsteady or abnormal walk, vaginal bleeding

Why should this drug not be prescribed?
If Celexa gives the patient an allergic reaction, it cannot be used. Also remember that Celexa must never be combined with an MAO inhibitor (see "Most important fact about this drug," above).

Special warnings about this medication
In recommended doses, Celexa does not seem to impair judgment or motor skills. However, a theoretical possibility of such problems

remains, so caution is advisable when driving or operating dangerous equipment until Celexa's effect is known.

There is a slight chance that Celexa will trigger a manic episode. Celexa should be used with caution in patients who suffer from bipolar disorder. Caution is also warranted in patients who are over 60 years old, have liver or kidney problems, suffer from heart disease or high blood pressure, or have ever had seizures.

Possible food and drug interactions when taking this medication

Celexa does not increase the effects of alcohol. Nevertheless, it's considered unwise to combine Celexa with alcohol or any other drug that affects the brain. (It's especially important to avoid MAO inhibitors.)

If Celexa is taken with certain other drugs, the effects of either could be increased, decreased, or altered. It's best to check with the doctor before combining any new prescription or over-the-counter drugs with Celexa. Here's an overview of the drugs most likely to cause a problem:

Carbamazepine (Tegretol)
Cimetidine (Tagamet)
Erythromycin (Eryc, Ery-Tab)
Fluconazole (Diflucan)
Itraconazole (Sporanox)
Ketoconazole (Nizoral)
Lithium (Eskalith, Lithobid)
Metoprolol (Lopressor)
Omeprazole (Prilosec)
Other antidepressants such as Elavil, Norpramin, Pamelor, and Tofranil
Sumatriptan (Imitrex)
Warfarin (Coumadin)

Special information about pregnancy and breastfeeding

The effects of Celexa during pregnancy have not been adequately studied, and the potential for harm has not been ruled out. Any patient who becomes pregnant or plans to become pregnant while on Celexa therapy should contact her doctor immediately.

Celexa appears in breast milk and will affect the nursing infant. Patients will need to choose between breastfeeding or continuing Celexa therapy.

Recommended dosage

ADULTS

The recommended starting dose is 20 milligrams once a day. Dosage is usually increased to 40 milligrams once daily after at least a week has passed. Doses above 40 milligrams a day are generally not recommended.

For older adults and those who have liver problems, the recommended dose is 20 milligrams once a day.

Overdosage

Any medication taken in excess can have serious consequences. If an overdose is suspected, seek medical attention immediately.

■ *Symptoms of Celexa overdose may include:*
Amnesia, bluish or purplish discoloration of the skin, coma, confusion, convulsions, dizziness, drowsiness, hyperventilation, nausea, rapid heartbeat, sweating, tremor, vomiting

Generic name:
Chlordiazepoxide

See Librium, page 94

Generic name:
Chlorpromazine

See Thorazine, page 201

Generic name:
Citalopram

See Celexa, page 25

Generic name:
Clomipramine

See Anafranil, page 11

Generic name:
Clonazepam

See Klonopin, page 90

Generic name:

Clorazepate

See *Tranxene, page 209*

Generic name:

Clozapine

See *Clozaril, page 29*

Brand name:

Clozaril

Pronounced: *KLOH-zah-ril*
Generic name: *Clozapine*

Why is this drug prescribed?

Clozaril is prescribed for people with severe schizophrenia who have failed to respond to standard treatments. Like all antipsychotic agents, Clozaril is not a cure, but it can help some people return to more normal lives.

Most important fact about this drug

Even though it does not produce some of the disturbing side effects of other antipsychotic medications, Clozaril may cause agranulocytosis, a potentially lethal disorder of the white blood cells. Because of the risk of agranulocytosis, anyone who takes Clozaril is required to have a blood test once a week for the first 6 months. The drug is carefully controlled so that those taking it must get their weekly blood test before receiving the following week's supply of medication. After 6 months of acceptable blood counts, patients are allowed to switch to an every-other-week testing schedule. Anyone whose blood test results are abnormal will be taken off Clozaril either temporarily or permanently, depending on the results of an additional 4 weeks of testing.

How should this medication be taken?

It is important to take Clozaril exactly as directed. Because of the significant risk of serious side effects associated with this drug, patients should be periodically reassessed for continuation of Clozaril therapy. Clozaril is distributed only through the Clozaril Patient Management System, which ensures regular white blood cell testing, monitoring, and pharmacy services prior to delivery of the next supply.

Clozaril may be taken with or without food.

■ *Missed dose...*

Generally, the forgotten dose should be taken as soon as remembered. However, if it is almost time for the next dose, patients should skip the one they missed and go back to their regular schedule. Doses should never be doubled.

If the patient stops taking Clozaril for more than 2 days, it should not be started again without first consulting the physician.

■ *Storage instructions...*

Clozaril may be stored at room temperature.

What side effects may occur?

Side effects cannot be predicted. If any develop or change in intensity, patients should inform their doctor as soon as possible.

The most feared side effect is agranulocytosis, a dangerous drop in the number of a certain kind of white blood cells. Symptoms include fever, lethargy, sore throat, and weakness. If not caught in time, agranulocytosis can be fatal. That is why all people who take Clozaril must have a blood test every week. About 1 percent develop agranulocytosis and must stop taking the drug.

Seizures are another potential side effect, occurring in some 5 percent of people who take Clozaril. The higher the dosage, the greater the risk of seizures.

■ *More common side effects may include:*

Abdominal discomfort, agitation, confusion, constipation, disturbed sleep, dizziness, drowsiness, dry mouth, fainting, fever, headache, heartburn, high blood pressure, inability to sit down, loss or slowness of muscle movement, low blood pressure, nausea, nightmares, rapid heartbeat and other heart conditions, restlessness, rigidity, salivation, sedation, sweating, tremors, vertigo, vision problems, vomiting, weight gain

■ *Less common side effects may include:*

Anemia, angina (severe, crushing chest pain), anxiety, appetite increase, blocked intestine, blood clots, bloodshot eyes, bluish tinge in the skin, breast pain or discomfort, bronchitis, bruising, chest pain, chills or chills and fever, constant involuntary eye movement, coughing, delusions, depression, diarrhea, difficult or labored breathing, difficulty swallowing, dilated pupils, disorientation, dry throat, ear disorders, ejaculation problems, excessive movement, eyelid disorder, fast, fluttery heartbeat, fatigue, fluid retention, frequent urination, glaucoma (high pressure in the eye), hallucinations, heart problems, hives, hot flashes, impacted stool, impotence, inability to fall asleep or stay asleep, inability to hold urine, inability to urinate, increase or decrease in sex drive, involuntary movement, irritability, itching, jerky movements, joint pain, lack of coordination, laryngitis, lethargy, light-headedness (especially when rising quickly from a seated or lying position), loss of appetite, loss of speech, low body temperature, memory loss, muscle pain or ache, muscle spasm, muscle weakness, nosebleed, numbness, pain in back, neck, or legs, painful menstruation, pallor, paranoia, pneumonia or pneumonia-like symptoms, poor coordination, rapid breathing, rash, runny nose, shakiness, shortness of breath, skin inflammation, redness, scaling, slow heartbeat, slurred speech, sneezing, sore or numb tongue, speech difficulty, stomach pain, stuffy nose, stupor, stuttering, swollen salivary glands, thirst, throat discomfort, tics, twitching, urination problems, vaginal infection, vaginal itch, a vague feeling of being sick, weakness, wheezing, yellow skin and eyes

Why should this drug not be prescribed?

Clozaril is considered a somewhat risky medication because of its potential to cause agranulocytosis and seizures. It should be taken only by people whose condition is serious, and who have not been helped by more traditional antipsychotic medications such as Haldol or Mellaril. Clozaril should not be used if the patient:

Has a bone marrow disease or disorder;

Has epilepsy that is not controlled;

Has ever developed an abnormal white blood cell count while taking Clozaril;

Is currently taking some other drug, such as Tegretol, that could cause a decrease in white blood cell count or a drug that could affect the bone marrow;

Has ever had an allergic reaction to any of Clozaril's ingredients.

Special warnings about this medication

Clozaril can cause drowsiness, especially at the start of treatment. For this reason, and also because of the potential for seizures, patients should not drive, swim, climb, or operate dangerous machinery while taking this medication, at least in the early stages of treatment.

Even though blood tests are done weekly for the first 6 months of treatment and every other week after that, patients need to stay alert for early symptoms of agranulocytosis: weakness, lethargy, fever, sore throat, a general feeling of illness, a flu-like feeling, or ulcers of the lips, mouth, or other mucous membranes. If any such symptoms develop, they should contact their doctor immediately.

Especially during the first 3 weeks of treatment, a fever may develop. If this happens, the patient should notify the doctor.

Instruct patients to check with their doctor before drinking alcohol or using drugs of any kind, including over-the-counter medicines.

Patients with an enlarged prostate or the eye condition called narrow-angle glaucoma must be closely monitored by the doctor. Clozaril could make these conditions worse.

On rare occasions, Clozaril can cause intestinal problems—constipation, impaction, or blockage—that can, in extreme cases, be fatal.

In very rare cases, Clozaril has been known to cause a potentially fatal inflammation of the heart. This problem is most likely to surface during the first month of treatment, but has also occurred later. Warning signs include unexplained fatigue, shortness of breath, fever, chest pain, and a rapid or pounding heartbeat. Patients should see their doctor immediately if they develop these symptoms. Even a suspicion of heart inflammation warrants discontinuation of Clozaril.

Especially when starting Clozaril therapy, patients may be troubled by a dramatic drop in blood pressure whenever they first stand up. This can lead to light-headedness, fainting, or even total collapse and cardiac arrest. Clozaril also tends to increase the heart rate. Both problems are more dangerous for someone with a heart problem. If a patient suffers from heart disease, make sure the doctor knows about it.

Patients with kidney, liver, or lung disease, or a history of seizures or prostate problems, should discuss the problem with their doctor before taking Clozaril. Nausea, vomiting, loss of appetite, and a yellow tinge to the skin and eyes are signs of liver trouble. The doctor should be contacted immediately if a patient develops these symptoms.

Drugs such as Clozaril can sometimes cause a set of symptoms called Neuroleptic Malignant Syndrome. Symptoms include high fever, muscle rigidity, irregular pulse or blood pressure, rapid heartbeat, excessive perspiration, and changes in heart rhythm. The patient will be taken off Clozaril while this condition is being treated.

There is also a risk of developing tardive dyskinesia, a condition of involuntary, slow, rhythmical movements. This happens more often in older adults, especially older women.

Clozaril has been known to occasionally raise blood sugar levels, causing unusual hunger, thirst, and weakness, along with excessive urination. Patients should alert their doctor if they develop these symptoms. They may have to switch to a different medication.

In very rare instances, Clozaril may also cause a blood clot in the lungs. Patients should call their doctor immediately if they develop severe breathing problems or chest pain.

Possible food and drug interactions when taking this medication

If Clozaril is taken with certain other drugs, the effects of either could be increased, decreased, or altered. Here's an overview of the drugs that can cause a problem:

Alcohol
Antidepressants such as Paxil, Prozac, and Zoloft
Antipsychotic drugs such as Thorazine and Mellaril
Blood pressure medications such as Aldomet and Hytrin

Caffeine
Chemotherapy drugs
Cimetidine (Tagamet)
Digitoxin (Crystodigin)
Digoxin (Lanoxin)
Drugs that depress the central nervous system such as phenobarbital and Seconal
Drugs that contain atropine such as Donnatal and Levsin
Epilepsy drugs such as Tegretol and Dilantin
Epinephrine (EpiPen)
Erythromycin (E-Mycin, Eryc, others)
Fluvoxamine (Luvox)
Heart rhythm stabilizers such as Rythmol, Quinidex, and Tambocor
Nicotine
Rifampin (Rifadin)
Tranquilizers such as Valium and Xanax
Warfarin (Coumadin)

Special information about pregnancy and breastfeeding

The effects of Clozaril during pregnancy have not been adequately studied. Patients who are pregnant or plan to become pregnant should inform their doctor immediately. Clozaril treatment should be continued during pregnancy only if absolutely necessary.

Breastfeeding is not recommended during Clozaril therapy, since the drug may appear in breast milk.

Recommended dosage

ADULTS

Dosage should be carefully individualized and monitored. The usual recommended initial dose is half of a 25-milligram tablet (12.5 milligrams) 1 or 2 times daily. The doctor may increase the dosage in increments of 25 to 50 milligrams a day to achieve a daily dose of 300 to 450 milligrams by the end of 2 weeks. Dosage increases after that will be made only once or twice a week and will be no more than 100 milligrams each time. Dosage is increased gradually because rapid increases and higher doses are more likely to cause seizures and changes in heart rhythm. The highest recommended dosage is 900 milligrams a day divided into 2 or 3 doses.

CHILDREN

Safety and efficacy have not been established for children up to 16 years of age.

Overdosage

Any medication taken in excess can have serious consequences. If an overdose is suspected, seek emergency medical attention immediately.

■ *Symptoms of overdose with Clozaril may include:*
Coma, delirium, drowsiness, excess salivation, low blood pressure, faintness, pneumonia, rapid heartbeat, seizures, shallow breathing or absence of breathing

Brand name:

Cognex

Pronounced: COG-necks
Generic name: Tacrine hydrochloride

Why is this drug prescribed?

Cognex is used for the treatment of mild to moderate Alzheimer's disease. This progressive, degenerative disorder causes physical changes in the brain that disrupt the flow of information and affect memory, thinking, and behavior. Like other Alzheimer's drugs (Aricept, Exelon, and Reminyl), Cognex can temporarily improve brain function in some Alzheimer's sufferers, although it does not halt the progress of the underlying disease.

Most important fact about this drug

Cognex treatment should not be stopped, or the dosage reduced, without consulting the doctor. A sudden reduction can cause the patient to become more disturbed and forgetful. Giving more Cognex than the doctor advises can also cause serious problems. Dosage should not be changed without instructions from the doctor.

How should this medication be taken?

This medication will work better if taken at regular intervals, usually 4 times a day. Cognex is best taken between meals. However, if it is irritating to the stomach, the doctor may advise taking it with meals. If Cognex is not taken regularly, as the doctor directs, the condition may get worse.

■ *Missed dose...*
Generally, the forgotten dose should be given as soon as possible. If it is within 2 hours of the next dose, caregivers should skip the missed dose and go back to the regular schedule. Doses should never be doubled.

■ *Storage instructions...*
Cognex should be stored at room temperature away from moisture.

What side effects may occur?

Side effects cannot be predicted. If any develop or change in intensity, caregivers should tell the doctor as soon as possible.

■ *More common side effects may include:*
Abdominal pain, abnormal thinking, agitation, anxiety, chest pain, clumsiness or unsteadiness, confusion, constipation, coughing, depression, diarrhea, dizziness, fatigue, flushing, frequent urination, gas, headache, inflamed nasal passages, insomnia, indigestion, liver function disorders, loss of appetite, muscle pain, nausea, rash, sleepiness, upper respiratory infection, urinary tract infection, vomiting, weight loss

■ *Less common side effects may include:*
Back pain, hallucinations, hostile attitude, purple or red spots on the skin, skin discoloration, tremor, weakness

Caregivers should report any symptoms that develop while on Cognex therapy. They should alert the doctor if the patient develops nausea, vomiting, loose stools, or diarrhea at the start of therapy or when the dosage is increased. Later in therapy, they should be on the lookout for rash or fever, yellowing of the eyes and skin, or changes in the color of the stool.

Why should this drug not be prescribed?

People who are sensitive to or have ever had an allergic reaction to Cognex (including symptoms such as rash or fever) should not take this medication. If during previous Cognex therapy the patient developed jaundice (yellow skin and eyes), which signals that something is wrong with the liver, Cognex should not be used again.

Special warnings about this medication

Cognex should be used with caution if the patient has a history of liver disease, certain heart disorders, stomach ulcers, or asthma.

Because of the risk of liver problems when taking Cognex, the doctor will schedule blood tests to monitor liver function every other week from at least the fourth week to the sixteenth week of treatment. After 16 weeks, blood tests will be given monthly for 2 months and every 3 months after that. If the patient develops any liver problems, the doctor may temporarily discontinue Cognex treatment until further testing shows that the liver has returned to normal. If the doctor resumes Cognex treatment, regular blood tests will be conducted again.

Before having any surgery, including dental surgery, caregivers should tell the doctor that the patient is being treated with Cognex.

Cognex can cause seizures, and may cause problems with urination.

Possible food and drug interactions when taking this medication

If Cognex is taken with certain other drugs, the effects of either could be increased, decreased, or altered. Here is an overview of drugs that can cause a problem:

Drugs that quell spasms, including Bentyl and Levsin

Bethanechol chloride (Urecholine)

Cimetidine (Tagamet)

Fluvoxamine (Luvox)

Muscle stimulants such as Mestinon, Mytelase, and Prostigmin

Nonsteroidal anti-inflammatory drugs such as Aleve, Motrin, and Naprosyn

The Parkinson's medications Artane and Cogentin

Theophylline (Theo-Dur)

Special information about pregnancy and breastfeeding

The effects of Cognex during pregnancy have not been studied; and it is not known whether Cognex appears in breast milk.

Recommended dosage

ADULTS

The usual starting dose is 10 milligrams 4 times a day, for at least 4 weeks. The dose should not be increased during this 4-week period unless the doctor directs.

Depending on the patient's tolerance of the drug, dosage may then be increased at 4-week intervals, first to 20 milligrams, then to 30, and finally to 40, always taken 4 times a day.

CHILDREN

The safety and effectiveness of Cognex have not been established in children.

Overdosage

Any medication taken in excess can have serious consequences. If an overdose is suspected, seek medical attention immediately.

■ *Symptoms of Cognex overdose include:*
Collapse, convulsions, extreme muscle weakness, possibly ending in death (if breathing muscles are affected), low blood pressure, nausea, salivation, slowed heart rate, sweating, vomiting.

Brand name:

Compazine

Pronounced: KOMP-ah-zeen
Generic name: Prochlorperazine

Why is this drug prescribed?

Compazine is used to treat symptoms of mental disorders such as schizophrenia, and is occasionally prescribed for anxiety. It is also used to control severe nausea and vomiting.

Most important fact about this drug

Compazine may cause tardive dyskinesia—involuntary muscle spasms and twitches in the face and body. This condition may be permanent. It appears to be most common among the elderly, especially women. Patients should see their doctor immediately at the first sign of this problem (spasms in the tongue may be an early warning). Antipsychotic medications usually must be discontinued if these symptoms appear.

How should this medication be taken?

Patients should never take more Compazine than prescribed. Doing so can increase the risk of serious side effects.

If patients are using the suppository form of Compazine and find it is too soft to insert, they can chill it in the refrigerator for about 30 minutes or run cold water over it before removing the wrapper.

To insert a suppository, patients should first remove the wrapper and moisten the suppository with cold water. They should then lie down on their side and use a finger to push the suppository well up into the rectum.

■ *Missed dose...*

Generally, the forgotten dose should be taken as soon as remembered. However, if it is almost time for the next dose, patients should skip the one they missed and go back to their regular schedule. Doses should never be doubled.

■ *Storage instructions...*

Compazine may be stored at room temperature. Protect from heat and light.

What side effects may occur?

Side effects cannot be predicted. If any develop or change in intensity, patients should inform their doctor as soon as possible.

■ *Side effects may include:*

Abnormal muscle rigidity, abnormal secretion of milk, abnormal sugar in urine, abnormalities of posture and movement, agitation, anemia, appetite changes, asthma, blurred vision, breast development in males, chewing movements, constipation, convulsions, difficulty swallowing, discolored skin tone, dizziness, drooling, drowsiness, dry mouth, ejaculation problems, exaggerated reflexes, fever, fluid retention, head arched backward, headache, heart attack, heels bent back on legs, high or low blood sugar, hives, impotence, inability to urinate, increased psychotic symptoms, increased weight, infection, insomnia, intestinal obstruction, involuntary movements (of arms, hands, legs, and feet), involuntary movements (of face, tongue, and jaw), irregular movements, jerky movements, jitteriness, light sensitivity, low blood pressure, mask-like face, menstrual irregularities, narrowed or dilated pupils, nasal congestion, nausea, pain in the shoulder and neck area, painful muscle spasm, Parkinson's-like symptoms, persistent, painful erections, pill-rolling motion, protruding tongue, puckering of the mouth, puffing of the cheeks, rigidity (in arms, feet, head, and muscles), rotation of eyeballs or state of fixed gaze, shock, shuffling gait, skin peeling, rash and inflammation, sore throat, mouth, and gums, spasms (in back, feet and ankles, jaw, and neck), swelling and itching skin, swelling in throat, tremors, yellowed eyes and skin

Why should this drug not be prescribed?

Compazine must be avoided by anyone who is sensitive to or has ever had an allergic reaction to prochlorperazine or other phenothiazine drugs such as Thorazine, Prolixin, Triavil, Mellaril, or Stelazine.

Special warnings about this medication

Patients should never take large amounts of alcohol, barbiturates, or narcotics when taking Compazine. Serious problems can result.

If Compazine is stopped suddenly, patients may experience a change in appetite, dizziness, nausea, vomiting, and tremors. Patients should follow their doctor's instructions closely when discontinuing this drug.

Make sure the doctor knows if the patient is being treated for a brain tumor, intestinal blockage, heart disease, glaucoma, or an abnormal blood condition such as leukemia, or has been exposed to extreme heat or pesticides.

This drug may impair the ability to drive a car or operate potentially dangerous machinery. Patients should avoid any activities that require full alertness if they are unsure about their ability.

Patients should try to stay out of the sun while taking Compazine. They should use sunblock and wear protective clothing. Their eyes may become more sensitive to sunlight, too, so they should keep sunglasses handy.

Compazine interferes with the body's ability to shed extra heat. Caution is warranted in hot weather.

Compazine may cause false-positive pregnancy tests.

Possible food and drug interactions when taking this medication

If Compazine is taken with certain other drugs, the effects of either could be increased, decreased, or altered. Here is an overview of drugs that may cause a problem:

Antiseizure drugs such as Dilantin and Tegretol
Anticoagulants such as Coumadin
Guanethidine
Lithium (Lithobid, Eskalith)
Narcotic painkillers such as Demerol and Tylenol with Codeine
Other central nervous system depressants such as Xanax, Valium,

Seconal, and Halcion
Propranolol (Inderal)
Thiazide diuretics such as Dyazide

Special information about pregnancy and breastfeeding

Compazine is not usually recommended for pregnant women, although it is sometimes prescribed for severe nausea and vomiting if the potential benefits of the drug outweigh the potential risks.

Compazine appears in breast milk and may affect a nursing infant. Patients are typically instructed to stop breastfeeding until their treatment is finished.

Recommended dosage

ADULTS

For Non-psychotic Anxiety
Tablets: The usual dose is 5 milligrams, taken 3 or 4 times a day.
"Spansule" Capsule: The usual starting dose is one 15-milligram capsule on getting up or one 10-milligram capsule every 12 hours.

Treatment should not continue for longer than 12 weeks, and daily doses should not exceed 20 milligrams.

Relatively Mild Psychotic Disorders
The usual dose is 5 or 10 milligrams, taken 3 or 4 times daily.

Moderate to Severe Psychotic Disorders
Dosages usually start at 10 milligrams, taken 3 or 4 times a day. If needed, dosage may be gradually increased; 50 to 75 milligrams daily has been helpful for some people.

More Severe Psychotic Disorders
Dosages may range from 100 to 150 milligrams per day.

To Control Severe Nausea and Vomiting
Tablets: The usual dosage is one 5-milligram or 10-milligram tablet 3 or 4 times a day.
"Spansule" Capsules: The usual starting dose is one 15-milligram capsule on getting out of bed or one 10-milligram capsule every 12 hours.

The usual rectal dosage (suppository) is 25 milligrams, taken 2 times a day.

CHILDREN

Children under 2 years of age or weighing less than 20 pounds should not be given Compazine. If a child becomes restless or excited after taking Compazine, the child should not get another dose.

For Psychotic Disorders
Children 2 to 5 Years Old
The starting oral or rectal dose is 2-1/2 milligrams 2 or 3 times daily. Do not exceed 10 milligrams the first day and 20 milligrams thereafter.
Children 6 to 12 Years Old
The starting oral or rectal dose is 2-1/2 milligrams 2 or 3 times daily. Do not exceed 10 milligrams the first day and 25 milligrams thereafter.

For Severe Nausea and Vomiting
An oral or rectal dose of Compazine is usually not needed for more than 1 day.
Children 20 to 29 Pounds
The usual dose is 2-1/2 milligrams 1 or 2 times daily. Total daily amount should not exceed 7.5 milligrams.
Children 30 to 39 Pounds
The usual dose is 2-1/2 milligrams 2 or 3 times daily. Total daily amount should not exceed 10 milligrams.
Children 40 to 85 Pounds
The usual dose is 2-1/2 milligrams 3 times daily, or 5 milligrams 2 times daily. Total daily amount should not exceed 15 milligrams.

OLDER ADULTS

In general, older people take lower dosages of Compazine. Because they may develop low blood pressure while taking the drug, the doctor should monitor them closely. Older people (especially women) may be more susceptible to tardive dyskinesia.

Overdosage
An overdose of Compazine can be fatal. If an overdose is suspected, seek medical help immediately.

■ *Symptoms of Compazine overdose may include:*
Agitation, coma, convulsions, dry mouth, extreme sleepiness, fever, intestinal blockage, irregular heart rate, restlessness

Brand name:
Concerta

See Ritalin, page 172

Brand name:

Cylert

Pronounced: SIGH-lert
Generic name: Pemoline

Why is this drug prescribed?

Cylert is used to help treat children who have Attention Deficit Hyperactivity Disorder (ADHD). Because it has been known to cause liver damage, it is usually prescribed only when other drugs have failed. Drugs such as Cylert should be used as part of a comprehensive treatment plan offering psychological and educational support to help the child become more stable.

Most important fact about this drug

Although cases of liver damage are rare, some have been serious enough to be fatal. Children taking Cylert should have their liver function tested every 2 weeks. If the child develops any signs of liver damage, the doctor should be called immediately. Warning signs include fatigue, loss of appetite, digestive problems, yellow skin or eyes, and pain in the upper right section of the abdomen.

How should this medication be taken?

Cylert should be taken once a day, in the morning.

■ *Missed dose...*
The child should take it as soon as remembered, then go back to the regular schedule. If it's not remembered until the next day, it should be skipped and the child should go back to the regular schedule. Doses should never be doubled.

■ *Storage instructions...*
Cylert may be stored at room temperature.

What side effects may occur?

Side effects cannot be predicted. If any develop or change in intensity, caregivers should inform the child's doctor as soon as possible.

■ *The most common side effect is:*
Insomnia

■ *Less common side effects may include:*
Depression, dizziness, drowsiness, hallucinations, headache, hepatitis and other liver problems, increased irritability, involuntary, fragmented movements of the face, eyes, lips, tongue, arms, and legs, loss of appetite, mild depression, nausea, seizures, skin rash, stomachache, suppressed growth, uncontrolled vocal outbursts (such as grunts, shouts, and obscene language), weight loss, yellowing of skin or eyes

■ *Rare side effects may include:*
A rare form of anemia with symptoms such as bleeding gums, bruising, chest pain, fatigue, headache, nosebleeds, and abnormal paleness

Why should this drug not be prescribed?

Cylert cannot be used if the child is allergic to it or has liver problems.

Special warnings about this medication

Cylert may cause dizziness. Patients should be careful climbing stairs or participating in activities that require mental alertness.

Although there have been no reports that Cylert is physically addictive, it is chemically similar to a class of drugs that are potentially addictive. It is important that the child be given no more than the prescribed dosage.

Children who take this drug on a long-term basis should be carefully monitored for signs of stunted growth.

The doctor will be extra cautious if the child has kidney problems.

Children who have a psychiatric illness and take Cylert may experience increasingly disordered thoughts and behavioral disturbances.

Possible food and drug interactions when taking this medication

If Cylert is taken with certain other drugs, the effects of either could be increased, decreased, or altered. Here is an overview of drugs that may cause a problem:

Seizure medications such as Tegretol
Other drugs that affect the central nervous system, such as Ritalin

Special information about pregnancy and breastfeeding

This drug is for use only in children, and its effects in pregnancy have not been adequately studied. Cylert should be used during pregnancy only if it is clearly necessary. It is not known whether the drug appears in breast milk, but caution is advised.

Recommended dosage

The recommended beginning dose is 37.5 milligrams daily. Dosages may be gradually increased if needed. Most children take doses ranging from 56.25 to 75 milligrams a day. The maximum recommended daily dose of Cylert is 112.5 milligrams. Significant improvement is gradual and may not be apparent until the third or fourth week of treatment with Cylert.

The doctor may occasionally stop treatment with Cylert to see whether behavioral problems return and whether further treatment with Cylert is necessary.

Overdosage

Any medication taken in excess can have serious consequences. If an overdose is suspected, seek medical help immediately.

■ *Symptoms of Cylert overdose may include:*

Agitation, coma, confusion, convulsions, delirium, dilated pupils, exaggerated feeling of well-being, extremely high temperature, flushing, hallucinations, headache, high blood pressure, increased heart rate, increased reflex reactions, muscle twitches, sweating, tremors, vomiting

Brand name:

Dalmane

Pronounced: DAL-main
Generic name: Flurazepam hydrochloride

Why is this drug prescribed?

Dalmane is used for the relief of insomnia—difficulty falling asleep, waking up frequently at night, or waking up early in the morning. It can be used by people whose insomnia keeps coming back and in those who have poor sleeping habits. It belongs to a class of drugs known as benzodiazepines.

Most important fact about this drug

Tolerance and dependence can occur with the use of Dalmane. Patients may experience withdrawal symptoms if they stop using this drug abruptly. They should discontinue or change their dose only in consultation with their doctor.

How should this medication be taken?

Dalmane is taken in a single dose at bedtime. It is important to take this medication exactly as prescribed.

■ *Missed dose...*

Dalmane should be taken only as needed. Doses should never be doubled.

■ *Storage instructions...*

Dalmane should be stored away from heat, light, and moisture.

What side effects may occur?

Side effects cannot be predicted. If any develop or change in intensity, patients should inform their doctor as soon as possible.

■ *More common side effects may include:*

Dizziness, drowsiness, falling, lack of muscular coordination, lightheadedness, staggering

■ *Less common or rare side effects may include:*
Apprehension, bitter taste, blurred vision, body and joint pain, burning eyes, chest pains, confusion, constipation, depression, diarrhea, difficulty in focusing, dry mouth, exaggerated feeling of well-being, excessive salivation, excitement, faintness, flushes, genital and urinary tract disorders, hallucinations, headache, heartburn, hyperactivity, irritability, itching, loss of appetite, low blood pressure, nausea, nervousness, rapid, fluttery heartbeat, restlessness, shortness of breath, skin rash, slurred speech, stimulation, stomach and intestinal pain, stomach upset, sweating, talkativeness, vomiting, weakness

■ *Side effects due to rapid decrease or abrupt withdrawal from Dalmane:*
Abdominal and muscle cramps, convulsions, depressed mood, inability to fall asleep or stay asleep, sweating, tremors, vomiting

Why should this drug not be prescribed?

Dalmane cannot be used by anyone who is sensitive to or has had an allergic reaction to it or similar drugs such as Valium.

Special warnings about this medication

Patients should avoid driving, operating dangerous machinery, or participating in any hazardous activity that requires full mental alertness after taking Dalmane.

This drug should be used with caution in patients who are severely depressed, or have suffered from severe depression.

Caution is also warranted in patients who have decreased kidney or liver function or chronic respiratory or lung disease.

Possible food and drug interactions when taking this medication

Alcohol intensifies the effects of Dalmane. Patients should avoid drinking alcohol while taking this medication.

If Dalmane is taken with certain other drugs, the effects of either could be increased, decreased, or altered. Here is an overview of drugs that may cause a problem:

Antidepressants such as Elavil and Tofranil
Antihistamines such as Benadryl and Tavist
Barbiturates such as Seconal and phenobarbital
Major tranquilizers such as Mellaril and Thorazine
Narcotic painkillers such as Demerol and Tylenol with Codeine
Sedatives such as Xanax and Halcion
Tranquilizers such as Librium and Valium

Special information about pregnancy and breastfeeding

Dalmane should not be used during pregnancy. There is an increased risk of birth defects. This drug may appear in breast milk and could affect a nursing infant. It may be advisable to discontinue breastfeeding until treatment with Dalmane is finished.

Recommended dosage

ADULTS

The usual recommended dose is 30 milligrams at bedtime; however 15 milligrams may be all that is necessary. The doctor should adjust the dose to the patient's needs.

CHILDREN

Safety and effectiveness of Dalmane have not been established in children under 15 years of age.

OLDER ADULTS

The doctor will limit the dosage to the smallest effective amount to avoid oversedation, dizziness, confusion, or lack of muscle coordination. The usual starting dose is 15 milligrams.

Overdosage

Any medication taken in excess can have serious consequences. If an overdose is suspected, seek medical attention immediately.

■ *The symptoms of Dalmane overdose may include:*
Coma, confusion, low blood pressure, sleepiness

Brand name:

Depakote

Pronounced: DEP-uh-coat
Generic name: Divalproex sodium (Valproic acid)

Why is this drug prescribed?

Depakote, in both delayed-release tablet and capsule form, is used to treat certain types of seizures and convulsions. It may be prescribed alone or with other epilepsy medications.

The delayed-release tablets are also used to control the manic episodes that occur in bipolar disorder.

An extended-release form of this drug, Depakote ER, is prescribed to prevent migraine headaches. The delayed-release tablets are also used for this purpose.

Most important fact about this drug

Depakote can cause serious or even fatal liver damage, especially during the first 6 months of treatment. Children under 2 years of age are the most vulnerable, especially if they are also taking other anticonvulsant medicines and have certain other disorders such as mental retardation.

The risk of liver damage decreases with age; but patients should always be alert for the following symptoms: loss of seizure control, weakness, dizziness, drowsiness, a general feeling of ill health, facial swelling, loss of appetite, vomiting, and yellowing of the skin and eyes. The doctor should be alerted immediately if a liver problem is suspected.

Depakote has also been known to cause life-threatening damage to the pancreas. This problem can surface at any time, even after years of treatment. Patients should call the doctor immediately if they develop any of the following warning signs: abdominal pain, loss of appetite, nausea, or vomiting.

How should this medication be taken?

Patients should take the Depakote tablet with water and swallow it whole (don't chew it or crush it). It has a special coating to avoid upsetting the stomach.

The sprinkle capsule can be swallowed whole or opened and sprinkled on a teaspoon of soft food such as applesauce or pudding. The food should be swallowed immediately, without chewing. The sprinkle capsules are large enough to be opened easily.

Depakote can be taken with meals or snacks to avoid stomach upset.

■ *Missed dose...*

If a patient takes Depakote once a day, the missed dose should be taken as soon as remembered. If it isn't remembered until the next day, the patient should skip the missed dose and return to the regular schedule.

If a patient takes more than one dose a day, the missed dose should be taken right away if it's within 6 hours of the scheduled time, and the rest of the day's doses should be taken at equal intervals during the remainder of the day. Doses should never be doubled.

■ *Storage instructions...*

Depakote may be stored at room temperature.

What side effects may occur?

Side effects cannot be predicted. If any develop or change in intensity, patients should inform their doctor as soon as possible. Because Depakote is often used with other antiseizure drugs, it may not be possible to determine whether a side effect is due to Depakote alone. Only the doctor can determine if it is safe to continue taking Depakote.

■ *More common side effects may include:*

Abdominal pain, abnormal thinking, breathing difficulty, bronchitis, bruising, constipation, depression, diarrhea, dizziness, emotional changeability, fever, flu symptoms, hair loss, headache, incoordination, indigestion, infection, insomnia, loss of appetite, memory loss, nasal inflammation, nausea, nervousness, ringing in the ears, sleepiness, sore throat, tremor, vision problems, vomiting, weakness, weight loss or gain

■ *Less common or rare side effects may include:*
Abnormal dreams, abnormal milk secretion, abnormal walk, aggression, anemia, anxiety, back pain, behavior problems, belching, bleeding, blood disorders, bone pain, breast enlargement, chest pain, chills, coma, confusion, coughing up blood, dental abscess, drowsiness, dry skin, ear inflammation, excessive urination (mainly children) or other urination problems, eye problems, feeling of illness, gas, growth failure in children, hallucinations, hearing problems, heart palpitations, high blood pressure, hostility, increased appetite, increased cough, involuntary rapid movement of eyeball, irregular or painful menstruation, itching, jerky movements, joint pain, lack of muscular coordination, leg cramps, liver problems, loss of bladder or bowel control, muscle or joint pain, muscle weakness, muscle pain, neck pain, nosebleed, overactivity, pneumonia, rapid heartbeat, rickets (mainly children), sedation, seeing "spots before your eyes," sensitivity to light, sinus inflammation, skin eruptions or peeling, skin rash, speech difficulties, stomach and intestinal disorders, swelling of arms and legs due to fluid retention, swollen glands, taste changes, tingling or pins and needles, twitching, urinary problems, vertigo, vision problems

Why should this drug not be prescribed?

This medication must be avoided by anyone with liver disease or poor liver function. It is also contraindicated for those who are sensitive to or have ever had an allergic reaction to Depakote.

Special warnings about this medication

This medication can severely damage the liver (see "Most important fact about this drug"). The doctor should test the patient's liver function before starting therapy with this medication and at regular intervals thereafter.

Also remember that the drug can damage the pancreas (see "Most important fact about this drug"). This problem can worsen very rapidly. Patients should contact their doctor without delay if they develop any symptoms.

Depakote causes some people to become drowsy or less alert. Patients should not drive, operate dangerous machinery, or participate in any hazardous activity that requires full mental alertness until they are certain the drug does not effect them this way.

This medication should not be stopped abruptly. A gradual reduction in dosage is usually required under a physician's supervision.

Depakote prolongs the time it takes blood to clot, which increases the chances of serious bleeding.

This drug can also increase the effect of painkillers and anesthetics. Before any surgery or dental procedure, the doctor should be informed that the patient is taking Depakote.

Patients taking Depakote to prevent migraine should remember that it will not cure a headache once it has started.

Some coated particles from the capsules may appear in the stool. This is to be expected, and is not a cause for worry.

Possible food and drug interactions when taking this medication

Depakote depresses activity of the central nervous system, and may increase the effects of alcohol. Patient's should not drink alcohol while taking this medication.

If Depakote is taken with certain other drugs, the effects of either could be increased, decreased, or altered. Here is an overview of drugs that can cause a problem:

Amitriptyline (Elavil)
Aspirin
Barbiturates such as phenobarbital and Seconal
Blood thinners such as Coumadin
Cyclosporine (Sandimmune, Neoral)
Notriptyline (Pamelor)
Oral contraceptives
Other seizure medications, including carbamazepine (Tegretol), clo-
    nazepam (Klonopin), ethosuximide (Zarontin), felbamate (Felbatol),
    lamotrigine (Lamictal), phenytoin (Dilantin), and Primidone
    (Mysoline)
Rifampin (Rifater)
Sleep aids such as Halcion
Tolbutamide (Orinase)
Tranquilizers such as Valium and Xanax
Zidovudine (Retrovir)

Special information about pregnancy and breastfeeding

Depakote may produce birth defects when taken during pregnancy. Patients who are pregnant or plan to become pregnant should inform their doctor immediately. Depakote should be used during pregnancy only if it is essential for seizure control.

Depakote appears in breast milk and could affect a nursing infant. If Depakote is essential to the patient's health, the doctor may advise her to discontinue breastfeeding until her treatment with this medication is finished.

Recommended dosage

EPILEPSY

Dosage for adults and children 10 years of age or older is determined by body weight. The usual recommended starting dose is 10 to 15 milligrams per 2.2 pounds per day, depending on the type of seizure. The doctor may increase the dose at 1-week intervals by 5 to 10 milligrams per 2.2 pounds per day until the seizures are controlled or the side effects become too severe. The maximum dose is 60 milligrams per 2.2 pounds per day. If the total dosage is more than 250 milligrams a day, the doctor will divide it into smaller individual doses.

Older adults usually begin taking this medication at lower dosages, and the dosage is increased more slowly.

MANIC EPISODES

The usual starting dose for those aged 18 and over is 750 milligrams a day, divided into smaller doses. The doctor will adjust the dose for best results.

MIGRAINE PREVENTION

Delayed-Release Tablets
The usual starting dose for those aged 16 and over is 250 milligrams twice a day. The doctor will adjust the dose, up to a maximum of 1,000 milligrams a day.

Extended-Release Tablets
The usual starting dose is 500 milligrams once a day for 1 week. The dose may then be increased to 1,000 milligrams once a day.

Depakote delayed-release and extended-release tablets work differently and cannot be substituted for each other.

Researchers have not established the safety and effectiveness of Depakote for prevention of migraines in children or adults over 65.

Overdosage
An overdose of Depakote can be fatal. If an overdose is suspected, seek medical attention immediately.

■ *Symptoms of Depakote overdose may include:*
Coma, extreme sleepiness, heart problems

Generic name:
Desipramine

See Norpramin, page 126

Brand name:

Desoxyn

Pronounced: des-OK-sin
Generic name: Methamphetamine hydrochloride

Why is this drug prescribed?

Desoxyn is used to treat Attention Deficit Hyperactivity Disorder (ADHD). This drug is given as part of a total treatment program that includes psychological, educational, and social measures.

Desoxyn also may be used for a short time as part of an overall diet plan for weight reduction. Desoxyn is given only when other weight loss drugs and weight loss programs have been unsuccessful.

Most important fact about this drug?

Excessive doses of this medication can produce addiction. Individuals who stop taking this medication after taking high doses for a long time may suffer withdrawal symptoms, including extreme tiredness, depression, and sleep disorders. Signs of excessive use of Desoxyn include severe skin inflammation, difficulty sleeping, irritability, hyperactivity, personality changes, and psychiatric problems.

Desoxyn can lose its effectiveness in decreasing the appetite after a few weeks. If this happens, the medication should be stopped. Patients should never take more than the recommended dose in an attempt to increase the drug's effect.

How should this medication be taken?

It is important to follow the doctor's directions carefully. The doctor will prescribe the lowest effective dose of Desoxyn; it should never be increased without approval.

Patients should avoid taking this medication late in the evening; it can cause difficulty sleeping.

■ *Missed dose . . .*
Generally, the forgotten dose should be taken as soon as remembered. However, if it is almost time for the next dose, the patient should skip the missed dose and return to the regular schedule. Doses should never be doubled.

■ *Storage instructions . . .*
Desoxyn may be stored at room temperature.

What side effects may occur?

Side effects cannot be predicted. If any develop or change in intensity, patients should inform their doctor as soon as possible.

■ Side effects may include:
Changes in sex drive, constipation, diarrhea, dizziness, dry mouth,

exaggerated feeling of well-being, feeling of unwellness or unhappiness, headache, hives, impaired growth, impotence, increased blood pressure, overstimulation, rapid or irregular heartbeat, restlessness, sleeplessness, stomach or intestinal problems, tremor, unpleasant taste, worsening of tics and Tourette's syndrome (severe twitching)

Why should this drug not be prescribed?

Desoxyn must never be combined with a monoamine oxidase (MAO) inhibitor drug such as Nardil or Parnate. Patients should allow 14 days between stopping an MAO inhibitor and beginning therapy with Desoxyn.

Desoxyn should not be taken by anyone who has high pressure in the eyes (glaucoma), advanced hardening of the arteries, heart disease, moderate to severe high blood pressure, thyroid problems, or sensitivity to this type of drug. This medication should also be avoided by anyone who suffers from tics (repeated, involuntary twitches) or Tourette's syndrome or who has a family history of these conditions.

People who are in an agitated state or who have a history of drug abuse should not take this medication.

Desoxyn should not be used to treat children whose symptoms may be caused by stress or a psychiatric disorder.

Special warnings about this medication

Desoxyn is not appropriate for all children with symptoms of ADHD. The doctor will do a complete history and evaluation before prescribing this medication. The doctor will take into account the duration and severity of the symptoms as well as the child's age.

This type of medication can affect the growth of children, so the doctor will monitor them carefully while they are taking this drug. The long-term effects of this type of medication in children have not been established.

Desoxyn should be used with caution by people with mild high blood pressure.

Desoxyn may affect the patient's ability to perform potentially hazardous activities, such as operating machinery or driving a car.

Desoxyn should not be used to combat fatigue or to replace rest.

Possible food and drug interactions when taking this medication

If Desoxyn is taken with certain other drugs, the effects of either could be increased, decreased, or altered. Here is an overview of drugs that may cause a problem:

Antidepressants classified as "tricyclics," such as Elavil, Pamelor, and Tofranil

Drugs classified as monoamine oxidase (MAO) inhibitors, such as the antidepressants Nardil and Parnate

Drugs classified as phenothiazines, such as the antipsychotic medications Compazine and Thorazine
Guanethidine
Insulin

Special information about pregnancy and breastfeeding

Infants born to women taking this type of drug have a risk of prematurity and low birth weight. Drug dependence may occur in newborns when the mother has taken this drug prior to delivery. Patients who are pregnant or plan to become pregnant should tell their doctor immediately.

Desoxyn makes its way into breast milk. Women should not breastfeed while taking this medication.

Recommended dosage

ATTENTION DEFICIT HYPERACTIVITY DISORDER

For children 6 years and older, the usual starting dose is 5 milligrams of Desoxyn taken once or twice a day. The doctor may increase the dose by 5 milligrams a week until the child responds to the medication. The typical effective dose is 20 to 25 milligrams a day, usually divided into two doses.

The doctor may periodically discontinue this drug in order to reassess the child's condition and see whether therapy is still needed.

Desoxyn should not be given to children under 6 years of age to treat attention deficit disorder; the safety and effectiveness in this age group have not been established.

WEIGHT LOSS

For adults and children 12 years and older, the usual starting dose is 5 milligrams taken one-half hour before each meal. Treatment should not continue for longer than a few weeks. The safety and effectiveness of Desoxyn for weight loss have not been established in children under age 12.

Overdosage

Any drug taken in excess can have dangerous consequences. If an overdose is suspected, seek medical attention immediately.

■ *Symptoms of Desoxyn overdose may include:*
Abdominal cramps, agitation, blood pressure changes, confusion, convulsions (may be followed by coma), depression, diarrhea, exaggerated reflexes, fatigue, hallucinations, high fever, irregular heartbeat, kidney failure, muscle aches and weakness, nausea, panic attacks, rapid breathing, restlessness, shock, tremor, vomiting

Brand name:

Desyrel

Pronounced: DES-ee-rel
Generic name: Trazodone hydrochloride

Why is this drug prescribed?

Desyrel is prescribed for the treatment of depression.

Most important fact about this drug

Desyrel does not provide immediate relief. It may take up to 4 weeks before its benefits are felt, although most patients notice improvement within 2 weeks.

How should this medication be taken?

Desyrel should be taken shortly after a meal or light snack. Patients are more apt to feel dizzy or light-headed if they take the drug before eating.

Desyrel may cause dry mouth. Sucking on a hard candy, chewing gum, or melting bits of ice in the mouth can relieve the problem.

■ *Missed dose...*

Generally, patients should take a forgotten dose as soon as they remember. However, if it is within 4 hours of their next dose, they should skip the one they missed and go back to their regular schedule. Doses should never be doubled.

■ *Storage instructions...*

Desyrel should be stored at room temperature in a tightly closed container away from light and excessive heat.

What side effects may occur?

Side effects cannot be predicted. If any develop or change in intensity, patients should inform their doctor as soon as possible.

■ *More common side effects may include:*

Abdominal or stomach disorder, aches or pains in muscles and bones, anger or hostility, blurred vision, brief loss of consciousness, confusion, constipation, decreased appetite, diarrhea, dizziness or light-headedness, drowsiness, dry mouth, excitement, fainting, fast or fluttery heartbeat, fatigue, fluid retention and swelling, headache, inability to fall or stay asleep, low blood pressure, nasal or sinus congestion, nausea, nervousness, nightmares or vivid dreams, tremors, uncoordinated movements, vomiting, weight gain or loss

■ *Less common or rare side effects may include:*

Allergic reactions, anemia, bad taste in mouth, blood in the urine, chest pain, delayed urine flow, decreased concentration, decreased sex drive, disorientation, ejaculation problems, excess salivation, gas, general feeling of illness, hallucinations or delusions, high blood pressure, impaired memory, impaired speech, impotence, increased appetite, increased sex drive, menstrual problems, more frequent urination, muscle twitches, numbness, prolonged erections, red, tired, itchy eyes, restlessness, ringing in the ears, shortness of breath, sweating or clammy skin, tingling or pins and needles

Why should this drug not be prescribed?

Anyone who is sensitive to or has ever had an allergic reaction to Desyrel or similar drugs cannot take this medication.

Special warnings about this medication

Desyrel may cause patients to become drowsy or less alert and may affect judgment. They should avoid driving, operating dangerous machinery, or participating in any hazardous activity that requires full mental alertness until they know how this drug affects them.

Desyrel has been associated with priapism, a persistent, painful erection of the penis. Men who experience prolonged or inappropriate erections should stop taking this drug and consult their doctor.

In a medical emergency, and before surgery or dental treatment, patients should notify the doctor or dentist that they are taking this drug. The doctor will ask them to stop using the drug if they are going to have elective surgery.

Caution is warranted in patients with heart disease. Desyrel can cause irregular heartbeats.

Possible food and drug interactions when taking this medication

Desyrel may intensify the effects of alcohol. Patient should avoid drinking alcohol while taking this medication.

If Desyrel is taken with certain other drugs, the effects of either could be increased, decreased, or altered. Here is an overview of drugs that may cause a problem:

Drugs classified as MAO inhibitors, including the antidepressants Nardil and Parnate
Barbiturates such as Seconal
Central nervous system depressants such as Demerol and Halcion
Chlorpromazine (Thorazine)
Digoxin (Lanoxin)
Drugs for high blood pressure such as Aldomet and Catapres
Other antidepressants such as Prozac and Norpramin
Phenytoin (Dilantin)
Warfarin (Coumadin)

Special information about pregnancy and breastfeeding

The effects of Desyrel during pregnancy have not been adequately studied. Patients should inform their doctor immediately if they are pregnant or planning to become pregnant. This medication may appear in breast milk. If treatment with this drug is essential to the patient's health, the doctor may advise her to discontinue breastfeeding until her treatment is finished.

Recommended dosage

ADULTS

The usual starting dosage is a total of 150 milligrams per day, divided into 2 or more smaller doses. The doctor may increase the dose by 50 milligrams per day every 3 or 4 days. Total dosage should not exceed 400 milligrams per day, divided into smaller doses. Once a patient has responded well to the drug, the doctor may gradually reduce the dose. Because this medication causes drowsiness, the doctor may schedule the largest dose at bedtime.

CHILDREN

The safety and effectiveness of Desyrel have not been established in children below 18 years of age.

Overdosage

Any medication taken in excess can have serious consequences. An overdose of Desyrel in combination with other drugs can be fatal. If an overdose is suspected, seek medical attention immediately.

■ *Symptoms of a Desyrel overdose may include:*
   Breathing failure, drowsiness, irregular heartbeat, prolonged, painful erection, seizures, vomiting

Brand name:

Dexedrine

Pronounced: DEX-eh-dreen
Generic name: Dextroamphetamine sulfate

Why is this drug prescribed?

Dexedrine, a stimulant drug available in tablet or sustained-release capsule form, is prescribed to help treat the following conditions:

1. Narcolepsy (recurrent "sleep attacks")
2. Attention Deficit Hyperactivity Disorder (The total treatment program should include social, psychological, and educational guidance along with Dexedrine.)

Most important fact about this drug

Because it is a stimulant, this drug has high abuse potential. The stimulant effect may give way to a letdown period of depression and fatigue.

Although the letdown can be relieved by taking another dose, this soon becomes a vicious circle.

Patients should be aware that if they habitually take Dexedrine in doses higher than recommended, or if they take it over a long period of time, they may eventually become dependent on the drug and suffer withdrawal symptoms when it is unavailable.

How should this medication be taken?

It is important to take Dexedrine exactly as prescribed. If it is prescribed in tablet form, patients may need up to 3 doses a day. The first dose should be taken upon awakening; the next 1 or 2 doses should be taken at intervals of 4 to 6 hours. The sustained-release capsules are taken only once a day.

It is best to avoid taking Dexedrine late in the day, since this could cause insomnia. If patients experience insomnia or loss of appetite while taking this drug, they should notify their doctor; they may need a lower dosage.

The doctor is likely to periodically take the patient off Dexedrine to determine whether the drug is still needed.

Patients should avoid chewing or crushing the sustained-release form, Dexedrine Spansules. They should never increase the dosage, except on their doctor's advice. Dexedrine should not be used to improve mental alertness or to stay awake. It should not be shared with others.

■ *Missed dose...*
Patients who take 1 dose a day should take it as soon as they remember, but not within 6 hours of going to bed. If they do not remember until the next day, they should skip the missed dose and go back to their regular schedule.

Patients who take 2 or 3 doses a day should take the missed dose immediately if it is within an hour or so of the scheduled time. Otherwise, they should skip the dose and go back to their regular schedule. Warn against taking 2 doses at once.

■ *Storage instructions...*
Dexedrine should be stored at room temperature in a tightly closed container, away from light.

What side effects may occur?

Side effects cannot be predicted. If any develop or change in intensity, patients should inform their doctor as soon as possible.

■ *More common side effects may include:*
Excessive restlessness, overstimulation

■ *Other side effects may include:*
Changes in sex drive, constipation, diarrhea, dizziness, dry mouth, exaggerated feeling of well-being or depression, headache, heart pal-

pitations, high blood pressure, hives, impotence, loss of appetite, rapid heartbeat, sleeplessness, stomach and intestinal disturbances, tremors, uncontrollable twitching or jerking, unpleasant taste in the mouth, weight loss

■ *Effects of chronic heavy abuse of Dexedrine may include:*
Hyperactivity, irritability, personality changes, schizophrenia-like thoughts and behavior, severe insomnia, severe skin disease

Why should this drug not be prescribed?

Dexedrine must not be taken by anyone who is sensitive to or has ever had an allergic reaction to it. It should be avoided for at least 14 days after taking a monoamine oxidase inhibitor (MAO inhibitor) such as the antidepressants Nardil and Parnate. Dexedrine and MAO inhibitors may interact to cause a sharp, potentially life-threatening rise in blood pressure.

Dexedrine must also be avoided by anyone suffering from one of the following conditions:
Agitation
Cardiovascular disease
Glaucoma
Hardening of the arteries
High blood pressure
Overactive thyroid gland
Substance abuse

Special warnings about this medication

Patients should be aware that one of the inactive ingredients in Dexedrine is a yellow food coloring called tartrazine (Yellow No. 5). In a few people, particularly those who are allergic to aspirin, tartrazine can cause a severe allergic reaction.

Dexedrine may impair judgment or coordination. Patients should avoid driving or operating dangerous machinery until they know how they react to the medication.

There is some concern that Dexedrine may stunt a child's growth. For the sake of safety, any child who takes Dexedrine should have his or her growth monitored.

Possible food and drug interactions when taking this medication

If Dexedrine is taken with certain foods or drugs, the effects of either could be increased, decreased, or altered. Here is an overview of drugs that may cause a problem:

■ *Substances that dampen the effects of Dexedrine:*
Ammonium chloride

Chlorpromazine (Thorazine)
Fruit juices
Glutamic acid hydrochloride
Guanethidine
Haloperidol (Haldol)
Lithium (Eskalith)
Methenamine (Urised)
Reserpine
Sodium acid phosphate
Vitamin C (as ascorbic acid)

■ *Substances that boost the effects of Dexedrine:*
Acetazolamide (Diamox)
MAO inhibitors such as Nardil and Parnate
Propoxyphene (Darvon)
Sodium bicarbonate (baking soda)
Thiazide diuretics such as Diuril

■ *Substances that have decreased effect when taken with Dexedrine:*
Antihistamines such as Benadryl
Blood pressure medications such as Catapres, Hytrin, and Minipress
Ethosuximide (Zarontin)
Veratrum alkaloids (found in certain blood pressure drugs)

■ *Substances that have increased effect when taken with Dexedrine:*
Antidepressants such as Norpramin
Meperidine (Demerol)
Norepinephrine (Levophed)
Phenobarbital
Phenytoin (Dilantin)

Special information about pregnancy and breastfeeding

If a patient is pregnant or plans to become pregnant, she should inform her doctor immediately. Babies born to women taking Dexedrine may be premature or have low birth weight. They may also be depressed, agitated, or apathetic due to withdrawal symptoms.

Since Dexedrine appears in breast milk, it should not be taken by a nursing mother.

Recommended dosage

Patients should take no more Dexedrine than prescribed. Intake should be kept to the lowest level that proves effective.

NARCOLEPSY

Adults

The usual dose is 5 to 60 milligrams per day, divided into smaller, equal doses.

Children

Narcolepsy seldom occurs in children under 12 years of age; however, when it does, Dexedrine may be used.

The suggested initial dose for children between 6 and 12 years of age is 5 milligrams per day. The doctor may increase the daily dose in increments of 5 milligrams at weekly intervals until it becomes effective.

Children 12 years of age and older will be started with 10 milligrams daily. The daily dosage may be raised in increments of 10 milligrams at weekly intervals until effective. If side effects such as insomnia or loss of appetite appear, the dosage will probably be reduced.

ATTENTION DEFICIT HYPERACTIVITY DISORDER

This drug is not recommended for children under 3 years of age.

Children from 3 to 5 Years of Age

The usual starting dose is 2.5 milligrams daily, in tablet form. The doctor may raise the daily dosage by 2.5 milligrams at weekly intervals until the drug becomes effective.

Children 6 Years of Age and Older

The usual starting dose is 5 milligrams once or twice a day. The doctor may raise the dose by 5 milligrams at weekly intervals until he or she is satisfied with the response. Only in rare cases will the child take more than 40 milligrams per day.

The child should take the first dose upon awakening; the remaining 1 or 2 doses are taken at intervals of 4 to 6 hours. Alternatively, the doctor may prescribe "Spansule" capsules that are taken once a day. The doctor may interrupt the schedule occasionally to see if behavioral symptoms come back enough to require continued therapy.

Overdosage

An overdose of Dexedrine can be fatal. If an overdose is suspected, seek medical attention immediately.

■ *Symptoms of an acute Dexedrine overdose may include:*

Abdominal cramps, assaultiveness, coma, confusion, convulsions, depression, diarrhea, fatigue, hallucinations, high fever, heightened reflexes, high or low blood pressure, irregular heartbeat, nausea, panic, rapid breathing, restlessness, tremor, vomiting

Generic name:
Dexmethylphenidate

See Focalin, page 76

Generic name:
Dextroamphetamine

See Dexedrine, page 55

Generic name:
Diazepam

See Valium, page 220

Generic name:
Divalproex

See Depakote, page 45

Generic name:
Donepezil

See Aricept, page 15

Brand name:
Doral

Pronounced: DOHR-al
Generic name: Quazepam

Why is this drug prescribed?
Doral, a sleeping medication available in tablet form, is taken as short-term treatment for insomnia. Symptoms of insomnia may include difficulty falling asleep, frequent awakenings throughout the night, or very early morning awakening.

Most important fact about this drug
Doral is a chemical cousin of Valium and is potentially addictive. Over time, the body will get used to the prescribed dosage of Doral, and a

patient will no longer derive any benefit from it. If the patient were to increase the dosage against medical advice, the drug would again work as a sleeping pill–but only until the body adjusted to the higher dosage. This is a vicious circle that can lead to addiction. To avoid this danger, Doral must be used only as prescribed.

How should this medication be taken?
Doral must be used exactly as prescribedone dose per day, at bedtime. Patients should keep in touch with their doctor. If they respond very well, it may be possible to cut their dosage in half after the first few nights. The older or more run-down the patient is, the more desirable it is to try for this early dosage reduction.

After taking Doral regularly for 6 weeks or so, patients may experience withdrawal symptoms if they stop suddenly, or even if they reduce the dosage without specific instructions on how to do it. They should see their doctor for instructions on how to taper off gradually from Doral.

■ *Missed dose...*
This medication should be taken only if needed.

■ *Storage instructions...*
Doral should be stored at room temperature, away from moisture.

What side effects may occur?
Side effects cannot be predicted. If any develop or change in intensity, patients should inform their doctor as soon as possible.

■ *More common side effects may include:*
Drowsiness during the day, headache

■ *Less common side effects may include:*
Changes in sex drive, dizziness, dry mouth, fatigue, inability to urinate, incontinence, indigestion, irregular menstrual periods, irritability, muscle spasms, slurred or otherwise abnormal speech, yellowed eyes and skin

In rare instances, Doral produces agitation, sleep disturbances, hallucinations, or stimulation—exactly the opposite of the desired effect. If this should happen, the patient should see the doctor, who will stop the medication.

Why should this drug not be prescribed?
Doral cannot be used by anyone who is sensitive to it or has ever had an allergic reaction to it or to another Valium-type medication.

Doral should not be used by patients with known or suspected sleep apnea (short periods of interrupted breathing that occur during sleep).

Doral must not be taken during pregnancy.

Special warnings about this medication

Because Doral may decrease daytime alertness, patients should not drive, climb, or operate dangerous machinery until they find out how the drug affects them. In some cases, Doral's sedative effect may last for several days after the last dose.

Doral may aggravate depression in patients with depressive disorders.

Patients with a history of alcohol or drug abuse are at special risk for addiction to Doral. It is important for patients to avoid increasing the dosage of Doral on their own. They should tell the doctor right away if the medication no longer seems to be working.

Possible food and drug interactions when taking this medication

If Doral is taken with certain other drugs, the effects of either could be increased, decreased, or altered. Here is an overview of drugs that may cause a problem:

Antihistamines such as Benadryl
Antiseizure medications such as Dilantin and Tegretol
Mood-altering medications such as Thorazine and Clozaril
Other central nervous system depressants such as Xanax and Valium

Patients should avoid drinking alcohol while taking Doral; it can increase the drug's effects.

Special information about pregnancy and breastfeeding

Because Doral may cause harm to the unborn child, it should not be taken during pregnancy. Patients should discontinue Doral before getting pregnant.

Babies whose mothers are taking Doral at the time of birth may experience withdrawal symptoms from the drug. Such babies may be "floppy" (flaccid) instead of having normal muscle tone.

Since Doral finds its way into breast milk, patients should not take this medication while nursing a baby.

Recommended dosage

ADULTS

The recommended initial dose is 15 milligrams daily. The doctor may later reduce this dosage to 7.5 milligrams.

CHILDREN

Safety and efficacy of Doral in children under 18 years old have not been established.

OLDER ADULTS

Older patients may be more sensitive to this drug, and the doctor may reduce the dosage after only 1 or 2 nights.

Overdosage

Any medication taken in excess can have serious consequences. If an overdose of Doral is suspected, seek medical attention immediately.

■ *Symptoms of an overdose of Doral may include:*
   Coma, confusion, extreme sleepiness

Generic name:

Doxepin

See Sinequan, page 188

Brand name:

Effexor

Pronounced: ef-ECKS-or
Generic name: Venlafaxine hydrochloride
Other brand name: Effexor XR

Why is this drug prescribed?

Effexor is prescribed for the treatment of depression. Effexor XR is also prescribed to relieve generalized anxiety disorder. The drug is thought to work by boosting levels of serotonin and norepinephrine, two important chemical messengers in the brain.

Most important fact about this drug

Serious, sometimes fatal reactions have occurred when Effexor is used in combination with drugs classified as MAO inhibitors, including the antidepressants Nardil and Parnate. Effexor must never be taken with one of these drugs; or within 14 days of discontinuing treatment with one of them. It is also important to allow at least 7 days between the last dose of Effexor and the first dose of an MAO inhibitor.

How should this medication be taken?

Effexor should be taken with food, exactly as prescribed. It may take several weeks before an effect is seen.

Effexor must be taken 2 or 3 times daily. The extended-release form, Effexor XR, permits once-a-day dosing. (It should be taken at the same time each day.) The capsule should be swallowed whole with water. It must not be divided, crushed, or chewed.

■ *Missed dose...*
   It is not necessary to make up a forgotten dose. Patients should skip the missed dose and continue with the next scheduled dose. They should never take 2 doses at once.

■ *Storage instructions...*
Effexor should be stored in a tightly closed container at room temperature and protected from excessive heat and moisture.

What side effects may occur?

Side effects cannot be predicted. If any develop or change in intensity, patients should inform their doctor as soon as possible.

■ *More common side effects may include:*
Abnormal dreams, abnormal ejaculation or orgasm, anxiety, appetite loss, blurred vision, chills, constipation, diarrhea, dizziness, dry mouth, frequent urination, flushing, gas, headache, impotence, infection, insomnia, muscle tension, nausea, nervousness, rash, sleepiness, sweating, tingling feeling, tremor, upset stomach, vomiting, weakness, yawning

■ *Less common side effects may include:*
Abnormal taste, abnormal thinking, agitation, chest pain, confusion, decreased sex drive, depression, dilated pupils, dizziness upon standing up, high blood pressure, itching, loss of identity, rapid heartbeat, ringing in the ears, trauma, twitching, urinary problems, weight loss

Why should this drug not be prescribed?

Remember that Effexor must never be combined with an MAO inhibitor. (See "Most important fact about this drug.") This drug should also be avoided by anyone who has had an allergic reaction to it.

Special warnings about this medication

Effexor should be used with caution in patients with high blood pressure; heart, liver, or kidney disease; or a history of seizures or mania. It's important for patients to discuss all of their medical problems with their doctor before taking Effexor.

Effexor sometimes causes an increase in blood pressure. If this happens, the doctor may need to reduce the dose or discontinue the drug.

Effexor also tends to increase the heart rate, especially at higher doses. Effexor must be used cautiously in patients who have recently had a heart attack, suffer from heart failure, or have an overactive thyroid gland.

Antidepressants such as Effexor may cause fluid retention, especially in older adults.

Effexor may cause patients to feel drowsy or less alert and may affect their judgment. They should avoid driving or operating dangerous machinery, or participating in any hazardous activity that requires full mental alertness, until they know how this drug affects them.

The doctor should regularly check any patient who has glaucoma (high pressure in the eye), or is at risk of developing it.

This drug should be discontinued only under supervision of a doctor. If it is stopped suddenly, patients may have withdrawal symptoms, even though Effexor does not seem to be habit-forming. The doctor will have them taper off gradually. If they have ever been addicted to drugs, they should tell the doctor before starting Effexor.

Patients who develop a skin rash or hives while taking Effexor should notify their doctor immediately. Effexor may also cause bleeding or bruising of the skin.

The safety and effectiveness of Effexor have not been established in children under 18 years of age.

Possible food and drug interactions when taking this medication

Combining Effexor with MAO inhibitors could cause a fatal reaction. (See "Most important fact about this drug.")

Although Effexor does not interact with alcohol, the manufacturer recommends avoiding alcohol while taking this medication.

Patients who have high blood pressure or liver disease, or are elderly, should check with their doctor before combining Effexor with cimetidine (Tagamet).

Effexor does not interact with Lithium or Valium. However, patients should consult their doctor before combining Effexor with other drugs that affect the central nervous system, including narcotic painkillers, sleep aids, tranquilizers, antipsychotic medicines such as Haldol, and other antidepressants such as Tofranil.

Effexor has been found to reduce blood levels of the HIV drug Crixivan. It's best for patients to check with their doctor before combining Effexor with any other drug or herbal product.

Special information about pregnancy and breastfeeding

The effects of Effexor during pregnancy have not been adequately studied. Patients should consult their doctor immediately if they are pregnant or are planning to become pregnant. Effexor should be used during pregnancy only if clearly needed.

If Effexor is taken shortly before delivery, the baby may suffer withdrawal symptoms. It's also known that Effexor appears in breast milk and could cause serious side effects in a nursing infant. Patients will need to choose between nursing their baby or continuing their treatment with Effexor.

Recommended dosage

EFFEXOR

The usual starting dose is 75 milligrams a day, divided into 2 or 3 smaller doses, and taken with food. If needed, the doctor may gradually increase the daily dose in steps of no more than 75 milligrams at a time up to a maximum of 375 milligrams per day.

If the patient has kidney or liver disease or is taking other medications, the doctor will adjust the dosage accordingly.

EFFEXOR XR

For both depression and anxiety the usual starting dose is 75 milligrams once daily, although some people begin with a dose of 37.5 milligrams for the first 4 to 7 days. The doctor may gradually increase the dose, in steps of no more than 75 milligrams, up to a maximum of 225 milligrams daily. As with regular Effexor, the doctor will make adjustments in the dosage for patients with kidney or liver disease.

Overdosage
An overdose of Effexor, combined with other drugs or alcohol, can be fatal. If an overdose is suspected, seek medical attention immediately.

■ *Symptoms of Effexor overdose include:*
Sleepiness, vertigo, rapid or slow heartbeat, low blood pressure, seizures, coma

Brand name:
Elavil

Pronounced: ELL-uh-vil
Generic name: Amitriptyline hydrochloride

Why is this drug prescribed?
Elavil is prescribed for the relief of major depression. It is a member of the group of drugs called tricyclic antidepressants. Some doctors also prescribe Elavil to treat bulimia (an eating disorder), to control chronic pain, to prevent migraine headaches, and to treat a pathological weeping and laughing syndrome associated with multiple sclerosis.

Most important fact about this drug
Elavil must be taken regularly for several weeks before it becomes fully effective. It's important that patients not skip any doses, even if they seem to make no difference or don't seem necessary.

How should this medication be taken?
Elavil must be taken exactly as prescribed. Patients may experience side effects, such as mild drowsiness, early in therapy. However, these problems usually disappear after a few days.

Elavil may cause dry mouth. Sucking a hard candy, chewing gum, or melting bits of ice in the mouth can provide relief.

■ *Missed dose...*
Generally, the forgotten dose should be taken as soon as remembered. However, if it is almost time for their next dose, patients should skip

the one they missed and go back to their regular schedule. Doses should never be doubled.

Patients who take a single daily dose at bedtime should not make up for it in the morning. It may cause side effects during the day.

■ *Storage instructions...*
Elavil should be stored at room temperature in a tightly closed container, and protected from light and excessive heat.

What side effects may occur?
Side effects cannot be predicted. If any develop or change in intensity, patients should inform their doctor as soon as possible.

Older adults are especially liable to certain side effects of Elavil, including rapid heartbeat, constipation, dry mouth, blurred vision, sedation, and confusion, and are in greater danger of sustaining a fall.

■ *Side effects may include:*
Abnormal movements, anxiety, black tongue, blurred vision, breast development in males, breast enlargement, coma, confusion, constipation, delusions, diarrhea, difficult or frequent urination, difficulty in speech, dilation of pupils, disorientation, disturbed concentration, dizziness on getting up, dizziness or light-headedness, drowsiness, dry mouth, excessive or spontaneous flow of milk, excitement, fatigue, fluid retention, hair loss, hallucinations, headache, heart attack, hepatitis, high blood pressure, high fever, high or low blood sugar, hives, impotence, inability to sleep, increased or decreased sex drive, increased perspiration, increased pressure within the eye, inflammation of the mouth, intestinal obstruction, irregular heartbeat, lack or loss of coordination, loss of appetite, low blood pressure, nausea, nightmares, numbness, rapid and/or fast, fluttery heartbeat, rash, red or purple spots on the skin, restlessness, ringing in the ears, seizures, sensitivity to light, stomach upset, strange taste, stroke, swelling due to fluid retention in the face and tongue, swelling of testicles, swollen glands, tingling and pins and needles in the arms and legs, tremors, vomiting, weakness, weight gain or loss, yellowed eyes and skin

■ *Side effects due to rapid decrease or abrupt withdrawal from Elavil include:*
Headache, nausea, vague feeling of bodily discomfort

■ *Side effects due to gradual dosage reduction may include:*
Dream and sleep disturbances, irritability, restlessness

These side effects do not signify an addiction to the drug.

Why should this drug not be prescribed?
Anyone who is sensitive to or has ever had an allergic reaction to Elavil or similar drugs such as Norpramin and Tofranil should not take this

medication. Patients should be careful to make the doctor aware of any drug reactions they have experienced.

Elavil cannot be used by anyone taking an MAO inhibitor such as the antidepressants Nardil and Parnate. Unless the doctor says otherwise, it should also be avoided by patients recovering from a heart attack.

Special warnings about this medication

Elavil should not be stopped abruptly, especially if the patient has been taking large doses for a long time. The doctor will schedule a gradual reduction in dosage that will help prevent a possible relapse and will reduce the possibility of withdrawal symptoms.

Elavil may make the skin more sensitive to sunlight. Patients should stay out of the sun, wear protective clothing, and apply a sunblock.

Elavil can make patients drowsy or less alert. They should avoid driving, operating dangerous machinery, or participating in any hazardous activity that requires full mental alertness until they know how this drug affects them.

While taking this medication, patients may feel dizzy or light-headed or actually faint when getting up from a lying or sitting position. If getting up slowly doesn't help or if this problem continues, the doctor should be notified.

Elavil should be used with caution in patients with a history of seizures, urinary retention, glaucoma or other chronic eye conditions, a heart or circulatory system disorder, or liver problems. Caution is also warranted in patients who are receiving thyroid medication. The doctor should be apprised of all the patient's medical problems before the start of Elavil therapy.

Patients should tell doctors they are taking Elavil before having surgery, dental treatment, or any diagnostic procedure. Certain drugs used during surgery, such as anesthetics and muscle relaxants, and drugs used in certain diagnostic procedures may react badly with Elavil.

Possible food and drug interactions when taking this medication

Elavil may intensify the effects of alcohol. Patients should avoid drinking alcohol while taking this medication.

If Elavil is taken with certain other drugs, the effects of either could be increased, decreased, or altered. Here is an overview of drugs that may cause a problem:

Airway-opening drugs such as Sudafed and Proventil
Antidepressants that raise serotonin levels, such as Paxil, Prozac, and Zoloft
Other antidepressants, such as amoxapine
Antihistamines such as Benadryl and Tavist
Antipsychotic medications such as Mellaril and Thorazine

Barbiturates such as phenobarbital
Certain blood pressure medicines such as Catapres
Cimetidine (Tagamet)
Disulfiram (Antabuse)
Drugs that control spasms, such as Bentyl and Donnatal
Estrogen drugs such as Premarin and oral contraceptives
Ethchlorvynol (Placidyl)
MAO inhibitors, such as Nardil and Parnate
Medications for irregular heartbeat, such as Tambocor and Rythmol
Painkillers such as Demerol and Percocet
Parkinson's drugs such as Cogentin and Larodopa
Quinidine (Quinidex)
Seizure medications such as Tegretol and Dilantin
Sleep medicines such as Halcion and Dalmane
Thyroid hormones (Synthroid)
Tranquilizers such as Librium and Xanax
Warfarin (Coumadin)

Special information about pregnancy and breastfeeding

The effects of Elavil during pregnancy have not been adequately studied. Patients should inform their doctor immediately if they are pregnant or are planning to become pregnant.

This medication appears in breast milk. If Elavil is essential to a patient's health, the doctor may advise her to discontinue breastfeeding until treatment is finished.

Recommended dosage

ADULTS

The usual starting dosage is 75 milligrams per day divided into 2 or more smaller doses. The doctor may gradually increase this dose to 150 milligrams per day. The total daily dose is generally never higher than 200 milligrams.

Alternatively, the doctor may start patients with 50 milligrams to 100 milligrams at bedtime. This bedtime dose may be gradually increased by 25 or 50 milligrams up to a total of 150 milligrams a day.

For long-term use, the usual dose ranges from 40 to 100 milligrams taken once daily, usually at bedtime.

CHILDREN

Use of Elavil is not recommended for children under 12 years of age.

The usual dose for adolescents 12 years of age and over is 10 milligrams, 3 times a day, with 20 milligrams taken at bedtime.

OLDER ADULTS

The usual dose is 10 milligrams taken 3 times a day, with 20 milligrams taken at bedtime.

Overdosage

An overdose of Elavil can prove fatal.

■ *Symptoms of Elavil overdose may include:*
Abnormally low blood pressure, confusion, convulsions, dilated pupils and other eye problems, disturbed concentration, drowsiness, hallucinations, impaired heart function, rapid or irregular heartbeat, reduced body temperature, stupor, unresponsiveness or coma

■ *Symptoms contrary to the usual effect of this medication are:*
Agitation, extremely high body temperature, overactive reflexes, rigid muscles, vomiting

If an overdose is suspected, seek medical attention immediately.

Brand name:

Eskalith

Pronounced: ESS-kuh-lith
Generic name: Lithium carbonate
Other brand names: Eskalith CR, Lithobid

Why is this drug prescribed?

Eskalith is used to treat the manic episodes of bipolar disorder. Once the mania subsides, Eskalith treatment may be continued over the long term, at a somewhat lower dosage, to prevent or reduce the intensity of future manic episodes.

Some doctors also prescribe lithium for premenstrual tension, eating disorders such as bulimia, certain movement disorders, and sexual addictions.

Most important fact about this drug

If the Eskalith dosage is too low, patients derive no benefit; if it is too high, they could suffer lithium poisoning. Patient and doctor must work together to find the correct dosage. Initially, this means frequent blood tests to find out how much of the drug is actually circulating in the patient's bloodstream. Later, the patient must stay alert for side effects. Signs of lithium poisoning include vomiting, unsteady walking, diarrhea, drowsiness, tremor, and weakness. If any of these symptoms develop, the patient should stop taking the drug and call the doctor.

How should this medication be taken?

To avoid stomach upset, Eskalith should be taken immediately after meals or with food or milk.

It is unwise to change from one brand of lithium to another without consulting a doctor or pharmacist. The drug should be taken exactly as prescribed.

While taking Eskalith, patients should drink 10 to 12 glasses of water or fluid a day. To minimize the risk of harmful side effects, they should eat a balanced diet that includes some salt and lots of liquids. Patients who have been sweating a great deal or have had diarrhea should be sure to get extra liquids and salt.

Patients should keep in close touch with their doctor if they develop an infection with a fever. They may need to cut back on their Eskalith dosage or even quit taking it temporarily.

Long-acting forms of lithium, such as Eskalith CR or Lithobid, should be swallowed whole. They should not be chewed, crushed, or broken.

■ *Missed dose...*
Patients need to check with the doctor; requirements vary for each individual. Doses should never be doubled.

■ *Storage instructions...*
Eskalith may be stored at room temperature.

What side effects may occur?
The possibility of side effects varies with the level of lithium in the bloodstream. Patients should inform their doctor as soon as possible if they experience unfamiliar symptoms of any kind.

■ *Side effects that may occur when lithium is started include:*
Discomfort, frequent urination, hand tremor, mild thirst, nausea

■ *Other side effects may include:*
Abdominal pain, blackout spells, cavities, changes in taste perception, coma, confusion, dehydration, dizziness, dry hair, dry mouth, fatigue, gas, hair loss, hallucinations, increased salivation, indigestion, involuntary tongue movements, involuntary urination or bowel movements, irregular heartbeat, itching, loss of appetite, low blood pressure, muscle rigidity, muscle twitching, painful joints, poor memory, restlessness, ringing in ears, seizures, sexual dysfunction, skin problems, sleepiness, slowed thinking, slurred speech, startle response, swelling, thinning hair, tightness in chest, vision problems, vomiting, weakness, weight gain, weight loss

Why should this drug not be prescribed?
Although doctors are cautious under certain conditions, lithium may be prescribed for anyone.

Special warnings about this medication
Eskalith may affect judgment or coordination. Patients should avoid driving, climbing, or performing hazardous tasks until they find out how this drug affects them.

Eskalith should be used with extra caution in patients who have a heart or kidney problem, brain or spinal cord disease, or a weak, run-down, or dehydrated condition. It's important for patients to make sure the doctor is aware of any medical problems they may have, including diabetes, epilepsy, thyroid problems, Parkinson's disease, and difficulty urinating.

Patients should avoid activities that cause heavy sweating. They should also avoid drinking large amounts of coffee, tea, or cola, which can cause dehydration through increased urination. It is unwise for patients to make a major change in eating habits or to go on a weight loss diet without consulting the doctor. The loss of water and salt from the body could lead to lithium poisoning.

Possible food and drug interactions when taking this medication

If Eskalith is taken with certain other drugs, the effects of either could be increased, decreased, or altered. Here is an overview of drugs that may cause a problem:

ACE-inhibitor blood pressure drugs such as Capoten or Vasotec
Acetazolamide (Diamox)
Amphetamines such as Dexedrine
Antidepressant drugs that boost serotonin levels, including Paxil, Prozac, and Zoloft
Anti-inflammatory drugs such as Indocin and Feldene
Antipsychotic medications such as Haldol and Thorazine
Bicarbonate of soda
Caffeine (No-Doz)
Calcium-blocking blood pressure drugs such as Calan and Cardizem
Carbamazepine (Tegretol)
Diuretics such as Lasix or HydroDIURIL
Iodine-containing preparations such as potassium iodide (Quadrinal)
Methyldopa (Aldomet)
Metronidazole (Flagyl)
Phenytoin (Dilantin)
Sodium bicarbonate
Tetracyclines such as Achromycin V and Sumycin
Theophylline (Theo-Dur, Quibron, others)

Special information about pregnancy and breastfeeding

The use of Eskalith during pregnancy can harm the developing baby. Patients should inform the doctor immediately if they are pregnant or plan to become pregnant.

Eskalith appears in breast milk and is considered potentially harmful to a nursing infant. If this medication is essential to the patient's health, the doctor may advise her to discontinue breastfeeding while she is taking it.

Recommended dosage

ADULTS

Acute Episodes

The usual dosage is a total of 1,800 milligrams per day. Immediate-release forms are taken in 3 or 4 doses per day; long-acting forms are taken twice a day.

Dosage is individualized according to the levels of the drug in the patient's blood. Blood levels will be checked at least twice a week when the drug is first prescribed and on a regular basis thereafter.

Long-term Control

Dosage will vary from one individual to another, but a total of 900 milligrams to 1,200 milligrams per day is typical. Immediate-release forms are taken in 3 or 4 doses per day; long-acting forms are taken twice a day. Blood levels in most cases should be checked every 2 months.

CHILDREN

Safety and effectiveness of Eskalith in children under 12 years of age have not been established.

OLDER ADULTS

Older people often need less Eskalith and may show signs of overdose at a dosage that younger people can handle well.

Overdosage

Any medication taken in excess can have serious consequences. If an overdose of Eskalith is suspected, seek medical attention immediately.

The harmful levels are close to those needed for treatment. Patients need to watch for early signs of overdose, such as diarrhea, drowsiness, lack of coordination, vomiting, and weakness. If they develop any of these signs, they should stop taking the drug and call the doctor.

Generic name:

Estazolam

See ProSom, page 154

Brand name:

Etrafon

See Triavil, page 212

Brand name:

Exelon

Pronounced: ECKS-ell-on
Generic name: Rivastigmine tartrate

Why is this drug prescribed?

Exelon is used in the treatment of mild to moderate Alzheimer's disease. Alzheimer's disease causes physical changes in the brain that disrupt the flow of information and interfere with memory, thinking, and behavior. By boosting levels of the chemical messenger acetylcholine, Exelon can temporarily improve brain function in some Alzheimer's sufferers, though it does not halt the progress of the underlying disease. Like other drugs for Alzheimer's (Aricept, Cognex, and Reminyl), Exelon may become less effective as the disease progresses.

Most important fact about this drug

Patience is in order when starting this drug. It can take up to 12 weeks before Exelon's full benefits appear.

How should this medication be taken?

Exelon should be taken with food in the morning and in the evening.

■ *Missed dose...*
  Generally, the forgotten dose should be given as soon as remembered. However, if it is almost time for the next dose, caregivers should skip the one they missed and go back to the regular schedule. Doses should never be doubled.
■ *Storage instructions...*
  Exelon should be stored at room temperature in a tightly closed container.

What side effects may occur?

Side effects cannot be predicted. If any develop or change in intensity, caregivers should inform the doctor as soon as possible.

■ *More common side effects may include:*
  Abdominal pain, accidental injury, anxiety, aggression, confusion, constipation, depression, diarrhea, dizziness, drowsiness, fainting, fatigue, flu-like symptoms, gas, hallucinations, headache, high blood pressure, increased sweating, indigestion, inflamed nasal passages, insomnia, loss of appetite, nausea, tremor, unwell feeling, urinary infection, vomiting, weakness, weight loss

■ *Less common side effects may include:*
  Belching

Why should this drug not be prescribed?

Exelon cannot be used if it causes an allergic reaction.

Special warnings about this medication

Exelon often causes nausea and vomiting, especially at the beginning of treatment. The problem is more likely in women, but it can lead to significant weight loss in both women and men. The doctor should be informed immediately if these side effects occur.

The chance of severe vomiting increases when Exelon is given after an interruption of several days. Caregivers should check with the doctor before starting to give the drug again. Dosage may need to be reduced to the lowest starting level.

Exelon may aggravate asthma and other breathing problems and can increase the risk of seizures. Other drugs of its type are also known to increase the chance of ulcers, stomach bleeding, and urinary obstruction, although these problems have not been noted with Exelon. Drugs in this category can also slow the heartbeat, possibly causing fainting in people who have a heart condition. The doctor should be alerted if any of these problems occur.

Exelon has not been tested in children.

Possible food and drug interactions when taking this medication

If Exelon is taken with certain other drugs, the effects of either could be increased, decreased, or altered. Here is an overview of drugs that may cause a problem:

Bethanechol (Urecholine)
Drugs that control spasms, such as Bentyl, Donnatal, and Levsin.

Special information about pregnancy and breastfeeding

Exelon is not intended for women of child-bearing age, and its effects during pregnancy and breastfeeding have not been studied.

Recommended dosage

ADULTS

The usual starting dose is 1.5 milligrams 2 times a day for at least 2 weeks. At 2-week intervals, the doctor may then increase the dose to 3 milligrams, 4.5 milligrams, and finally 6.0 milligrams 2 times a day. Higher doses tend to be more effective. The maximum dosage is 12 milligrams daily.

If side effects such as nausea and vomiting begin to develop, the doctor may recommend skipping a few doses, then starting again at the same or the next lowest dosage.

Overdosage

Any medication taken in excess can have serious consequences. If an overdose is suspected, seek emergency medical attention immediately.

■ *Symptoms of Exelon overdose may include:*
Collapse, convulsions, breathing difficulty, extreme muscle weakness (possibly ending in death if breathing muscles are affected), low blood pressure, salivation, severe nausea, slow heartbeat, sweating, vomiting

Generic name:

Fluoxetine

See Prozac, page 157

Generic name:

Fluphenazine

See Prolixin, page 150

Generic name:

Flurazepam

See Dalmane, page 43

Generic name:

Fluvoxamine

See Luvox, page 104

Brand name:

Focalin

Pronounced: FOKE-ah-lin
Generic name: Dexmethylphenidate hydrochloride

Why is this drug prescribed?
Focalin is a mild central nervous system stimulant used to treat Attention Deficit Hyperactivity Disorder (ADHD) in children. The drug is a modified version of Ritalin (a common medication for attention disorders) and contains only the most active component of Ritalin. Because of this special formulation, the usual dose of Focalin is half the amount of the Ritalin dose. Focalin should be given as part of a total treatment program that includes psychological, educational, and social measures.

Most important fact about this drug

Excessive doses of Focalin over a long period of time can produce addiction. It is also possible to develop tolerance to the drug, so that larger doses are needed to produce the original effect. Because of these dangers, the doctor should be consulted before making any change in dosage; and the drug should be withdrawn only under a doctor's supervision.

How should this medication be taken?

Focalin can be taken with or without food. The drug is usually taken twice a day, at least 4 hours apart, but the doctor may adjust the schedule depending on the child's response.

■ *Missed dose...*
The dose should be given to the child as soon as it's remembered. If it is almost time for the next dose, the missed dose should be skipped and the child should return to the regular schedule. Doses should never be doubled.

■ *Storage instructions...*
Like all drugs, this one should be kept out of reach of children. It should be stored below 86 degrees Fahrenheit in a tightly closed, light-resistant container. It should not be stored in hot, damp, or humid places.

What side effects may occur?

Side effects cannot be predicted. If any develop or change in intensity, the caregiver should inform the child's doctor as soon as possible.

■ *More common side effects may include:*
Fever, loss of appetite, nausea, and stomach pain

The most common side effects reported for drugs that are similar to Focalin (including Ritalin) are nervousness and the inability to fall asleep or stay asleep. In children, loss of appetite, stomach pain, weight loss during long-term treatment, inability to fall asleep or stay asleep, and abnormally fast heartbeat are the more common side effects.

■ *Less common or rare side effects may include:*
Abnormal heartbeat, abnormal muscular movements, allergic reactions including skin rash, anemia, blood pressure changes, blood vessel inflammation or blockage in the brain, chest pain, depression, dizziness, drowsiness, emotional instability marked by abnormal thinking or hallucinations, hair loss, headache, hives, inability to fall asleep or stay asleep, jerking or twitching body movements, joint pain, palpitations, pulse changes, purplish skin spots or bruises, severe skin rash, skin inflammation with peeling, Tourette's syndrome (severe twitching), vomiting

Why should this drug not be prescribed?

Focalin should not be used by people who suffer from anxiety, tension, and agitation, since the drug may aggravate these symptoms.

If Focalin, or similar drugs such as Ritalin, cause an allergic reaction, the drug should be avoided. It should not be taken by anyone with the eye condition known as glaucoma. It should also be avoided by anyone who suffers from motion tics (repeated, uncontrollable twitches) or verbal tics (uncontrollable repetition of words or sounds), or someone who suffers from, or has a family history of, Tourette's syndrome (severe and multiple tics).

Focalin should not be taken with drugs classified as monoamine oxidase (MAO) inhibitors, such as the antidepressants Nardil and Parnate, or within 14 days of stopping this type of medication.

Special warnings about this medication

The doctor will do a complete history and evaluation before prescribing Focalin. It is important to remember that the drug is only part of the overall management of ADHD, and that the doctor should also recommend counseling or other therapy.

There is no information about the safety and effectiveness of long-term Focalin treatment in children. However, suppression of growth has been seen with the long-term use of stimulants, so it's important to watch the child carefully while he or she is taking this drug. If the child is not growing or gaining weight as expected, the doctor may have to stop Focalin treatment. This drug should not be given to children under 6 years of age; safety and effectiveness in this age group have not been established.

Blood pressure should be monitored in anyone taking Focalin, especially those with high blood pressure or abnormal heart rate or rhythm. Caution is also advised in those with heart or thyroid problems.

The doctor should be alerted if the child develops blurred vision while taking Focalin; some people have reported visual disturbances while taking stimulants similar to this drug.

The use of Focalin by anyone with a seizure disorder or psychosis is not recommended. Caution is also advisable for anyone with a history of emotional instability or substance abuse, due to the danger of addiction. Focalin should not be used for the prevention or treatment of normal fatigue, nor should it be used for the treatment of severe depression.

Focalin should not be shared with anyone else, and the child should be given only the number of tablets prescribed by the doctor. Caregivers should keep track of the number of tablets in a bottle so they can tell if any are missing. Incorrect use of Focalin can lead to dependence. The doctor should be consulted *immediately* if the drug is being used in more than the prescribed amount.

Possible food and drug interactions when taking this medication

If Focalin is taken with certain other drugs, the effects of either can be increased, decreased, or altered. Here is an overview of drugs that may cause a problem:

Antidepressant drugs, including MAO inhibitors (Nardil, Parnate), tricyclics (Elavil, Tofranil), and serotonin reuptake inhibitors (Prozac, Paxil)

Antiseizure drugs such as phenobarbital, Dilantin, and Mysoline

Blood pressure drugs such as Catapres

Blood thinners such as Coumadin

Herbal remedies such as Ephedra and St. John's Wort

Special information about pregnancy and breastfeeding

The effects of Focalin during pregnancy have not been adequately studied. Caregivers should tell the doctor immediately if the patient becomes pregnant. Focalin should be used during pregnancy only if clearly needed.

It is not known whether Focalin appears in breast milk. Caution is advised if the patient is nursing a baby.

Recommended dosage

For patients who are not currently taking Ritalin, the usual starting dose is 5 milligrams a day. For those who are switching from Ritalin, the starting Focalin dose is half the amount of the Ritalin dose. In either case, the total daily dose of Focalin should be divided into 2 doses taken at least 4 hours apart.

Depending on the response, the doctor may increase the dose by 2.5 to 5 milligrams a day, up to a maximum daily dose of 20 milligrams (10 milligrams twice a day). Increases are usually made at weekly intervals.

Overdosage

If an overdose is suspected, seek medical attention immediately.

■ *Symptoms of Focalin overdose may include:*
Abnormal reflexes, agitation, confusion, convulsions (may be followed by coma), delirium, dryness of mucous membranes, enlarged pupils in the eyes, exaggerated feeling of elation, extremely elevated body temperature, flushing, hallucinations, headache, high blood pressure, irregular or rapid heartbeat, muscle twitching, palpitations, sweating, tremors, vomiting

Generic name:

Galantamine

See Reminyl, page 163

Brand name:

Geodon

Pronounced: GEE-oh-dahn
Generic name: Ziprasidone hydrochloride

Why is this drug prescribed?

Geodon is used in the treatment of schizophrenia. Researchers believe that it works by opposing the action of serotonin and dopamine, two of the brain's major chemical messengers. Because of its potentially serious side effects, Geodon is typically prescribed only after other medications have proved inadequate. An intramuscular injection is available for use in agitated patients.

Most important fact about this drug

In some people with heart problems or a slow heartbeat, Geodon can cause serious and potentially fatal heartbeat irregularities. The chance of a problem is greater if the patient is taking a water pill (diuretic) or a medication that prolongs a part of the heartbeat known as the QT interval. Many of the drugs prescribed for heartbeat irregularities prolong the QT interval and should never be combined with Geodon. Other drugs to avoid when taking Geodon include Anzemet, Avelox, Halfan, Inapsine, Lariam, Mellaril, Nebupent, Orap, Orlaam, Pentam, Probucol, Prograf, Serentil, Tequin, Thorazine, Trisenox, and Zagam. Patients should check with their doctor before combining Geodon with any drug they're unsure of.

How should this medication be taken?

Geodon capsules should be taken twice a day with food.

■ *Missed dose...*
Generally, the forgotten dose should be taken as soon as remembered. However, if it is almost time for the next dose, patients should skip the one they missed and go back to their regular schedule. Doses should never be doubled.

■ *Storage instructions...*
Geodon may be stored at room temperature.

What side effects may occur?

Side effects cannot be predicted. If any develop or change in intensity, patients should inform their doctor as soon as possible.

■ *More common side effects may include:*
Accidental injury, cold symptoms, constipation, cough, diarrhea, dizziness, drowsiness, dry mouth, indigestion, muscle tightness, nausea, rash, stuffy and runny nose, upper respiratory infection, vision problems, weakness

■ *Other side effects may include:*
Abdominal pain, abnormal body movements, abnormal ejaculation, abnormal secretion of milk, abnormal walk, abnormally low cholesterol, agitation, amnesia, anemia, bleeding gums, bleeding in the eye, blood clots, blood disorders, blood in urine, body spasms, breast development in males, bruising or purple spots, cataracts, chest pain, chills, clogged bowels, confusion, conjunctivitis (pinkeye), coordination problems, decreased blood flow to the heart, delirium, difficulty breathing, difficulty swallowing, difficulty with orgasm, double vision, dry eyes, enlarged heart, eyelid inflammation, female sexual problems, fever, flank pain, flu-like symptoms, fungal infections, gout, hair loss, heavy menstruation, heavy uterine or vaginal bleeding, high blood pressure, high blood sugar, hives, hostility, impotence, increased reflexes, increased sensitivity to touch or sound, inflammation of the cornea, inflammation of the heart, involuntary or jerky movements, irregular heartbeat, liver problems, lockjaw, loss of appetite, loss of menstruation, low blood sugar, low blood pressure, low body temperature, lymph disorders, male sexual problems, muscle disorders, muscle pain, muscle weakness, nighttime urination, nosebleed, pneumonia, prickling or tingling sensation, rapid heartbeat, rectal bleeding, rigid muscle movement, ringing in ears, rolling of the eyeballs, sensitivity to sunlight, skin problems, slow heartbeat, slowed movement, speech problems, stroke, sudden drop in blood pressure upon standing up, swelling in the arms and legs, swelling in the face, swollen lymph nodes, swollen tongue, tarry stools, tendon inflammation, thirst, throat spasms, thyroid disorders, tremor, twitching, uncontrolled eye movement, urination decrease or increase, vaginal bleeding, vein inflammation, vertigo, vision disorders, vomiting, vomiting or spitting blood, yellowed skin and eyes, weight gain, white spots in the mouth

Why should this drug not be prescribed?
Geodon cannot be taken by anyone who has the heartbeat irregularity known as QT prolongation, has had a recent heart attack, or suffers from heart failure. This drug should also be avoided if it causes an allergic reaction.

Special warnings about this medication
Remember that Geodon can cause dangerous—even fatal—heartbeat irregularities. Warning signs include dizziness, palpitations, and faint-

ing. The doctor should be consulted immediately if any of these symptoms develop.

Particularly during the first few days of therapy, Geodon can cause low blood pressure, with accompanying dizziness, fainting, and rapid heartbeat. The doctor should be notified of any of these side effects. To minimize such problems, the doctor will increase the dose gradually. If a patient is prone to low blood pressure, takes blood pressure medicine, becomes dehydrated, or has heart disease or poor circulation in the brain, Geodon should be used with caution.

Geodon may cause drowsiness and can impair judgment, thinking, and motor skills. Patients should use caution while driving and should avoid operating potentially dangerous machinery until they know how this drug affects them.

Geodon poses a very slight risk of seizures, especially if a patient is over age 65, has a history of seizures, or has Alzheimer's disease.

Drugs such as Geodon sometimes cause a condition called Neuroleptic Malignant Syndrome. Symptoms include high fever, muscle rigidity, irregular pulse or blood pressure, rapid heartbeat, excessive perspiration, and changes in heart rhythm. If these symptoms appear, the doctor should be informed immediately. The patient will need to stop taking Geodon while the condition is under treatment.

There also is the risk of developing tardive dyskinesia, a condition marked by slow, rhythmical, involuntary movements. This problem is more likely to occur in mature adults, especially older women. When it does, use of Geodon is usually stopped.

Geodon can suppress the cough reflex, making it difficult to clear the airway. Some people taking Geodon also develop a rash. If this happens, the doctor should be informed. If the rash doesn't clear up with treatment, the drug may have to be discontinued.

Other antipsychotic medications have been known to interfere with the body's temperature-regulating mechanism, causing the body to overheat. Although this problem has not occurred with Geodon, caution is still advisable. Patients should avoid exposure to extreme heat, strenuous exercise, and dehydration. There also is a remote chance that this medication may cause abnormal, prolonged and painful erections.

Possible food and drug interactions when taking this medication

Patients should be careful to avoid drugs that prolong the QT interval of the heartbeat. They should check with their doctor before combining any other medication with Geodon.

If Geodon is taken with certain other drugs, the effects of either could be increased, decreased, or altered. Here is an overview of drugs that may cause a problem:

Carbamazepine (Tegretol)

Certain blood pressure medications

Drugs that boost the effects of dopamine such as Mirapex, Parlodel, Permax, and Requip

Drugs that affect the brain and nervous system, such as sedatives, tranquilizers, and antidepressants

Ketoconazole (Nizoral)

Levodopa (Larodopa, Sinemet)

Special information about pregnancy and breastfeeding

Geodon has caused fetal harm when tested in animals. It should be taken during pregnancy only if the benefits outweigh the potential risk. Patients should notify their doctor as soon as they become pregnant or plan to become pregnant.

It is not known whether Geodon appears in breast milk, and breastfeeding is not recommended.

Recommended dosage

The usual starting dose is 20 milligrams twice a day. If needed, the dosage may be increased at several-week intervals up to a maximum of 80 milligrams twice a day. Intramuscular injections of 10 milligrams may be given every 2 hours. Injections of 20 milligrams may be given every 4 hours. The maximum daily dose by injection is 40 milligrams.

Overdosage

Any medication taken in excess can have serious consequences. If an overdose is suspected, seek medical help immediately.

■ *Symptoms of Geodon overdose may include:*
  Drowsiness, slurred speech, high blood pressure

Brand name:

Halcion

Pronounced: HAL-see-on
Generic name: Triazolam

Why is this drug prescribed?

Halcion is used for short-term treatment of insomnia. It is a member of the benzodiazepine class of drugs, many of which are used as tranquilizers.

Most important fact about this drug

Sleep problems are usually temporary, requiring treatment for only a short time, usually 1 or 2 days and no more than 1 to 2 weeks. Insomnia that lasts longer than this may be a sign of another medical problem. If patients find they need this medicine for more than 7 to 10 days, they should check with their doctor.

How should this medication be taken?

This medication must be taken exactly as directed. It is important to never take more than the doctor has prescribed.

■ *Missed dose...*
Halcion should be taken only as needed.

■ *Storage instructions...*
This medication should be kept in the container it came in, tightly closed, and out of reach of children. It may be stored at room temperature.

What side effects may occur?

Side effects cannot be predicted. If any develop or change in intensity, patients should inform their doctor as soon as possible.

■ *More common side effects may include:*
Coordination problems, dizziness, drowsiness, headache, lightheadedness, nausea/vomiting, nervousness

■ *Less common or rare side effects may include:*
Aggressiveness, agitation, behavior problems, burning tongue, changes in sexual drive, chest pain, confusion, congestion, constipation, cramps/pain, delusions, depression, diarrhea, disorientation, dreaming abnormalities, drowsiness, dry mouth, exaggerated sense of well-being, excitement, fainting, falling, fatigue, hallucinations, impaired urination, inappropriate behavior, incontinence, inflammation of the tongue and mouth, irritability, itching, loss of appetite, loss of sense of reality, memory impairment, memory loss (e.g. traveler's amnesia), menstrual irregularities, morning "hangover" effects, muscle spasms in the shoulders or neck, nightmares, rapid heart rate, restlessness, ringing in the ears, skin inflammation, sleep disturbances including insomnia, sleepwalking, slurred or difficult speech, stiff awkward movements, taste changes, tingling or pins and needles, tiredness, visual disturbances, weakness, yellowing of the skin and whites of the eyes

Why should this drug not be prescribed?

Halcion should not be taken during pregnancy. Patients should also avoid it if they have had an allergic reaction to it or to other benzodiazepine drugs such as Valium. It should never be combined with the antifungal medications Nizoral or Sporanox, or the antidepressant Serzone.

Special warnings about this medication

When Halcion is used every night for more than a few weeks, it loses its effectiveness. This is known as tolerance. Also, it can cause dependence, especially when it is used regularly for longer than a few weeks or at high doses.

Abrupt discontinuation of Halcion should be avoided, since it has been associated with withdrawal symptoms (convulsions, cramps, tremor, vomiting, sweating, feeling ill, perceptual problems, and insomnia). A gradual dosage tapering schedule is usually recommended for patients taking more than the lowest dose of Halcion for longer than a few weeks. The usual treatment period is 7 to 10 days.

If patients develop unusual and disturbing thoughts or behavior—including increased anxiety or depression—during treatment with Halcion, they should discuss them with their doctor immediately.

"Traveler's amnesia" has been reported by patients who took Halcion to induce sleep while traveling. To avoid this condition, patients should not take Halcion on an overnight airplane flight of less than 7 to 8 hours.

Some people suffer increased anxiety during the daytime while taking Halcion.

Because Halcion could have a "carry over" effect the next day, patients first starting therapy should use extreme care while doing anything that requires complete alertness, such as driving a car or operating machinery.

After discontinuing the drug, patients may experience a "rebound insomnia" for the first 2 nights.

They should be aware that anterograde amnesia (forgetting events after an injury) has been associated with benzodiazepine drugs such as Halcion.

Halcion should be used with caution by anyone who has liver or kidney problems, lung problems, or a tendency to temporarily stop breathing while asleep.

Possible food and drug interactions when taking this medication

Patients should avoid alcoholic beverages and grapefruit juice while taking Halcion.

If Halcion is taken with certain other drugs, the effects of either could be increased, decreased, or altered. Here is an overview of drugs that may cause a problem:

Amiodarone (Cordarone)
Antidepressant medications, including "tricyclic" drugs such as Elavil and such MAO inhibitors as Nardil and Parnate
Antihistamines such as Benadryl and Tavist
Antipsychotic medications such as Mellaril and Thorazine
Barbiturates such as phenobarbital and Seconal
Cimetidine (Tagamet)
Clarithromycin (Biaxin)
Cyclosporine (Sandimmune, Neoral)
Diltiazem (Cardizem)
Ergotamine (Cafergot)

Erythromycin (E.E.S., PCE, E-Mycin, others)
Fluvoxamine (Luvox)
Isoniazid (Nydrazid)
Itraconazole (Nizoral)
Ketoconazole (Sporanox)
Narcotic painkillers such as Demerol
Nefazodone (Serzone)
Nicardipine (Cardene)
Nifedipine (Adalat)
Other tranquilizers such as BuSpar, Valium, and Xanax
Oral contraceptives
Paroxetine (Paxil)
Ranitidine (Zantac)
Seizure medications such as Dilantin and Tegretol
Sertraline (Zoloft)
Verapamil (Calan)

Special information about pregnancy and breastfeeding

Since benzodiazepines have been associated with damage to the developing baby, women should not take Halcion if they are pregnant, think they may be pregnant, or are planning to become pregnant. Halcion must also be avoided while breastfeeding.

Recommended dosage

ADULTS

The usual dose is 0.25 milligram before bedtime. The dose should never be more than 0.5 milligram.

CHILDREN

Safety and effectiveness for children under the age of 18 have not been established.

OLDER ADULTS

To decrease the possibility of oversedation, dizziness, or impaired coordination, the usual starting dose is 0.125 milligram. This may be increased to 0.25 milligram if necessary.

Overdosage

Any medication taken in excess can have serious consequences. Severe overdosage of Halcion can be fatal. If an overdose is suspected, seek medical help immediately.

■ *Symptoms of Halcion overdose may include:*
Apnea (temporary cessation of breathing), coma, confusion, excessive sleepiness, problems in coordination, seizures, shallow or difficult breathing, slurred speech

Brand name:

Haldol

Pronounced: HAL-dawl
Generic name: Haloperidol

Why is this drug prescribed?

Haldol is used to reduce the symptoms of mental disorders such as schizophrenia. It is also prescribed to control tics (uncontrolled muscle contractions of face, arms, or shoulders) and the unintended utterances that mark Gilles de la Tourette's syndrome. It is used in the short-term treatment of children with severe behavior problems such as combative hyperexcitability. It is also prescribed for the short-term treatment of hyperactive children with conduct disorders marked by some or all of the following symptoms: impulsivity, difficulty sustaining attention, aggressivity, mood lability, and poor frustration tolerance.

Some doctors also prescribe Haldol to relieve severe nausea and vomiting caused by cancer drugs, to treat drug problems such as LSD flashback and PCP intoxication, and to control symptoms of hemiballismus, a condition that causes involuntary writhing of one side of the body.

Most important fact about this drug

Haldol may cause tardive dyskinesia—a condition characterized by involuntary muscle spasms and twitches in the face and body. This condition can be permanent, and appears to be most common among the elderly, especially women.

How should this medication be taken?

Haldol may be taken with food or after eating. If taking Haldol in a liquid concentrate form, patients will need to dilute it with milk or water.

Haldol should not be taken with coffee, tea, or other caffeinated beverages, or with alcohol.

Haldol causes dry mouth. Sucking on a hard candy or ice chips may help alleviate the problem.

■ *Missed dose...*
The forgotten dose should be taken as soon as remembered. The rest of the doses for that day should follow at equally spaced intervals. Doses should never be doubled.

■ *Storage instructions...*
Haldol should be stored away from heat, light, and moisture in a tightly closed container. The liquid should be protected from freezing.

What side effects may occur?

Side effects cannot be predicted. If any develop or change in intensity, patients should inform their doctor as soon as possible.

■ *Side effects may include:*

Abnormal secretion of milk, acne-like skin reactions, agitation, anemia, anxiety, blurred vision, breast pain, breast development in males, cataracts, catatonic state, chewing movements, confusion, constipation, coughing, deeper breathing, dehydration, depression, diarrhea, dizziness, drowsiness, dry mouth, epileptic seizures, exaggerated feeling of well-being, exaggerated reflexes, excessive perspiration, excessive salivation, hair loss, hallucinations, headache, heat stroke, high fever, high or low blood pressure, high or low blood sugar, impotence, inability to urinate, increased sex drive, indigestion, involuntary movements, irregular menstrual periods, irregular pulse, lack of muscular coordination, liver problems, loss of appetite, muscle spasms, nausea, Parkinson-like symptoms, persistent abnormal erections, physical rigidity and stupor, protruding tongue, puckering of mouth, puffing of checks, rapid heartbeat, restlessness, rigid limbs and muscles, rotation of eyeballs, sensitivity to light, skin rash, skin eruptions, sleeplessness, sluggishness, swelling of breasts, twitching in the body, neck, shoulders, and face, vertigo, visual problems, vomiting, wheezing or asthma-like symptoms, yellowing of skin and whites of eyes

Why should this drug not be prescribed?

Haldol should be avoided by anyone who has Parkinson's disease or is sensitive to or allergic to the drug.

Special warnings about this medication

Haldol should be used with caution by patients who have had or currently have breast cancer, a severe heart or circulatory disorder, chest pain, the eye condition known as glaucoma, seizures, or any drug allergies.

Temporary muscle spasms and twitches may occur if Haldol is stopped abruptly. Patients need to follow the doctor's instructions closely when discontinuing the drug.

This drug may impair the ability to drive a car or operate potentially dangerous machinery. Patients should avoid any activities that require full alertness if they are unsure of their reaction to Haldol.

Haldol may make the skin more sensitive to sunlight. Patients should use a sunscreen or wear protective clothing when spending time in the sun.

Patients should avoid exposure to extreme heat or cold. Haldol interferes with the body's temperature-regulating mechanism, so they could become overheated or suffer severe chills.

Possible food and drug interactions when taking this medication

Extreme drowsiness and other potentially serious effects can result if Haldol is combined with alcohol, narcotics, painkillers, sleeping medications, or other drugs that slow down the central nervous system.

If Haldol is taken with certain other drugs, the effects of either could be increased, decreased, or altered. Here is an overview of drugs that may cause a problem:

Antiseizure drugs such as Dilantin or Tegretol
Blood-thinning medications such as Coumadin
Certain antidepressants, including Elavil, Tofranil, and Prozac
Drugs that quell spasms, such as Bentyl and Cogentin
Epinephrine (EpiPen)
Lithium (Eskalith, Lithobid)
Methyldopa (Aldomet)
Propranolol (Inderal)
Rifampin (Rifadin)

Special information about pregnancy and breastfeeding

The effects of Haldol during pregnancy have not been adequately studied. Pregnant women should use Haldol only if clearly needed. Patients should inform their doctor immediately if they are pregnant or plan to become pregnant. Haldol should not be used by women who are breastfeeding an infant.

Recommended dosage

ADULTS

Moderate Symptoms
The usual dosage is 1 to 6 milligrams daily. This amount should be divided into 2 or 3 smaller doses.

Severe Symptoms
The usual dosage is 6 to 15 milligrams daily, divided into 2 or 3 smaller doses.

CHILDREN

Children younger than 3 years old should not take Haldol. For children between the ages of 3 and 12, weighing approximately 33 to 88 pounds, doses should start at 0.5 milligram per day. The doctor will increase the dose if needed.

For Psychotic Disorders
The daily dose may range from 0.05 milligram to 0.15 milligram for every 2.2 pounds of body weight.

For Non-Psychotic Behavior Disorders and Tourette's Syndrome
The daily dose may range from 0.05 milligram to 0.075 milligram for every 2.2 pounds of body weight.

OLDER ADULTS

In general, older people take dosages of Haldol in the lower ranges. Older adults (especially older women) may be more susceptible to tardive dyskinesia. Doses may range from 1 to 6 milligrams daily.

Overdosage

Any medication taken in excess can have serious consequences. If an overdose is suspected, seek medical help immediately.

■ *Symptoms of Haldol overdose may include:*
Catatonic (unresponsive) state, coma, decreased breathing, low blood pressure, rigid muscles, sedation, tremor, weakness

Generic name:

Haloperidol

See Haldol, page 87

Generic name:

Hydroxyzine

See Atarax, page 18

Generic name:

Imipramine

See Tofranil, page 205

Brand name:

Klonopin

Pronounced: KLON-uh-pin
Generic name: Clonazepam

Why is this drug prescribed?

Klonopin has two major uses. In the mental health field it is prescribed for panic disorder. In neurology it is used, alone or along with other medications, to treat convulsive disorders such as epilepsy. Klonopin belongs to the class of drugs known as benzodiazepines.

Most important fact about this drug

Klonopin works best when there is a constant amount in the bloodstream. It is important for patients to take their doses at regularly spaced intervals and to avoid missing any if possible.

How should this medication be taken?

Klonopin should be taken exactly as prescribed. If patients are taking it for panic disorder and find it makes them sleepy, the doctor may recommend a single dose at bedtime.

■ *Missed dose...*
If it is within an hour after the scheduled time, the dose should be taken as soon as remembered. If it's not remembered until later, the patient should skip it and go back to the regular schedule. Doses should never be doubled.

■ *Storage instructions...*
Klonopin should be stored at room temperature away from heat, light, and moisture.

What side effects may occur?

Side effects cannot be predicted. If any develop or change in intensity, patients should inform their doctor as soon as possible.

■ *More common side effects in panic disorder may include:*
Allergic reaction, constipation, coordination problems, depression, dizziness, fatigue, inflamed sinuses or nasal passages, flu, memory problems, menstrual problems, nervousness, reduced thinking ability, respiratory infection, sleepiness, speech problems

■ *Less common or rare side effects in panic disorder may include:*
Abdominal pain/discomfort, abnormal hunger, acne, aggressive reaction, anxiety, apathy, asthma attack, bleeding from the skin, blood clots, bronchitis, burning sensation, changes in appetite, changes in sex drive, confusion, coughing, difficulty breathing, dizziness when standing, ear problems, emotional changeability, excessive dreaming, excitement, fever, flushing, fluttery or throbbing heartbeat, frequent bowel movements, gas, general feeling of illness, gout, hair loss, hemorrhoids, hoarseness, increased salivation, indigestion, infections, inflamed stomach and intestines, lack of attention, lack of sensation, leg cramps, loss of taste, male sexual problems, migraine, motion sickness, muscle pain/cramps, nightmares, nosebleed, overactivity, pain (anywhere in the body), paralysis, pneumonia, shivering, skin problems, sleep problems, sneezing, sore throat, swelling with fluid retention, swollen knees, thick tongue, thirst, tingling/pins and needles, tooth problems, tremor, twitching, upset stomach, urinary problems, vertigo, vision problems, weight gain or loss, yawning

■ *More common side effects in seizure disorders may include:*
Behavior problems, drowsiness, lack of muscular coordination

■ *Less common or rare side effects in seizure disorders may include:*

Abnormal eye movements, anemia, bed-wetting, chest congestion, coated tongue, coma, confusion, constipation, dehydration, depression, diarrhea, double vision, dry mouth, excess hair, fever, fluttery or throbbing heartbeat, "glassy-eyed" appearance, hair loss, hallucinations, headache, inability to fall or stay asleep, inability to urinate, increased sex drive, involuntary rapid movement of the eyeballs, loss of or increased appetite, loss of voice, memory loss, muscle and bone pain, muscle weakness, nausea, nighttime urination, painful or difficult urination, partial paralysis, runny nose, shortness of breath, skin rash, slowed breathing, slurred speech, sore gums, speech difficulties, stomach inflammation, swelling of ankles and face, tremor, uncontrolled body movement or twitching, vertigo, weight loss or gain

Klonopin can also cause aggressive behavior, agitation, anxiety, excitability, hostility, irritability, nervousness, nightmares, sleep disturbances, and vivid dreams.

■ *Side effects due to rapid decrease or abrupt withdrawal from Klonopin may include:*

Abdominal and muscle cramps, behavior disorders, convulsions, depressed feeling, hallucinations, restlessness, sleeping difficulties, tremors

Why should this drug not be prescribed?

This medication should be avoided by anyone who is sensitive to or has ever had an allergic reaction to it or to similar drugs, such as Librium and Valium. Klonopin also cannot be used in patients with severe liver disease or the eye condition known as acute narrow-angle glaucoma.

Special warnings about this medication

Klonopin makes some people drowsy or less alert. Patients should avoid driving, operating dangerous machinery, or participating in any hazardous activity that requires full mental alertness until they know how this drug affects them.

If a patient suffers from several types of seizures, this drug may increase the possibility of grand mal seizures (epilepsy). Patients should inform their doctor immediately if this occurs. The doctor may wish to prescribe an additional anticonvulsant drug or increase the dose of Klonopin.

Klonopin can be habit-forming and can lose its effectiveness as patients build up a tolerance to it. They may experience withdrawal symptoms—such as convulsions, hallucinations, tremor, and abdominal and muscle cramps—if they stop using this drug abruptly. Patients should discontinue or change their dose only in consultation with their doctor.

Possible food and drug interactions when taking this medication

Klonopin slows the nervous system, and its effects may be intensified by alcohol. Patients should avoid alcohol while taking this medication.

If Klonopin is taken with certain other drugs, the effects of either could be increased, decreased, or altered. Here is an overview of drugs that may cause a problem:

Antianxiety drugs such as Valium
Antidepressant drugs such as Elavil, Nardil, Parnate, and Tofranil
Antipsychotic medications such as Haldol, Navane, and Thorazine
Barbiturates such as phenobarbital
Carbamazepine (Tegretol)
Narcotic pain relievers such as Demerol and Percocet
Oral antifungal drugs such as Fungizone, Mycelex, and Mycostatin
Other anticonvulsants such as Dilantin, Depakene, and Depakote
Sedatives such as Halcion

Special information about pregnancy and breastfeeding

Klonopin should be avoided if at all possible during the first 3 months of pregnancy; there is a risk of birth defects. When taken later in pregnancy, the drug can cause other problems, such as withdrawal symptoms in the newborn. Patients who are pregnant or plan to become pregnant should inform their doctor immediately.

Klonopin appears in breast milk and could affect a nursing infant. Mothers taking this drug should not breastfeed.

Recommended dosage

PANIC DISORDER

Adults

The starting dose is 0.25 milligram twice a day. After 3 days, the doctor may increase the dose to 1 milligram daily. Some people need as much as 4 milligrams a day.

Children

For panic disorder, safety and effectiveness have not been established in children under age 18.

SEIZURE DISORDERS

Adults

The starting dose should be no more than 1.5 milligrams per day, divided into 3 doses. The doctor may increase the daily dosage by 0.5 to 1 milligram every 3 days until the patient's seizures are controlled or the side effects become too bothersome. The maximum daily dosage is 20 milligrams.

Children

The starting dose for infants and children up to 10 years old or up to 60 pounds should be 0.01 to 0.03 milligram—no more than 0.05 milligram—per 2.2 pounds of body weight daily. The daily dosage should be given in 2 or 3 smaller doses. The doctor may increase the dose by 0.25 to 0.5 milligram every 3 days until seizures are controlled or side effects become too bad. If the dose cannot be divided into 3 equal doses, the largest dose should be given at bedtime. The maximum maintenance dose is 0.1 to 0.2 milligram per 2.2 pounds daily.

Older Adults

Klonopin tends to build up in the body if the kidneys are weak—a common problem among older adults. Higher doses of the drug also tend to cause more drowsiness and confusion in older patients. People over age 65 are therefore started on low doses of Klonopin and watched with extra care.

Overdosage

Any medication taken in excess can have serious consequences. If an overdose is suspected, seek medical attention immediately.

■ *The symptoms of Klonopin overdose may include:*
Coma, confusion, sleepiness, slowed reaction time

Brand name:

Librium

Pronounced: LIB-ree-um
Generic name: Chlordiazepoxide

Why is this drug prescribed?

Librium is used in the treatment of anxiety disorders. It is also prescribed for short-term relief of the symptoms of anxiety, symptoms of withdrawal in acute alcoholism, and anxiety and apprehension before surgery. It belongs to a class of drugs known as benzodiazepines.

Most important fact about this drug

Librium is habit-forming and can lead to dependency. Warn patients that they could experience withdrawal symptoms if they stopped taking the drug abruptly (See "What side effects may occur?"). They should discontinue or change their dose only on advice of their doctor.

How should this medication be taken?

Instruct patients to take this medication exactly as prescribed.

■ *Missed dose...*
Patients should take the forgotten dose as soon as they remember if it

is within an hour or so of the scheduled time. If they do not remember until later, they should skip the missed dose and go back to their regular schedule. Warn against taking 2 doses at once.

■ *Storage instructions...*
Librium should be stored away from heat, light, and moisture.

What side effects may occur?

Side effects cannot be predicted. If any develop or change in intensity, patients should inform their doctor as soon as possible.

■ *Side effects may include:*
Confusion, constipation, drowsiness, fainting, increased or decreased sex drive, liver problems, lack of muscle coordination, minor menstrual irregularities, nausea, skin rash or eruptions, swelling due to fluid retention, yellow eyes and skin

■ *Side effects due to rapid decrease or abrupt withdrawal from Librium include:*
Abdominal and muscle cramps, convulsions, exaggerated feeling of depression, sleeplessness, sweating, tremors, vomiting

Why should this drug not be prescribed?

This medication should be avoided by anyone who is sensitive to or has ever had an allergic reaction to Librium or similar tranquilizers.

Anxiety or tension related to everyday stress usually does not require treatment with Librium. Patients should discuss their symptoms thoroughly with the doctor.

Special warnings about this medication

Librium may cause patients to become drowsy or less alert. They should not drive or operate dangerous machinery or participate in any hazardous activity that requires full mental alertness until they know how they react to this drug.

Patients who are severely depressed or have suffered from severe depression should consult with their doctor before taking this medication.

If Librium has been prescribed for a hyperactive, aggressive child, the doctor should be informed of contrary reactions such as excitement, stimulation, or acute rage.

Patients should check with their doctor before taking Librium if they are being treated for porphyria (a rare metabolic disorder) or kidney or liver disease.

Possible food and drug interactions when taking this medication

Librium is a central nervous system depressant and may intensify the effects of alcohol or have an additive effect. Warn patients against drinking alcohol while taking this medication.

If Librium is taken with certain other drugs, the effects of either can be increased, decreased, or altered. Here is an overview of drugs that may cause a problem:

Antacids such as Maalox and Mylanta
Drugs classified as MAO inhibitors, including the antidepressants Nardil and Parnate
Barbiturates such as phenobarbital
Blood-thinning drugs such as Coumadin
Cimetidine (Tagamet)
Disulfiram (Antabuse)
Levodopa (Larodopa)
Antipsychotic medications such as Stelazine and Thorazine
Narcotic pain relievers such as Demerol and Percocet
Oral contraceptives

Special information about pregnancy and breastfeeding

Women should not take Librium if they are pregnant or planning to become pregnant. There may be an increased risk of birth defects.

This drug may appear in breast milk and could affect a nursing infant. If the medication is essential to the patient's health, her doctor may advise her to discontinue breastfeeding until her treatment with the drug is finished.

Recommended dosage

ADULTS

Mild or Moderate Anxiety
The usual dose is 5 or 10 milligrams, 3 or 4 times a day.

Severe Anxiety
The usual dose is 20 to 25 milligrams, 3 or 4 times a day.

Apprehension and Anxiety before Surgery
On days preceding surgery, the usual dose is 5 to 10 milligrams, 3 or 4 times a day.

Withdrawal Symptoms of Acute Alcoholism
The usual starting oral dose is 50 to 100 milligrams; the doctor will repeat this dose, up to a maximum of 300 milligrams per day, until agitation is controlled. The dose will then be reduced as much as possible.

CHILDREN

The usual dose for children 6 years of age and older is 5 milligrams, 2 to 4 times per day. Some children may need to take 10 milligrams 2 or 3 times per day. The drug is not recommended for children under 6.

OLDER ADULTS

The doctor will limit the dose to the smallest effective amount in order to avoid oversedation or lack of coordination. The usual dose is 5 milligrams, 2 to 4 times per day.

Overdosage

Any medication taken in excess can cause symptoms of overdose. If an overdose is suspected, seek medical attention immediately.

■ *The symptoms of Librium overdose may include:*
   Coma, confusion, sleepiness, slow reflexes

Brand name:

Limbitrol

Pronounced: LIM-bit-roll
Generic ingredients: Chlordiazepoxide, Amitriptyline hydrochloride
Other brand names: Limbitrol DS

Why is this drug prescribed?

Limbitrol is a combination of an antidepressant and an antianxiety drug. It is used in the treatment of moderate to severe depression associated with moderate to severe anxiety.

Most important fact about this drug

Limbitrol is habit-forming and can lead to dependency. Patients could experience withdrawal symptoms if they stopped taking it abruptly (see "What side effects may occur?"). They should discontinue or change their dose only on advice of the doctor.

How should this medication be taken?

It is important that this medication be taken exactly as prescribed.

■ *Missed dose...*
   Patients should skip the missed dose and go back to their regular schedule. They should never take 2 doses at once.

■ *Storage instructions...*
   Limbitrol should be stored away from heat, light, and moisture.

What side effects may occur?

Side effects cannot be predicted. If any develop or change in intensity, patients should inform their doctor as soon as possible.

■ *More common side effects may include:*
   Bloating, blurred vision, constipation, dizziness, drowsiness, dry mouth

■ *Less common or rare side effects may include:*
Confusion, fatigue, impotence, lack or loss of appetite, liver problems, nasal congestion, restlessness, sluggishness, unresponsiveness, tremors, vivid dreams, weakness, yellow eyes and skin

■ *Side effects from rapid decrease in or abrupt withdrawal from Limbitrol include:*
Abdominal and muscle cramps, convulsions, exaggerated feeling of depression, headache, inability to fall asleep or stay asleep, nausea, restlessness, sweating, tremors, vague bodily discomfort, vomiting

Why should this drug not be prescribed?

Limbitrol should be avoided by anyone who is sensitive to or has ever had an allergic reaction to related drugs—benzodiazepine tranquilizers and tricyclic antidepressants.

Limbitrol should not be used by patients who have just had a heart attack.

Patients who are taking an antidepressant drug classified as an MAO inhibitor (Nardil, Parnate) should not take Limbitrol. Convulsions and death have occurred when the drugs were combined. (MAO inhibitors are long-lasting. A minimum of 14 days should be allowed between stopping an MAO inhibitor and starting Limbitrol.)

Special warnings about this medication

Limbitrol may cause patients to become drowsy or less alert. They should not drive or participate in any hazardous activity that requires full mental alertness until they know how this drug affects them.

This drug, especially when given in high doses, can cause irregular heartbeat, an increase in heart rate, heart attack, or stroke. Patients who are being treated for a heart or circulatory disorder should consult their doctor before taking Limbitrol.

Patients who are severely depressed or have been treated for severe depression should check with their doctor before taking this medication.

They should also double check with the doctor before taking this medication if they are being treated for the eye condition known as angle-closure glaucoma or for inability to pass urine. The doctor should also be alerted if they have a thyroid condition or liver or kidney problems, or if they have ever had seizures.

Before elective surgery, the doctor will discontinue Limbitrol several days prior to the operation. Limbitrol should be used with caution in patients who are getting electroconvulsive therapy.

Possible food and drug interactions when taking this medication

Limbitrol is a central nervous system depressant and may intensify the effects of alcohol. Patients should not drink alcohol while taking this medication.

If Limbitrol is taken with certain other drugs, the effects of either could be increased, decreased, or altered. Here is an overview of drugs that may cause a problem:

Any type of antidepressant drug
Barbiturates such as phenobarbital
Cimetidine (Tagamet)
Disulfiram (Antabuse)
Flecainide (Tambocor)
Levodopa (Larodopa)
Antipsychotic medications such as Thorazine and Mellaril
Oral contraceptives
Other mood-altering drugs
Propafenone (Rythmol)
Quinidine (Quinidex)
The blood-pressure medication guanethidine
Thyroid medication such as Synthroid

Severe constipation may occur if Limbitrol is combined with spasm-quelling drugs such as Donnatal or Bentyl.

Special information about pregnancy and breastfeeding

Women who are pregnant or plan to become pregnant should avoid Limbitrol. There is an increased risk of birth defects.

This drug may appear in breast milk and could affect a nursing infant. If this medication is essential to the patient's health, the doctor may advise her to discontinue breastfeeding until her treatment is finished.

Recommended dosage

ADULTS

Limbitrol Tablets

The usual starting dosage is a total of 3 or 4 tablets per day in several small doses. The larger portion of the daily dose may be taken at bedtime. A single bedtime dose may be sufficient.

Limbitrol DS (Double-strength)

The usual starting dosage is a total of 3 or 4 tablets per day divided into smaller doses. The doctor may increase the dose to 6 tablets per day or decrease it to 2 tablets per day, depending on response.

CHILDREN

Safety and effectiveness have not been established in children under 12 years old.

OLDER ADULTS

The doctor will prescribe the smallest amount possible in order to avoid side effects such as oversedation, confusion, and loss of muscle control.

Overdosage

Any medication taken in excess can cause symptoms of overdose. If an overdose is suspected, seek medical attention immediately.

■ *The symptoms of Limbitrol overdose may include:*
Abnormally fast heart rate, agitation, coma, confusion, congestive heart failure, convulsions, dilated pupils, disturbed concentration, drowsiness, exaggerated reflexes, hallucinations, high fever, irregular heartbeat, muscle rigidity, reduction of body temperature, severe low blood pressure, stupor, vomiting

Generic name:
Lithium

See Eskalith, page 70

Brand name:
Lithobid

See Eskalith, page 70

Generic name:
Lorazepam

See Ativan, page 20

Brand name:
Ludiomil

Pronounced: LOO-dee-oh-mill
Generic name: Maprotiline hydrochloride

Why is this drug prescribed?
Ludiomil is used to treat depression and anxiety associated with depres-

sion. It is also used for depression in people with manic-depressive illness.

Ludiomil is classified as a tetracyclic antidepressant. It is thought to work by boosting sensitivity at nerve junctions in the brain.

Most important fact about this drug

Seizures have been associated with Ludiomil, particularly when the drug was taken in amounts larger than prescribed, the dosage was increased too fast, or it was taken with certain other drugs such as Stelazine and Thorazine. To reduce the risk of seizures, patients should be sure to follow the doctor's instructions for taking this medication.

How should this medication be taken?

The doctor may prescribe a single daily dose or several smaller doses.

Improvement may not be evident for 2 to 3 weeks. Patients should not let this discourage them. They should continue Ludiomil therapy until instructed otherwise by the doctor.

■ *Missed dose...*
Patients who take 1 dose at bedtime should check with their doctor. Taking it in the morning may cause side effects during the day.

Patients who take more than 1 dose a day should take the forgotten dose as soon as they remember. If it is almost time for the next dose, they should skip the one they missed and go back to their regular schedule. They should never try to "catch up" by doubling the dose.

■ *Storage instructions...*
Ludiomil should be stored at room temperature in a tightly closed container.

What side effects may occur?

Side effects cannot be predicted. If any develop or change in intensity, patients should inform the doctor as soon as possible.

■ *More common side effects may include:*
Anxiety, blurred vision, constipation, dizziness, drowsiness, dry mouth, fatigue, headache, nervousness, tremors, weakness

■ *Less common or rare side effects may include:*
Abdominal cramps, agitation, allergies, bitter taste in the mouth, black tongue, bleeding sores, blocked intestine, breast development in the male, breast enlargement in the female, confusion (especially in older adults), decreased memory, delusions, diarrhea, difficulty swallowing, difficulty urinating, dilated pupils, disorientation, excessive or spontaneous milk excretion, excessive sweating, fainting, feeling of unreality, fever, flushing, frequent urination, hair loss, hallucinations, heart attack, high blood pressure, impotence, inability to fall or stay asleep, increased or decreased sex drive, increased psychotic symptoms,

increased salivation, inflammation of the mouth, involuntary movement, irregular heart rate, itching, low blood pressure, low or high blood sugar, mania, nasal congestion, nausea, nightmares, numbness, overactivity, palpitations, rapid heartbeat, red, black and blue, or purple spots on skin, restlessness, ringing in the ears, seizures, sensitivity to light, skin itching, skin rash, speech disorder, stomach pain, stroke, swelling due to fluid retention, swelling of testicles, tingling, twitches, unstable movements and gait, visual problems, vomiting, weight loss or gain, yellowish skin tone

Why should this drug not be prescribed?

Ludiomil should not be used by anyone who has had a recent heart attack. It should be avoided by patients who have taken one of the antidepressant drugs known as MAO inhibitors, including Parnate and Nardil, within the preceding 14 days. It should not be used by people who have had seizures. It should not be taken by individuals known to be hypersensitive to it.

Special warnings about this medication

Ludiomil should be used cautiously if the patient has ever had glaucoma (excessive pressure in the eyes), heart disease, heart attacks, irregular heartbeats, strokes, thyroid disease, or difficulty urinating.

This drug may impair patients' ability to drive a car or operate potentially dangerous machinery. They should not participate in any activities that require full alertness if they are unsure of their response to the drug.

Ludiomil may cause sensitivity to light. Patients should avoid prolonged exposure to the sun; they should use sunscreens and wear protective clothing until they learn their tolerance.

Possible food and drug interactions when taking this medication

Ludiomil should not be combined with MAO inhibitors such as Nardil.

If Ludiomil is taken with certain other drugs, the effects of either could be increased, decreased, or altered. Here is an overview of drugs that may cause a problem:

Airway-opening drugs such as Ventolin
Antipsychotic medications such as Stelazine and Thorazine
Choline
Cimetidine (Tagamet)
Drugs that control spasms, such as Bentyl
Fluoxetine (Prozac)
Guanethidine
Phenytoin (Dilantin)
Thyroid medications such as Synthroid
Tranquilizers such as Valium and Xanax

Extreme drowsiness and other potentially serious effects can result if Ludiomil is combined with alcohol, sleeping medications such as Seconal, and other drugs that depress the central nervous system.

Special information about pregnancy or breastfeeding

The effects of Ludiomil during pregnancy have not been adequately studied. Pregnant women should use Ludiomil only if clearly needed.

Ludiomil appears in breast milk and could affect a nursing infant. Women who nurse infants should use the drug cautiously and only when the potential benefits clearly outweigh the potential risks.

Recommended dosage

ADULTS

For Mild to Moderate Depression
Dosages usually start at 75 milligrams a day, taken as a single daily dose or divided into smaller doses. The doctor may increase the dose gradually to a maximum of 150 milligrams daily.

For Moderate to Severe Depression
For those who are hospitalized, dosages as high as 225 milligrams daily may be prescribed.

CHILDREN

Safety and effectiveness for children under 18 years old have not been established.

OLDER ADULTS

For Mild to Moderate Depression
Dosages usually start at 25 milligrams a day and may range up to 50 to 75 milligrams daily.

Overdosage

An overdose of Ludiomil can be fatal. If an overdose is suspected, seek medical help immediately.

■ *Symptoms of Ludiomil overdose may include:*
Agitation, bluish skin, coma, convulsions, dilated pupils, drowsiness, heart failure, high fever, irregular heart rate, lack of coordination, loss of consciousness, muscle rigidity, rapid heartbeat, restlessness, severely low blood pressure, shock, vomiting, writhing movement of the hands

Brand name:

Luvox

Pronounced: LOO-voks
Generic name: Fluvoxamine maleate

Why is this drug prescribed?
Luvox is prescribed for obsessive-compulsive disorder.

Most important fact about this drug
Before starting therapy with Luvox, patients should tell the doctor what medications they are taking—both prescription and over-the-counter—since combining Luvox with certain drugs may cause serious or even life-threatening effects. Luvox should never be combined with thioridazine (Mellaril) or pimozide (Orap). In addition, it should not be used within 14 days of taking any antidepressant drug classified as an MAO inhibitor, including Nardil and Parnate.

How should this medication be taken?
This medication should be taken only as directed by the doctor. It may be taken with or without food.

■ *Missed dose...*
Patients who are taking 1 dose a day should skip the missed dose and go back to their regular schedule. If they are taking 2 doses a day, they should take the missed dose as soon as possible, then go back to the regular schedule. They should never take 2 doses at the same time.

■ *Storage instructions...*
Luvox should be stored at room temperature and protected from humidity.

What side effects may occur?
Side effects cannot be predicted. If any develop or change in intensity, patients should tell the doctor immediately.

■ *More common side effects may include:*
Abnormal ejaculation, abnormal tooth decay and toothache, anxiety, blurred vision, constipation, decreased appetite, diarrhea, dizziness, dry mouth, feeling "hot or flushed," "flu-like" symptoms, frequent urination, gas and bloating, headache, heart palpitations, inability to fall asleep, indigestion, nausea, nervousness, sleepiness, sweating, taste alteration, tremor, unusual tiredness or weakness, upper respiratory infection, vomiting

■ *Less common side effects may include:*
Abnormal muscle tone, agitation, chills, decreased sex drive, depression, difficult or labored breathing, difficulty swallowing, extreme

excitability, impotence, inability to urinate, lack of orgasm, persistent erection, yawning

Why should this drug not be prescribed?

Patients who are sensitive to or have ever had an allergic reaction to Luvox or similar drugs, such as Prozac and Zoloft, should not take this medication.

Luvox should never be combined with Mellaril or Orap, or taken within 14 days of taking an MAO inhibitor such as Nardil or Parnate. (See "Most important fact about this drug.")

Special warnings about this medication

Patients should discuss all their medical problems with their doctor before starting therapy with Luvox, as certain physical conditions or diseases may affect their reaction to Luvox.

If they suffer from seizures, this medication should be used cautiously. Patients who experience a seizure while taking Luvox should stop taking the drug and call the doctor immediately.

The dosage of Luvox may need adjustment if the patient has ever had suicidal thoughts. The drug should be used with caution by patients who have a history of mania.

The doctor will need to adjust the dosage if the patient has liver disease.

Luvox may cause patients to become drowsy or less alert and may affect their judgment. They should avoid driving, operating dangerous machinery, or participating in any hazardous activity that requires full mental alertness until they know how this medication affects them.

Luvox can also deplete the body's supply of salt, especially in older adults and people who take diuretics or suffer from dehydration. Under these conditions, the doctor will check salt levels regularly.

If the patient develops a rash or hives, or any other allergic-type reaction, the physician should be notified immediately.

Possible food and drug interactions when taking this medication

Patients should not drink alcohol while taking this medication. If they smoke, they should tell the doctor before starting Luvox therapy, as their dosage may need adjustment.

If Luvox is taken with certain other drugs, the effects of either could be increased, decreased, or altered. Here is an overview of drugs that may cause a problem:

Anticoagulant drugs such as Coumadin

Antidepressant medications such as Anafranil, Elavil, and Tofranil, as well as the MAO inhibitors Nardil and Parnate

Blood pressure medications known as beta blockers, including Inderal and Lopressor

Carbamazepine (Tegretol)
Clozapine (Clozaril)
Diltiazem (Cardizem)
Lithium (Eskalith, Lithobid)
Methadone (Dolophine)
Phenytoin (Dilantin)
Pimozide (Orap)
Quinidine (Quinidex)
Sumatriptan (Imitrex)
Tacrine (Cognex)
Theophylline (Theo-Dur)
Thioridazine (Mellaril)
Tranquilizers and sedatives such as Halcion, Valium, Versed, and Xanax
Tryptophan

Special information about pregnancy and breastfeeding

The effects of Luvox in pregnancy have not been adequately studied. Patients who are pregnant or plan to become pregnant should consult their doctor immediately. Luvox passes into breast milk and may cause serious reactions in a nursing baby. If this medication is essential to the mother's health, her doctor may advise her to discontinue breastfeeding until her treatment with Luvox is finished.

Recommended dosage

ADULTS

The usual starting dose is one 50-milligram tablet taken at bedtime. The doctor may increase the dose, depending on response. The maximum daily dose is 300 milligrams. If the patient takes more than 100 milligrams a day, the doctor will divide the total amount into 2 doses; if the doses are not equal, the larger dose is taken at bedtime.

CHILDREN

For children aged 8 to 17, the recommended starting dose is 25 milligrams taken at bedtime. The dose may be increased to a maximum of 200 milligrams daily for children under 11, and 300 milligrams for children aged 11 to 17. Young girls sometimes respond to lower doses than boys do. Larger daily dosages are divided in two, as for adults.

OLDER ADULTS

Older adults and people with liver problems may need a reduced dosage.

Overdosage

An overdose of Luvox can be fatal. If an overdose is suspected, seek medical help immediately.

■ *Common symptoms of Luvox overdose include:*
  Coma, breathing difficulties, sleepiness, rapid heartbeat, nausea, vomiting

Other possible symptoms include convulsions, tremor, diarrhea, exaggerated reflexes, and slow or irregular heartbeat. After recovery, some overdose victims have been left with kidney complications, bowel damage, an unsteady gait, or dilated pupils.

Generic name:

Maprotiline

See Ludiomil, page 100

Brand name:

Mellaril

Pronounced: MEL-ah-rill
Generic name: Thioridazine hydrochloride

Why is this drug prescribed?

Mellaril combats schizophrenia. Because Mellaril has been known to cause dangerous heartbeat irregularities, it is usually prescribed only when at least two other medications have failed. Patients should receive an electrocardiogram before the drug is prescribed and periodically during Mellaril therapy.

Most important fact about this drug

The danger of potentially fatal cardiac irregularities increases when Mellaril is combined with any medication that prolongs a part of the heartbeat known as the QT interval. Many of the drugs prescribed for heartbeat irregularities (including Cordarone, Inderal, Quinaglute, Quinidex, and Rythmol) prolong the QT interval and should never be combined with Mellaril. Other drugs to be avoided during Mellaril therapy include Luvox, Norvir, Paxil, Pindolol, Prozac, Rescriptor, and Tagamet. Patients should make sure the doctor knows they are taking Mellaril whenever a new drug is prescribed.

How should this medication be taken?

Patients taking Mellaril in a liquid concentrate form can dilute it with a liquid such as distilled water, soft tap water, or juice just before taking it.

Patients should not change from one brand of thioridazine to another without consulting their doctor.

■ *Missed dose...*
Patients who take 1 dose a day and remember later in the day should take the dose immediately. If they don't remember until the next day, they should skip the dose and go back to their regular schedule.
Patients who take more than 1 dose a day and remember the forgotten

dose within an hour or so after its scheduled time should take it immediately. If they don't remember until later, they should skip the dose and go back to their regular schedule.

Patients should never try to "catch up" by doubling a dose.

■ *Storage instructions...*
Mellaril should be stored at room temperature, tightly closed, in the container the medication came in.

What side effects may occur?
Side effects cannot be predicted. If any develop or change in intensity, patients should inform the doctor as soon as possible.

■ *Side effects may include:*
Abnormal and excessive secretion of milk, agitation, anemia, asthma, blurred vision, body spasm, breast development in males, changed mental state, changes in sex drive, chewing movements, confusion (especially at night), constipation, diarrhea, discolored eyes, drowsiness, dry mouth, excitement, eyeball rotation, fever, fluid accumulation and swelling, headache, inability to hold urine, inability to urinate, inhibition of ejaculation, intestinal blockage, involuntary movements, irregular blood pressure, pulse, and heartbeat, irregular or missed menstrual periods, jaw spasm, loss of appetite, loss of muscle movement, mouth puckering, muscle rigidity, nasal congestion, nausea, overactivity, painful muscle spasm, paleness, pinpoint pupils, protruding tongue, psychotic reactions, puffing of cheeks, rapid heartbeat, redness of the skin, restlessness, rigid and masklike face, sensitivity to light, skin pigmentation and rash, sluggishness, stiff, twisted neck, strange dreams, sweating, swelling in the throat, swelling or filling of breasts, swollen glands, tremors, vomiting, weight gain, yellowing of the skin and whites of eyes

Why should this drug not be prescribed?
Due to the danger of cardiac irregularities, Mellaril must never be combined with drugs that increase its effects or prolong the part of the heartbeat known as the QT interval. (See "Most important fact about this drug.") It is also important to avoid combining Mellaril with excessive amounts of central nervous system depressants such as alcohol, barbiturates, or narcotics. It should not be used by anyone who has heart disease accompanied by severe high or low blood pressure.

Special warnings about this medication
Warning signs of the heartbeat irregularities that may be triggered by Mellaril include dizziness, palpitations, and fainting. Any patient who develops these symptoms should check with the doctor immediately.
Mellaril may cause tardive dyskinesia–a condition marked by involuntary muscle spasms and twitches in the face and body. This condition

may be permanent, and appears to be most common among the elderly, especially women.

Drugs such as Mellaril are also known to cause a potentially fatal condition known as Neuroleptic Malignant Syndrome. Symptoms of this problem include high fever, rigid muscles, altered mental status, sweating, fast or irregular heartbeat, and changes in blood pressure. Patients who develop these symptoms should see their doctor immediately. Mellaril therapy may have to be permanently discontinued.

In rare cases, Mellaril has been known to trigger blood disorders and seizures. It can cause dizziness or faintness upon first standing up. High doses can also cause vision problems, including blurring, brownish coloring of vision, and poor night vision.

This drug may impair the ability to drive a car or operate potentially dangerous machinery. Patients should not participate in any activities that require full alertness until they are certain the drug will not interfere.

If the patient has ever had breast cancer, the doctor should be made aware of it.

Mellaril may cause false positive results in tests for pregnancy.

Possible food and drug interactions when taking this medication

Remember that combining Mellaril with certain drugs can increase the danger of potentially fatal heartbeat irregularities. Among the drugs to avoid are the following:

Amiodarone (Cordarone)
Cimetidine (Tagamet)
Delavirdine (Rescriptor)
Fluoxetine (Prozac)
Fluvoxamine (Luvox)
Paroxetine (Paxil)
Pindolol
Propafenone (Rythmol)
Propranolol (Inderal)
Quinidine (Quinaglute, Quinidex)
Ritonavir (Norvir)

Extreme drowsiness and other potentially serious effects can result if Mellaril is combined with alcohol or other central nervous system depressants such as narcotics, painkillers, and sleeping medications. Patients should check with their doctor before adding any new drug to their regimen.

Special information about pregnancy and breastfeeding

Pregnant women should use Mellaril only if clearly needed. Patients who are pregnant or plan to become pregnant should inform their doctor immediately.

Recommended dosage

The doctor will tailor the dose to the patient's needs, using the smallest effective amount.

ADULTS

The starting dose ranges from 50 to 100 milligrams 3 times a day. The doctor may gradually increase the dosage to as much as 800 milligrams a day, taken in 2 to 4 small doses. Once the symptoms improve, the doctor will decrease the dosage to the lowest effective amount.

CHILDREN

The usual starting dose for schizophrenic children is 0.5 milligrams per 2.2 pounds of body weight per day, divided into smaller doses. The dose may be gradually increased to a maximum of 3 milligrams per 2.2 pounds per day.

Overdosage

An overdose of Mellaril can be fatal. If an overdose is suspected, seek medical help immediately.

■ *Symptoms of Mellaril overdose may include:*
Agitation, blurred vision, coma, confusion, constipation, difficulty breathing, dilated or constricted pupils, diminished flow of urine, dry mouth, dry skin, excessively high or low body temperature, extremely low blood pressure, fluid in the lungs, heart abnormalities, inability to urinate, intestinal blockage, nasal congestion, restlessness, sedation, seizures, shock

Generic name:

Meprobamate

See Miltown, page 111

Generic name:

Mesoridazine

See Serentil, page 178

Brand name:
Metadate

See Ritalin, page 172

Generic name:
Methamphetamine

See Desoxyn, page 50

Brand name:
Methylin

See Ritalin, page 172

Generic name:
Methylphenidate

See Ritalin, page 172

Brand name:
Miltown

Pronounced: MILL-town
Generic name: Meprobamate

Why is this drug prescribed?
Miltown is a tranquilizer used in the treatment of anxiety disorders and for short-term relief of the symptoms of anxiety.

Most important fact about this drug
Miltown can be habit-forming. Patients can develop tolerance and dependence, and may experience withdrawal symptoms if they stop using this drug abruptly. They should discontinue this drug or change the dose only on their doctor's advice.

How should this medication be taken?
Miltown should be taken exactly as prescribed.

■ *Missed dose...*
The dose should be taken as soon as remembered if it is within an hour of the scheduled time. If it's not remembered until later, the

patient should skip it and go back to the regular schedule. Doses should never be doubled.

■ *Storage instructions...*
Miltown should be stored at room temperature in a tightly closed container.

What side effects may occur?
Side effects cannot be predicted. If any develop or change in intensity, patients should inform their doctor as soon as possible.

■ *More common side effects may include:*
Allergic reactions, blood disorders, bruises, diarrhea, dizziness, drowsiness, exaggerated feeling of well-being, fainting, fast throbbing heartbeat, fever, headache, inappropriate excitement, itchy rash, loss of muscle coordination, nausea, rapid or irregular heartbeat, skin eruptions, slurred speech, small, purplish spots on the skin, sudden severe drop in blood pressure, swelling due to fluid retention, tingling sensation or numbness, vertigo, vision problems, vomiting, weakness

■ *Less common or rare side effects may include:*
Breathing difficulty, chills, high fever, inflammation of mouth, inflammation of the rectum, little or no urine, redness and swelling of skin, severe allergic reaction, skin inflammation and flaking, Stevens-Johnson syndrome (blisters in the mouth and eyes)

■ *Side effects due to rapid decrease in dose or abrupt withdrawal from Miltown:*
Anxiety, confusion, convulsions, hallucinations, inability to fall or stay asleep, loss of appetite, loss of coordination, muscle twitching, tremors, vomiting

Withdrawal symptoms usually become apparent within 12 to 48 hours after discontinuation of this medication and should disappear in another 12 to 48 hours.

Why should this drug not be prescribed?
Miltown should be avoided by anyone who is sensitive to or has ever had an allergic reaction to it or related drugs such as carisoprodol (Soma).

Miltown should not be taken by individuals with acute intermittent porphyria, an inherited disease of the body's metabolism. It can make the symptoms worse.

Anxiety or tension related to everyday stress usually does not require treatment with Miltown.

Special warnings about this medication

Patients who develop a skin rash, sore throat, fever, or shortness of breath should contact their doctor immediately. They may be having an allergic reaction to the drug.

Miltown may cause patients to become drowsy or less alert. They should not drive, operate dangerous machinery, or participate in any hazardous activity that requires full mental alertness until they know how this drug affects them.

Long-term use of this drug should be evaluated by the doctor periodically for its usefulness.

If the patient has liver or kidney disorders, the doctor should be made aware of these conditions before therapy begins.

Use of this drug may bring on seizures in people with epilepsy. They need to consult with their doctor before taking this medication.

Possible food and drug interactions when taking this medication

Miltown may intensify the effects of alcohol. Patients should not drink alcohol while taking this medication.

If Miltown is taken with certain other drugs, the effects of either could be increased, decreased, or altered. Interactions are particularly likely with mood-altering drugs and central nervous system depressants such as the following:

Antidepressant drugs such as Elavil, Nardil, and Tofranil
Barbiturates such as Seconal and phenobarbital
Major tranquilizers such as Thorazine and Mellaril
Narcotics such as Percocet or Demerol
Tranquilizers such as Halcion, Restoril, and Valium

Special information about pregnancy and breastfeeding

Miltown should not be taken by patients who are pregnant or are planning to become pregnant. There is an increased risk of birth defects.

Miltown appears in breast milk and could affect a nursing infant. If this medication is essential to the mother's health, the doctor may advise her to discontinue breastfeeding until her treatment is finished.

Recommended dosage

ADULTS

The usual dosage is 1,200 milligrams to 1,600 milligrams per day divided into 3 or 4 doses. The maximum dosage is 2,400 milligrams a day.

CHILDREN

The usual dose for children 6 to 12 years of age is 200 to 600 milligrams per day divided into 2 or 3 doses.

Miltown is not recommended for children under age 6.

OLDER ADULTS

The doctor will limit the dose to the smallest effective amount to avoid oversedation.

Overdosage
Any medication taken in excess can cause symptoms of overdose. If an overdose is suspected, seek emergency medical attention immediately.

■ *The symptoms of Miltown overdose may include:*
Coma, drowsiness, loss of muscle control, severely impaired breathing, shock, sluggishness, and unresponsiveness

Generic name:
Mirtazapine

See Remeron, page 161

Brand name:
Moban

Pronounced: MOW-ban
Generic name: Molindone hydrochloride

Why is this drug prescribed?
Moban is used in the treatment of schizophrenia.

Most important fact about this drug?
Moban can cause tardive dyskinesia, a condition marked by involuntary movements in the face and body, including chewing movements, puckering, puffing the cheeks, and sticking out the tongue. This condition may be permanent and appears to be most common among the elderly, especially elderly women.

How should this medication be taken?
Moban should be taken exactly as prescribed. It should not be taken with alcohol.

■ *Missed dose...*
Generally, the forgotten dose should be taken as soon as remembered. However, if it is almost time for the next dose, the missed dose should be skipped and the patient should return to the regular schedule. Doses should never be doubled.

■ *Storage instructions...*
Moban should be stored at room temperature and protected from light.

What side effects may occur?

Side effects cannot be predicted. If any develop or change in intensity, patients should inform their doctor as soon as possible.

■ *The most common side effect is:*
Drowsiness (especially at the start of therapy)

■ *Other side effects may include:*
Abnormal secretion of breast milk, blood disorders, blurred vision, breast development in men, changed mental state, changes in sex drive, constipation, depression, difficulty urinating, drooling, dry mouth, exaggerated sense of well being, excessive sweating, high fever, hyperactivity, irregular or rapid heartbeat, irregular or missed menstrual periods, liver problems, loss of muscle movement, low or irregular blood pressure, muscle contractions, muscle rigidity, nausea, painful erection, rash, restlessness, tardive dyskinesia, tremor, vision problems, weight change

Why should this drug not be prescribed?

Moban should not be combined with alcohol, barbiturates (sleep aids), narcotics (painkillers), or other substances that slow down the nervous system, nor should it be given to anyone in a comatose state. Moban cannot be used by anyone who is hypersensitive to the drug. The concentrate form of Moban contains a sulfite that may cause life-threatening allergic reactions in some people, especially in those with asthma.

Special warnings about this medication

Drugs such as Moban can cause a potentially fatal condition called Neuroleptic Malignant Syndrome (NMS). Symptoms include high fever, rigid muscles, irregular pulse or blood pressure, rapid heartbeat, excessive perspiration, and changes in heart rhythm. If patients develop these symptoms, they need to contact their doctor immediately. Moban should be discontinued.

Moban should be used with caution by anyone who has ever had breast cancer. The drug stimulates production of a hormone that promotes the growth of certain types of tumors.

Because this drug may cause drowsiness, patients should not participate in activities that require full alertness, such as driving or operating machinery, until they are sure how this medicine effects them.

Moban may mask signs of a brain tumor or intestinal blockage. It causes increased activity in some people. On rare occasions, it causes seizures.

Possible food and drug interactions when taking this medication

Remember that Moban must never be combined with alcohol, barbiturates, or narcotics. In addition, Moban tablets contain calcium, which may interfere with the absorption of tetracycline antibiotics (Achromycin V, Sumycin) and phenytoin (Dilantin).

Special information about pregnancy and breastfeeding

The safety and effectiveness of Moban during pregnancy have not been adequately studied. Patients who are pregnant or planning to become pregnant should tell their doctor immediately. Moban should be used during pregnancy only if the benefits outweigh the potential risks.

It is not known whether Moban appears in breast milk. Patients should check with their doctor before deciding to breastfeed.

Recommended dosage

ADULTS

The usual starting dose is 50 to 75 milligrams a day. The doctor may increase the dose to 100 milligrams a day after 3 or 4 days of treatment.

The long-term maintenance dose depends on the patient's response to the medication. The usual maintenance dose for treatment of mild symptoms is 5 milligrams to 15 milligrams taken 3 or 4 times a day. For moderate symptoms it is 10 milligrams to 25 milligrams taken 3 or 4 times a day. For severe symptoms, up to 225 milligrams a day may be prescribed. Older adults generally take lower dosages of Moban.

CHILDREN

The safety and effectiveness of Moban in children under age 12 have not been established.

Overdosage

Any medication taken in excess can have serious consequences. If an overdose of Moban is suspected, seek medical help immediately.

Generic name:

Molindone

See Moban, page 114

Brand name:

Nardil

Pronounced: NAHR-dill
Generic name: Phenelzine sulfate

Why is this drug prescribed?

Nardil is a monoamine oxidase (MAO) inhibitor used to treat depression as well as anxiety or phobias mixed with depression. MAO is an enzyme responsible for breaking down certain neurotransmitters in the brain. By inhibiting MAO, Nardil boosts the levels of these neurotransmitters and helps restore more normal mood states. Unfortunately, MAO inhibitors such as Nardil also block MAO activity throughout the body, an action that can have serious, even fatal, side effects—especially if MAO inhibitors are combined with certain foods or drugs.

Most important fact about this drug

It is essential that patients avoid the following foods, beverages, and medications while taking Nardil and for 2 weeks thereafter:

Beer (including alcohol-free or reduced-alcohol beer)
Caffeine (in excessive amounts)
Cheese (except for cottage cheese and cream cheese)
Chocolate (in excessive amounts)
Dry sausage (including Genoa salami, hard salami, pepperoni, and Lebanon bologna)
Fava bean pods
Liver
Meat extract
Pickled herring
Pickled, fermented, aged, or smoked meat, fish, or dairy products
Sauerkraut
Spoiled or improperly stored meat, fish, or dairy products
Wine (including alcohol-free or reduced-alcohol wine)
Yeast extract (including large amounts of brewer's yeast)
Yogurt

Medications to avoid:
Amphetamines
Appetite suppressants such as Redux and Tenuate
Antidepressants and related medications such as Prozac, Effexor, Luvox, Paxil, Remeron, Serzone, Wellbutrin, Zoloft, Elavil, Triavil, Tegretol, and Flexeril
Asthma inhalants such as Proventil and Ventolin
Cold and cough preparations including those with dextromethorphan, such as Robitussin DM
Hay fever medications such as Contac and Dristan
L-tryptophan-containing products
Nasal decongestants in tablet, drop, or spray form such as Sudafed
Sinus medications such as Sinutab

Taking Nardil with any of the above foods, beverages, or medications can cause serious, potentially fatal, high blood pressure. When taking Nardil patients should immediately report the occurrence of a headache, heart palpitations, or any other unusual symptom. In addition, patients should be sure to inform any physician or dentist they see that they are currently taking Nardil or have taken Nardil within the last 2 weeks.

How should this medication be taken?

Nardil may be taken with or without food. It can take up to 4 weeks for the drug to begin working.

Use of Nardil may complicate other medical treatment. Patients should carry a card that says they are taking Nardil, or wear a Medic Alert bracelet.

■ *Missed dose...*

Generally, the dose should be taken as soon as remembered. However if it is within 2 hours of the next dose, the patient should skip the missed dose and go back to the regular schedule. Doses should never be doubled.

■ *Storage instructions...*

Nardil may be stored at room temperature.

What side effects may occur?

Side effects cannot be predicted. If any develop or change in intensity, patients should inform their doctor as soon as possible.

■ *More common side effects may include:*

Constipation, disorders of the stomach and intestines, dizziness, drowsiness, dry mouth, excessive sleeping, fatigue, headache, insomnia, itching, low blood pressure (especially when rising quickly from lying down or sitting up), muscle spasms, sexual difficulties, strong reflexes, swelling due to fluid retention, tremors, twitching, weakness, weight gain

■ *Less common or rare side effects may include:*

Anxiety, blurred vision, coma, convulsions, delirium, exaggerated feeling of well-being, fever, glaucoma, inability to urinate, involuntary eyeball movements, jitteriness, lack of coordination, liver damage, mania, muscular rigidity, onset of schizophrenia, rapid breathing, rapid heart rate, repetitious use of words and phrases, skin rash or lupus-like disease, sweating, swelling in the throat, tingling sensation, yellowed skin and whites of eyes

Why should this drug not be prescribed?

This drug cannot be taken by anyone with pheochromocytoma (a tumor of the adrenal gland), congestive heart failure, a history of liver disease, or an allergy to the drug's ingredients.

Nardil should not be combined with medications that may increase blood pressure (such as amphetamines, cocaine, allergy and cold medications, or Ritalin), other MAO inhibitors, L-dopa, methyldopa (Aldomet), phenylalanine, L-tryptophan, L-tyrosine, fluoxetine (Prozac), buspirone (BuSpar), bupropion (Wellbutrin), guanethidine (Ismelin), meperidine (Demerol), dextromethorphan, or substances that slow the central nervous system such as alcohol and narcotics. It is also important to avoid foods, beverages, or medications listed above in the "Most important fact about this drug" section.

Special warnings about this medication

Patients *must* follow the food and drug limitations established by the physician; failure to do so may lead to potentially fatal side effects. While taking Nardil, they should promptly report the occurrence of a headache or any other unusual symptoms.

The doctor should prescribe Nardil with caution if the patient has diabetes, since it is not clear how MAO inhibitors affect blood sugar levels.

Patients need to tell the doctor that they are taking Nardil before deciding to have elective surgery.

Abrupt discontinuation of Nardil may trigger withdrawal symptoms. They may include nightmares, agitation, strange behavior, and convulsions.

Possible food and drug interactions when taking this medication

If Nardil is taken with certain other drugs, the effects of either could be increased, decreased, or altered. It is important for patients to closely follow the doctor's dietary and medication limitations when taking Nardil. Consult the "Most important fact about this drug" and "Why should this drug not be prescribed?" sections for lists of the foods, beverages, and medications that should be avoided while taking Nardil.

In addition, blood pressure medications (including water pills and beta blockers) should be used with caution by anyone taking Nardil, since excessively low blood pressure may result. Symptoms of low blood pressure include dizziness when rising from a lying or sitting position, fainting, and tingling in the hands or feet.

Special information about pregnancy and breastfeeding

The effects of Nardil during pregnancy have not been adequately studied. Nardil should be used during pregnancy only if the benefits of therapy clearly outweigh the potential risks to the fetus. If a patient is pregnant or plans to become pregnant, she should inform her doctor immediately. Nursing mothers should use Nardil only after consulting their physician, since it is not known whether Nardil appears in human milk.

Recommended dosage

ADULTS

The usual starting dose is 15 milligrams (1 tablet) 3 times a day. The doctor may increase the dosage to 90 milligrams per day.

It may be 4 weeks before the drug starts to work. Once the patient responds, the doctor may gradually reduce the dose, possibly to as low as 15 milligrams daily or every 2 days.

OLDER ADULTS

Because older people are more likely to have poor liver, kidney, or heart function, or other diseases that could increase the likelihood of side effects, a relatively low dose of Nardil is usually recommended at the start.

CHILDREN

Nardil is not recommended, since safety and efficacy for children under the age of 16 have not been determined.

Overdosage

An overdose of Nardil can be fatal. If an overdose is suspected, seek medical help immediately.

■ *Symptoms of overdose may include:*
Agitation, backward arching of the head, neck, and back, cool, clammy skin, coma, convulsions, difficult breathing, dizziness, drowsiness, faintness, hallucinations, high blood pressure, high fever, hyperactivity, irritability, jaw muscle spasms, low blood pressure, pain in the heart area, rapid and irregular pulse, rigidity, severe headache, sweating

Brand name:

Navane

Pronounced: NA-vain
Generic name: Thiothixene

Why is this drug prescribed?

Navane is used to treat psychotic disorders. Researchers theorize that this type of antipsychotic medication works by lowering levels of dopamine, a neurotransmitter in the brain.

Most important fact about this drug

Navane may cause tardive dyskinesia–a condition marked by involuntary muscle spasms and twitches in the face and body. This condition can be permanent and appears to be most common among the elderly, especially women.

How should this medication be taken?

Navane may be taken in liquid or capsule form. For the liquid form, a dropper is supplied.

■ *Missed dose...*

Generally, it should be taken as soon as remembered. However, if it is within 2 hours of the next dose, patients can skip the missed dose and go back to their regular schedule. Doses should never be doubled.

■ *Storage instructions...*

Navane should be stored at room temperature away from heat, light, and moisture. The liquid form should not be allowed to freeze.

What side effects may occur?

Side effects cannot be predicted. If any develop or change in intensity, patients should inform their doctor as soon as possible.

■ *Side effects may include:*

Abnormal muscle rigidity, abnormal secretion of milk, abnormalities in movements and posture, agitation, anemia, blurred vision, breast development in males, chewing movements, constipation, diarrhea, dizziness, drowsiness, dry mouth, excessive thirst, eyeball rotation or state of fixed gaze, fainting, fatigue, fluid accumulation and swelling, headache, high fever, high or low blood sugar, hives, impotence, insomnia, intestinal blockage, involuntary movements of the arms and legs, irregular menstrual periods, itching, light-headedness, loss or increase of appetite, low blood pressure, narrow or dilated pupils of the eye, nasal congestion, nausea, painful muscle spasm, protruding tongue, puckering of mouth, puffing of cheeks, rapid heartbeat, rash, restlessness, salivation, sedation, seizures, sensitivity to light, severe allergic reaction, skin inflammation and peeling, strong reflexes, sweating, swelling of breasts, tremors, twitching in the body, neck, shoulders, and face, visual problems, vomiting, weakness, weight increase, worsening of psychotic symptoms

Why should this drug not be prescribed?

Navane should not be given to comatose individuals. It should be avoided by anyone known to be hypersensitive to it. Also, it should not be used when the activity of the central nervous system is slowed down for any—example, by a sleeping medication, circulatory system collapse, or an abnormal bone marrow or blood condition.

Special warnings about this medication

Navane may hide symptoms of brain tumor and intestinal obstruction. The doctor will prescribe Navane cautiously if the patient has or has ever had a brain tumor, breast cancer, a convulsive disorder, the eye condition called glaucoma, intestinal blockage, or heart disease. It should also be avoided by patients exposed to extreme heat and those recovering from alcohol addiction.

This drug may impair the ability to drive a car or operate potentially dangerous machinery. Patients should not participate in any activities that require full alertness if they are unsure of their ability.

Possible food and drug interactions when taking this medication

If Navane is taken with certain other drugs, the effects of either could be increased, decreased, or altered. Here is an overview of drugs that may cause a problem:

Antihistamines such as Benadryl
Barbiturates such as phenobarbital
Drugs that contain atropine, such as Donnatal

Extreme drowsiness and other potentially serious effects can result if Navane is combined with alcohol or other central nervous system depressants such as painkillers, narcotics, or sleeping medications.

Special information about pregnancy and breastfeeding

If a patient is pregnant or plans to become pregnant, she should inform her doctor immediately; pregnant women should use Navane only if clearly needed. The doctor may also advise her to avoid breastfeeding while she is taking Navane.

Recommended dosage

Dosages of Navane are tailored to the individual. Usually treatment begins with a small dose, which is increased if needed.

ADULTS

For Milder Conditions
The usual starting dosage is a daily total of 6 milligrams, divided into doses of 2 milligrams and taken 3 times a day. The doctor may increase the dose to a total of 15 milligrams a day.

For More Severe Conditions
The usual starting dosage is a daily total of 10 milligrams, taken in 2 doses of 5 milligrams each. The doctor may increase this dose to a total of 60 milligrams a day.

Taking more than 60 milligrams a day rarely increases the benefits of Navane.

Some people are able to take Navane once a day. Patients should check with their doctor to see whether they can follow this schedule.

CHILDREN

Navane is not recommended for children younger than 12 years old.

OLDER ADULTS

In general, older adults are prescribed dosages of Navane in the lower ranges. Because older adults may develop low blood pressure while taking Navane, their doctors will monitor them closely. Older adults (especially women) may be more susceptible to such side effects as involuntary muscle spasms and twitches in the face and body.

Overdosage

Any medication taken in excess can have serious consequences. If an overdose is suspected, seek medical help immediately.

■ *Symptoms of Navane overdose may include:*
Central nervous system depression, coma, difficulty swallowing, dizziness, drowsiness, head tilted to the side, low blood pressure, muscle twitching, rigid muscles, salivation, tremors, walking disturbances, weakness

Generic name:
Nefazodone

See Serzone, page 185

Brand name:
Nembutal

Pronounced: NEM-byoo-tall
Generic name: Pentobarbital sodium

Why is this drug prescribed?
Nembutal is used as a sedative. It is prescribed on a short-term basis to help people fall asleep. After 2 weeks, it appears to lose its effectiveness as a sleep aid.

Most important fact about this drug
If taken for a long enough time, Nembutal can cause physical and psychological addiction. An overdose can be fatal. Nembutal should be used in the smallest possible amount, and it should always be stored in child-resistant containers.

How should this medication be taken?
Nembutal should be taken at bedtime, only as prescribed.

■ *Missed dose...*
This drug is for use only at bedtime. The dose should never be doubled.

■ *Storage instructions...*
Nembutal may be stored at room temperature.

What side effects may occur?

Side effects cannot be predicted. If any develop or change in intensity, patients should inform their doctor as soon as possible.

■ *More common side effects may include:*
Extreme sleepiness

■ *Less common or rare side effects may include:*
Agitation, anemia, anxiety, central nervous system depression, confusion, constipation, difficulty breathing, disturbed thinking, dizziness, fainting, fever, hallucinations, headache, insomnia, lack of coordination, low blood pressure, nausea, nervousness, nightmares, overactivity, skin inflammation and flaking, skin rash, slow heartbeat, temporary failure to breathe, vomiting

Why should this drug not be prescribed?

People with the rare blood disorder porphyria and those who are allergic or sensitive to barbiturates must avoid Nembutal.

Special warnings about this medication

Nembutal must not be stopped abruptly. Doing so can result in withdrawal symptoms and even death. To reduce any possible withdrawal symptoms, patients should follow the doctor's instructions closely when stopping Nembutal.

Minor withdrawal symptoms may include increased dreams or nightmares. Other minor withdrawal symptoms usually occur in the following order: anxiety, muscle twitching, tremors of hands and fingers, progressive weakness, dizziness, visual problems, nausea, vomiting, insomnia, and light-headedness on standing up. Major withdrawal symptoms may include convulsions and delirium.

The doctor will prescribe Nembutal cautiously if the patient has had liver disease or has a history of depression or substance abuse.

Patients should tell the doctor if they suffer from pain. Nembutal may hide pain-causing symptoms that require treatment.

Older adults may become confused, depressed, or excited while taking Nembutal, and should be prescribed lower doses. People with kidney or liver problems should also use lower doses.

Nembutal may lessen the effectiveness of oral contraceptives. Women who take Nembutal may need to consider another type of birth control.

This drug may impair the ability to drive a car or operate potentially dangerous machinery. Patients should not participate in any activities that require full alertness if they are unsure of their ability.

Nembutal may lose its effect when taken regularly. Patients should not increase the dose in an effort to get the drug to work again. Instead, they should contact the doctor.

Possible food and drug interactions when taking this medication

If Nembutal is taken with certain other drugs, the effects of either could be increased, decreased, or altered. Here is an overview of drugs that may cause a problem:

Antidepressant drugs classified as MAO inhibitors, including Nardil and Parnate
Antihistamines such as Benadryl
Blood-thinning medications such as Coumadin
Doxycycline (Vibramycin)
Epilepsy drugs such as Dilantin and Depakene Griseofulvin (Gris-PEG)
Hormonal medications such as Premarin
Oral contraceptives
Sedatives such as Halcion and Dalmane
Steroids such as prednisone
Tranquilizers such as Xanax and Valium

Extreme drowsiness and other potentially serious effects can result if Nembutal is combined with alcohol or drugs that slow down the central nervous system such as Percocet and Demerol.

Special information about pregnancy and breastfeeding

Nembutal causes damage to developing babies and withdrawal symptoms in newborns. Patients who are pregnant or plan to become pregnant should inform their doctor immediately.

This drug appears in breast milk and should be used with caution by nursing mothers.

Recommended dosage

ADULTS

For Insomnia
The usual intramuscular dose is 150 to 200 milligrams.

CHILDREN

Dosages for children should be based on the child's age and weight.

OLDER ADULTS

Because older adults may be more sensitive to Nembutal, it will be prescribed at lower dosages.

Overdosage

An overdose of Nembutal can be fatal. If an overdose is suspected, seek medical help immediately.

■ *Symptoms of Nembutal overdose may include:*
Coma, constriction (or sometimes dilation) of pupils, difficulty
breathing, fluid in the lungs, heart failure, kidney failure, lack of
reflexes, low blood pressure, low body temperature, pneumonia, rapid
or irregular heartbeat, reduced flow of urine

Brand name:

Norpramin

Pronounced: NOR-pram-in
Generic name: Desipramine hydrochloride

Why is this drug prescribed?

Norpramin is used in the treatment of depression. It is one of a family of
drugs called tricyclic antidepressants. Drugs in this class are thought to
work by affecting the levels of neurotransmitters in the brain, and adjusting the brain's response to them.

Norpramin has also been used to treat bulimia and attention deficit
disorders, and to help with cocaine withdrawal.

Most important fact about this drug

Serious, sometimes fatal, reactions have been known to occur when
drugs such as Norpramin are taken with another type of antidepressant
called an MAO inhibitor. Drugs in this category include Nardil and
Parnate. Norpramin cannot be taken within two weeks of taking one of
these drugs.

How should this medication be taken?

Patients should continue taking Norpramin even if they feel no immediate effect. It can take up to 2 or 3 weeks for improvement to begin.

Norpramin can cause dry mouth. Sucking hard candy or chewing
gum can help this problem.

■ *Missed dose...*
Patients who take several doses per day should take the forgotten dose
as soon as they remember, then take any remaining doses for the day
at evenly spaced intervals. If the patient takes Norpramin once a day
at bedtime and doesn't remember until morning, the missed dose
should be skipped. Doses should never be doubled in an effort to
"catch up."

■ *Storage instructions...*
Norpramin can be stored at room temperature. It should be protected
from excessive heat.

What side effects may occur?

Side effects cannot be predicted. If any develop or change in intensity, patients should inform their doctor as soon as possible.

■ *Side effects may include:*

Abdominal cramps, agitation, anxiety, black tongue, black, red, or blue spots on skin, blurred vision, breast development in males, breast enlargement in females, confusion, constipation, delusions, diarrhea, dilated pupils, disorientation, dizziness, drowsiness, dry mouth, excessive or spontaneous flow of milk, fatigue, fever, flushing, frequent urination or difficulty or delay in urinating, hallucinations, headache, heart attack, heartbeat irregularities, hepatitis, high or low blood pressure, high or low blood sugar, hives, impotence, increased or decreased sex drive, inflammation of the mouth, insomnia, intestinal blockage, lack of coordination, light-headedness (especially when rising from lying down), loss of appetite, loss of hair, mild elation, nausea, nightmares, odd taste in mouth, painful ejaculation, palpitations, purplish spots on the skin, rapid heartbeat, restlessness, ringing in the ears, seizures, sensitivity to light, skin itching and rash, sore throat, stomach pain, stroke, sweating, swelling due to fluid retention (especially in face or tongue), swelling of testicles, swollen glands, tingling, numbness and pins and needles in hands and feet, tremors, urinating at night, visual problems, vomiting, weakness, weight gain or loss, worsening of psychosis, yellowed skin and whites of eyes

Why should this drug not be prescribed?

Norpramin should not be used by anyone known to be hypersensitive to it, or by someone who has had a recent heart attack.

People who take antidepressant drugs known as MAO inhibitors (including Nardil and Parnate) should not take Norpramin.

Special warnings about this medication

Norpramin should be used with caution in patients who have heart or thyroid disease, a seizure disorder, a history of being unable to urinate, or high pressure in the eyes (glaucoma).

Nausea, headache, and uneasiness can result if Norpramin is discontinued abruptly. Patients should consult their doctor and follow instructions closely when discontinuing Norpramin.

This drug may impair the ability to drive a car or operate potentially dangerous machinery. Patients should not participate in any activities that require full alertness if they are unsure about their ability.

Norpramin may increase the skin's sensitivity to sunlight. Overexposure could cause rash, itching, redness, or sunburn. Patients should avoid direct sunlight or wear protective clothing.

Patients planning to have elective surgery should make sure that the doctor is aware that they are taking Norpramin. It should be discontinued as soon as possible prior to surgery.

The doctor should be alerted if a fever and sore throat develop during Norpramin therapy. He may want to do some blood tests.

Possible food and drug interactions when taking this medication

People who take antidepressant drugs known as MAO inhibitors (including Nardil and Parnate) should not take Norpramin.

If Norpramin is taken with certain other drugs, the effects of either could be increased, decreased, or altered. Here is an overview of drugs that may cause a problem:

Cimetidine (Tagamet)
Drugs that improve breathing, such as Proventil
Drugs that quell spasms, such as Bentyl
Fluoxetine (Prozac)
Guanethidine
Paroxetine (Paxil)
Sedatives/hypnotics (Halcion, Valium)
Sertraline (Zoloft)
Thyroid medications (Synthroid)

Extreme drowsiness and other potentially serious effects can result if Norpramin is combined with alcohol or other depressants, including narcotic painkillers such as Percocet and Demerol, sleeping medications such as Halcion and Nembutal, and tranquilizers such as Valium and Xanax.

Special information about pregnancy and breastfeeding

Pregnant women or mothers who are nursing an infant should use Norpramin only when the potential benefits clearly outweigh the potential risks. If a patient is pregnant or planning to become pregnant, she should inform her doctor immediately.

Recommended dosage

Doses are tailored to individual needs.

ADULTS

The usual dosage ranges from 100 to 200 milligrams per day, taken in 1 dose or divided into smaller doses. If needed, dosage may gradually be increased to 300 milligrams a day. Dosages above 300 milligrams per day are not recommended.

CHILDREN

Norpramin is not recommended for children.

OLDER ADULTS AND ADOLESCENTS

The usual dose ranges from 25 to 100 milligrams per day. If needed, dosage may gradually be increased to 150 milligrams a day. Dosages above 150 milligrams per day are not recommended.

Overdosage

An overdose of Norpramin can be fatal. If an overdose is suspected, seek medical help immediately.

■ *Symptoms of overdose may include:*
Agitation, coma, confusion, convulsions, dilated pupils, disturbed concentration, drowsiness, extremely low blood pressure, hallucinations, high fever, irregular heart rate, low body temperature, overactive reflexes, rigid muscles, stupor, vomiting

Generic name:

Nortriptyline

See Pamelor, page 132

Generic name:

Olanzapine

See Zyprexa, page 238

Generic name:

Oxazepam

Pronounced: oks-AS-eh-pam

Why is this drug prescribed?

Oxazepam is used in the treatment of anxiety disorders, including anxiety associated with depression.

This drug seems to be particularly effective for anxiety, tension, agitation, and irritability in older people. It is also prescribed to relieve symptoms of acute alcohol withdrawal.

Oxazepam belongs to a class of drugs known as benzodiazepines.

Most important fact about this drug

Oxazepam can be habit-forming or addicting and can lose its effectiveness over time as patients develop a tolerance for it. They may experience withdrawal symptoms if they stop using the drug abruptly. When discontinuing the drug, the doctor will reduce the dose gradually.

How should this medication be taken?

Oxazepam should be taken exactly as prescribed.

■ *Missed dose...*
If remembered within an hour or so, the dose should be taken immediately. If not remembered until later, the dose should be skipped and the patient should return to the regular schedule. Doses should never be doubled.

■ *Storage instructions...*
Oxazepam should be stored at room temperature in a tightly closed container.

What side effects may occur?

Side effects cannot be predicted. If any develop or change in intensity, patients should inform their doctor as soon as possible. The doctor should periodically reassess the need for this drug.

■ *More common side effects may include:*
Drowsiness

■ *Less common or rare side effects may include:*
Blood disorders, change in sex drive, dizziness, excitement, fainting, headache, hives, liver problems, loss or lack of muscle control, nausea, skin rashes or eruptions, sluggishness or unresponsiveness, slurred speech, swelling due to fluid retention, tremors, vertigo, yellowed eyes and skin

■ *Side effects due to rapid decrease or abrupt withdrawal from Serax:*
Abdominal and muscle cramps, convulsions, depressed mood, inability to fall or stay asleep, sweating, tremors, vomiting

Why should this drug not be prescribed?

Anyone who is sensitive to or has ever had an allergic reaction to Oxazepam or other tranquilizers such as Valium should not take this medication. Patients should make sure the doctor is aware of any drug reactions they have experienced.

Anxiety or tension related to everyday stress usually does not require treatment with Oxazepam. Patients should discuss their symptoms thoroughly with their doctor.

Oxazepam should not be prescribed for people who are being treated for mental disorders more serious than anxiety.

Special warnings about this medication

Oxazepam may cause patients to become drowsy or less alert. They should not drive, operate dangerous machinery, or participate in any hazardous activity that requires full mental alertness until they know how this drug affects them.

This medication may cause a drop in blood pressure. People with heart problems should check with their doctor before taking this medication.

Possible food and drug interactions when taking this medication

Oxazepam may intensify the effects of alcohol. It may be best to avoid alcohol while taking this medication.

If Oxazepam is taken with certain other drugs, the effects of either could be increased, decreased, or altered. Here is an overview of drugs that may cause a problem:

Antihistamines such as Benadryl
Narcotic painkillers such as Percocet and Demerol
Sedatives such as Seconal and Halcion
Tranquilizers such as Valium and Xanax

Special information about pregnancy and breastfeeding

Patients should not take Oxazepam if they are pregnant or planning to become pregnant. There is an increased risk of birth defects.

Oxazepam may appear in breast milk and could affect a nursing infant. If this drug is essential to the patient's health, the doctor may advise her to stop breastfeeding until her treatment with this medication is finished.

Recommended dosage

ADULTS

Mild to Moderate Anxiety with Tension, Irritability, Agitation
The usual dose is 10 to 15 milligrams 3 or 4 times per day.

Severe Anxiety, Depression with Anxiety, or Alcohol Withdrawal
The usual dose is 15 to 30 milligrams 3 or 4 times per day.

CHILDREN

Safety and effectiveness have not been established for children under 6 years of age, nor have dosage guidelines been established for children 6 to 12 years old. Doctors adjust the dosage to fit the child's needs.

OLDER ADULTS

The usual starting dose is 10 milligrams 3 times a day. The doctor may increase the dose to 15 milligrams 3 or 4 times a day, if needed.

Overdosage

An overdose of Oxazepam can be fatal. If an overdose is suspected, seek medical attention immediately.

■ *Symptoms of mild Oxazepam overdose may include:*
Confusion, drowsiness, lethargy

■ *Symptoms of more serious overdose may include:*
Coma, hypnotic state, lack of coordination, limp muscles, low blood pressure

Brand name:

Pamelor

Pronounced: PAM-eh-lore
Generic name: Nortriptyline hydrochloride
Other brand name: Aventyl

Why is this drug prescribed?

Pamelor is prescribed to relieve the symptoms of depression. It is one of the drugs known as tricyclic antidepressants.

Some doctors also prescribe Pamelor to treat chronic hives, premenstrual depression, Attention Deficit Hyperactivity Disorder in children, and bed-wetting.

Most important fact about this drug

Pamelor must be taken regularly to be effective, and it may be several weeks before the patient begins to feel better. It's important to keep taking regular doses, even if they seem to make no difference.

How should this medication be taken?

Pamelor should be taken exactly as prescribed. This drug can make the mouth dry. Sucking on hard candy, chewing gum, or melting ice chips in the mouth can provide relief.

■ *Missed dose...*
A forgotten dose should be taken as soon as remembered, unless it is almost time for the next dose. If that's the case, the missed dose should be skipped and the patient should return to the regular schedule. Patients who take Pamelor once a day at bedtime and miss a dose should not take it in the morning, since disturbing side effects could occur. Doses should never be doubled.

■ *Storage instructions...*
Pamelor should be kept in the container it came in, tightly closed and away from light. It is especially important to keep this drug out of reach of children; an overdose is particularly dangerous in the young. Pamelor may be stored at room temperature.

What side effects may occur?

Side effects cannot be predicted. If any develop or change in intensity, patients should inform their doctor as soon as possible.

■ *Side effects may include:*
Abdominal cramps, agitation, anxiety, black tongue, blurred vision, breast development in males, breast enlargement, confusion, constipation, delusions, diarrhea, dilation of pupils, disorientation, dizziness, drowsiness, dry mouth, excessive or spontaneous flow of milk, excessive urination at night, fatigue, fever, fluid retention, flushing, frequent urination, hair loss, hallucinations, headache, heart attack, high or low blood pressure, high or low blood sugar, hives, impotence, inability to sleep, inability to urinate, increased or decreased sex drive, inflammation of the mouth, intestinal blockage, itching, loss of appetite, loss of coordination, nausea, nightmares, numbness, panic, perspiration, pins and needles in the arms and legs, rapid, fluttery, or irregular heartbeat, rash, reddish or purplish spots on skin, restlessness, ringing in the ears, seizures, sensitivity to light, stomach upset, strange taste, stroke, swelling of the testicles, swollen glands, tingling, tremors, vision problems, vomiting, weakness, weight gain or loss, yellow eyes and skin

■ *Side effects due to rapid decrease or abrupt withdrawal from Pamelor after a long term of treatment include:*
Headache, nausea, vague feeling of bodily discomfort

These side effects do not indicate addiction to this drug.

Why should this drug not be prescribed?

Anyone who is sensitive to or has ever had an allergic reaction to Pamelor or similar drugs should not take this medication.

Pamelor must be avoided by people who are taking—or have taken within the past 14 days—a drug classified as an MAO inhibitor. Drugs in this category include the antidepressants Nardil and Parnate. Combining these drugs with Pamelor can cause fever and convulsions, and could even be fatal.

Unless directed to do so by a doctor, patients should not take this medication while recovering from a heart attack or taking any other antidepressant drugs.

Patients who have been taking Prozac typically have to wait at least 5 weeks before beginning therapy with Pamelor. Otherwise, a drug interaction could result.

Special warnings about this medication

Pamelor may cause patients to become drowsy or less alert. They should not drive, operate dangerous machinery, or participate in any hazardous activity that requires full mental alertness until they know how this drug affects them.

Pamelor should be used with caution in people who have a history of seizures, difficulty urinating, diabetes, or chronic eye conditions such as glaucoma. Caution is also warranted with patients who have heart disease, high blood pressure, or an overactive thyroid, and with those who are receiving thyroid medication.

If a patient is being treated for a severe mental disorder (schizophrenia or manic depression), the doctor should be made aware of this before Pamelor therapy begins.

Pamelor may make the skin more sensitive to sunlight. Patients should stay out of the sun, wear protective clothing, and apply a sunblock.

Before any surgery, dental treatment, or diagnostic procedure is undertaken, the doctor should be informed that the patient is taking Pamelor. Certain drugs used during these procedures, such as anesthetics and muscle relaxants, may interact with Pamelor.

Possible food and drug interactions when taking this medication

Combining Pamelor and MAO inhibitors can be fatal.

Pamelor may intensify the effects of alcohol. Patients should avoid alcohol while taking this medication.

If Pamelor is taken with certain other drugs, the effects of either can be increased, decreased, or altered. Here is an overview of drugs that may cause a problem:

Airway-opening drugs such as Ventolin and Proventil
Antidepressants such as Wellbutrin and Desyrel
Antidepressants that act on serotonin, such as Prozac, Paxil, and Zoloft
Antipsychotic medications such as Thorazine and Mellaril
Blood pressure medications such as Catapres
Cimetidine (Tagamet)
Chlorpropamide (Diabinese)
Drugs for heart irregularities, such as Tambocor and Rythmol
Drugs that control spasms, such as Donnatal and Bentyl
Levodopa (Larodopa)
Quinidine (Quinidex)
Reserpine (Diupres)
Stimulants such as Dexedrine
Thyroid medications such as Synthroid
Warfarin (Coumadin)

Special information about pregnancy and breastfeeding

The effects of Pamelor during pregnancy have not been adequately studied. Patients who are pregnant or planning to become pregnant should inform their doctor immediately. The doctor should also be consulted about breastfeeding.

Recommended dosage

This medication is available in tablet and liquid form. Only tablet dosages are listed. For liquid dosages, check with the doctor.

ADULTS

Doctors monitor response to this medication carefully, and gradually increase or decrease the dose to suit the patient's needs. Some doctors use blood tests to help determine the ideal dose.

The usual starting dosage is 25 milligrams, 3 or 4 times per day. Alternatively, the doctor may instruct that the total daily dose be taken once a day. Doses above 150 milligrams per day are not recommended.

CHILDREN

The safety and effectiveness of Pamelor have not been established for children and its use is not recommended. However, adolescents may be given 30 to 50 milligrams per day, either in a single dose or divided into smaller doses, as determined by the doctor.

OLDER ADULTS

The usual dose is 30 to 50 milligrams taken in a single dose or divided into smaller doses, as determined by the doctor.

Overdosage

An overdose of this type of antidepressant can be fatal. If an overdose is suspected, seek medical help immediately.

■ *Symptoms of Pamelor overdose may include:*
Agitation, coma, confusion, congestive heart failure, convulsions, dilated pupils, disturbed concentration, drowsiness, excessive reflexes, extremely high fever, fluid in the lungs, hallucinations, irregular heartbeat, low body temperature, restlessness, rigid muscles, severely low blood pressure, shock, stupor, vomiting.

Brand name:

Parnate

Pronounced: PAR-nate
Generic name: Tranylcypromine sulfate

Why is this drug prescribed?

Parnate is prescribed for the treatment of major depression. A member of the class of drugs known as monoamine oxidase (MAO) inhibitors, it works by increasing concentrations of the brain chemicals epinephrine, norepinephrine, and serotonin.

Most important fact about this drug

Parnate is a potent drug with the capability of producing serious side effects. It is typically prescribed only if other antidepressants fail, and then only for adults who are under close medical supervision. It is considered especially risky because it can interact with a long list of drugs and foods to produce life-threatening side effects (see "Possible food and drug interactions when taking this medication taking this medication").

How should this medication be taken?

Dosage is adjusted according to the patient's individual needs and response. The drug usually produces improvement within 48 hours to 3 weeks after starting therapy.

■ *Missed dose...*

Generally, the forgotten dose should be taken as soon as remembered. However, if it is within 2 hours of the next dose, the missed dose should be skipped and the patient should return to the regular schedule. Doses should never be doubled.

■ *Storage instructions...*

Parnate should be stored at room temperature.

What side effects may occur?

Side effects cannot be predicted. If any develop or change in intensity, patients should inform their doctor as soon as possible.

■ *Side effects may include:*

Abdominal pain, agitation, altered touch sensation, anxiety, appetite loss, blood disorders, blurred vision, chills, constipation, diarrhea, dizziness, drowsiness, dry mouth, hair loss, headaches, hepatitis, impotence, insomnia, irregular or rapid heartbeat, mania, muscle spasms and jerks, nausea, numbness, overstimulation, restlessness, retarded ejaculation, ringing in ears, reduced urination, skin rashes, tremors, swelling, water retention, weakness

Why should this drug not be prescribed?

Parnate should be avoided by anyone in danger of a stroke, by those who have heart or liver disease, high blood pressure, or a history of headaches, by individuals who have a type of tumor known as pheochromocytoma, and by anyone who will be undergoing elective surgery requiring general anesthesia.

Special warnings about this medication

The most dangerous reaction to Parnate is a surge in blood pressure, which has sometimes been fatal. For this reason, patients should report promptly to their doctor any of the following symptoms: constriction or pain in the throat or chest, dizziness, fever, headache, irregular heartbeat, light sensitivity, nausea, neck stiffness or soreness, palpitations, pupil dilation, sweating, or vomiting.

A number of people who take Parnate experience low blood pressure, faintness, or drowsiness. Great care should be exercised when performing potentially hazardous tasks, such as driving a car or operating machinery.

Some people become physically dependent on Parnate and experience withdrawal symptoms when the drug is stopped, including restlessness, anxiety, depression, confusion, hallucinations, headache, weakness, and diarrhea.

If the patient has kidney problems, the doctor should be made aware of it. The doctor may need to reduce the dosage of Parnate to avoid a buildup of the drug. Parnate should also be used with caution by people who have an overactive thyroid gland.

MAO inhibitors can suppress heart pain that would otherwise serve as a warning sign of a heart attack. For this reason and others, it should be used with caution by older adults. Also, it should be used with caution by diabetics and people with epilepsy or other convulsive disorders because it can alter the level of drugs used to treat these conditions.

Possible food and drug interactions when taking this medication

Parnate should never be combined with the following drugs; the combination can trigger seizures or a dangerous spike in blood pressure:

Other MAO inhibitors such as Nardil
Antidepressant drugs classified as "tricyclics," such as Anafranil, Elavil, and Tofranil
Carbamazepine (Tegretol)
Cyclobenzaprine (Flexeril)

When switching from one of these drugs to Parnate, or vice versa, patients must allow an interval of at least 1 week between medications.

Parnate should also be avoided by people taking any of the following:

Antidepressant drugs classified as "selective serotonin reuptake inhibitors," such as Paxil, Prozac, and Zoloft
Amphetamines such as Adderall and Dexedrine
Anesthetics
Antihistamines such as Allegra, Benadryl, and Clarinex
Blood pressure medications such as Accupril, Lotensin, and Prinivil
Bupropion (Wellbutrin)
Buspirone (BuSpar)
Cold and hay fever remedies that constrict blood vessels
Cough remedies containing dextromethorphan
Demerol and other narcotic painkillers such as Percodan, OxyContin, and Vicodin
Disulfiram (Antabuse)
Guanethidine
Methyldopa
Over-the-counter weight reduction aids
Parkinson's disease medications such as Parlodel, Requip, and Sinemet
Reserpine
Sedatives such as Halcion, Nembutal, and Seconal

Tryptophan
Water pills such as HydroDIURIL

While taking Parnate, patients should also avoid foods that contain a high amount of a substance called tyramine, including:

Anchovies
Avocados
Bananas
Beer (including nonalcoholic beer)
Caviar
Cheese (especially strong and aged varieties)
Chianti wine
Chocolate
Dried fruits (including raisins, prunes, and figs)
Liqueurs
Liver
Meat extracts or meat prepared with tenderizers
Overripe fruit
Pickled herring
Pods of broad beans like fava beans
Raspberries
Sauerkraut
Sherry
Sour cream
Soy sauce
Yeast extracts
Yogurt

Likewise, patients taking Parnate should avoid alcohol and large amounts of caffeine.

Special information about pregnancy and breastfeeding

Patients who are pregnant or plan to become pregnant should inform their doctor immediately. Parnate should be used during pregnancy only if its benefits outweigh potential risks.

Parnate makes its way into breast milk. If the drug is essential to the patient's health, the doctor may advise her to stop nursing until her treatment is finished.

Recommended dosage

ADULTS

The usual dosage is 30 milligrams per day, divided into smaller doses. If ineffective, the dosage may be slowly increased under the doctor's supervision to a maximum of 60 milligrams per day.

Overdosage
If an overdose of Parnate is suspected, seek medical help immediately.

■ *Symptoms of Parnate overdose may include:*
Agitation, confusion, coma, dizziness, drowsiness, high fever, incoherence, rigid muscles, severe headache, twitching, weakness

Generic name:
Paroxetine
See Paxil, page 139

Brand name:
Paxil

Pronounced: PACKS-ill
Generic name: Paroxetine hydrochloride

Why is this drug prescribed?
Paxil relieves a variety of emotional problems. It can be prescribed for major depressive disorder, obsessive-compulsive disorder (OCD), panic disorder, generalized anxiety disorder, social anxiety disorder (also known as social phobia), and posttraumatic stress disorder.

Most important fact about this drug
Improvement may be noted within 1 to 4 weeks after treatment begins. Patients should continue taking the medication even if they begin to feel better.

How should this medication be taken?
Paxil is taken once a day, with or without food, usually in the morning. The oral suspension must be thoroughly shaken before each use.

■ *Missed dose...*
Patients should skip the forgotten dose and go back to their regular schedule with the next dose. They should not take a double dose to make up for the one they missed.

■ *Storage instructions...*
Paxil tablets and suspension can be stored at room temperature.

What side effects may occur?
Side effects cannot be predicted. If any develop or change in intensity, patients should inform their doctor as soon as possible.

Over a 4 to 6 week period, patients may find some side effects less troublesome (nausea and dizziness, for example) than others (dry mouth, drowsiness, and weakness).

■ *More common side effects may include:*
Abnormal ejaculation, abnormal orgasm, constipation, decreased appetite, decreased sex drive, diarrhea, dizziness, drowsiness, dry mouth, gas, impotence, male and female genital disorders, nausea, nervousness, sleeplessness, sweating, tremor, weakness, vertigo

■ *Less common side effects may include:*
Abdominal pain, abnormal dreams, abnormal vision, agitation, altered taste sensation, blurred vision, burning or tingling sensation, drugged feeling, emotional instability, headache, increased appetite, infection, itching, joint pain, muscle tenderness or weakness, pounding heart-beat, rash, ringing in ears, sinus inflammation, tightness in throat, twitching, upset stomach, urinary disorders, vomiting, yawning, weight gain, vertigo

■ *Rare side effects may include:*
Abnormal thinking, acne, alcohol abuse, allergic reaction, asthma, belching, blood and lymph abnormalities, breast pain, bronchitis, chills, colitis, difficulty swallowing, dry skin, ear pain, exaggerated sense of well-being, eye pain or inflammation, face swelling, fainting, generally ill feeling, hair loss, hallucinations, heart and circulation problems, high blood pressure, hostility, hyperventilation, increased salivation, increased sex drive, inflamed gums, inflamed mouth or tongue, lack of emotions, menstrual problems, migraine, movement disorders, neck pain, nosebleeds, paranoid and manic reactions, poor coordination, respiratory infections, sensation disorders, shortness of breath, skin disorders, stomach inflammation, swelling, teeth grind-ing, thirst, urinary disorders, vaginal inflammation, vision problems, weight loss

Why should this drug not be prescribed?
Dangerous and even fatal reactions are possible when Paxil is combined with thioridazine (Mellaril) or drugs classified as monoamine oxidase (MAO) inhibitors, such as the antidepressants Nardil and Parnate. Paxil must not be taken with any of these medications, or within 2 weeks of starting or stopping use of an MAO inhibitor. Paxil must also be avoided if it causes an allergic reaction.

Special warnings about this medication
Paxil should be used cautiously by people with a history of manic disor-ders and those with high pressure in the eyes (glaucoma). Caution is also warranted if the patient has a disease or condition that affects the metab-olism or blood circulation.

If the patient has a history of seizures, the doctor should be informed about it. Paxil must be used with caution in this situation. If the patient develops seizures once therapy has begun, the drug should be discontinued.

Paxil may impair judgment, thinking, or motor skills. Patients should not drive, operate dangerous machinery, or participate in any hazardous activity that requires full mental alertness until they are sure the medication is not affecting them in this way.

It's best to avoid an abrupt discontinuation of Paxil therapy. It can lead to symptoms such as dizziness, abnormal dreams, and tingling sensations. To prevent such problems, the dosage is reduced gradually.

Possible food and drug interactions when taking this medication

Remember that Paxil must never be combined with Mellaril or MAO inhibitors such as Nardil and Parnate.

If Paxil is taken with certain other drugs, the effects of either could be increased, decreased, or altered. Here is an overview of drugs that may cause a problem:

Alcohol
Antidepressants such as Elavil, Tofranil, Norpramin, Pamelor, Prozac
Cimetidine (Tagamet)
Diazepam (Valium)
Digoxin (Lanoxin)
Flecainide (Tambocor)
Lithium (Eskalith)
Phenobarbital
Phenytoin (Dilantin)
Procyclidine (Kemadrin)
Propafenone (Rythmol)
Propranolol (Inderal, Inderide)
Quinidine (Quinaglute)
Sumatriptan (Imitrex)
Tryptophan
Warfarin (Coumadin)

Special information about pregnancy and breastfeeding

The effects of Paxil during pregnancy have not been adequately studied. Patients who are pregnant or plan to become pregnant should inform their doctor immediately.

Paxil appears in breast milk and could affect a nursing infant. If this medication is essential to the patient's health, the doctor may advise her to discontinue breastfeeding until her treatment with Paxil is finished.

Recommended dosage
DEPRESSION

The usual starting dose is 20 milligrams a day, taken as a single dose, usually in the morning. At intervals of at least 1 week, the dosage may be increased by 10 milligrams a day, up to a maximum of 50 milligrams a day.

OBSESSIVE-COMPULSIVE DISORDER

The usual starting dose is 20 milligrams a day, typically taken in the morning. At intervals of at least 1 week, the dosage may be increased by 10 milligrams a day. The recommended long-term dosage is 40 milligrams daily. The maximum is 60 milligrams a day.

PANIC DISORDER

The usual starting dose is 10 milligrams a day, taken in the morning. At intervals of 1 week or more, the dosage may be increased by 10 milligrams a day. The target dose is 40 milligrams daily; dosage should never exceed 60 milligrams.

GENERALIZED ANXIETY DISORDER

The recommended dose is 20 milligrams taken once a day, usually in the morning.

SOCIAL ANXIETY DISORDER

The recommended dose is 20 milligrams taken once a day, usually in the morning.

POSTTRAUMATIC STRESS DISORDER

The recommended dose is 20 milligrams taken once a day, usually in the morning.

For older adults, the weak, and those with severe kidney or liver disease, starting doses are reduced to 10 milligrams daily, and later doses are limited to no more than 40 milligrams a day. Safety and effectiveness in children have not been established.

Overdosage
Any medication taken in excess can have serious consequences. If an overdose is suspected, seek medical attention immediately.

■ *Symptoms of Paxil overdose may include:*
Coma, dizziness, drowsiness, facial flushing, nausea, sweating, tremor, vomiting

Generic name:

Pemoline

See Cylert, page 41

Generic name:

Pentobarbital

See Nembutal, page 123

Generic name:

Perphenazine

See Trilafon, page 216

Generic name:

Phenelzine

See Nardil, page 116

Brand name:

Phenergan

Pronounced: FEN-er-gan
Generic name: Promethazine hydrochloride

Why is this drug prescribed?

Phenergan is an antihistamine. Because antihistamines of this type cause drowsiness, the drug is used as a sedative and sleep aid for both children and adults.

Like other antihistamines, Phenergan is also prescribed to relieve the nasal stuffiness and inflammation and red, inflamed eyes caused by hay fever and other allergies. It is used to treat itching, swelling, and redness from hives and other rashes; allergic reactions to blood transfusions; and, with other medications, anaphylactic shock (severe allergic reaction). It is prescribed to prevent and control nausea and vomiting before and after surgery and to prevent and treat motion sickness. It is also used, with other medications, for pain after surgery.

Antihistamines work by decreasing the effects of histamine, a chemical the body releases in response to certain irritants. Histamine narrows air passages in the lungs and contributes to inflammation. Antihistamines reduce itching and swelling and dry up secretions from the nose, eyes, and throat.

Most important fact about this drug

Because Phenergan may cause considerable drowsiness, patients should not drive, operate dangerous machinery, or participate in any hazardous activity that requires full mental alertness until they know how they react to Phenergan. Children should be carefully supervised while they are bike-riding, roller-skating, or playing until the drug's effect on them is established.

How should this medication be taken?

Phenergan should be taken exactly as prescribed.

■ *Missed dose...*

If Phenergan is being taken on a regular schedule, the forgotten dose should be taken as soon as remembered. If it is almost time for the next dose, patients should skip the one they missed and go back to their regular schedule. Doses should never be doubled.

■ *Storage instructions...*

Tablets should be stored at room temperature, away from light. Suppositories should be stored in the refrigerator, in a tightly closed container.

What side effects may occur?

Side effects cannot be predicted. If any develop or change in intensity, patients should inform their doctor as soon as possible.

■ *Side effects may include:*

Abnormal eye movements, agitation, asthma, blood disorders, blurred vision, changes in blood pressure, confusion, disorientation, dizziness, double vision, dry mouth, excitement, faintness, fatigue, fever, hallucinations, hives, hysteria, impaired or interrupted breathing, insomnia, irregular heartbeat, lack of coordination, lack of energy, loss of movement, nasal stuffiness, nausea, nervousness, nightmares, protruding tongue, rapid heartbeat, rash, rigid muscles, ringing in the ears, sedation (extreme calm), seizures, sensitivity to light, sleepiness, slow heartbeat, stiff neck, sweating, swollen face and throat, tremors, unnaturally good mood, vomiting, yellow skin and eyes

Why should this drug not be prescribed?

Phenergan should be avoided by anyone who has ever had an allergic reaction to it or to related medications, such as Thorazine, Mellaril, Stelazine, or Prolixin. Phenergan is not for use in comatose patients, and should not be used to treat asthma or other breathing problems.

Special warnings about this medication

If the patient is taking other medications that cause sedation, the doctor may reduce the dosage of these medications or eliminate them during Phenergan therapy.

In people who have a seizure disorder, Phenergan may cause seizures to occur more often.

Phenergan can cause a serious—even fatal—decline in the breathing function. This medication should be avoided by people with chronic breathing problems such as emphysema, and those who suffer from sleep apnea (periods during sleep when breathing stops).

Phenergan can also cause a potentially fatal condition called Neuroleptic Malignant Syndrome. Symptoms include high fever, rigid muscles, sweating, and a rapid or irregular heartbeat. Patients who develop these symptoms should stop taking Phenergan and see their doctor immediately.

Phenergan should be used with caution by anyone who has heart disease, high blood pressure or circulatory problems, liver problems, the eye condition called narrow-angle glaucoma, peptic ulcer or other abdominal obstructions, or urinary bladder obstruction due to an enlarged prostate.

Phenergan may affect the results of pregnancy tests and can raise blood sugar.

Some people have developed jaundice (yellow eyes and skin) while on this medication.

The doctor should be notified if the patient develops any uncontrolled movements or seems to be unusually sensitive to sunlight.

Remember that Phenergan can cause drowsiness.

Phenergan should not be given to children under two years of age, and should be used with caution in older children, due to the danger of impaired breathing. Large doses have been known to cause hallucinations, seizures, and sudden death, especially in children who are dehydrated. Drugs such as Phenergan are not recommended for the treatment of vomiting in children unless the problem is severe. Phenergan should also be avoided if the child has the serious neurological disease known as Reye's syndrome or any disease of the liver.

Possible food and drug interactions when taking this medication

Phenergan may increase the effects of alcohol. Patients should avoid alcohol, or at least substantially reduce the amount they drink, while taking this medication.

If Phenergan is taken with certain other drugs, the effects of either could be increased, decreased, or altered. Here is an overview of drugs that may cause a problem:

Certain antidepressant drugs, including Elavil and Tofranil

Drugs that control spasms, such as Cogentin

Drugs that reduce bone-marrow function (certain cancer drugs)

MAO inhibitors such as the antidepressants Nardil and Parnate

Narcotic pain relievers such as Demerol and Dilaudid

Sedatives such as Halcion, Dalmane, and Seconal

Tranquilizers such as Xanax and Valium

Special information about pregnancy and breastfeeding

The effects of Phenergan during pregnancy have not been adequately studied. If the patient is pregnant or plans to become pregnant, she should inform her doctor immediately.

Although it is not known whether Phenergan appears in breast milk, there is a chance that it could cause a nursing infant serious harm. If possible, the use of Phenergan should be discontinued during breastfeeding.

Recommended dosage

Phenergan is available in tablet, syrup, and suppository form. The suppositories are for rectal use only. Phenergan tablets and suppositories are not recommended for children under 2 years of age.

INSOMNIA

Adults

The usual dose is 25 to 50 milligrams for nighttime sedation.

Children

The usual dose is 12.5 to 25 milligrams by tablets or rectal suppository at bedtime.

Older Adults

The dosage is usually reduced for people over 60.

ALLERGY

Adults

The average oral dose is 25 milligrams taken before bed. However, the doctor may prescribe 12.5 milligrams before meals and before bed.

Children

The usual dose is a single 25-milligram dose at bedtime, or 6.25 to 12.5 milligrams 3 times daily.

MOTION SICKNESS

Adults

The average adult dose is 25 milligrams taken twice daily. The first dose should be taken one-half to 1 hour before the patient plans to travel, and the second dose 8 to 12 hours later, if necessary. On travel days after that, the recommended dose is 25 milligrams upon arising and again before the evening meal.

Children
The usual dose of Phenergan tablets, syrup, or rectal suppositories is 12.5 to 25 milligrams taken twice a day.

NAUSEA AND VOMITING

The average dose of Phenergan for nausea and vomiting in children or adults is 25 milligrams. When oral medication cannot be tolerated, use the rectal suppository. The doctor may prescribe 12.5 to 25 milligrams every 4 to 6 hours, if necessary.

For nausea and vomiting in children, the dose is usually calculated at 0.5 milligram per pound of body weight and will also be based on the age of the child and the severity of the condition being treated. Phenergan and other anti-vomiting drugs should not be given to children if the cause of the problem is unknown.

Overdosage
An overdose of Phenergan can be fatal. If an overdose is suspected, seek medical treatment immediately.

■ *Symptoms of Phenergan overdose may include:*
Difficulty breathing, dry mouth, fixed, and dilated pupils, flushing, heightened reflexes, loss of consciousness, muscle tension, poor coordination, seizures, slowdown in brain activity, slowed heartbeat, stomach and intestinal problems, very low blood pressure, writhing movements

Children may become overstimulated and have nightmares. Older adults may also become overstimulated.

Generic name:

Phenobarbital

Pronounced: fee-noe-BAR-bi-tal

Why is this drug prescribed?
Phenobarbital, a barbiturate, is used as a sleep aid and in the treatment of certain types of epilepsy, including generalized or grand mal seizures and partial seizures.

Most important fact about this drug
Phenobarbital can be habit-forming. One can become tolerant (needing more and more of the drug to achieve the same effect) and physically and psychologically dependent with continued use. Patients should never increase the amount of phenobarbital they take without first checking with their doctor.

How should this medication be taken?

It is important to take this medication exactly as prescribed.

Patients taking phenobarbital for seizures should not discontinue it abruptly.

■ *Missed dose...*

Generally, a forgotten dose should be taken as soon as remembered. However, if it is almost time for the next dose, patients should skip the one they missed and go back to their regular schedule. Doses should never be doubled.

■ *Storage instructions...*

Phenobarbital may be stored at room temperature in a tightly closed container.

What side effects may occur?

Side effects cannot be predicted. If any develop or change in intensity, patients should notify their doctor as soon as possible.

■ *Side effects may include:*

Abnormal thinking, aggravation of existing emotional disturbances and phobias, agitation, anemia, angioedema (swelling of the face around lips, tongue, and throat, swollen arms and legs, difficulty breathing), allergic reactions (localized swelling, especially of the eyelids, cheeks, or lips, skin redness and inflammation), anxiety, confusion, constipation, decreased breathing, delirium, difficulty sleeping, dizziness, drowsiness, excitement, fainting, fever, hallucinations, headache, increased physical activity and muscle movement, irritability and hyperactivity in children, lack of muscle coordination, low blood pressure, muscle, nerve, or joint pain, especially in people with insomnia, nausea, nervousness, nightmares, psychiatric disturbances, rash, residual drowsiness, restlessness, excitement, and delirium when taken for pain, shallow breathing, sleepiness, slow heartbeat, slowdown of the nervous system, sluggishness, softening of bones, temporary cessation of breathing, vertigo, vomiting

Why should this drug not be prescribed?

Phenobarbital should not be used by anyone suffering from porphyria (an inherited metabolic disorder), liver disease, or a lung disease that causes blockages or breathing difficulties, or by anyone who has ever had an allergic reaction to or is sensitive to phenobarbital or other barbiturates.

Special warnings about this medication

Remember that phenobarbital may be habit-forming. It must be taken exactly as prescribed.

Phenobarbital should be used with extreme caution, or not at all, by people who are depressed, or have a history of drug abuse.

Patients should tell the doctor if they are in pain, or if they have constant pain, before they take phenobarbital.

Phenobarbital may cause excitement, depression, or confusion in elderly or weakened individuals, and excitement in children.

People with liver disease or poorly functioning adrenal glands should use phenobarbital with extra caution.

Barbiturates such as phenobarbital can cause people to become tired or less alert. Patients should be careful driving, operating machinery, or doing any activity that requires full mental alertness until they know how they react to this medication.

Possible food and drug interactions when taking this medication

Phenobarbital may increase the effects of alcohol. Patients should avoid alcoholic beverages while taking phenobarbital.

If phenobarbital is taken with certain other drugs, the effects of either could be increased, decreased, or altered. Here is an overview of drugs that may cause a problem:

Antihistamines such as Benadryl
Blood-thinning medications such as Coumadin
Doxycycline (Doryx, Vibramycin)
Griseofulvin (Fulvicin-P/G, Grifulvin V)
MAO inhibitors, including the antidepressants Nardil and Parnate
Narcotic pain relievers such as Percocet
Oral contraceptives
Other epilepsy drugs such as Dilantin, Depakene, and Depakote
Other sedatives such as Nembutal and Seconal
Steroids such as Medrol and Deltasone
Tranquilizers such as Xanax and Valium

Special information about pregnancy and breastfeeding

Barbiturates such as phenobarbital may cause damage to the developing baby during pregnancy. Withdrawal symptoms may occur in an infant whose mother took barbiturates during the last 3 months of pregnancy. Patients who are pregnant or plan to become pregnant should inform their doctor immediately.

Phenobarbital appears in breast milk and could affect a nursing infant. If phenobarbital is essential to the patient's health, the doctor may advise her to stop breastfeeding until her treatment is finished.

Recommended dosage

ADULTS

Sedation

The usual initial dose of phenobarbital is a single dose of 30 to 120 milligrams. The doctor may repeat this dose at intervals, depending on the patient's response to this medication. The maximum amount allowable during a 24-hour period is 400 milligrams.

Daytime Sedation
The usual dose is 30 to 120 milligrams a day, divided into 2 to 3 doses.

To Induce Sleep
The usual dose is 100 to 200 milligrams.

Anticonvulsant Use
Phenobarbital dosage must be individualized on the basis of specific laboratory tests. The usual dose is 60 to 200 milligrams daily.

CHILDREN

Anticonvulsant Use
The phenobarbital dosage must be individualized on the basis of specific laboratory tests. The usual dose is 3 to 6 milligrams per 2.2 pounds of body weight per day.

OLDER ADULTS

For the old or debilitated, the dose may be lower than the regular adult dose. People who have liver or kidney disease may also require a lower dose of phenobarbital.

Overdosage

Barbiturate overdose can be fatal. If an overdose is suspected, seek medical treatment immediately.

■ *Symptoms of phenobarbital overdose may include:*
Congestive heart failure, diminished breathing, extremely low body temperature, fluid in lungs, involuntary eyeball movements, irregular heartbeat, kidney failure, lack of muscle coordination, low blood pressure, poor reflexes, skin reddening or bloody blisters, slowdown of the central nervous system

Generic name:

Prochlorperazine

See Compazine, page 36

Brand name:

Prolixin

Pronounced: pro-LICKS-inn
Generic name: Fluphenazine hydrochloride

Why is this drug prescribed?

Prolixin is used to reduce the symptoms of severe mental disturbances such as schizophrenia.

Most important fact about this drug

Prolixin may cause tardive dyskinesia—a condition marked by involuntary muscle spasms and twitches in the face and body. This condition may be permanent and appears to be most common among the elderly, especially women.

How should this medication be taken?

The elixir form of Prolixin should be examined before it's taken. The flavoring oils may have separated from the solution, causing globs or a wispy appearance. If this happens, the bottle should be gently shaken. The oil should blend in, and the solution should look clear. If the solution is not clear, it should not be used.

Prolixin Concentrate can be mixed with homogenized milk, noncaffeinated soft drinks, or fruit juice. It should not be mixed with caffeine-containing beverages, tea, or apple juice.

■ *Missed dose...*

Patients who take 1 dose a day should take the forgotten dose as soon as they remember, then go back to their regular schedule. If they do not remember until the next day, they should skip the dose they missed and go back to their regular schedule.

If they take more than 1 dose a day, they should take the forgotten dose as soon as they remember if it is within an hour or so of their scheduled time. If they do not remember until later, they should skip the dose they missed and go back to their regular schedule. Doses should never be doubled.

■ *Storage instructions...*

Prolixin should be stored at room temperature in a tightly closed container, away from light. The liquid forms should not be frozen. The tablets should be protected from excessive heat.

What side effects may occur?

Side effects cannot be predicted. If any develop or change in intensity, patients should inform their doctor as soon as possible.

■ *Side effects may include:*

Abnormal muscle rigidity, abnormal secretion of milk, abnormalities of movements and posture, asthma, blood disorders, blurred vision, body rigidly arched backward, breast development in males, changed mental state, chewing movements, complete or almost complete loss of movement, constipation, dizziness, drowsiness, dry mouth, excessive or spontaneous flow of milk, excessive urine, excitement, eye problems, eyeball rotation or state of fixed gaze, fluid accumulation and swelling, fluid accumulation in the brain, glaucoma, headache, heart attack, high blood pressure, high fever, hives, impotence, inability to sit still, increased sex drive in women, intestinal blockage, irregular blood pressure, pulse, and heartbeat, irregular menstrual periods, loss of appetite, mask-like face and rigidity, muscle spasms, nasal congestion, nausea, oily scalp, painful muscle spasm, protruding tongue, puckering of mouth, puffing of cheeks, purple or red spots on the skin, rapid heartbeat, red blood spots, restlessness, salivation, sensitivity to light, severe allergic reactions, skin inflammation and peeling, skin itching or rash, skin lesions or crusts, sluggishness, sore throat, mouth and gums, strange dreams, sweating, swelling of the throat, twitching in the body, neck, shoulders, and face, visual problems, weight change, yellowing of skin and whites of eyes

Why should this drug not be prescribed?

Do not give Prolixin to someone in a comatose state. This drug should not be taken by anyone who is also taking large doses of hypnotic drugs such as Seconal, Halcion, and phenobarbital, who is very depressed, who has had brain or liver damage, or who has an abnormal bone marrow or blood condition. It should also be avoided by anyone who has ever had an allergic reaction to it or similar major tranquilizers.

Special warnings about this medication

Prolixin should be used with caution by anyone who has ever had breast cancer; convulsive disorders; heart or kidney disease; or certain tumors. Caution is warranted, too, if the patient is exposed to extreme heat or certain pesticides.

Stomach inflammation, dizziness, nausea, vomiting, and tremors can result if Prolixin is suddenly stopped. Patients must follow their doctor's instructions closely when discontinuing Prolixin.

Prolixin can cause a collection of symptoms called Neuroleptic Malignant Syndrome. If the patient develops high fever, rigid muscles, changed mental state, irregular pulse or blood pressure, rapid or abnormal heartbeat, or excessive perspiration, the doctor should be notified immediately.

The doctor will periodically check your liver, kidneys, and blood during Prolixin therapy.

This drug may impair the ability to drive a car or operate potentially dangerous machinery. Patients should not participate in any activities that require full alertness if they are unsure of their ability.

Prolixin 2.5-, 5-, and 10-milligram tablets contain a coloring agent that can cause an allergic reaction in some people, especially those who are also allergic to aspirin.

Possible food and drug interactions when taking this medication

Prolixin should not be used with epinephrine (EpiPen). Extreme drowsiness and other potentially serious effects can result if Prolixin is combined with alcohol, narcotic pain relievers such as Percocet, sleeping medications such as Seconal, antihistamines such as Benadryl, or tranquilizers such as Valium. Prolixin may also interact with Atropine.

Special information about pregnancy and breastfeeding

Pregnant women should use Prolixin only if clearly needed. Patients who are pregnant or plan to become pregnant should inform their doctor immediately.

Prolixin may appear in breast milk and could affect a nursing infant. If this medication is essential to the patient's health, the doctor may advise her not to breastfeed while taking it.

Recommended dosage

ADULTS

The usual beginning total daily dose is 2.5 to 10 milligrams. This amount is divided into 3 or 4 equal doses and taken 6 or 8 hours apart.

If necessary, the doctor may increase the total dosage to 40 milligrams daily. When symptoms are under control, the doctor may decrease the dose. A daily maintenance dose may range from 1 to 5 milligrams, usually taken once daily.

CHILDREN

Safety and efficacy of Prolixin in children have not been established.

OLDER ADULTS

Older people may start with a daily dose of 1 to 2.5 milligrams. In general, they will take dosages of Prolixin in the lower ranges. Older people (especially older women) may be more susceptible to tardive dyskinesia—a possibly permanent condition characterized by involuntary muscle spasms and twitches in the face and body.

Overdosage

Any medication taken in excess can have serious consequences. If an overdose of Prolixin is suspected, seek medical help immediately.

Generic name:

Promethazine

See Phenergan, page 143

Brand name:

ProSom

Pronounced: PROE-som
Generic name: Estazolam

Why is this drug prescribed?

ProSom, a sleeping pill, is given for the short-term treatment of insomnia. Insomnia may involve difficulty falling asleep, frequent awakenings during the night, or too-early awakening in the morning.

Most important fact about this drug

As a chemical cousin of Valium and similar tranquilizers, ProSom is potentially addictive. It should be used only as a temporary sleeping aid. Even after relatively short-term use of ProSom, withdrawal symptoms may occur when the medication is stopped.

How should this medication be taken?

ProSom must be taken exactly as prescribed. A typical schedule is 1 tablet at bedtime. For small, physically run-down, or older people, one-half a tablet may be a safer starting dose.

■ *Missed dose...*
ProSom should be taken at bedtime only as needed. It is not necessary to make up a missed dose.

■ *Storage instructions...*
ProSom may be stored at room temperature.

What side effects may occur?

Side effects cannot be predicted. If any develop or change in intensity, patients should inform their doctor as soon as possible.

■ *More common side effects may include:*
Abnormal coordination, decreased movement or activity, dizziness, general feeling of illness, hangover, headache, leg and foot pain, nausea, nervousness, sleepiness, weakness

■ *Less common or rare side effects may include:*
Abdominal pain, abnormal dreaming, abnormal thinking, abnormal vision, acne, agitation, allergic reaction, altered taste, anxiety, apathy, arm and hand pain, arthritis, asthma, back pain, black stools, blood in urine, body pain, chest pain, chills, confusion, constant, involuntary eye movement, constipation, cough, decreased appetite, decreased hearing, decreased reflexes, decreased sex drive, depression, difficult/labored breathing, double vision, dry mouth, dry skin, ear pain, emotional changeability, eye irritation, fainting, fever, fluid retention, flushing, frequent urination, gas, hallucinations, hostility,

inability to hold urine, inability to urinate, increased appetite, indigestion, inflamed sinuses, intestinal upset, itching, joint pain, lack of coordination, little or no urine flow, loss of memory, menstrual cramps, mouth sores, muscle stiffness, nasal inflammation, neck pain, nighttime urination, nosebleed, numbness or tingling around the mouth, purple or reddish spots on the skin, rapid, heavy breathing, rash, ringing in the ears, seizure, sensitivity to light, sinus problems, sleep problems, sore throat, stupor, sweating, swollen breast, swollen lymph glands, thirst, throbbing or fluttering heartbeat, tingling or "pins and needles," tremor, twitch, urgent need to urinate, vaginal discharge/itching, vomiting, weight gain or loss

Why should this drug not be prescribed?

ProSom should not be taken by anyone who is sensitive or allergic to it, or by anyone who has ever had an adverse reaction to another Valium-type medication.

ProSom should be avoided during pregnancy. Drugs in this class may cause damage to the unborn child.

Special warnings about this medication

Since ProSom may cloud thinking, impair judgment, or interfere with normal physical coordination, patients should not drive, climb, or perform hazardous tasks until they know their reaction to this medication. It is important to remember that a tablet taken in the evening may continue to have effects well into the following day.

People who are older or physically run-down and those who have liver or kidney damage or breathing problems are particularly vulnerable to side effects from ProSom. They should use this medication with special caution.

Patients who have ever had seizures should not abruptly stop taking ProSom, even if they are taking antiseizure medication. Instead, they should taper off from ProSom under their doctor's supervision.

Even if a patient has never had a seizure, it is better to taper off from ProSom than to stop taking the medication abruptly. Experience suggests that tapering off can help prevent drug withdrawal symptoms.

Typically, the only withdrawal symptoms caused by ProSom are mild and temporary insomnia or irritability. Occasionally, however, withdrawal can involve considerable discomfort or even danger, with symptoms such as abdominal and muscle cramps, convulsions, sweating, tremors, and vomiting.

Possible food and drug interactions when taking this medication

Patients should not drink alcohol while taking ProSom; this combination could make them comatose or dangerously slow their breathing.

For the same reason, it is unwise to combine ProSom with any other medication that might calm or slow the functioning of the central nervous system. Among such drugs are:

Antipsychotic medications such as Haldol and Mellaril
Antiseizure drugs such as Dilantin, Tegretol, and Depakene
Antihistamines such as Benadryl and Chlor-Trimeton
Barbiturates such as phenobarbital
MAO inhibitors such as the antidepressants Nardil and Parnate
Narcotics such as Percodan and Tylox
Tranquilizers such as Valium and Xanax

Smokers tend to process and eliminate ProSom fairly quickly compared with nonsmokers.

Special information about pregnancy and breastfeeding

ProSom should not be used during pregnancy; it could cause birth defects in the developing baby.

When a pregnant woman takes ProSom or a similar medication shortly before giving birth, her baby is likely to have poor muscle tone (flaccidity) and/or experience drug withdrawal symptoms.

Because ProSom is thought to pass into breast milk, this medication should not be used while breastfeeding.

Recommended dosage

ADULTS

The recommended initial dose is 1 milligram at bedtime. Some people may need a 2-milligram dose.

CHILDREN

There is no information on the safety and effectiveness of ProSom in people under age 18.

OLDER ADULTS

The recommended usual dosage for older adults is 1 milligram. Some may require only 0.5 milligram.

Overdosage

Any medication taken in excess can have serious consequences. If an overdose is suspected, seek medical attention immediately.

■ *Symptoms of a ProSom overdose may include:*
Confusion, depressed breathing, drowsiness and eventually coma, lack of coordination, slurred speech.

Generic name:

Protriptyline

See Vivactil, page 223

Brand name:

Prozac

Pronounced: PRO-zak
Generic name: Fluoxetine hydrochloride
Other brand name: Sarafem

Why is this drug prescribed?

Prozac is prescribed for the treatment of major depression and obsessive-compulsive disorder. The drug is also used in the treatment of bulimia and has been used to treat other eating disorders and obesity.

Under the brand name Sarafem, the active ingredient in Prozac is also prescribed for the treatment of premenstrual dysphoric disorder (PMDD), formerly known as premenstrual syndrome (PMS). Symptoms of PMDD include mood problems such as anxiety, depression, irritability or persistent anger, mood swings, and tension. Physical problems that accompany PMDD include bloating, breast tenderness, headache, and joint and muscle pain. Symptoms typically begin 1 to 2 weeks before a woman's menstrual period and are severe enough to interfere with day-to-day activities and relationships.

Prozac is a member of the family of drugs called "selective serotonin re-uptake inhibitors." Serotonin is one of the chemical messengers believed to govern moods. Ordinarily, it is quickly reabsorbed after its release at the junctures between nerves. Re-uptake inhibitors such as Prozac slow this process, thereby boosting the levels of serotonin available in the brain.

Most important fact about this drug

Serious, sometimes fatal, reactions have been known to occur when Prozac is used in combination with drugs known as MAO inhibitors, including the antidepressants Nardil and Parnate; and when Prozac is discontinued and an MAO inhibitor is started. Prozac should never be taken with one of these drugs or within at least 14 days of discontinuing therapy with one of them; and 5 weeks or more should be allowed between stopping Prozac and starting an MAO inhibitor. Caution is especially warranted if the patient has been taking Prozac in high doses or for a long time.

Patients who are taking any prescription or nonprescription drugs should notify their doctor before taking Prozac.

How should this medication be taken?

Prozac should be taken exactly as prescribed. It usually is taken once or twice a day. To be effective, it should be taken regularly. Patients should make a habit of taking it at the same time they do some other daily activity.

It may be 4 weeks before a patient feels any relief from depression, but the drug's effects should last about 9 months after a 3-month treatment regimen. For obsessive-compulsive disorder, the full effect may take 5 weeks to appear.

■ *Missed dose...*
The forgotten dose should be taken as soon as the patient remembers. If several hours have passed, the dose should be skipped. Patients should never try to "catch up" by doubling the dose.

■ *Storage instructions...*
Store at room temperature.

What side effects may occur?

Side effects cannot be predicted. If any develop or change in intensity, patients should inform their doctor as soon as possible.

■ *More common side effects may include:*
Abnormal dreams, abnormal ejaculation, abnormal vision, anxiety, diminished sex drive, dizziness, dry mouth, flu-like symptoms, flushing, gas, headache, impotence, insomnia, itching, loss of appetite, nausea, nervousness, rash, sinusitis, sleepiness, sore throat, sweating, tremors, upset stomach, vomiting, weakness, yawning

■ *Less common side effects may include:*
Abnormal taste, agitation, bleeding problems, chills, confusion, ear pain, emotional instability, fever, frequent urination, high blood pressure, increased appetite, loss of memory, palpitations, ringing in the ears, sleep disorders, weight gain

A wide variety of other very rare reactions have been reported during Prozac therapy. Patients who develop any new or unexplained symptoms should tell their doctor without delay.

Why should this drug not be prescribed?

This drug should be avoided by anyone who is sensitive to or has ever had an allergic reaction to it or to similar drugs such as Paxil and Zoloft. Remember, too, that Prozac should never be combined with an MAO inhibitor. (See "Most important fact about this drug.")

Special warnings about this medication

Unless the doctor directs, this medication should not be taken by anyone who is recovering from a heart attack or has liver disease or diabetes.

Prozac may cause patients to become drowsy or less alert and may affect their judgment. Therefore, driving, operating dangerous machinery, or participating in any hazardous activity that requires full mental alertness is not recommended.

While taking this medication, some people may feel dizzy or light-headed or actually faint when getting up from a lying or sitting position. If getting up slowly doesn't help, or if this problem continues, the doctor should be notified.

Patients who develop a skin rash or hives while taking Prozac should discontinue use of the medication and notify the doctor immediately.

Prozac should be used with caution if the patient has a history of seizures. All the patient's medical conditions should be discussed with the doctor before this medication is taken.

The safety and effectiveness of Prozac have not been established in children.

Possible food and drug interactions when taking this medication

Remember that combining Prozac with MAO inhibitors is dangerous. Alcohol should also be avoided by people on Prozac.

If Prozac is taken with certain other drugs, the effects of either could be increased, decreased, or altered. Here is an overview of drugs that may cause a problem:

Alprazolam (Xanax)
Carbamazepine (Tegretol)
Clozapine (Clozaril)
Diazepam (Valium)
Digitoxin (Crystodigin)
Drugs that impair brain function, such as Xanax
Flecainide (Tambocor)
Haloperidol (Haldol)
Lithium (Eskalith)
Other antidepressants (Elavil)
Phenytoin (Dilantin)
Pimozide (Orap)
Tryptophan
Vinblastine (Velban)
Warfarin (Coumadin)

Special information about pregnancy and breastfeeding

The effects of Prozac during pregnancy have not been adequately studied. Patients who are pregnant or plan to become pregnant should inform their doctor immediately. This medication appears in breast milk, and breastfeeding is not recommended during Prozac therapy.

Recommended dosage
ADULTS

The usual starting dose is 20 milligrams per day, taken in the morning. The doctor may increase your dose after several weeks if no improvement is observed. People with kidney or liver disease, the elderly, and those taking other drugs may have their dosages adjusted by their doctor.

Dosages above 20 milligrams daily should be taken once a day in the morning or in 2 smaller doses taken in the morning and at noon.

The usual daily dose for depression ranges from 20 to 60 milligrams. For obsessive-compulsive disorder the customary range is 20 to 60 milligrams per day, though a maximum of 80 milligrams is sometimes prescribed. For bulimia nervosa, the usual dose is 60 milligrams, taken in the morning. The doctor may start with less and build up to this dosage. The usual dose for premenstrual dysphoric disorder is 20 milligrams a day.

Patients taking a 20-milligram daily dose of Prozac for depression may be switched to a delayed-release formulation called Prozac Weekly. To make the change, patients are asked to skip their daily dose for 7 days, then take their first weekly capsule.

Overdosage
An overdose of Prozac can be fatal. In addition, combining Prozac with certain other drugs can cause symptoms of overdose. If an overdose is suspected, seek medical attention immediately.

■ *Common symptoms of Prozac overdose include:*
Nausea, rapid heartbeat, seizures, sleepiness, vomiting

■ *Other symptoms of Prozac overdose include:*
Coma, delirium, fainting, high fever, irregular heartbeat, low blood pressure, mania, rigid muscles, sweating, stupor

Generic name:

Quazepam

See Doral, page 60

Generic name:

Quetiapine

See Seroquel, page 181

Brand name:

Remeron

Pronounced: REM-ur-on
Generic name: Mirtazapine

Why is this drug prescribed?

Remeron is prescribed for the treatment of major depression. The drug is thought to work by adjusting the balance of the brain's natural chemical messengers, especially norepinephrine and serotonin.

Most important fact about this drug

Remeron makes some people drowsy or less alert, and may affect judgment and thinking. Patients should avoid driving or participating in any hazardous activity that requires full mental alertness until they know whether Remeron has this effect on them.

How should this medication be taken?

Remeron may be taken with or without food. It is preferable to take it in the evening before going to bed. Even though improvement may begin in 1 to 4 weeks, it is important for the patient to continue taking this medication exactly as prescribed. Regular daily doses are needed for the drug to work properly.

Patients using Remeron SolTabs, an orally disintegrating form of the drug, should make sure their hands are dry before removing the tablet from the blister pack and should immediately place the tablet on their tongue. They should not attempt to split the tablet; it will fall apart rapidly and can be swallowed with saliva.

■ *Missed dose...*
   If the forgotten dose is remembered within a few hours, it should be taken immediately. Otherwise, it should be skipped. Doses should never be doubled.

■ *Storage instructions...*
   Remeron should be stored at room temperature in a tight, light-resistant container.

What side effects may occur?

Side effects cannot be predicted. If any develop or change in intensity, patients should tell their doctor as soon as possible.

■ *More common side effects may include:*
   Abnormal dreams and thinking, constipation, dizziness, dry mouth, "flu-like" symptoms, increased appetite, sleepiness, weakness, weight gain

■ *Less common side effects may include:*

Back pain, confusion, difficult or labored breathing, fluid retention, frequent urination, muscle pain, nausea, swelling of ankles or hands, tremors

Why should this drug not be prescribed?

Anyone who has ever had an allergic reaction to Remeron or similar drugs such as Ludiomil and Desyrel should not take this medication. It is important for patients to tell the doctor about any drug reactions they have experienced.

Remeron must also be avoided by anyone taking the antidepressants Nardil or Parnate (see "Special warnings about this medication").

Special warnings about this medication

Serious, sometimes fatal, reactions have been known to occur when drugs such as Remeron are taken in combination with other drugs known as MAO inhibitors, including the antidepressants Nardil and Parnate. Remeron should never be taken with one of these drugs or within 14 days of discontinuing therapy with one of them. Patients should also allow at least 14 days between stopping Remeron and starting an MAO inhibitor.

Patients who develop "flu-like" symptoms, a sore throat, chills or fever, mouth sores, or any other signs of infection should call their doctor; these symptoms may signal a serious underlying condition.

Remeron tends to raise cholesterol levels in some people. If the patient has a cholesterol problem, it should be mentioned to the doctor before Remeron therapy begins.

Remeron should be used with caution by people with active liver or kidney disease, or heart or blood pressure problems. The doctor should also be alerted if the patient has a history of seizures, mania, hypomania (mild excitability), drug use, or any other physical or emotional problems.

While first taking this medication, some people feel dizzy or light-headed, especially when getting up from a lying or sitting position. If getting up slowly doesn't help, or if this problem continues, the doctor should be notified.

People who must avoid phenylalanine should not use the SolTab form of Remeron, which contains this substance.

Possible food and drug interactions when taking this medication

Remeron should never be combined with an MAO inhibitor; and patients should not drink alcohol while taking this medication. If Remeron is taken with certain other drugs, the effects of either could be increased, decreased, or altered. It is especially important for patients to check with the doctor before combining Remeron with tranquilizers such as Valium, Xanax, and Ativan.

Special information about pregnancy and breastfeeding

The effects of Remeron during pregnancy have not been adequately studied. If the patient is pregnant or plans to become pregnant, she should tell her doctor immediately. It is not known whether Remeron appears in breast milk. However, because many drugs do make their way into breast milk, caution is advised.

Recommended dosage

ADULTS

The usual starting dose is 15 milligrams taken daily before going to sleep. Depending upon the patient's response, the dosage may be increased to as much as 45 milligrams a day.

CHILDREN

The safety and effectiveness of Remeron have not been established in children.

Overdosage

Any medication taken in excess can have serious consequences. If you suspect an overdose, seek medical attention immediately.

■ *Symptoms of Remeron overdose include:*
Drowsiness, impaired memory, mental confusion, rapid heartbeat

Brand name:

Reminyl

Pronounced: REM-in-ill
Generic name: Galantamine

Why is this drug prescribed?

Reminyl can delay or even reverse mental decline in some patients with mild to moderate Alzheimer's disease. It is thought to work by boosting levels of the chemical messenger acetylcholine in the brain. (In Alzheimer's disease, the cells that produce acetylcholine slowly deteriorate.)

Like other Alzheimer's drugs (Aricept, Cognex, and Exelon), Reminyl is a temporary remedy. It doesn't work for everyone, and it doesn't halt the underlying disease.

Most important fact about this drug

Reminyl therapy starts at a low dose and increases over several months. It is important to wait 4 weeks between dosage adjustments. If treatment with Reminyl is interrupted for several days or longer, the patient will need to start over again at the lowest dose, increasing the dose at 4-week intervals until the former dose is achieved.

How should this medication be taken?

Reminyl should be taken twice a day, preferably with the morning and evening meals. The drug is available in tablet form and as an oral solution. If the solution is used, the required amount should be drawn into the measuring pipette that comes with the bottle and emptied into 3 to 4 ounces of a non-alcoholic beverage. The mixture should be stirred well and administered immediately.

■ *Missed dose...*
Generally, it should be given as soon as remembered. However, if it is almost time for the next dose, the missed dose should be skipped and the next dose given on schedule. Doses should never be doubled.

■ *Storage instructions...*
Both the tablets and the oral solution may be stored at room temperature. The solution should be protected from freezing.

What side effects may occur?

Side effects cannot be predicted. If any develop or change in intensity, caregivers should inform the doctor as soon as possible.

■ *More common side effects may include:*
Abdominal pain, anemia, blood in urine, depression, diarrhea, dizziness, fatigue, headache, inability to sleep, indigestion, loss of appetite, nausea, runny nose, sleepiness, tremor, abdominal pain, urinary tract infection, vomiting, weight loss

■ *Less common side effects may include:*
Chest pain, dizziness, fainting, gas, incontinence, slow heartbeat

■ *Rare side effects may include:*
Apathy, black stools, convulsions, delirium, difficulty swallowing, drooling, dry mouth, frequent urination, heart failure, hiccup, inability to comprehend language, increased sex drive, kidney stones, low blood pressure, movement and muscle disorders, nighttime urination, nosebleed, paranoia, purple or red discoloration of the skin, rapid or irregular heartbeat, rectal bleeding, stomach upset, swelling, tingling or prickly sensation, urinary retention, vertigo, weakness

Why should this drug not be prescribed?

Reminyl cannot be used if it gives the patient an allergic reaction. This drug is not recommended for patients with severe liver disease or kidney disease.

Special warnings about this medication

Reminyl should be used with caution if the patient has severe asthma, obstructive lung disease, or a history of stomach ulcers.

Reminyl can slow the heart rate and cause fainting episodes. Caution is especially important if the patient has a heart irregularity.

Before surgery, the doctor should be made aware of the use of Reminyl.

Possible food and drug interactions when taking this medication

If Reminyl is taken with certain other drugs, the effect of either may be increased, decreased, or altered. Here is an overview of drugs that may cause a problem:

Certain Parkinson's drugs such as Artane and Cogentin
Cimetidine (Tagamet)
Erythromycin (E.E.S., Eryc, PCE)
Ketoconazole (Nizoral)
Meclizine (Antivert)
Nonsteroidal anti-inflammatory drugs such as Motrin and Voltaren
Paroxetine (Paxil)
Urinary tract medications such as Urispas and Urecholine.

Special information about pregnancy and breastfeeding

Reminyl is not usually prescribed for women of childbearing age. It should be used during pregnancy only if the potential benefit justifies the risk to the developing baby. Reminyl should not be used by nursing mothers.

Recommended dosage

ADULTS

The recommended starting dose of Reminyl is 4 milligrams twice a day. Four weeks later, the dose should be increased to 8 milligrams twice a day. After waiting an additional four weeks, the doctor may increase the dose to 12 milligrams twice a day if necessary.

For patients with mild to moderate liver problems and kidney problems, dosage should not exceed 16 milligrams per day.

Overdosage

Any medication taken in excess can have serious consequences. A massive overdose of Reminyl could prove fatal. If you suspect an overdose, seek medical attention immediately.

■ *Symptoms of Reminyl overdose may include:*
Convulsions, drooling, fainting, incontinence, low blood pressure, muscle weakness, severe nausea, slow heartbeat, stomach cramps, sweating, teary eyes, twitching, weak breathing, vomiting

Brand name:

Restoril

Pronounced: RES-tah-rill
Generic name: Temazepam

Why is this drug prescribed?

Restoril is used for the relief of insomnia (difficulty in falling asleep, waking up frequently at night, or waking up early in the morning). It belongs to a class of drugs known as benzodiazepines.

Most important fact about this drug

Sleep problems are usually temporary, requiring treatment for only a short time, usually 1 or 2 days and no more than 2 to 3 weeks. Insomnia that lasts longer than this may be a sign of another medical problem. Needing this medicine for more than 7 to 10 days is a signal to check with the doctor.

How should this medication be taken?

It is important to take this medication exactly as directed, and in no more than the prescribed amount.

■ *Missed dose...*
Restoril should be taken only as needed.

■ *Storage instructions...*
This medication should be kept in the container it came in, tightly closed, and out of the reach of children. It may be stored at room temperature.

What side effects may occur?

Side effects cannot be predicted. If any develop or change in intensity, patients should inform their doctor as soon as possible.

■ *More common side effects may include:*
Dizziness, drowsiness, fatigue, headache, nausea, nervousness, sluggishness

■ *Less common or rare side effects may include:*
Abdominal discomfort, abnormal sweating, agitation, anxiety, backache, blurred vision, burning eyes, confusion, constant, involuntary movement of the eyeball, depression, diarrhea, difficult or labored breathing, dry mouth, exaggerated feeling of well-being, fluttery or throbbing heartbeat, hallucinations, hangover, increased dreaming, lack of coordination, loss of appetite, loss of equilibrium, loss of memory, nightmares, overstimulation, restlessness, tremors, vertigo, vomiting, weakness

■ *Side effects due to rapid decrease in or abrupt withdrawal
from Restoril:*
Abdominal and muscle cramps, convulsions, feeling of discomfort,
inability to fall asleep or stay asleep, sweating, tremors, vomiting

Why should this drug not be prescribed?
Women who are pregnant or plan to become pregnant should not take
this medication. It poses a potential risk to the developing baby.

Special warnings about this medication
When Restoril is used every night for more than a few weeks, it loses its
effectiveness to promote sleep. This is known as tolerance. Patients can
also develop physical dependence on this drug, especially if they take it
regularly for more than a few weeks, or take high doses.

When patients first start taking Restoril, until they know whether the
medication will have any "carry over" effect the next day, they should
use extreme care while doing anything that requires complete alertness
such as driving a car or operating machinery.

Patients who are severely depressed, or have suffered from severe
depression in the past, should double-check with their doctor before
taking this medication. They should also make sure the doctor is aware
of any kidney ailments, liver problems, or chronic lung disease they may
have.

After stopping Restoril, patients may have more trouble sleeping than
they had before they started taking it. This is called "rebound insomnia"
and should clear up after 1 or 2 nights.

Possible food and drug interactions when taking this medication
Restoril may intensify the effects of alcohol. Patients should avoid
alcohol while taking this medication.

If Restoril is taken with certain other drugs, the effects of either
could be increased, decreased, or altered. Here is an overview of drugs
that may cause a problem:
Antidepressant drugs such as Elavil, Nardil, Parnate, and Tofranil
Antihistamines such as Benadryl
Antipsychotic medications such as Mellaril and Thorazine
Barbiturates such as phenobarbital and Seconal
Narcotic pain relievers such as Percocet and Demerol
Oral contraceptives
Tranquilizers such as Valium and Xanax

Special information about pregnancy and breastfeeding
Women who are pregnant—or are planning to become pregnant—should
avoid Restoril. There is an increased risk of birth defects.

This drug may appear in breast milk and could affect a nursing
infant. If this medication is considered essential to a woman's health, her

doctor may advise her to discontinue breastfeeding until her treatment with this medication is finished.

Recommended dosage

ADULTS

The usual recommended dose is 15 milligrams at bedtime. However, 7.5 milligrams may be all that is necessary, while some people may need 30 milligrams. Your doctor will tailor your dose to your needs.

CHILDREN

The safety and effectiveness of Restoril have not been established in children under 18 years of age.

OLDER ADULTS

The doctor will prescribe the smallest effective amount in order to avoid side effects such as oversedation, dizziness, confusion, and lack of muscle coordination. The usual starting dose is 7.5 milligrams.

Overdosage

Any medication taken in excess can cause symptoms of overdose. If an overdose is suspected, seek medical attention immediately.

■ *The symptoms of Restoril overdose may include:*
Coma, confusion, diminished reflexes, loss of coordination, low blood pressure, labored or difficult breathing, seizures, sleepiness, slurred speech

Brand name:

Risperdal

Pronounced: RIS-per-dal
Generic name: Risperidone

Why is this drug prescribed?

Risperdal is prescribed for the treatment of schizophrenia. It is thought to work by muting the impact of dopamine and serotonin, two of the brain's key chemical messengers.

Most important fact about this drug

Risperdal may cause tardive dyskinesia, a condition that causes involuntary muscle spasms and twitches in the face and body. This condition can become permanent and is most common among older people, especially women. Patients should see their doctor immediately if they begin to have any involuntary movements. They may need to discontinue Risperdal therapy.

How should this medication be taken?

It is important for patients to take exactly the amount of Risperdal prescribed. Higher doses are more likely to cause unwanted side effects.

Risperdal may be taken with or without food.

Risperdal oral solution comes with a calibrated pipette to use for measuring. The oral solution can be taken with water, coffee, orange juice, and low-fat milk, but not with cola drinks or tea.

■ *Missed dose...*

Generally, the dose should be taken as soon as remembered. However, if it is almost time for the next dose, patients should skip the one they missed and go back to their regular schedule. Doses should never be doubled.

■ *Storage instructions...*

Risperdal may be stored at room temperature. The tablets should be protected from light and moisture; the oral solution should be protected from light and freezing.

What side effects may occur?

Side effects cannot be predicted. If any develop or change in intensity, patients should inform their doctor as soon as possible.

■ *More common side effects may include:*

Abdominal pain, abnormal walk, agitation, aggression, anxiety, chest pain, constipation, coughing, decreased activity, diarrhea, difficulty with orgasm, diminished sexual desire, dizziness, dry skin, erection and ejaculation problems, excessive menstrual bleeding, fever, headache, inability to sleep, increased dreaming, increased duration of sleep, indigestion, involuntary movements, joint pain, lack of coordination, nasal inflammation, nausea, overactivity, rapid heartbeat, rash, reduced salivation, respiratory infection, sleepiness, sore throat, tremor, underactive reflexes, urination problems, vomiting, weight gain

■ *Less common side effects may include:*

Abnormal vision, back pain, dandruff, difficult or labored breathing, increased saliva, sinus inflammation, toothache

Why should this drug not be prescribed?

Risperdal cannot be taken by anyone who is sensitive to or has ever had an allergic reaction to it or to other antipsychotic medications.

Special warnings about this medication

Risperdal should be used with caution in patients who have kidney, liver, or heart disease, seizures, breast cancer, thyroid disorders, or any other diseases that affect the metabolism. Caution is also warranted in patients exposed to extremes of temperature.

Be aware that Risperdal may mask signs and symptoms of drug overdose and of conditions such as intestinal obstruction, brain tumor, and Reye's syndrome (a dangerous neurological condition that may follow viral infections, usually occurring in children).

Risperdal may cause Neuroleptic Malignant Syndrome (NMS), a condition marked by muscle stiffness or rigidity, fast heartbeat or irregular pulse, increased sweating, high fever, and high or low blood pressure. Unchecked, this condition can prove fatal. Patients should call their doctor immediately if they notice any of these symptoms. Risperdal therapy should be discontinued.

This drug may impair the ability to drive a car or operate potentially dangerous machinery. Patients should avoid participating in any activities that require full alertness if they are unsure of their ability.

Risperdal can cause orthostatic hypotension (low blood pressure when rising to a standing position), with dizziness, rapid heartbeat, and fainting, especially at the start of therapy. This problem should be reported to the doctor if it develops. The dosage can be adjusted to reduce the symptoms.

Possible food and drug interactions when taking this medication

If Risperdal is taken with certain other drugs, the effects of either can be increased, decreased, or altered. Here is an overview of drugs that may cause a problem:

Blood pressure medicines such as Aldomet, Procardia, and Vasotec
Bromocriptine mesylate (Parlodel)
Carbamazepine (Tegretol)
Clozapine (Clozaril)
Levodopa (Sinemet, Larodopa)
Quinidine (Quinidex)

Risperdal tends to increase the effect of blood pressure medicines.

Patients may experience drowsiness and other potentially serious effects if Risperdal is combined with alcohol and other drugs that slow the central nervous system such as Valium, Percocet, Demerol, or Haldol.

Patients should check with their doctor before taking any new medications.

Special information about pregnancy and breastfeeding

The safety and effectiveness of Risperdal during pregnancy have not been adequately studied. Patients who are pregnant or plan to become pregnant should tell their doctor immediately.

Risperdal makes its way into breast milk, so women taking Risperdal must avoid breastfeeding.

Recommended dosage

ADULTS

Doses of Risperdal can be taken once a day, or divided in half and taken twice daily. The usual dose on the first day is 2 milligrams or 2 milliliters of oral solution. On the second day, the dose increases to 4 milligrams or milliliters, and on the third day rises to 6 milligrams or milliliters. Further dosage adjustments can be made at intervals of 1 week. Over the long term, typical daily doses range from 2 to 8 milligrams or milliliters.

For patients with liver or kidney disease, the doctor will start with one-half of a 1-milligram tablet or 0.5 milliliter of oral solution twice daily and may then increase the dosage by one-half tablet or 0.5 milliliter per dose. Increases above the 1.5-milligram level are typically made at 1 week intervals.

CHILDREN

The safety and effectiveness of Risperdal in children have not been established.

OLDER ADULTS

Older adults generally take Risperdal at lower doses. The usual starting dose is one-half of a 1-milligram tablet or 0.5 milliliter of oral solution twice daily. The doctor may increase the dose gradually and possibly switch the patient to a once-a-day dosing schedule after the first 2 to 3 days of drug therapy.

Overdosage

Any medication taken in excess can have serious consequences. If an overdose of Risperdal is suspected, seek medical attention immediately.

■ *Symptoms of Risperdal overdose may include:*
   Drowsiness, low blood pressure, rapid heartbeat, sedation

Generic name:

Risperidone

See Risperdal, page 168

Brand name:

Ritalin

Pronounced: RIT-ah-lin
Generic name: Methylphenidate hydrochloride
Other brand names: Concerta, Metadate, Methylin

Why is this drug prescribed?

Ritalin and other brands of methylphenidate are mild central nervous system stimulants used in the treatment of Attention Deficit Hyperactivity Disorder (ADHD) in children. With the exception of Concerta and Metadate CD, these products are also used in adults to treat narcolepsy.

When given for ADHD, this drug should be an integral part of a total treatment program that includes psychological, educational, and social measures.

Most important fact about this drug

Excessive doses of this drug over a long period of time can produce addiction. It is also possible to develop tolerance to the drug, so that larger doses are needed to produce the original effect. Because of these dangers, dosage should be changed only as directed, and the drug should be withdrawn only under a doctor's supervision.

How should this medication be taken?

The doctor's directions should be followed carefully. It is recommended that methylphenidate be taken 30 to 45 minutes before meals. If the drug interferes with sleep, the child should receive the last dose before 6 p.m. Ritalin-SR, Metadate CD, Methylin ER, and Concerta are long-acting forms of the drug, taken less frequently. They should be swallowed whole, never crushed or chewed.

■ *Missed dose...*
It should be given as soon as remembered. The remaining doses for the day should then be administered at regularly spaced intervals. Doses should never be doubled.

■ *Storage instructions...*
This drug should be kept out of reach of children and stored below 86 degrees Fahrenheit in a tightly closed, light-resistant container. Ritalin-SR should be protected from moisture.

What side effects may occur?

Side effects cannot be predicted. If any develop or change in intensity, patients should inform their doctor as soon as possible.

■ *More common side effects may include:*
Inability to fall or stay asleep, nervousness

These side effects can usually be controlled by reducing the dosage and omitting the drug in the afternoon or evening.

In children, loss of appetite, abdominal pain, weight loss during long-term therapy, inability to fall or stay asleep, and abnormally fast heart-beat are more common side effects.

■ *Less common or rare side effects may include:*
Abdominal pain, abnormal heartbeat, abnormal muscular movements, blood pressure changes, chest pain, dizziness, drowsiness, fever, hair loss, headache, hives, jerking, joint pain, loss of appetite, nausea, palpitations (fluttery or throbbing heartbeat), pulse changes, rapid heartbeat, reddish or purplish skin spots, skin reddening, skin inflammation with peeling, skin rash, Tourette's syndrome (severe twitching), weight loss during long-term treatment

Why should this drug not be prescribed?
This drug should not be prescribed for anyone experiencing anxiety, tension, and agitation, since the drug may aggravate these symptoms.

Anyone sensitive or allergic to this drug should not take it.

This medication should not be taken by anyone with the eye condition known as glaucoma, anyone who suffers from tics (repeated, involuntary twitches), or someone with a family history of Tourette's syndrome (severe and multiple tics).

This drug is not intended for use in children whose symptoms may be caused by stress or a psychiatric disorder.

This medication should not be used for the prevention or treatment of normal fatigue, nor should it be used for the treatment of severe depression.

This drug should not be taken during treatment with drugs classified as monoamine oxidase inhibitors, such as the antidepressants Nardil and Parnate, nor for the 2 weeks following discontinuation of these drugs.

Special warnings about this medication
The doctor should do a complete history and evaluation before prescribing this drug. He or she will take into account the severity of the symptoms, as well as the child's age.

This drug should not be given to children under 6 years of age; safety and effectiveness in this age group have not been established.

There is no information regarding the safety and effectiveness of long-term treatment in children. However, suppression of growth has been seen with the long-term use of stimulants, so the child should be monitored carefully while taking this drug.

Blood pressure should be monitored in anyone taking this drug, especially those with high blood pressure.

Some people have had visual disturbances such as blurred vision while being treated with this drug.

The use of this drug by anyone with a seizure disorder is not recommended. Make sure the doctor is aware of any problem in this area. Caution is also advisable for anyone with a history of emotional instability or substance abuse, due to the danger of addiction.

Possible food and drug interactions when taking this medication

If this medication is taken with certain other drugs, the effects of either can be increased, decreased, or altered. Here is an overview of drugs that may cause a problem:

Antiseizure drugs such as phenobarbital, Dilantin, and Mysoline
Antidepressant drugs such as Tofranil, Anafranil, Norpramin, and Effexor
Blood thinners such as Coumadin
Clonidine (Catapres-TTS)
Drugs that restore blood pressure, such as EpiPen
Guanethidine
MAO inhibitors (drugs such as the antidepressants Nardil and Parnate)
Phenylbutazone

Special information about pregnancy and breastfeeding

The effects of this drug during pregnancy have not been adequately studied. Patients who are pregnant or plan to become pregnant should inform their doctor immediately.

It is not known if this drug appears in breast milk. If this medication is essential to a patient's health, the doctor may advise her to discontinue nursing until her treatment with this medication is finished.

Recommended dosage

ADULTS

Ritalin and Methylin Tablets
The average dosage is 20 to 30 milligrams a day, divided into 2 or 3 doses, preferably taken 30 to 45 minutes before meals. Some people may need 40 to 60 milligrams daily, others only 10 to 15 milligrams. The doctor will determine the best dose.

Ritalin-SR, Methylin ER, and Metadate ER Tablets
These tablets keep working for 8 hours. They may be used in place of Ritalin tablets if they deliver a comparable dose over an 8-hour period.

CHILDREN

This drug should not be given to children under 6 years of age.

Ritalin and Methylin Tablets
The usual starting dose is 5 milligrams taken twice a day, before breakfast and lunch. The doctor will increase the dose by 5 to 10 milligrams a

week, up to a maximum of 60 milligrams a day. If improvement fails to appear after 1 month, the doctor may decide to discontinue the drug.

Ritalin-SR, Methylin ER, and Metadate ER Tablets
These tablets continue working for 8 hours. The doctor will decide if they should be used in place of the regular tablets.

Concerta Tablets
The recommended starting dose is 18 milligrams once daily in the morning. At weekly intervals, the doctor may increase the dose in 18-milligram steps, up to a maximum of 54 milligrams each morning.

Metadate CD Capsules
The recommended starting dose is 20 milligrams once daily before breakfast. If necessary, the doctor may increase the dose in 20-milligram steps to a maximum of 60 milligrams once a day.

The doctor will periodically discontinue the drug in order to reassess the child's condition. Drug treatment should not, and need not, be indefinite, and usually can be discontinued after puberty.

Overdosage

If an overdose is suspected, seek medical attention immediately.

■ *Symptoms of Ritalin overdose may include:*
Agitation, confusion, convulsions (may be followed by coma), delirium, dryness of mucous membranes, enlarging of the pupil of the eye, exaggerated feeling of elation, extremely elevated body temperature, flushing, hallucinations, headache, high blood pressure, irregular or rapid heartbeat, muscle twitching, sweating, tremors, vomiting

---

Generic name:

Rivastigmine

See Exelon, page 74

Brand name:

Sarafem

See Prozac, page 157

Generic name:

Secobarbital

See Seconal, page 176

Brand name:

Seconal

Pronounced: SEK-oh-nal
Generic name: Secobarbital sodium

Why is this drug prescribed?

Seconal is a barbiturate used to treat insomnia on a short-term basis. After 2 weeks, Seconal appears to lose its effectiveness as a sleep aid.

Most important fact about this drug

If taken for a long enough time, Seconal can cause physical addiction. Taken in a large enough amount, it can cause death.

How should this medication be taken?

Seconal should be taken only at bedtime, and only in the prescribed amount. It should not be taken with alcohol.

■ *Missed dose...*

Seconal is taken only as needed. It is not necessary to make up for a missed dose. Doses should never be doubled.

■ *Storage instructions...*

Seconal should be stored at room temperature in a tightly closed container.

What side effects may occur?

Side effects cannot be predicted. If any develop or change in intensity, patients should inform their doctor as soon as possible.

■ *Side effects may include:*

Agitation, anemia, anxiety, confusion, constipation, difficulty breathing, disturbed thinking, dizziness, fainting, fever, fluid retention, hallucinations, headache, insomnia, lack of coordination, low blood pressure, nausea, nervousness, nightmares, overactivity, slow heartbeat, skin rash, inflammation, and/or peeling, temporary interruptions of breathing, vomiting

Why should this drug not be prescribed?

Seconal should be avoided by anyone who has the rare blood disorder porphyria, liver damage, or a lung disease that makes breathing difficult. The drug cannot be used by people who have ever had an allergic reaction to barbiturates.

Special warnings about this medication

Seconal should not be stopped suddenly, since this may result in severe withdrawal symptoms and even death. To reduce the possibility of withdrawal symptoms, patients should follow the doctor's instructions closely when discontinuing Seconal.

Minor withdrawal symptoms include (in order of occurrence): anxiety, muscle twitching, tremors of hands and fingers, progressive weakness, dizziness, visual problems, nausea, vomiting, insomnia, and light-headedness upon first standing up. Major withdrawal symptoms include convulsions and delirium.

Seconal should be used with caution by people who have had liver disease or have a history of depression or substance abuse.

Patients should inform the doctor if they have any pain. Seconal may hide pain-causing disorders that require treatment.

Children may become excited while taking Seconal. Elderly people may become confused, depressed, or excited.

Seconal may lessen the effectiveness of oral contraceptives. Women who take Seconal may need to consider another type of birth control.

This drug may impair the ability to drive a car or operate potentially dangerous machinery. Patients should not participate in any activities that require full alertness if they are unsure about their ability.

Possible food and drug interactions when taking this medication

If Seconal is taken with certain other drugs, the effects of either could be increased, decreased, or altered. Here is an overview of drugs that may cause a problem:

Antihistamines such as Benadryl
Blood thinners such as Coumadin
Doxycycline (Vibramycin)
Griseofulvin (Gris-PEG)
Drugs classified as MAO inhibitors, such as the antidepressant drugs Nardil and Parnate
Oral contraceptives
Phenytoin (Dilantin)
Sedatives such as Halcion
Sodium valproate (Depakote)
Steroids such as prednisone
Tranquilizers such as Xanax and Valium
Valproic acid (Depakene)

Extreme drowsiness and other potentially serious effects can result if Seconal is combined with alcohol and other drugs that slow the activity of the brain.

Special information about pregnancy and breastfeeding

Studies have shown Seconal to have a potentially harmful effect on the unborn child. Patients who are pregnant or plan to become pregnant should inform their doctor immediately. This drug should be used during pregnancy only if clearly needed and only if potential benefits outweigh possible risks.

Small amounts of Seconal appear in breast milk. The doctor should be consulted before breastfeeding is undertaken.

Recommended dosage

ADULTS

For Insomnia
The usual dosage is 100 milligrams, taken at bedtime.

CHILDREN

Dosages for children, generally given before an operation, are based on the child's weight.

OLDER ADULTS

Because older people may be more sensitive to Seconal, they should take lower dosages; this is also true for people whose kidneys are not functioning properly and those who have liver disease.

Overdosage

An overdose of Seconal can be fatal. If an overdose is suspected, seek medical help immediately.

■ *Symptoms of Seconal overdose may be seen within 15 minutes and may include:*
Blood blisters, difficulty breathing, extreme drowsiness, extreme low body temperature, fluid in the lungs, irregular heartbeat, low blood pressure

Brand name:

Serentil

Pronounced: seh-REN -til
Generic name: Mesoridazine besylate

Why is this drug prescribed?

Serentil is prescribed to treat schizophrenia. Because of its dangerous side effects, this medication is recommended only after at least two other drugs have failed to provide relief.

Most important fact about this drug?

Serentil may cause dangerous and even fatal cardiac irregularities by prolonging a part of the heartbeat known as the QT interval. The likelihood of such irregularities increases when Serentil is combined with other medications known to prolong the QT interval, such as the heart medications Cordarone, Inderal, Quinaglute, Quinidex, and Rythmol. These drugs must never be taken with Serentil, and it's advisable for patients to check with their doctor before taking any new medications.

Symptoms of a possible heart irregularity include palpitations, dizziness, and fainting. Patients should call the doctor immediately if they experience any of these symptoms.

How should this medication be taken?

It is important to take Serentil exactly as prescribed. Patients taking Serentil in a liquid concentrate form can dilute it with distilled water, orange juice, or grape juice just before swallowing it.

If Serentil is given by injection, the patient should remain lying down for at least one-half hour after the injection.

■ *Missed dose . . .*

Generally, the forgotten dose should be taken as soon as remembered. However, if it is almost time for the next dose, the patient should skip the missed dose and return to the regular schedule. Doses should never be doubled.

■ *Storage instructions . . .*

Serentil should be stored at room temperature in a tightly closed container and protected from light.

What side effects may occur?

Side effects cannot be predicted. If any develop or change in intensity, patients should inform their doctor as soon as possible. Side effects generally occur when high doses are given early in treatment.

■ *The most common side effects include:*

Drowsiness, low blood pressure

■ *Other side effects may include:*

Abnormal posture, abnormal secretion of milk, agitation, allergic reaction, asthma, blood problems, blurred vision, breast development in men, changes in sex drive, confusion, constipation, disturbing dreams, dizziness, dry mouth, ejaculation problems, enlarged tongue, excitement, eye spasms, fainting, false positive pregnancy tests, fluid accumulation and swelling, high fever, heartbeat irregularities, hyperactivity, impotence, inability to urinate, intestinal blockage, involuntary urination, itching, large hives, light sensitivity, lockjaw, loss of appetite, loss of coordination, loss of muscle movement, Lupus-like symptoms, menstrual irregularities, muscle rigidity, muscle spasms, narrowed pupils, nausea, painful erections, Parkinson-like symptoms, pigmentation changes in skin and eyes, psychotic reactions, rash, restlessness, skin inflammation and peeling, slurring, strange dreams, stuffy nose, tardive dyskinesia (see "Special warnings"), throat swelling, tremor, twisted neck, vomiting, weakness, weight gain, whole body spasms, yellowed skin and whites of eyes

Why should this drug not be prescribed?

Serentil must be avoided by anyone who has a history of heartbeat irregularities, and all those who are taking other medications that may cause an irregular heartbeat (see "Most important fact about this drug"). Serentil should not be combined with other substances that slow the nervous system, such as alcohol, barbiturates (sleep aids), and narcotics (painkillers), nor should it be given to anyone in a comatose state. People who have shown a hypersensitivity to Serentil cannot take this drug.

Special warnings about this medication

Before using Serentil, patients should tell the doctor if they have a history of heart problems. The doctor will perform tests to check the health of their heart before prescribing this medication.

Serentil can cause tardive dyskinesia, a condition marked by involuntary muscle spasms and twitches in the face and body, including chewing movements, puckering, puffing the cheeks, and sticking out the tongue. This condition may be permanent and appears to be most common among older adults, especially older women.

Drugs such as Serentil can also cause a potentially fatal condition called Neuroleptic Malignant Syndrome (NMS). Symptoms include high fever, rigid muscles, irregular pulse or blood pressure, rapid heartbeat, excessive perspiration, and changes in heart rhythm. If a patient develops these symptoms, the doctor should be alerted immediately. Serentil therapy should be discontinued.

This type of drug can cause vision problems. If patients suffer a change in vision while taking this medication, they should inform the doctor.

Serentil may impair the ability to drive a car or operate machinery. Patients should not participate in any activities that require full alertness until they are sure of their reaction to this drug.

Serentil should be used with caution by anyone who has ever had breast cancer. The drug stimulates production of a hormone that promotes the growth of certain types of tumors.

Serentil may cause a condition called agranulocytosis, a dangerous drop in the number of certain kinds of white blood cells. Symptoms include fever, lethargy, sore throat, and weakness.

Possible food and drug interactions when taking this medication

Remember that Serentil must never be combined with alcohol, barbiturates, or narcotics. It's also best to avoid combining it with other drugs prescribed for schizophrenia, depression, or anxiety, or with the spasm-quelling drug atropine (Donnatal). Be careful, too, to avoid exposure to phosphorus insecticides.

Special information about pregnancy and breastfeeding

The effects of Serentil during pregnancy have not been adequately studied. Patients who are pregnant or plan to become pregnant should tell the doctor immediately. Pregnant women should use Serentil only if clearly needed.

It is not known whether Serentil appears in breast milk. Patients should talk with their doctor before deciding to breastfeed.

Recommended dosage

The doctor will tailor the dose of Serentil to the patient's needs. Once symptoms improve, the doctor will gradually reduce the dosage to the lowest effective dose.

ADULTS

Tablets and Oral Soulution

The usual starting dose of Serentil tablets or oral solution is 50 milligrams taken 3 times daily. Over the long term, the usual daily dose ranges from 100 to 400 milligrams per day.

CHILDREN

The safety and effectiveness of Serentil in children have not been established.

Overdosage

An overdose of Serentil can be fatal. If an overdose is suspected, seek medical attention immediately.

■ *Symptoms of Serentil overdose include:*

Absence of reflexes, agitation, blurred vision, coma, confusion, convulsions, difficulty breathing, disorientation, drowsiness, dry mouth, enlarged pupils, heartbeat irregularities, heart failure or arrest, high temperature, nasal congestion, overactive reflexes, rigid muscles, stupor, swollen throat, throat spasms, vomiting

Brand name:

Seroquel

Pronounced: SER-oh-kwell
Generic name: Quetiapine fumarate

Why is this drug prescribed?

Seroquel combats the symptoms of schizophrenia. It is the first in a new class of antipsychotic medications. Researchers believe that it works by diminishing the action of dopamine and serotonin, two of the brain's chief chemical messengers.

Most important fact about this drug

Seroquel may cause tardive dyskinesia—a condition characterized by uncontrollable muscle spasms and twitches in the face and body. This problem can be permanent, and appears to be most common among older adults, especially women.

How should this medication be taken?

Dosage is increased gradually until the drug takes effect. Patients who stop taking Seroquel for more than 1 week will need to build up to their ideal dosage once again.

■ *Missed dose...*

Generally, a missed dose should be taken as soon as remembered. However, if it is almost time for the next dose, patients should skip the one they missed and go back to their regular schedule. Doses should never be doubled.

■ *Storage instructions...*

Seroquel should be stored at room temperature.

What side effects may occur?

Side effects cannot be predicted. If any develop or change in intensity, patients should inform their doctor as soon as possible.

■ *More common side effects may include:*

Abdominal pain, constipation, diminished movement, dizziness, drowsiness, dry mouth, excessive muscle tone, headache, indigestion, low blood pressure, nasal inflammation, neck rigidity, rapid heartbeat, rash, tremor, uncontrollable movements, weakness

■ *Less common side effects may include:*

Back pain, cough, difficulty breathing, difficulty speaking, ear pain, fever, flu, loss of appetite, palpitations, sore throat, sweating, swelling, weight gain

■ *Rare side effects may include:*

Abnormal dreams, abnormal ejaculation, abnormal vision, abnormal gait, abnormal thinking, acne, alcohol intolerance, amnesia, arthritis, asthma, bleeding gums, bone pain, bruising, chills, confusion, conjunctivitis (pinkeye), dehydration, delusions, diabetes, difficulty swallowing, dry eyes, ear ringing, eczema, eye pain, face swelling, fungal infection, gas, gum inflammation, hallucinations, heavy menstruation, hemorrhoids, impotence, increased appetite, increased sex drive, increased salivation, irregular pulse, itching, jerky or irregular movement, joint pain, lack of emotion, lack of coordination, leg cramps, loss of menstruation, low blood sugar, manic reaction, migraine, mouth sores, muscle weakness, neck pain, nosebleeds, painful menstruation, painful urination, paralysis, paranoia, pelvic pain, pneumonia, rash, rectal bleeding, seborrhea, sensitivity to light, skin inflammation or ulcer, slow heart rate, stomach and intestinal inflammation, stupor, swollen testicles, taste disturbances, teeth grinding, thirst, tongue swelling, twitching, uncontrollable bowel movements, underactive thyroid, urinary frequency or incontinence, urinary retention, urinary tract infection, vaginal bleeding, vaginal inflammation, vaginal yeast infection, vertigo, weight loss

Why should this drug not be prescribed?

If Seroquel causes an allergic reaction, the patient will not be able to use this drug.

Special warnings about this medication

Patients who develop muscle stiffness, confusion, irregular or rapid heartbeat, excessive sweating, and high fever should call their doctor immediately. These are signs of a serious—and potentially fatal—reaction to the drug. Patients should be especially wary if they have a history of heart attack, heart disease, heart failure, circulation problems, or irregular heartbeat.

Particularly during the first few days of therapy, Seroquel can cause low blood pressure, with accompanying dizziness, fainting, and rapid heartbeat. To minimize these effects, the doctor will increase the dose gradually. People who are prone to low blood pressure, take blood pressure medication, or become dehydrated should use Seroquel with caution.

Seroquel also tends to cause drowsiness, especially at the start of therapy, and can impair judgment, thinking, and motor skills. Until patients are certain of the drug's effect, they need to use caution when operating machinery or driving a car.

Patients should report any vision problems to the doctor. There is a chance that Seroquel may cause cataracts, and some people may be asked to see an eye doctor when they start Seroquel therapy, and every 6 months thereafter.

Seroquel poses a very slight risk of seizures, especially in people who are over 65 or have epilepsy or Alzheimer's disease. The drug can also suppress an underactive thyroid, and generally causes a minor increase in cholesterol levels. There is also a remote chance that it will trigger a prolonged and painful erection.

Other antipsychotic medications have been known to interfere with the body's temperature-regulating mechanism, causing patients to overheat. Although this problem has not occurred with Seroquel, caution is still advisable. Patients should avoid exposure to extreme heat, strenuous exercise, and dehydration.

Possible food and drug interactions when taking this medication

Seroquel increases the effects of alcohol. Patients should avoid alcoholic beverages while on Seroquel therapy.

If Seroquel is taken with certain other drugs, the effects of either could be increased, decreased, or altered. Here is an overview of drugs that may cause a problem:

Barbiturates such as phenobarbital
Carbamazepine (Tegretol)
Cimetidine (Tagamet)
Erythromycin (Eryc, Ery-Tab)
Fluconazole (Diflucan)
Itraconazole (Sporanox)
Ketoconazole (Nizoral)
Levodopa (Sinemet)
Lorazepam (Ativan)
Phenytoin (Dilantin)
Rifampin (Rifadin, Rifamate, Rimactane)
Steroid medications such as hydrocortisone and prednisone
Thioridazine (Mellaril)

Special information about pregnancy and breastfeeding

The possibility of harm to a developing baby has not been ruled out. Women should take Seroquel during pregnancy only if the benefits outweigh this potential risk. They should notify their doctor as soon as they become pregnant or decide to become pregnant.

It is not known whether Seroquel appears in breast milk, and breastfeeding is not recommended.

Recommended dosage

ADULTS

On the first day of therapy, patients take 2 doses of 25 milligrams each. On the second and third day, doses are usually increased by 25 to 50 milligrams apiece. Frequency may be increased to 3 times daily.

Long-term, the usual dosage is 300 to 400 milligrams a day, taken as 2 or 3 smaller doses. Doses as low as 150 milligrams a day sometimes prove effective, and daily dosage rarely exceeds 750 milligrams. Doses of 800 milligrams or more per day have not been tested for safety.

Dosage is increased more gradually—and is maintained at a lower level—for older adults, those with liver disease, those prone to low blood pressure reactions, and the debilitated.

Overdosage

Any medication taken in excess can have serious consequences. If an overdose is suspected, seek medical help immediately.

■ *Symptoms of Seroquel overdose may include:*
Dizziness, drowsiness, fainting, rapid heartbeat

Generic name:

Sertraline

See Zoloft, page 234

Brand name:

Serzone

Pronounced: sur-ZONE
Generic name: Nefazodone hydrochloride

Why is this drug prescribed?

Serzone is prescribed for the treatment of major depression. Researchers believe it works by boosting levels of two of the brain's key chemical messengers, serotonin and norepinephrine. However, the drug is chemically unrelated to the family of serotonin-boosters that includes Prozac and Paxil.

Most important fact about this drug

It may be several weeks before patients feel the full antidepressant effect of Serzone. Once they do begin to feel better, it is important for them to keep taking the drug.

How should this medication be taken?

Patients must take Serzone exactly as prescribed, even if they no longer feel depressed.

■ *Missed dose...*
Generally, a missed dose should be taken as soon as remembered. However, if it is within 4 hours of the next dose, patients should skip the one they missed and go back to their regular schedule. Doses should never be doubled.

■ *Storage instructions...*
Serzone should be stored at room temperature in a tightly closed container.

What side effects may occur?

Side effects cannot be predicted. If any develop or change in intensity, patients should tell their doctor as soon as possible.

■ *More common side effects may include:*
Blurred or abnormal vision, confusion, constipation, dizziness, dry mouth, light-headedness, nausea, sleepiness, weakness

■ *Less common side effects may include:*
Abnormal dreams, cough, decreased concentration, diarrhea, dizziness on getting up, flu-like symptoms, headache, increased appetite, water retention

■ *Rare side effects may include:*
Abnormal bleeding, anxiety, blisters in mouth and eyes, breast pain, breast-milk discharge, breast enlargement in males, chills, coma, decreased sex drive, difficulty urinating, exaggerated reflexes, fever, frequent urination, lack of coordination, liver disease, prolonged erections, rigidity, ringing in ears, seizures, severe allergic reactions, spasms, stiff neck, sweating, taste change, thirst, tremors, urinary tract infection, vaginal inflammation

Why should this drug not be prescribed?

This medication should be avoided by anyone who is sensitive to or has ever had an allergic reaction to it or to similar drugs, such as Desyrel.

Serious, sometimes fatal reactions have occurred when Serzone is used in combination with drugs known as MAO inhibitors, including the antidepressants Nardil and Parnate. Serzone must never be taken with one of these drugs or within 14 days of discontinuing treatment with one of them. Also, patients should allow at least 7 days between the last dose of Serzone and the first dose of an MAO inhibitor.

Serzone should also be avoided by people taking Halcion or Tegretol, and should never be combined with Orap, as heart problems could result.

Special warnings about this medication

The doctor will prescribe Serzone with caution if the patient has a history of seizures or mania, or heart or liver disease. Serzone should also be used with caution in patients who have had a heart attack, stroke, or angina; take drugs for high blood pressure; or suffer from dehydration. Under these circumstances, Serzone could cause an unwanted drop in blood pressure. Patients should discuss all of their medical problems with the doctor before taking this drug.

Serzone may cause patients to become drowsy or less alert and may affect their judgment. They should not drive, operate dangerous machinery, or participate in any hazardous activity that requires full mental alertness until they know how the drug affects them.

Before having surgery, dental treatment, or any diagnostic procedure requiring anesthesia, patients should tell the doctor or dentist they are taking Serzone. If they develop an allergic reaction such as a skin rash or hives while taking Serzone, they should notify the doctor. Men who experience a prolonged or inappropriate erection while taking Serzone should discontinue the drug and call their doctor.

Serzone should be used with caution in people who have been addicted to drugs.

Possible food and drug interactions when taking this medication

If Serzone is taken with certain other drugs, the effects of either could be increased, decreased, or altered. Here is an overview of drugs that may cause a problem:

Alcohol
Alprazolam (Xanax)
Antidepressants that boost serotonin levels, including Celexa, Luvox, Paxil, Prozac, and Zoloft
Buspirone (BuSpar)
Carbamazepine (Tegretol)
Cyclosporine (Neoral and Sandimmune)
Digoxin (Lanoxin)
Haloperidol (Haldol)
MAO inhibitors, including Nardil and Parnate
Pimozide (Orap)
The cholesterol-lowering drugs Lipitor, Mevacor, and Zocor
Triazolam (Halcion)

Special information about pregnancy and breastfeeding

The effects of Serzone during pregnancy have not been adequately studied. Women who are pregnant or are planning to become pregnant should tell their doctor immediately. Serzone should be used during pregnancy only if clearly needed.

Serzone may appear in breast milk. If this medication is essential to the patient's health, the doctor may tell her to discontinue breastfeeding until treatment with Serzone is finished.

Recommended dosage

ADULTS

The usual starting dose for Serzone is 200 milligrams a day, divided into 2 doses. If needed, the doctor may increase the dose gradually to 300 to 600 milligrams a day.

CHILDREN

The safety and effectiveness of Serzone have not been established in children under 18 years of age.

OLDER ADULTS

The usual starting dose for older people and those in a weakened condition is 100 milligrams a day, taken in 2 doses. The doctor will adjust the dose according to the patient's response.

Overdosage

Any medication taken in excess can have serious consequences. If an overdose is suspected, seek medical attention immediately.

■ *Symptoms of Serzone overdose include:*
Nausea, sleepiness, vomiting

Brand name:

Sinequan

Pronounced: SIN-uh-kwan
Generic name: Doxepin hydrochloride

Why is this drug prescribed?

Sinequan is used in the treatment of depression and anxiety. It helps relieve tension, improve sleep, elevate mood, increase energy, and generally ease feelings of fear, guilt, apprehension, and worry. It is effective in treating people whose depression and/or anxiety is psychological, associated with alcoholism, or a result of another disease (cancer, for example). It is also prescribed for major depression and bipolar disorder. It is in the family of drugs called tricyclic antidepressants.

Most important fact about this drug

Serious, sometimes fatal, reactions have occurred when Sinequan is used in combination with drugs known as MAO inhibitors, including the antidepressants Nardil and Parnate. Any drug of this type should be discontinued at least 2 weeks prior to starting treatment with Sinequan, and the patient should be carefully monitored by the doctor.

Patients should consult their doctor before combining Sinequan with any other prescription or nonprescription drugs.

How should this medication be taken?

This medication must be taken exactly as prescribed. It may take several weeks for its beneficial effects to appear.

■ *Missed dose...*
Patients taking several doses a day should take the missed dose as soon as they remember, then take any remaining doses for that day at evenly spaced intervals. If it is almost time for the next dose, they should skip the one they missed and go back to their regular schedule.

Patients who take a single dose at bedtime and do not remember until the next morning should skip the dose. Doses should never be doubled.

■ *Storage instructions...*
Sinequan may be stored at room temperature.

What side effects may occur?
Side effects cannot be predicted. If any develop or change in intensity, patients should inform their doctor as soon as possible.

■ *The most common side effect is:*
Drowsiness.

■ *Less common or rare side effects may include:*
Blurred vision, breast development in males, bruises, buzzing or ringing in the ears, changes in sex drive, chills, confusion, constipation, diarrhea, difficulty urinating, disorientation, dizziness, dry mouth, enlarged breasts, fatigue, fluid retention, flushing, fragmented or incomplete movements, hair loss, hallucinations, headache, high fever, high or low blood sugar, inappropriate breast milk secretion, indigestion, inflammation of the mouth, itching and skin rash, lack of muscle control, loss of appetite, loss of coordination, low blood pressure, nausea, nervousness, numbness, poor bladder control, rapid heartbeat, red or brownish spots on the skin, seizures, sensitivity to light, severe muscle stiffness, sore throat, sweating, swelling of the testicles, taste disturbances, tingling sensation, tremors, vomiting, weakness, weight gain, yellow eyes and skin

Why should this drug not be prescribed?
Anyone who is sensitive to or has ever had an allergic reaction to Sinequan or similar antidepressants should not take this medication. Sinequan should also be avoided by patients with the eye condition known as glaucoma and by those who have difficulty urinating.

Special warnings about this medication
Sinequan may cause the patient to become drowsy or less alert. Driving, operating dangerous machinery, or participating in any hazardous activity that requires full mental alertness is not recommended.

In a medical emergency, and before surgery or dental treatment, the doctor or dentist should be made aware that the patient is taking Sinequan.

Possible food and drug interactions when taking this medication
Alcohol increases the danger in a Sinequan overdose. Patients should not drink alcohol while taking this medication.

Sinequan should never be combined with drugs known as MAO inhibitors. Medications in this category include the antidepressants Nardil and Parnate.

Patients switching from Prozac should wait at least 5 weeks after their last dose of Prozac before starting Sinequan.

If Sinequan is taken with certain other drugs, the effects of either could be increased, decreased, or altered. Here is an overview of drugs that may cause a problem:

Antidepressants that boost serotonin, such as Prozac, Zoloft, and Paxil
Other antidepressants such as Elavil and Serzone
Antipsychotic medications such as Compazine, Mellaril, and Thorazine
Carbamazepine (Tegretol)
Cimetidine (Tagamet)
Clonidine (Catapres)
Flecainide (Tambocor)
Guanethidine
Propafenone (Rythmol)
Quinidine (Quinidex)
Tolazamide (Tolinase)

Special information about pregnancy and breastfeeding
The effects of Sinequan during pregnancy have not been adequately studied. Women who are pregnant or are planning to become pregnant should inform their doctor immediately.

Sinequan may appear in breast milk and could affect a nursing infant. If this medication is essential to the patient's health, the doctor may advise her to discontinue breastfeeding until treatment is finished.

Recommended dosage
ADULTS

The starting dose for mild to moderate illness is usually 75 milligrams per day. This dose can be increased or decreased by the doctor according to individual need. The usual ideal dose ranges from 75 milligrams per day to 150 milligrams per day, although it can be as low as 25 to 50 milligrams per day. The total daily dose can be given once a day or divided into smaller doses. For people taking this drug once a day, the recommended dose is 150 milligrams at bedtime.

The 150-milligram capsule strength is intended for long-term therapy only and is not recommended as a starting dose.

For more severe illness, gradually increased doses of up to 300 milligrams may be required as determined by the doctor.

CHILDREN

Safety and effectiveness have not been established for use in children under 12 years of age.

OLDER ADULTS

Due to a greater risk of drowsiness and confusion, older people are usually started on a low dose.

Overdosage

◼ *Symptoms of Sinequan overdose may include:*
Agitation, coma, confusion, convulsions, dilated pupils, disturbed concentration, drowsiness, hallucinations, high or low body temperature, irregular heartbeat, overactive reflexes, rigid muscles, severely low blood pressure, stupor, vomiting

These symptoms signal the need for immediate medical attention. An overdose of this drug can be fatal.

Brand name:

Sonata

Pronounced: Sah-NAH-ta
Generic name: Zaleplon

Why is this drug prescribed?

Sonata is prescribed for people who have trouble falling asleep at bedtime. Because it has a short duration of action, it doesn't help those who suffer from frequent awakenings during the night or those who wake too early in the morning. It is intended only for short-term use (7 to 10 days).

Most important fact about this drug

Problems with sleep are usually temporary and require only short-term treatment with medication. Patients should call their doctor immediately if it seems the medication is making the problem worse, or if they notice any unusual changes in their thinking or behavior, such as hallucinations, amnesia, agitation, or a lack of inhibition. The emergence of new symptoms could be a sign of an undiagnosed medical or psychiatric condition.

How should this medication be taken?

Sonata is very fast-acting and should be taken only at bedtime.

◼ *Missed dose...*
Sonata should be taken only when the patient is ready to sleep. The dose should never be doubled.

◼ *Storage instructions...*
Sonata should be stored at room temperature in a light-resistant container.

What side effects may occur?

Side effects cannot be predicted. If any develop or change in intensity patients should inform their doctor as soon as possible.

■ *The most common side effect is:*
Headache

■ *Other common side effects may include:*
Abdominal pain, coordination problems, daytime sleepiness, dizziness, drowsiness, eye pain, memory loss, menstrual pain, muscle pain, nausea, stomach upset, weakness

■ *Less common side effects may include:*
Anxiety, burning or tingling sensation, decrease of sensation, ear pain, feeling of loss of identity or unreality, fever, hallucinations, loss of appetite, intestinal inflammation, nosebleed, sensitivity to light, sensitivity to noise, sensitivity to odors, swelling of the hands or feet, tiredness, tremor, vertigo, visual disturbances

A variety of other symptoms have been reported on very rare occasions. If Sonata is suspected of causing any sort of problem, it would be wise to check with the doctor.

Why should this drug not be prescribed?

There are no absolute restrictions on the use of Sonata, but it is not recommended for people with severe liver disease and is best avoided during pregnancy.

Special warnings about this medication

Sonata should not be used unless the patient plans to be in bed for at least four hours after taking it. Those who need to be alert and active in less than four hours may find that their performance is impaired. No one should attempt to drive a car or operate other dangerous machinery right after taking Sonata.

Sonata should be used only for temporary relief of insomnia; sleep medicines tend to lose their effect when taken for more than a few weeks. Remember, too, that taking sleeping pills for extended periods or in high doses can lead to physical dependence and the danger of a withdrawal reaction when the drug is abruptly stopped. Special caution is warranted for patients who have had addiction problems with alcohol or other drugs.

The safety and effectiveness of Sonata have not been established in children.

Possible food and drug interactions when taking this medication

Patients should avoid alcoholic beverages when taking Sonata; the drug increases alcohol's effect. They should also forego high-fat meals mmediately before taking Sonata; they tend to slow or reduce the drug's effect.

If Sonata is used with certain other drugs, the effects of either could be increased, decreased, or altered. Here is an overview of drugs that may cause a problem:

Carbamazepine (Tegretol)
Cimetidine (Tagamet)
Diphenhydramine (Benadryl)
Imipramine (Tofranil)
Phenobarbital
Rifampin (Rifadin)
Thioridazine (Mellaril)

Special information about pregnancy and breastfeeding

Sonata can affect a developing baby, especially during the last weeks before delivery, and is therefore not recommended for use during pregnancy. This drug also appears in breast milk and should not be used by nursing mothers.

Recommended dosage

ADULTS

The usual dose is 10 milligrams taken once daily at bedtime. The doctor may adjust the dose according to individual need, especially for those who are in a weakened condition or have a low body weight. A dose of 5 milligrams is recommended if the patient has liver disease or uses the drug cimetidine.

OLDER ADULTS

The usual dose for older adults is 5 milligrams, as they may be more sensitive to the effects of Sonata.

Overdosage

An overdose of drugs such as Sonata can be fatal. If an overdose is suspected, seek medical attention immediately.

■ *Symptoms of Sonata overdose may include:*
Drowsiness, mental confusion, grogginess, lack of coordination, flaccid muscles, labored breathing, coma

Brand name:

Stelazine

Pronounced: STEL-ah-zeen
Generic name: Trifluoperazine hydrochloride

Why is this drug prescribed?

Stelazine is used to treat severe mental disturbances as well as anxiety that does not respond to ordinary tranquilizers.

Most important fact about this drug

Stelazine may cause tardive dyskinesia–a condition marked by involuntary muscle spasms and twitches in the face and body. This condition may be permanent and appears to be most common among the elderly, especially women.

How should this medication be taken?

Patients taking Stelazine in a liquid concentrate form will need to dilute it with a liquid such as a carbonated beverage, coffee, fruit juice, milk, tea, tomato juice, or water. It can also be mixed with puddings, soups, and other semisolid foods. It should not be mixed with alcohol.

Stelazine should be diluted just before it's taken.

■ *Missed dose...*

Patients taking 1 dose a day should take the missed dose as soon as they remember. If they do not remember until the next day, they should skip the missed dose and go back to their regular schedule.

Patient who take more than 1 dose a day should take the missed dose if it is within an hour or so of the scheduled time. If they do not remember until later, they should skip the missed dose and go back to their regular schedule. Doses should never be doubled.

■ *Storage instructions...*

Stelazine may be stored at room temperature. The concentrate should be protected from light.

What side effects may occur?

Side effects cannot be predicted. If any develop or change in intensity, patients should inform their doctor as soon as possible.

■ *Side effects may include:*

Abnormal secretion of milk, abnormal sugar in urine, abnormalities in movement and posture, agitation, allergic reactions (sometimes severe), anemia, asthma, blood disorders, blurred vision, body rigidly arched backward, breast development in males, chewing movements, constipation, constricted pupils, difficulty swallowing, dilated pupils, dizziness, drooling, drowsiness, dry mouth, ejaculation problems, exaggerated or excessive reflexes, excessive or spontaneous flow of milk, eye problems causing a state of fixed gaze, eye spasms, fatigue, fever or high fever, flu-like symptoms, fluid accumulation and swelling (including the brain), fragmented movements, headache, heart attack, high or low blood sugar, hives, impotence, inability to urinate, increase in appetite and weight, infections, insomnia, intestinal blockage, involuntary movements of tongue, face, mouth, jaw, arms, and legs, irregular blood pressure, pulse, and heartbeat, irregular or no menstrual periods, jitteriness, light-headedness (especially when standing up), liver damage, lockjaw, loss of appetite, low blood pressure, mask-like face, muscle stiffness and rigidity, nasal congestion, nausea, persistent, painful erections, pill-rolling movement, protruding tongue, puckering of mouth, puffing of cheeks, purple or red spots on the skin, rapid heartbeat, restlessness, rigid arms, feet, head, and muscles, seizures, sensitivity to light, shuffling walk, skin inflammation and peeling, skin itching, pigmentation, reddening, or rash, spasms in jaw, face, tongue, neck, hands, feet, back, and mouth, sweating, swelling of the throat, totally unresponsive state, tremors, twisted neck, weakness, yellowing of skin and whites of eyes

Why should this drug not be prescribed?

Stelazine should be avoided by people with liver damage and those who are taking central nervous system depressants such as alcohol, barbiturates, or narcotic pain relievers. It is also contraindicated for people who have an abnormal bone marrow or blood condition.

Special warnings about this medication

Stelazine should be used with caution by anyone who has ever had a brain tumor, breast cancer, intestinal blockage, the eye condition called glaucoma, heart or liver disease, or seizures. Caution is warranted, too, if the patient is exposed to certain pesticides or extreme heat.

Stelazine may hide the signs of overdose of other drugs and may make it more difficult for the doctor to diagnose intestinal obstruction, brain tumor, and the dangerous neurological condition called Reye's syndrome.

Patients should inform the doctor if they have ever had an allergic reaction to any antipsychotic medication similar to Stelazine.

Dizziness, nausea, vomiting, and tremors can result if a patient suddenly stops taking Stelazine. The drug should be discontinued under a doctor's supervision.

The doctor should be alerted immediately if a patient experiences symptoms such as a fever or sore throat, mouth, or gums. These signs of infection may signal the need to stop Stelazine treatment. The doctor should be notified, too, of flu-like symptoms with fever.

This drug may impair the ability to drive a car or operate potentially dangerous machinery, especially during the first few days of treatment.

Patients should not participate in any activities that require full mental alertness if they are unsure about their ability.

Any vision problems that develop should be reported to the doctor.

Stelazine concentrate contains a sulfite that may cause allergic reactions in some people, especially in those with asthma.

Stelazine can cause a potentially fatal condition called Neuroleptic Malignant Syndrome. Signs are high body temperature, rigid muscles, irregular pulse or blood pressure, rapid or abnormal heartbeat, and excessive perspiration. These symptoms should be reported to the doctor immediately. Antipsychotic therapy will have to be discontinued.

Possible food and drug interactions when taking this medication

Extreme drowsiness and other potentially serious effects can result if Stelazine is combined with alcohol, tranquilizers such as Valium, narcotic painkillers such as Percocet, antihistamines such as Benadryl, and barbiturates such as phenobarbital.

If Stelazine is taken with certain other drugs, the effects of either could be increased, decreased, or altered. Here is an overview of drugs that may cause a problem:

Antiseizure drugs such as Dilantin
Atropine (Donnatal)
Blood thinners such as Coumadin
Guanethidine
Lithium (Eskalith, Lithobid)
Propranolol (Inderal)
Thiazide diuretics such as Dyazide

Special information about pregnancy and breastfeeding

Pregnant women should use Stelazine only if clearly needed. The effects of Stelazine during pregnancy have not been adequately studied.

Stelazine appears in breast milk and may affect a nursing infant. If this medication is essential to the patient's health, the doctor may have her discontinue breastfeeding while she is taking it.

Recommended dosage

ADULTS

Nonpsychotic Anxiety
Doses usually range from 2 to 4 milligrams daily. This amount should be divided into 2 equal doses and taken twice a day. The maximum dose is 6 milligrams a day. Treatment should continue for no more than 12 weeks.

Psychotic Disorders
The usual starting dose is 4 to 10 milligrams a day, divided into 2 equal doses; doses range from 15 to 40 milligrams daily.

CHILDREN

Doses are based on the child's weight and the severity of his or her symptoms.

Psychotic Children 6 to 12 Years Old Who Are Closely Monitored or Hospitalized
The starting dose is 1 milligram a day, taken all at once or divided into 2 doses. The doctor will increase the dosage gradually, up to 15 milligrams a day.

OLDER ADULTS

Older people usually take Stelazine at lower doses. Because they may develop low blood pressure while taking this drug, the doctor will watch them closely.

Overdosage

Any medication taken in excess can have serious consequences. If you suspect an overdose of Stelazine, seek medical help immediately.

■ *Symptoms of Stelazine overdose may include:*
Agitation, coma, convulsions, difficulty breathing, difficulty swallowing, dry mouth, extreme sleepiness, fever, intestinal blockage, irregular heart rate, low blood pressure, restlessness

Brand name:

Surmontil

Pronounced: SIR-mon-til
Generic name: Trimipramine maleate

Why is this drug prescribed?

Surmontil is used to treat depression. It is a member of the family of drugs known as tricyclic antidepressants.

Most important fact about this drug

Serious, sometimes fatal, reactions have been known to occur when drugs such as Surmontil are taken with drugs classified as MAO inhibitors. Drugs in this category include the antidepressants Nardil and Parnate. Surmontil must not be used within 2 weeks of taking one of these drugs.

How should this medication be taken?

Surmontil may be taken in 1 dose at bedtime. Alternatively, the total daily dosage may be divided into smaller amounts taken during the day. The single bedtime dose is preferred for people on long-term therapy with Surmontil.

It is important to take Surmontil exactly as prescribed, even if the drug seems to have no effect. It may take up to 4 weeks for its benefits to appear.

Surmontil can make the mouth dry. Sucking hard candy or chewing gum can help this problem.

■ *Missed dose...*

Generally, a missed dose should be taken as soon as remembered. However, if it is almost time for the next dose, patients should skip the one they missed and go back to their regular schedule. Doses should never be doubled.

Patients who take Surmontil once a day at bedtime and miss a dose should not take it in the morning. It could cause disturbing side effects during the day.

■ *Storage instructions...*

Surmontil should be stored at room temperature in a tightly closed container. Capsules in blister strips should be protected from moisture.

What side effects may occur?

Side effects cannot be predicted. If any develop or change in intensity, patients should inform their doctor as soon as possible.

■ *Side effects may include:*

Abdominal cramps, agitation, anxiety, black tongue, blocked intestine, blood disorders, blurred vision, breast development in men, confusion (especially in older adults), constipation, delusions, diarrhea, difficulty urinating, dilated pupils, disorientation, dizziness, drowsiness, dry mouth, excessive or spontaneous milk excretion, fatigue, fever, flushing, fluttery or throbbing heartbeat, frequent urination, hair loss, hallucinations, headache, heart attack, high blood pressure, high blood sugar, hives, impotence, increased or decreased sex drive, inflammation of the mouth, insomnia, irregular heart rate, lack of coordination, loss of appetite, low blood pressure, low blood sugar, nausea, nightmares, numbness, peculiar taste in mouth, purple or reddish-brown spots on skin, rapid heartbeat, restlessness, ringing in the ears, seizures, sensitivity to light, skin itching, skin rash, sore throat, stomach upset, stroke, sweating, swelling of breasts, swelling of face and tongue, swelling of testicles, swollen glands, tingling, pins and needles, tremors, visual problems, vomiting, weakness, weight gain or loss, yellowing of the skin and whites of the eyes

Why should this drug not be prescribed?

Surmontil should not be used by anyone recovering from a recent heart attack. It should not be taken by people who are sensitive to it or have ever had an allergic reaction to it or to similar drugs such as Tofranil.

Special warnings about this medication

Surmontil should be used with caution by patients who have a seizure disorder, the eye condition known as glaucoma, heart disease, or a liver disorder. Caution is also warranted if they have thyroid disease or are taking thyroid medication. People who have had problems urinating should also be careful about taking Surmontil.

Nausea, headache, and a general feeling of illness may result if Surmontil is stopped suddenly. This does not signify addiction, but the doctor's instructions should be followed closely when discontinuing the drug.

This drug may impair the ability to drive a car or operate potentially dangerous machinery. Patients should not participate in any activities that require full alertness if they are unsure of the drug's effect.

Possible food and drug interactions when taking this medication

People who are taking antidepressants known as MAO inhibitors (Parnate and Nardil) should not take Surmontil. They need to wait 2 weeks after stopping an MAO inhibitor before starting Surmontil.

If Surmontil is taken with certain other drugs, the effects of either could be increased, decreased, or altered. Here is an overview of drugs that may cause a problem:

Antidepressants such as Desyrel and Wellbutrin
Antidepressants that act on serotonin, such as Prozac, Paxil, and Zoloft
Antipsychotic medications such as Thorazine and Mellaril
Cimetidine (Tagamet)
Drugs for heart irregularities, such as Rythmol and Tambocor
Drugs that quell spasms, such as Donnatal and Cogentin
Guanethidine
Local anesthetics containing epinephrine
Local decongestants such as Dristan Nasal Spray
Quinidine (Quinidex, Quinaglute)
Stimulants such as Proventil, Sudafed, and EpiPen
Thyroid medications such as Synthroid

Extreme drowsiness and other potentially serious effects may result if the patient drinks alcoholic beverages while taking Surmontil.

Special information about pregnancy and breastfeeding

The effects of Surmontil in pregnancy have not been adequately studied. Pregnant women should use Surmontil only when the potential benefits clearly outweigh the potential risks.

Recommended dosage

ADULTS

The usual starting dose is 75 milligrams per day, divided into equal smaller doses. The doctor may gradually increase the dose to 150 milligrams per day, divided into smaller doses. Doses over 200 milligrams a day are not recommended. Doses in long-term therapy may range from 50 to 150 milligrams daily. This total daily dosage at bedtime can be taken at bedtime or spread out through the day.

CHILDREN

Safety and effectiveness of Surmontil in children have not been established.

OLDER ADULTS AND ADOLESCENTS

Dosages usually start at 50 milligrams per day. The doctor may increase the dose to 100 milligrams a day, if needed.

Overdosage

An overdose of Surmontil can be fatal. If an overdose is suspected, seek medical help immediately.

■ *Symptoms of Surmontil overdose may include:*
Agitation, coma, confusion, convulsions, dilated pupils, disturbed concentration, drowsiness, hallucinations, high fever, irregular heart rate, low body temperature, muscle rigidity, overactive reflexes, severely low blood pressure, stupor, vomiting

Also possible are any of the symptoms listed under "What side effects may occur?"

Generic name:

Tacrine

See Cognex, page 34

Generic name:

Temazepam

See Restoril, page 166

Generic name:

Thioridazine

See Mellaril, page 107

Generic name:

Thiothixene

See Navane, page 120

Brand name:

Thorazine

Pronounced: THOR-ah-zeen
Generic name: Chlorpromazine

Why is this drug prescribed?

Thorazine is used for the reduction of symptoms of psychotic disorders such as schizophrenia; for the short-term treatment of severe behavioral disorders in children, including explosive hyperactivity and combativeness; and for the manic phase of bipolar disorder.

Thorazine is also used to control nausea and vomiting, and to relieve restlessness and apprehension before surgery. It is used as an aid in the treatment of tetanus, and is prescribed for uncontrollable hiccups and acute intermittent porphyria (attacks of severe abdominal pain sometimes accompanied by psychiatric disturbances, cramps in the arms and legs, and muscle weakness).

Most important fact about this drug

Thorazine may cause tardive dyskinesia–a condition marked by involuntary muscle spasms and twitches in the face and body. This condition may be permanent, and appears to be most common among the elderly, especially women.

How should this medication be taken?

Patients taking Thorazine in a liquid concentrate form will need to dilute it with a liquid such as a carbonated beverage, coffee, fruit juice, milk, tea, tomato juice, or water. Puddings, soups, and other semisolid foods may also be used. Thorazine should not be mixed with alcoholic beverages. It will taste best if it is diluted immediately prior to use.

Antacids such as Gelusil should not be taken at the same time as Thorazine. At least 1 to 2 hours should be allowed between doses of the two drugs.

■ *Missed dose...*

Patients taking 1 dose a day should take the missed dose as soon as they remember. If they do not remember until the next day, they should skip the missed dose and go back to their regular schedule.

Patient who take more than 1 dose a day should take the missed dose if it is within an hour or so of the scheduled time. If they do not remember until later, they should skip the missed dose and go back to their regular schedule. Doses should never be doubled.

■ *Storage instructions...*

Thorazine should be stored away from heat, light, and moisture. The liquid should be protected from freezing. Since the liquid concentrate form of Thorazine is light-sensitive, it should be stored in a dark place, but it does not need to be refrigerated.

What side effects may occur?

Side effects cannot be predicted. If any develop or change in intensity, patients should inform their doctor as soon as possible.

■ *Side effects may include:*

Abnormal secretion of milk, abnormalities in movement and posture, agitation, anemia, asthma, blood disorders, breast development in males, chewing movements, constipation, difficulty breathing, difficulty swallowing, dizziness, drooling, drowsiness, dry mouth, ejaculation problems, eye problems causing fixed gaze, fainting, fever, flu-like symptoms, fluid accumulation and swelling, headache, heart attack, high or low blood sugar, hives, impotence, inability to urinate, inability to move or talk, increase of appetite, infections, insomnia, intestinal blockage, involuntary movements of arms and legs, tongue, face, mouth, or jaw, irregular blood pressure, pulse, and heartbeat, irregular or no menstrual periods, jitteriness, light-headedness (on standing up), lockjaw, mask-like face, muscle stiffness and rigidity, narrow or dilated pupils, nasal congestion, nausea, pain and stiffness in the neck, persistent, painful erections, pill-rolling motion, protruding tongue, puckering of the mouth, puffing of the cheeks, rapid heartbeat, red or purple spots on the skin, rigid arms, feet, head, and muscles (including the back), seizures, sensitivity to light, severe allergic reactions, shuffling walk, skin inflammation and peeling, sore throat, spasms in jaw, face, tongue, neck, mouth, and feet, sweating, swelling of breasts in women, swelling of the throat, tremors, twitching in the body, neck, shoulders and face, twisted neck, visual problems, weight gain, yellowed skin and whites of eyes

Why should this drug not be prescribed?

Thorazine should not be combined with large amounts of any substance that slows down mental function, such as alcohol, barbiturates, or narcotics. It should be avoided by anyone who has ever had an allergic reaction to a member of the phenothiazine family of antipsychotic medications.

Special warnings about this medication

Thorazine should be used with caution if the patient has asthma, a brain tumor, breast cancer, intestinal blockage, emphysema, the eye condition known as glaucoma, heart problems, kidney or liver disease, a severe respiratory infection, seizures, or an abnormal bone marrow or blood condition. Caution is also advisable if the patient is exposed to pesticides or extreme heat. Be aware that Thorazine can mask symptoms of brain tumor, intestinal blockage, and the neurological condition called Reye's syndrome.

Stomach inflammation, dizziness, nausea, vomiting, and tremors may result if Thorazine is stopped suddenly. Therapy should be discontinued only under a doctor's supervision.

This drug may impair the ability to drive a car or operate potentially dangerous machinery. Patients should not participate in any activities that require full alertness if they are unsure about their ability.

This drug can increase sensitivity to light. Patients should avoid being out in the sun too long.

Thorazine can cause a potentially fatal group of symptoms called Neuroleptic Malignant Syndrome. Symptoms include extremely high body temperature, rigid muscles, mental changes, irregular pulse or blood pressure, rapid heartbeat, sweating, and changes in heart rhythm. The doctor should be alerted immediately if these symptoms develop. Thorazine therapy will need to be discontinued.

Patients on Thorazine for a prolonged period should see their doctor for regular evaluations, since side effects can get worse over time.

Possible food and drug interactions when taking this medication

If Thorazine is taken with certain other drugs, the effects of either could be increased, decreased, or altered. Here is an overview of drugs that may cause a problem:

Anesthetics
Antacids such as Gelusil
Antiseizure drugs such as Dilantin
Antispasmodic drugs such as Cogentin
Atropine (Donnatal)
Barbiturates such as phenobarbital
Blood-thinning drugs such as Coumadin
Captopril (Capoten)
Cimetidine (Tagamet)
Diuretics such as Dyazide
Drugs classified as MAO inhibitors, such as the antidepressants Nardil and Parnate

Epinephrine (EpiPen)
Guanethidine
Lithium (Lithobid, Eskalith)
Narcotics such as Percocet
Propranolol (Inderal)

Extreme drowsiness and other potentially serious effects can result if Thorazine is combined with alcohol and other mental depressants such as narcotic painkillers like Demerol.

Because Thorazine prevents vomiting, it can hide the signs and symptoms of overdose of other drugs.

Special information about pregnancy and breastfeeding

The effects of Thorazine during pregnancy have not been adequately studied. Patients who are pregnant or plan to become pregnant should notify their doctor. Pregnant women should use Thorazine only if clearly needed.

Thorazine appears in breast milk and may affect a nursing infant. If this medication is essential to the mother's health, the doctor may advise her not to breastfeed until treatment is finished.

Recommended dosage

ADULTS

Psychotic Disorders

Your doctor will gradually increase the dosage until symptoms are controlled. Full improvement may not be seen for weeks or even months.

Initial dosages may range from 30 to 75 milligrams daily. The amount is divided into equal doses and taken 3 or 4 times a day. If needed, the doctor may increase the dosage by 20 to 50 milligrams at semiweekly intervals.

Nausea and Vomiting

The usual tablet dosage is 10 to 25 milligrams, taken every 4 or 6 hours, as needed.

One 100-milligram suppository can be used every 6 to 8 hours.

Uncontrollable Hiccups

Dosages may range from 75 to 200 milligrams daily, divided into 3 or 4 equal doses.

Acute Intermittent Porphyria

Dosages may range from 75 to 200 milligrams daily, divided into 3 or 4 equal doses.

CHILDREN

Thorazine is generally not prescribed for children younger than 6 months.

Severe Behavior Problems, Nausea, and Vomiting
Dosages are based on the child's weight.

Oral: The daily dose is one-quarter milligram for each pound of the child's weight, taken every 4 to 6 hours, as needed.

Rectal: The usual dose is one-half milligram per pound of body weight, taken every 6 to 8 hours, as necessary.

OLDER ADULTS

In general, older people take lower dosages of Thorazine, and any increase in dosage will be gradual. Because of a greater risk of low blood pressure, the doctor will watch the patient closely. Remember that older people (especially older women) may be more susceptible to tardive dyskinesia.

Overdosage

An overdose of Thorazine can be fatal. If an overdose is suspected, seek medical help immediately.

■ *Symptoms of Thorazine overdose may include:*
Agitation, coma, convulsions, difficulty breathing, difficulty swallowing, dry mouth, extreme sleepiness, fever, intestinal blockage, irregular heart rate, low blood pressure, restlessness

Brand name:

Tofranil

Pronounced: toe-FRAY-nil
Generic name: Imipramine hydrochloride

Why is this drug prescribed?

Tofranil is used to treat major depression. It is a member of the family of drugs called tricyclic antidepressants.

Tofranil is also used on a short term basis, along with behavioral therapies, to treat bed-wetting in children aged 6 and older. Its effectiveness may decrease with longer use.

Some doctors also prescribe Tofranil to treat bulimia, attention deficit disorder in children, obsessive-compulsive disorder, and panic disorder.

Most important fact about this drug

Serious, sometimes fatal, reactions have been known to occur when drugs such as Tofranil are taken with another type of antidepressant called an MAO inhibitor. Drugs in this category include Nardil and Parnate. Tofranil must not be taken within 2 weeks of taking one of these drugs.

How should this medication be taken?

Tofranil may be taken with or without food. It should not be combined with alcohol.

Patients should keep taking Tofranil even if they feel no immediate effect. It can take from 1 to 3 weeks for improvement to begin.

Tofranil can cause dry mouth. Sucking hard candy or chewing gum can help this problem.

■ *Missed dose...*

Patients who take 1 dose a day at bedtime should contact their doctor. They should not take the dose in the morning because of possible side effects.

If they take 2 or more doses a day, they should take the forgotten dose as soon as they remember. However, if it is almost time for the next dose, they should skip the one they missed and go back to their regular schedule. Doses should never be doubled.

■ *Storage instructions...*

Tofranil should be stored at room temperature in a tightly closed container.

What side effects may occur?

Side effects cannot be predicted. If any develop or change in intensity, patients should inform their doctor as soon as possible.

■ *Side effects may include:*

Abdominal cramps, agitation, anxiety, black tongue, bleeding sores, blood disorders, blurred vision, breast development in males, confusion, congestive heart failure, constipation or diarrhea, cough, fever, sore throat, delusions, dilated pupils, disorientation, dizziness, drowsiness, dry mouth, episodes of elation or irritability, excessive or spontaneous flow of milk, fatigue, fever, flushing, frequent urination or difficulty or delay in urinating, hair loss, hallucinations, headache, heart attack, heart failure, high blood pressure, high or low blood sugar, high pressure of fluid in the eyes, hives, impotence, increased or decreased sex drive, inflammation of the mouth, insomnia, intestinal blockage, irregular heartbeat, lack of coordination, light-headedness (especially when rising from lying down), loss of appetite, nausea, nightmares, odd taste in mouth, palpitations, purple or reddish-brown spots on skin, rapid heartbeat, restlessness, ringing in the ears, seizures, sensitivity to light, skin itching and rash, stomach upset, stroke, sweating, swelling due to fluid retention (especially in face or tongue), swelling of breasts, swelling of testicles, swollen glands, tendency to fall, tingling, pins and needles, and numbness in hands and feet, tremors, visual problems, vomiting, weakness, weight gain or loss, yellowed skin and whites of eyes

■ *The most common side effects in children being treated for bed-wetting are:*
Nervousness, sleep disorders, stomach and intestinal problems, tiredness

■ *Other side effects in children are:*
Anxiety, collapse, constipation, convulsions, emotional instability, fainting

Why should this drug not be prescribed?

Tofranil should not be used by anyone recovering from a recent heart attack.

People who take drugs known as MAO inhibitors, such as the antidepressants Nardil and Parnate, should not take Tofranil. The drug should also be avoided by those who are sensitive or allergic to it.

Special warnings about this medication

Tofranil should be used with caution by people who have or have ever had narrow-angle glaucoma (increased pressure in the eye); difficulty urinating; heart, liver, kidney, or thyroid disease; or seizures. Caution is also warranted for those taking thyroid medication.

General feelings of illness, headache, and nausea can result if Tofranil is stopped abruptly. Patients need to follow the doctor's instructions closely when discontinuing Tofranil.

The doctor should be alerted if a sore throat or fever develops during Tofranil therapy.

This drug may impair the ability to drive a car or operate potentially dangerous machinery. Patients should avoid any activities that require full alertness if they are unsure about their ability.

This drug can make people sensitive to light. Patients should stay out of the sun as much as possible.

Tofranil should be discontinued before elective surgery.

Possible food and drug interactions when taking this medication

Tofranil must never be combined with an MAO inhibitor. If Tofranil is taken with certain other drugs, the effects of either could be increased, decreased, or altered. Here is an overview of drugs that may cause a problem:

Albuterol (Proventil, Ventolin)
Antidepressants that act on serotonin, including Prozac, Paxil, and Zoloft
Other antidepressants such as Elavil and Pamelor
Antipsychotic medications such as Mellaril and Thorazine
Barbiturates such as Nembutal and Seconal
Blood pressure medications such as Catapres

Carbamazepine (Tegretol)
Cimetidine (Tagamet)
Decongestants such as Sudafed
Drugs that control spasms, such as Cogentin
Epinephrine (EpiPen)
Flecainide (Tambocor)
Methylphenidate (Ritalin)
Norepinephrine
Phenytoin (Dilantin)
Propafenone (Rythmol)
Quinidine (Quinaglute)
Thyroid medications such as Synthroid
Tranquilizers and sleep aids such as Halcion, Xanax, and Valium
Extreme drowsiness and other potentially serious effects can result if Tofranil is combined with alcohol or other mental depressants, such as narcotic painkillers (Percocet), sleeping medications (Halcion), or tranquilizers (Valium).

Patients switching from Prozac should wait at least 5 weeks after the last dose of Prozac before starting Tofranil.

Special information about pregnancy and breastfeeding

The effects of Tofranil during pregnancy have not been adequately studied. Pregnant women should use Tofranil only when the potential benefits clearly outweigh the potential risks. If a patient is pregnant or plans to become pregnant, she should inform her doctor immediately.

Tofranil may appear in breast milk and could affect a nursing infant. If this medication is essential to the patient's health, the doctor may advise her to stop breastfeeding until treatment is finished.

Recommended dosage

ADULTS

The usual starting dose is 75 milligrams a day. The doctor may increase this to 150 milligrams a day. The maximum daily dose is 200 milligrams.

CHILDREN

Tofranil is not to be used in children to treat any condition but bedwetting, and its use will be limited to short-term therapy. Safety and effectiveness in children under the age of 6 have not been established.

Total daily dosages for children should not exceed 2.5 milligrams for each 2.2 pounds of the child's weight.

Doses usually begin at 25 milligrams per day. This amount should be taken an hour before bedtime. If needed, this dose may be increased after 1 week to 50 milligrams (ages 6 through 11) or 75 milligrams (ages

12 and up), taken in one dose at bedtime or divided into 2 doses, 1 taken at mid-afternoon and 1 at bedtime.

OLDER ADULTS AND ADOLESCENTS

People in these two age groups should take lower doses. Dosage starts out at 30 to 40 milligrams per day and can go up to no more than 100 milligrams a day.

Overdosage

An overdose of Tofranil can be fatal. It has been reported that children are more sensitive than adults to overdoses of Tofranil. If an overdose is suspected, seek medical help immediately.

■ *Symptoms of Tofranil overdose may include:*
Agitation, bluish skin, coma, convulsions, difficulty breathing, dilated pupils, drowsiness, heart failure, high fever, involuntary writhing or jerky movements, irregular or rapid heartbeat, lack of coordination, low blood pressure, overactive reflexes, restlessness, rigid muscles, shock, stupor, sweating, vomiting.

Brand name:

Tranxene

Pronounced: TRAN-zeen
Generic name: Clorazepate dipotassium
Other brand names: Tranxene-SD, Tranxene-SD Half Strength

Why is this drug prescribed?

Tranxene belongs to a class of drugs known as benzodiazepines. It is used in the treatment of anxiety disorders and for short-term relief of the symptoms of anxiety.

It is also used to relieve the symptoms of acute alcohol withdrawal and to help in treating certain convulsive disorders such as epilepsy.

Most important fact about this drug

Tranxene can be habit-forming if taken regularly over a long period. Withdrawal symptoms may occur if this drug is stopped abruptly. Patients should consult the doctor before discontinuing Tranxene or making any change in their dose.

How should this medication be taken?

Tranxene should be taken exactly as prescribed.

■ *Missed dose...*
If it is within an hour or so of the scheduled time, the forgotten dose should be taken immediately. If it's not remembered until later, the patient should skip the dose and go back to the regular schedule.

Doses should never be doubled.

■ *Storage instructions...*
Tranxene should be stored at room temperature and protected from excessive heat.

What side effects may occur?
Side effects cannot be predicted. If any develop or change in intensity, patients should inform their doctor as soon as possible.

■ *More common side effects may include:*
Drowsiness

■ *Less common or rare side effects may include:*
Blurred vision, depression, difficulty in sleeping or falling asleep, dizziness, dry mouth, double vision, fatigue, genital and urinary tract disorders, headache, irritability, lack of muscle coordination, mental confusion, nervousness, tremors, skin rashes, slurred speech, stomach and intestinal disorders, tremor

■ *Side effects due to rapid decrease or abrupt withdrawal from Tranxene may include:*
Abdominal cramps, convulsions, diarrhea, difficulty in sleeping or falling asleep, hallucinations, impaired memory, irritability, muscle aches, nervousness, tremors, vomiting

Why should this drug not be prescribed?
Anyone who is sensitive to or has ever had an allergic reaction to Tranxene should not take this medication. It should also be avoided by people with the eye condition known as acute narrow-angle glaucoma.

Anxiety or tension related to everyday stress usually does not require treatment with such a strong drug. Patients should discuss their symptoms thoroughly with the doctor.

Tranxene is not recommended for use in more serious conditions such as depression or severe psychological disorders.

Special warnings about this medication
Tranxene may cause patients to become drowsy or less alert. They should not drive, operate dangerous machinery, or participate in any hazardous activity that requires full mental alertness until they know how this drug affects them.

For anxiety associated with depression, the dosage of this medication is usually reduced, and should not be increased without the doctor's approval.

The elderly and people in a weakened condition are more apt to become unsteady or oversedated when taking Tranxene.

Possible food and drug interactions when taking this medication

Tranxene slows down the central nervous system and may intensify the effects of alcohol. Patients should avoid alcohol while taking this medication.

If Tranxene is taken with certain other drugs, the effects of either could be increased, decreased, or altered. Here is an overview of drugs that may cause a problem:

Antidepressant drugs known as MAO inhibitors (Nardil, Parnate) and other antidepressants such as Elavil and Prozac
Antipsychotic medications such as Mellaril and Thorazine
Barbiturates such as Nembutal and Seconal
Narcotic pain relievers such as Demerol and Percodan

Special information about pregnancy and breastfeeding

The effects of Tranxene during pregnancy have not been adequately studied. However, because there is an increased risk of birth defects associated with this class of drug, its use during pregnancy should be avoided.

Tranxene may appear in breast milk and could affect a nursing infant. If this medication is essential to the patient's health, the doctor may advise her to discontinue breastfeeding until treatment with this medication is finished.

Recommended dosage

ANXIETY

Adults

The usual daily dosage is 30 milligrams divided into several smaller doses. A normal daily dose can be as little as 15 milligrams. The doctor may increase the dosage gradually to as much as 60 milligrams, according to the patient's individual needs.

Tranxene can also be taken in a single bedtime dose. The initial dose is 15 milligrams. The doctor may increase it if necessary.

Tranxene-SD, a 22.5-milligram tablet, and Tranxene-SD Half Strength, an 11.25-milligram tablet, can be taken once every 24 hours. The doctor may switch patients to this form of the drug after they have been taking Tranxene for several weeks.

Older Adults

The usual starting dose is 7.5 to 15 milligrams per day.

ACUTE ALCOHOL WITHDRAWAL

Tranxene can be used in a multi-day program for relief of the symptoms of acute alcohol withdrawal.

Dosages are usually increased in the first 2 days from 30 to 90 milligrams and then reduced over the next 2 days to lower levels. After that, the doctor will gradually lower the dose still further until the drug is no longer necessary.

WHEN USED WITH ANTIEPILEPTIC DRUGS

Tranxene can be used in conjunction with antiepileptic drugs. Recommended dosages must be followed carefully to avoid drowsiness.

Adults and Children over 12 Years Old
The starting dose is 7.5 milligrams 3 times a day. The doctor may increase the dosage by 7.5 milligrams per week to a maximum of 90 milligrams a day.

Children 9 to 12 Years Old
The starting dose is 7.5 milligrams twice a day. The doctor may increase the dosage by 7.5 milligrams a week to a maximum of 60 milligrams a day.
     Safety and effectiveness in children under 9 years of age have not been established.

Overdosage
Any medication taken in excess can have serious consequences. If an overdose is suspected, seek medical treatment immediately.

■ *Symptoms of Tranxene overdose may include:*
   Coma, low blood pressure, sedation

Generic name:
Tranylcypromine

See Parnate, page 135

Generic name:
Trazodone
See Desyrel, page 53

Brand name:
Triavil

Pronounced: TRY-uh-vill
Generic ingredients: Amitriptyline hydrochloride, Perphenazine
Other brand name: Etrafon

Why is this drug prescribed?
Triavil is used to treat anxiety, agitation, and depression. Triavil is a

combination of a tricyclic antidepressant (amitriptyline) and a tranquilizer (perphenazine).

Triavil can also help people with schizophrenia who are depressed and people with insomnia, fatigue, loss of interest, loss of appetite, or a slowing of physical and mental reactions.

Most important fact about this drug

Triavil may cause tardive dyskinesia—a condition marked by involuntary muscle spasms and twitches in the face and body. This condition may be permanent and appears to be most common among the elderly, especially women.

How should this medication be taken?

Triavil may be taken with or without food. It should not be taken with alcohol.

■ *Missed dose...*

Generally, a forgotten dose should be taken as soon as remembered. However, if it is within 2 hours of the next dose, patients should skip the one they missed and go back to their regular schedule. Doses should never be doubled.

■ *Storage instructions...*

Triavil should be stored at room temperature in a tightly closed container. Triavil 2-10 tablets should be protected from light.

What side effects may occur?

Side effects cannot be predicted. If any develop or change in intensity, patients should inform their doctor as soon as possible.

■ *Side effects may include:*

Abnormal secretion of milk, abnormalities of movements and posture, anxiety, asthma, black tongue, blood disorders, blurred vision, body rigidly arched backward, breast development in males, change in pulse rate, chewing movements, coma, confusion, constipation, convulsions, delusions, diarrhea, difficulty breathing, difficulty concentrating, difficulty swallowing, dilated pupils, disorientation, dizziness, drowsiness, dry mouth, eating abnormal amounts of food, ejaculation failure, episodes of elation or irritability, excessive or spontaneous flow of milk, excitement, exhaustion, eye problems, eye spasms, eyes in a fixed position, fatigue, fever, fluid accumulation and swelling (including throat and brain, face and tongue, arms and legs), frequent urination, hair loss, hallucinations, headache, heart attacks, hepatitis, high blood pressure, high fever, high or low blood sugar, hives, impotence, inability to stop moving, inability to urinate, increased or decreased sex drive, inflammation of the mouth, insomnia, intestinal blockage, intolerance to light, involuntary jerky movements of tongue, face, mouth, lips, jaw, body, or arms and legs, irregular blood pressure, pulse, and heartbeat, irregular menstrual periods, lack of coordination, light-headedness upon standing up, liver problems, lockjaw, loss or increase of appetite, low blood pressure, muscle stiffness, nasal congestion, nausea, nightmares, odd taste in the mouth, overactive reflexes, pain and stiffness around neck, palpitations, protruding tongue, puckering of the mouth, puffing of the cheeks, purple-reddish-brown spots on skin, rapid heartbeat, restlessness, rigid arms, feet, head, and muscles, ringing in the ears, salivation, sedation, seizures, sensitivity to light, severe allergic reactions, skin rash or inflammation, scaling, spasms in the hands and feet, speech problems, stomach upset, stroke, sweating, swelling of breasts, swelling of testicles, swollen glands, tingling, pins and needles, and numbness in hands and feet, tremors, twisted neck, twitching in the body, neck, shoulders, and face, uncontrollable and involuntary urination, urinary problems, visual problems, vomiting, weakness, weight gain or loss, writhing motions, yellowed skin and whites of eyes

Why should this drug not be prescribed?

Triavil must never be combined with drugs that slow down the central nervous system, including alcohol, barbiturates, analgesics, antihistamines, or narcotics.

It should not be used by anyone who is recovering from a recent heart attack or has an abnormal bone marrow condition. It should be avoided by patients who have had an allergic reaction to phenothiazines or amitriptyline.

People who are taking antidepressant drugs known as MAO inhibitors (including Nardil and Parnate) should not take Triavil.

Special warnings about this medication

Triavil should be used with caution by anyone who has ever had the eye condition known as glaucoma; difficulty urinating; breast cancer; seizures; or heart, liver, or thyroid disease. Caution is also in order if the patient is exposed to extreme heat or pesticides. Be aware that Triavil may mask signs of brain tumor, intestinal blockage, and overdose of other drugs.

Nausea, headache, and a general ill feeling can result if Triavil is stopped abruptly. Patients need to follow the doctor's instructions closely when discontinuing Triavil. If the dose is gradually reduced, they may still experience irritability, restlessness, and dream and sleep disturbances, but these effects will not last.

This drug may impair the ability to drive a car or operate potentially dangerous machinery. Patients should not participate in any activities that require full alertness if they are unsure about their ability.

Patients who develop a fever that has no other cause should stop taking Triavil and call their doctor.

Possible food and drug interactions when taking this medication

If Triavil is taken with certain other drugs, the effects of either could be increased, decreased, or altered. Here is an overview of drugs that may cause a problem:

Airway-opening drugs such as Proventil
Antiseizure drugs such as Dilantin
Antihistamines such as Benadryl
Atropine (Donnatal)
Barbiturates such as phenobarbital
Blood-thinning drugs such as Coumadin
Cimetidine (Tagamet)
Disulfiram (Antabuse)
Drugs classified as MAO inhibitors, including the antidepressants Nardil and Parnate
Drugs that quell spasms, such as Bentyl
Epinephrine (EpiPen)
Ethchlorvynol (Placidyl)
Fluoxetine (Prozac)
Furazolidone (Furoxone)
Guanethidine
Major tranquilizers such as Haldol
Narcotic analgesics such as Percocet
Thyroid medications such as Synthroid

Extreme drowsiness and other potentially serious effects can result if Triavil is combined with alcohol or other central nervous system depressants such as narcotics, painkillers, and sleep medications.

Special information about pregnancy and breastfeeding

Triavil may cause false-positive results on pregnancy tests. Triavil should not be used by pregnant women or mothers who are breastfeeding.

Recommended dosage

Each patient's dose must be individualized. The maximum dose is 8 tablets a day. It may be a few days to a few weeks before the patient notices any improvement.

ADULTS

For Non-Psychotic Anxiety and Depression

The usual dose is 1 tablet of Triavil 2-25 or 4-25 taken 3 or 4 times a day.

For Anxiety in People with Schizophrenia

The usual dose is 2 tablets of Triavil 4-25 taken 3 times a day. The doctor may prescribe another tablet of Triavil 4-25 at bedtime, if needed.

For patients who continue taking Triavil, the doctor will probably reduc
the dosage to 1 tablet of Triavil 2-25 or 4-25 from 2 to 4 times a day.

CHILDREN

Children should not use Triavil.

OLDER ADULTS AND ADOLESCENTS

For Anxiety
People in these age groups usually take Triavil at lower doses.

Overdosage

Any medication taken in excess can have serious consequences. A
overdose of Triavil can be fatal. If you suspect an overdose, seek medica
help immediately.

■ *Symptoms of Triavil overdose may include:*
Abnormalities of posture and movements, agitation, coma, convu
sions, dilated pupils, drowsiness, extreme low body temperature, ey
movement problems, high fever, heart failure, overactive reflexe:
rapid or irregular heartbeat, rigid muscles, stupor, very low bloo
pressure, vomiting.

Generic name:
Triazolam

See Halcion, page 83

Generic name:
Trifluoperazine

See Stelazine, page 194

Brand name:
Trilafon

Pronounced: TRILL-ah-fon
Generic name: Perphenazine

Why is this drug prescribed?

Trilafon is used to treat schizophrenia and to control severe nausea ar
vomiting in adults. It is a member of the phenothiazine family o
antipsychotic medications, which includes such drugs as Mellari
Stelazine, and Thorazine.

Most important fact about this drug

Trilafon can cause tardive dyskinesia, a condition marked by involuntary muscle spasms and twitches in the face and body, including chewing movements, puckering, puffing the cheeks, and sticking out the tongue. This condition may be permanent and appears to be most common among older adults, especially older women.

How should this medication be taken?

Trilafon should be taken exactly according to physician instructions and for no longer than necessary.

■ *Missed dose...*

If it is within an hour or so after the scheduled time, the forgotten dose should be taken as soon as remembered. If they do not remember until later, patients should skip the dose and go back to their regular schedule. They should never double the dose.

■ *Storage instructions...*

Trilafon should be stored at room temperature.

What side effects may occur?

Side effects cannot be predicted. If any develop or change in intensity, patients should inform their doctor as soon as possible.

■ *Side effects may include:*

Allergic reactions, asthma, bizarre dreams, blood disorders, blurred vision, body spasms, breast enlargement in males and females, breast milk production, cardiac arrest, changes in sex drive, confusion, constipation and intestinal problems, diarrhea, difficulty swallowing, dizziness, drowsiness, dry mouth, exaggerated reflexes, eye changes and disorders, faintness, false-positive pregnancy test results, fast or slow heartbeat, fever, fixed stare, headaches, high or low blood pressure, high or low blood sugar, high pressure in the eyes, hives, hyperactivity, inappropriate excitement, increased appetite and weight, inhibition of ejaculation, insomnia, irregular heartbeat, itching, large or small pupils, lethargy, light sensitivity, limb aches, liver problems, lockjaw, loss of appetite, loss of coordination, lupus-like symptoms, menstrual irregularities, muscle weakness, nasal congestion, nausea, numbness, pallor, paranoia, Parkinsonism (rigidity and tremors), protruding or aching tongue, restlessness, salivation, seizures, skin rash or redness, slurred speech, stupor, sweating, swelling of the arms and legs, swelling of the ear, swelling of the face or throat, tardive dyskinesia (see "Most important fact"), tics, throat tightness, twisting or spasms of the neck and mouth muscles, urinary problems, yellow skin or eyes, vomiting

Why should this drug not be prescribed?

People who are comatose or who are at reduced levels of consciousness or alertness should not take Trilafon. Nor should those who are taking large amounts of any substance that slows brain function, including barbiturates, alcohol, narcotics, pain killers, and antihistamines.

Trilafon should also be avoided by people who have blood disorders, liver problems, or brain damage It cannot be taken by anyone who is hypersensitive to its ingredients or to related drugs.

Special warnings about this medication

Drugs such as Trilafon are capable of triggering a potentially fatal condition known as Neuroleptic Malignant Syndrome. Symptoms include high fever, muscle rigidity, altered mental status, unstable blood pressure, a rapid or irregular heartbeat, and excessive sweating. If any of these symptoms develop, patients should see their doctor immediately; Trilafon therapy will need to be discontinued.

Any significant increase in body temperature should also be reported to the doctor. It could be an early warning that the drug cannot be tolerated.

Patients should alert their physician before taking Trilafon if they are going through alcohol withdrawal, suffer from convulsions or seizures, or have a depressive disorder. They will have to use the drug with caution.

Caution is also warranted for patients who have kidney problems or trouble breathing. The doctor will periodically monitor kidney and liver function and check patients' blood count for possible side effects.

Patient should be sure to tell the doctor if they've ever had breast cancer. Trilafon stimulates production of a hormone that promotes the growth of certain types of tumors.

Trilafon may impair the mental or physical abilities needed to drive a car or operate heavy machinery. Also, patients should avoid prolonged exposure to the sun since Trilafon may increase sensitivity to light.

Stomach inflammation, dizziness, nausea, vomiting, and tremors may result if Trilafon is stopped suddenly. Therapy should be discontinued only under a doctor's supervision.

Trilafon is not recommended for children under the age of 12 years.

Possible food and drug interactions when taking this medication

If Trilafon is taken with certain other drugs, the effects of either could be increased, decreased, or altered. Here is an overview of drugs that may cause a problem:

Antidepressants such as Elavil, Nardil, and Prozac

Antihistamines such as Benadryl and Tavist

Antipsychotic medications such as Mellaril and Thorazine

Antiseizure drugs such as Dilantin

Barbiturates such as Nembutal and Seconal
Drugs that quell spasms, such as Donnatal and Levsin
Narcotic painkillers such as Percodan and Vicodin
Phosphorus insecticides
Tranquilizers and sleep aids such as Halcion, Valium, and Xanax

Because Trilafon prevents vomiting, it can hide the signs and symptoms of overdose of other drugs.

Patients scheduled for an operation should inform the surgeon that they are taking Trilafon, since it may alter the amount of anesthesia they require.

Special information about pregnancy and breastfeeding

Safe use of Trilafon during pregnancy and breastfeeding has not been established. The possible benefits of taking Trilafon must be weighed against the possible hazards to mother and child.

Recommended dosage

The dosage of Trilafon is adjusted according to the severity of the condition and the drug's effect. Doctors aim for the lowest effective dose

SCHIZOPHRENIA

The usual initial dosage of Trilafon tablets is 4 to 8 milligrams 3 times daily, up to a maximum daily dose of 24 milligrams. Hospitalized patients are usually given 8 to 16 milligrams 2 to 4 times daily, up to a maximum daily dose of 64 milligrams.

SEVERE NAUSEA AND VOMITING IN ADULTS

For this problem, the usual dosage of Trilafon tablets is 8 to 16 milligrams daily divided into smaller doses. Up to 24 milligrams daily is occasionally necessary.

Overdosage

Anyone suspected of having taken on overdose of Trilafon should be hospitalized immediately for emergency treatment.

■ *Usual symptoms of Trilafon overdose include:*
  Stupor, coma, convulsions (in children)

Victims may also exhibit symptoms such as rigid muscles, twitches and involuntary movements, hair-trigger reflexes, loss of coordination, rolling eyeballs, and slurred speech.

Generic name:

Trimipramine

See Surmontil, page 197

Brand name:

Valium

Pronounced: VAL-ee-um
Generic name: Diazepam

Why is this drug prescribed?

Valium is used for treatment of anxiety disorders and for short-term relief of the symptoms of anxiety. It belongs to a class of drugs known as benzodiazepines.

Valium is also used to relieve the symptoms of acute alcohol withdrawal, to relax muscles, to relieve the uncontrolled muscle movements caused by disorders such as cerebral palsy, to control involuntary movement of the hands (athetosis), to relax tight, aching muscles, and, along with other medications, to treat convulsive disorders such as epilepsy.

Most important fact about this drug

Valium can be habit-forming or addictive. Some patients may experience withdrawal symptoms if they stop using this drug abruptly. Patients should consult their doctor before discontinuing the drug or making any change in their dose.

How should this medication be taken?

This medication must be taken exactly as prescribed. People taking the drug for epilepsy should be sure to take it at the same times every day.

■ *Missed dose...*

If it is within an hour or so of the scheduled time, the forgotten dose should be taken as soon as remembered. Otherwise, it should be skipped and the patient should return to the regular schedule. Doses should never be doubled.

■ *Storage instructions...*

Valium should be stored away from heat, light, and moisture.

What side effects may occur?

Side effects cannot be predicted. If any develop or change in intensity, patients should inform their doctor as soon as possible.

■ *More common side effects may include:*

Drowsiness, fatigue, light-headedness, loss of muscle coordination

■ *Less common or rare side effects may include:*

Anxiety, blurred vision, changes in salivation, changes in sex drive, confusion, constipation, depression, difficulty urinating, dizziness, double vision, hallucinations, headache, inability to hold urine, low blood pressure, nausea, overstimulation, rage, seizures (mild changes in brain wave patterns), skin rash, sleep disturbances, slow heartbeat, slurred speech and other speech problems, stimulation, tremors, vertigo, yellowing of eyes and skin

◼ *Side effects due to rapid decrease in dose or abrupt withdrawal from Valium:*
Abdominal and muscle cramps, convulsions, sweating, tremors, vomiting

Why should this drug not be prescribed?

Anyone who is sensitive to or has ever had an allergic reaction to Valium should not take this medication. It should also be avoided by those with the eye condition known as acute narrow-angle glaucoma.

Anxiety or tension related to everyday stress usually does not require treatment with such a powerful drug as Valium. Patients should discuss their symptoms thoroughly with the doctor.

Valium should not be prescribed for patients who are being treated for mental disorders more serious than anxiety.

Special warnings about this medication

Valium causes some people to become drowsy or less alert. Patients should not drive, operate dangerous machinery, or participate in any hazardous activity that requires full mental alertness until they know how this drug affects them.

This medication should be used cautiously by people with liver or kidney problems.

Possible food and drug interactions when taking this medication

Valium slows down the central nervous system and may intensify the effects of alcohol. Patients should avoid alcohol while taking this medication.

If Valium is taken with certain other drugs, the effects of either could be increased, decreased, or altered. Here is an overview of drugs that may cause a problem:

Antiseizure drugs such as Dilantin
Antidepressant drugs such as Elavil and Prozac
Antipsychotic medications such as Mellaril and Thorazine
Barbiturates such as phenobarbital
Cimetidine (Tagamet)
Digoxin (Lanoxin)
Disulfiram (Antabuse)
Isoniazid (Rifamate)
Levodopa (Larodopa, Sinemet)
MAO inhibitors such as the antidepressant drugs Nardil and Parnate
Narcotics such as Percocet
Omeprazole (Prilosec)

Oral contraceptives
Propoxyphene (Darvon)
Ranitidine (Zantac)
Rifampin (Rifadin)

Special information about pregnancy and breastfeeding

Valium should not be taken during pregnancy. There is an increased risk
of birth defects. The doctor may also advise against breastfeeding until
treatment with this drug is finished.

Recommended dosage

ADULTS

*Treatment of Anxiety Disorders and Short-Term Relief of the Symptoms
of Anxiety*
The usual dose ranges from 2 milligrams to 10 milligrams 2 to 4 times
daily, depending upon severity of symptoms.

Acute Alcohol Withdrawal
The usual dose is 10 milligrams 3 or 4 times during the first 24 hours,
then 5 milligrams 3 or 4 times daily as needed.

Relief of Muscle Spasm
The usual dose is 2 milligrams to 10 milligrams 3 or 4 times daily.

Convulsive Disorders
The usual dose is 2 milligrams to 10 milligrams 2 to 4 times daily.

CHILDREN

Valium should not be given to children under 6 months of age.

The usual starting dose for children over 6 months is 1 to 2.5 milligrams 3 or 4 times a day. The doctor may increase the dosage gradually
if needed.

OLDER ADULTS

The usual starting dose is 2 milligrams to 2.5 milligrams once or twice a
day. The doctor will increase the dose as needed, but will limit it to the
smallest effective amount because older people are more apt to become
oversedated or uncoordinated.

Overdosage

Any medication taken in excess can have serious consequences. If an
overdose is suspected, seek medical attention immediately.

■ *Symptoms of Valium overdose may include:*
  Coma, confusion, diminished reflexes, sleepiness

Generic name:

Venlafaxine

See Effexor, page 63

Brand name:

Vistaril

See Atarax, page 18

Brand name:

Vivactil

Pronounced: vi-VAC-til
Generic name: Protriptyline hydrochloride

Why is this drug prescribed?

Vivactil is used to treat the symptoms of mental depression in people who are under close medical supervision. It is particularly suitable for those who are inactive and withdrawn.

Vivactil is a member of the family of drugs called tricyclic antidepressants. Researchers don't know exactly how it works. Unlike the class of antidepressants known as monoamine oxidase inhibitors (MAOIs), it does not act primarily through stimulation of the central nervous system. It tends to work more rapidly than some other tricyclic antidepressants. Improvement sometimes begins within a week.

Most important fact about this drug

For patients prone to anxiety or agitation, Vivactil can make the problem worse. It can also exaggerate the symptoms of manic-depression and schizophrenia. If this seems to be happening, the doctor should be alerted immediately. The dose of Vivactil may need reduction, or addition of another drug may be required.

How should this medication be taken?

Vivactil should be taken exactly as prescribed. It should not be taken with alcohol.

■ *Missed dose . . .*
Generally, the forgotten dose should be taken as soon as remembered. However, if it is almost time for the next dose, the missed dose should be skipped and the patient should return to the regular schedule. Doses should never be doubled.

■ *Storage instructions . . .*
Vivactil should be stored at room temperature in a tightly closed container.

What side effects may occur?

Side effects cannot be predicted. If any develop or change in intensity, patients should inform their doctor as soon as possible.

■ *Side effects may include:*
Abdominal cramps, abnormally high or low blood pressure, abnormal touch sensation, agitation, anxiety, black tongue, blood disorders, blurred vision, breast enlargement in males and females, breast milk production, changes in taste, confusion, constipation, delusions, diarrhea, disorientation, dizziness, drowsiness, dry mouth, drug fever, exacerbation of psychoses, fatigue, fever, flushing, headache, hair loss, hallucinations, heart attack, heart block, high or low blood sugar, high pressure in the eyes, hives, hyperactivity, impotence, increased or decreased sex drive, inflammation of the mouth or tongue, insomnia, intestinal distress, intestinal paralysis, irregular or rapid heartbeat, itching, lack of coordination, light sensitivity, liver problems, loss of appetite, muscle weakness, nausea, nerve disturbances, nightmares, numbness, palpitations, panic, pupil dilation, rashes, restlessness, ringing in the ears, seizures, stroke, sweating, swelling (general or in the face and mouth), testicular swelling, tingling, tremors, urinary problems, visual focusing difficulties, vomiting, weakness, weight gain or loss, yellowing of skin or eyes

Why should this drug not be prescribed?

Due to the possibility of life-threatening side effects, Vivactil must never be taken with a drug classified as a monoamine oxidase inhibitor, such as the antidepressants Nardil and Parnate. At least 14 days should be allowed between the last dose of one of these drugs and the first dose of Vivactil.

Vivactil should not be used during recovery from a heart attack. It also cannot be used by anyone who has had an allergic reaction to it.

Special warnings about this medication

Drugs such as Vivactil sometimes cause heartbeat irregularities. Vivactil should be used with caution by people who have heart problems or a thyroid disorder. Caution is also advisable for those who have a history of seizures, tend to retain urine, have high pressure in the eyes, or use alcohol excessively. The drug is not recommended during shock therapy. It should be discontinued several days before any surgery.

Vivactil may impair the physical and/or mental abilities required to drive a car or operate heavy machinery.

Possible food and drug interactions when taking this medication

Remember that Vivactil must never be combined with monoamine inhibitors such as Nardil and Parnate.

If Vivactil is taken with certain other drugs, the effects of either could be increased, decreased, or altered. Here is an overview of drugs that may cause a problem.

Antidepressants that boost serotonin, including Paxil, Prozac, and Zoloft
Antipsychotic medications such as Mellaril and Thorazine
Barbiturates such as Nembutal and Seconal
Certain blood pressure medications such as guanethidine
Cimetidine (Tagamet)
Decongestants such as Sudafed
Drugs that quell spasms, such as Donnatal and Levsin
Epinephrine (EpiPen)
Flecainide (Tambocor)
Narcotic painkillers such as Percodan and Vicodin
Norepinephrine
Other antidepressants such as Elavil and Tofranil
Propafenone (Rythmol)
Quinidine (Quinaglute)
Tramadol (Ultram)
Tranquilizers and sleep aids such as Halcion, Valium, and Xanax

Special information about pregnancy and breastfeeding

The effects of Vivactil during pregnancy have not been adequately studied. It should be used during pregnancy only if its benefits outweigh the potential risk. Patients who are pregnant or planning to become pregnant should inform their doctor immediately.

It is not known whether Vivactil makes its way into breast milk. Patients should consult with their doctor before deciding to breastfeed.

Recommended dosage

The doctor will start with a low dose and increase it gradually, watching for side effects and a positive response

ADULTS

The usual adult dosage is 15 to 40 milligrams in 3 or 4 doses per day. The maximum dosage is 60 milligrams daily. Increases are made in the morning dose.

CHILDREN

The safety and efficacy of Vivactil in children have not been established.

OLDER ADULTS AND ADOLESCENTS

Lower dosages are recommended for adolescents and older adults. Five milligrams 3 times a day may be given initially, followed by a gradual increase if necessary. Heart function must be monitored in older adults who are taking 20 or more milligrams per day.

Overdosage

An overdose of Vivactil can be fatal. If an overdose is suspected, seek medical help immediately.

■ *Critical signs of Vivactil overdose may include:*
Convulsions, irregular heartbeat, severely low blood pressure, reduced level of consciousness or even coma

■ *Other signs of Vivactil overdose may include:*
Agitation, confusion, dilated pupils, disturbed concentration, drowsiness, fever, hyperactive reflexes, low body temperature, muscle rigidity, sporadic hallucinations, stupor, vomiting, or any of the other symptoms listed in the "side effects" section

Brand name:

Wellbutrin

Pronounced: Well-BEW-trin
Generic name: Bupropion hydrochloride
Other brand name: Wellbutrin SR

Why is this drug prescribed?

Wellbutrin is given to help relieve certain kinds of major depression. Unlike the more familiar tricyclic antidepressants, such as Elavil, Tofranil, and others, Wellbutrin tends to have a somewhat stimulating effect.

The drug is available in regular and sustained-release formulations (Wellbutrin SR).

Most important fact about this drug

Although Wellbutrin occasionally causes weight gain, a more common effect is weight loss Some 28 percent of people who take this medication lose 5 pounds or more. If depression has already caused a decline in weight, and if further weight loss would be detrimental to the patient's health, Wellbutrin may not be the best choice.

How should this medication be taken?

Wellbutrin should be taken exactly as prescribed. The usual dosing regimen is 3 equal doses spaced evenly throughout the day. At least 6 hours should elapse between doses. The doctor will probably start at a low dosage and gradually increase it; this helps minimize side effects.

Wellbutrin SR, the sustained-release form, should be taken in 2 doses at least 8 hours apart. Wellbutrin SR tablets must be swallowed whole; not chewed, divided, or crushed.

If Wellbutrin proves effective, the doctor will probably continue therapy for at least several months.

■ *Missed dose...*
Generally a forgotten dose should be taken as soon as remembered. However, if it is within 4 hours of the next dose, the missed dose should be skipped and the patient should go back to the regular schedule. Doses should never be doubled.

■ *Storage instructions...*
Wellbutrin should be stored at room temperature and should be protected from light and moisture.

What side effects may occur?

Side effects cannot be predicted. If any develop or change in intensity, patients should inform their doctor as soon as possible.

Seizures are perhaps the most worrisome side effect.

■ *More common side effects may include:*
Abdominal pain (Wellbutrin SR), agitation, anxiety (Wellbutrin SR), constipation, dizziness, dry mouth, excessive sweating, headache, loss of appetite (Wellbutrin SR), nausea, palpitations (Wellbutrin SR), vomiting, skin rash, sleep disturbances, sore throat (Wellbutrin SR), tremor

■ *Other side effects may include:*
Acne, allergic reactions (severe), bed-wetting, blisters in the mouth and eyes (Stevens-Johnson syndrome) blurred vision, breathing difficulty, chest pain, chills, complete or almost complete loss of movement, confusion, dry skin, episodes of over-activity, elation, or irritability, extreme calmness, fatigue, fever, fluid retention, flu-like symptoms, gum irritation and inflammation, hair color changes, hair loss, hives, impotence, incoordination and clumsiness, indigestion, itching, increased libido, menstrual complaints, mood instability, muscle rigidity, painful ejaculation, painful erection, retarded ejaculation, ringing in the ears, sexual dysfunction, suicidal ideation, thirst disturbances, toothache, urinary disturbances, weight gain or loss

Why should this drug not be prescribed?

Anyone who is sensitive to or has ever had an allergic reaction to Wellbutrin should avoid it

Since Wellbutrin causes seizures in some people, it should not be taken by anyone who has any type of seizure disorder. It should also be avoided by people who are taking another medication containing bupropion, such as Zyban, the quit-smoking aid.

Wellbutrin must be avoided by patients who currently have, or formerly had, an eating disorder. For some reason, people with a history of anorexia nervosa or bulimia seem to be more likely to experience Wellbutrin-related seizures.

Wellbutrin should not be used if, within the past 14 days, the patient has taken a monoamine oxidase inhibitor (MAO inhibitor) drug such as the antidepressants Nardil and Parnate. This particular drug combination could cause a sudden, dangerous rise in blood pressure.

Special warnings about this medication

Wellbutrin increases the risk of seizures if the dosage is too high or the patient has ever suffered brain damage or experienced seizures in the past. The danger of seizures is greater in people addicted to narcotics, cocaine, or stimulants, and in those using over-the-counter stimulants or diet pills. Alcohol abuse or withdrawal also increases the risk, as does the use of other antidepressants or major tranquilizers. The risk is higher, too, for people taking insulin or oral diabetes medication.

Because seizures are possible, patients who have been taking Valium or a similar tranquilizer but are ready to stop should taper off gradually rather than quitting abruptly.

Patients who have had any kind of heart trouble or liver or kidney disease should be sure to alert the doctor before they start taking this drug. It must be used with extreme caution by people with severe cirrhosis of the liver. A reduced dosage may be needed by those with any sort of liver or kidney problem.

Patients should stop taking Wellbutrin and call the doctor immediately if they have difficulty breathing or swallowing; notice swelling in the face, lips, tongue, or throat; develop swollen arms and legs; or break out with itchy eruptions. These are warning signs of a potentially severe allergic reaction.

Wellbutrin may impair coordination or judgment. Patients should not drive or operate dangerous machinery until they find out how the medication affects them.

Possible food and drug interactions when taking this medication

Patients should avoid alcohol while taking Wellbutrin; an interaction between alcohol and Wellbutrin could increase the possibility of a seizure.

If Wellbutrin is taken with certain other drugs, the effects of either could be increased, decreased, or altered. Here is an overview of drugs that may cause a problem:

Beta blockers (used for high blood pressure and heart conditions) such as Inderal, Lopressor, and Tenormin
Carbamazepine (Tegretol)
Cimetidine (Tagamet)
Cyclophosphamide (Cytoxan)
Heart-stabilizing drugs such as Rythmol and Tambocor
Levodopa (Larodopa)
Antipsychotic medications such as Haldol, Risperdal, Thorazine, and Mellaril
MAO inhibitors (such as the antidepressants Parnate and Nardil)
Nicotine patches such as Habitrol, NicoDerm CQ, and Nicotrol patch
Orphenadrine (Norgesic)
Other antidepressants such as Elavil, Norpramin, Pamelor, Paxil, Prozac, Tofranil, and Zoloft
Phenobarbital
Phenytoin (Dilantin)
Steroid medications such as Prednisone
Theophylline (Theo-Dur)

Special information about pregnancy and breastfeeding
Patients who are pregnant or plan to become pregnant should notify their doctor immediately. Wellbutrin should be taken during pregnancy only if clearly needed.

Wellbutrin does pass into breast milk and may cause serious reactions in a nursing baby. New mothers will need to choose between breastfeeding or continuing this medication.

Recommended dosage
No single dose of Wellbutrin should exceed 150 milligrams.

ADULTS

Wellbutrin

At the beginning, the dose will probably be 200 milligrams per day, taken as 100 milligrams 2 times a day. After at least 3 days at this dose, the doctor may increase the dosage to 300 milligrams per day, taken as 100 milligrams 3 times a day, with at least 6 hours between doses. This is the usual adult dose. The maximum recommended dosage is 450 milligrams per day taken in doses of no more than 150 milligrams each.

Wellbutrin SR

The usual starting dose is 150 milligrams in the morning. After 3 days, if the patient responds well, the doctor will prescribe another

150 milligrams at least 8 hours after the first dose. It may be 4 weeks before the patient feels the benefit and therapy may continue for several months. The maximum recommended dose is 400 milligrams a day, taken in doses of 200 milligrams each.

For people with severe cirrhosis of the liver, the dosage should be no more than 75 milligrams once a day. With less serious liver and kidney problems, the dosage will be somewhat reduced.

CHILDREN

The safety and effectiveness in children under 18 years old have not been established.

Overdosage

Any medication taken in excess can have serious consequences. If an overdose of Wellbutrin is suspected, seek medical attention immediately.

■ *Symptoms of Wellbutrin overdose may include:*
Hallucinations, heart failure, loss of consciousness, rapid heartbeat, seizures

■ *Symptoms of Wellbutrin SR overdose may include:*
Blurred vision, confusion, jitteriness, lethargy, light-headedness, nausea, seizures, vomiting

■ *An overdose that involves other drugs in combination with Wellbutrin may also cause these symptoms:*
Breathing difficulties, coma, fever, rigid muscles, stupor

Brand name:

Xanax

Pronounced: ZAN-ax
Generic name: Alprazolam

Why is this drug prescribed?

Xanax is a tranquilizer used for the treatment of anxiety disorders and the short-term relief of symptoms of anxiety. Xanax is also used in the treatment of panic disorder and anxiety associated with depression. Some doctors prescribe Xanax to treat alcohol withdrawal, fear of open spaces and strangers, depression, irritable bowel syndrome, and premenstrual syndrome.

Most important fact about this drug

Tolerance and dependence can occur with the use of Xanax. Withdrawal symptoms may occur if the drug is stopped abruptly. Patients should discontinue the drug or change the dose only under a doctor's supervision.

How should this medication be taken?

Xanax must be taken exactly as prescribed. It may be taken with or without food.

■ *Missed dose...*

If it is less than 1 hour late, the dose should be taken as soon as remembered. Otherwise it should be skipped and the patient should go back to the regular schedule. Doses should never be doubled.

■ *Storage instructions...*

Store Xanax at room temperature.

What side effects may occur?

Side effects cannot be predicted. If any develop or change in intensity, patients should inform their doctor as soon as possible.

Side effects of Xanax are usually seen at the beginning of treatment and disappear with continued medication. However, if dosage is increased, side effects will be more likely.

■ *More common side effects may include:*

Abdominal discomfort, abnormal involuntary movement, agitation, allergies, anxiety, blurred vision, chest pain, confusion, constipation, decreased or increased sex drive, depression, diarrhea, difficult urination, dream abnormalities, drowsiness, dry mouth, fainting, fatigue, fluid retention, headache, hyperventilation (too frequent or too deep breathing), inability to fall asleep, increase or decrease in appetite, increased or decreased salivation, impaired memory, irritability, lack of coordination, light-headedness, low blood pressure, menstrual problems, muscular twitching, nausea and vomiting, nervousness, palpitations, rapid heartbeat, rash, restlessness, ringing in the ears, sexual dysfunction, skin inflammation, speech difficulties, stiffness, stuffy nose, sweating, tiredness/sleepiness, tremors, upper respiratory infections, weakness, weight gain or loss

■ *Less common or rare side effects may include:*

Abnormal muscle tone, concentration difficulties, decreased coordination, dizziness, double vision, fear, hallucinations, inability to control urination or bowel movements, infection, itching, loss of appetite, muscle cramps, muscle spasticity, rage, sedation, seizures, sleep disturbances, slurred speech, stimulation, talkativeness, taste alterations, temporary memory loss, tingling or pins and needles, uninhibited behavior, urine retention, warm feeling, weakness in muscle and bone, weight gain or loss, yellow eyes and skin

■ *Side effects due to decrease or withdrawal from Xanax:*

Blurred vision, decreased concentration, decreased mental clarity, diarrhea, heightened awareness of noise or bright lights, impaired sense of smell, loss of appetite, loss of weight, muscle cramps, seizures, tingling sensation, twitching

Why should this drug not be prescribed?

Anyone who is sensitive to or has ever had an allergic reaction to Xanax or other antianxiety agents should not take this medication. It should be avoided by people who have the eye condition called narrow-angle glaucoma. It must not be combined with the antifungal drugs Sporanox or Nizoral.

Anxiety or tension related to everyday stress usually does not require treatment with Xanax. Patients should discuss their symptoms thoroughly with the doctor. The doctor should periodically reassess the need for this drug.

Special warnings about this medication

Xanax may cause patients to become drowsy or less alert. Driving, operating dangerous machinery, or participating in any hazardous activity that requires full mental alertness is not recommended.

Individuals being treated for panic disorder may need a higher dose of Xanax than those being treated for anxiety alone. High doses—more than 4 milligrams a day—taken for long intervals may cause emotional and physical dependence. The doctor should monitor such patients carefully.

Possible food and drug interactions when taking this medication

Xanax may intensify the effect of alcohol. Patients should avoid alcohol while taking this medication.

Xanax should never be combined with Sporanox or Nizoral. These drugs cause a buildup of Xanax in the body.

If Xanax is taken with certain other drugs, the effects of either could be increased, decreased, or altered. Here is an overview of drugs that may cause a problem:

Amiodarone (Cordarone)
Antihistamines such as Benadryl and Tavist
Antipsychotic medications such as Mellaril and Thorazine
Carbamazepine (Tegretol)
Certain antibiotics such as Biaxin and erythromycin
Certain antidepressant drugs, including Elavil, Norpramin, and Tofranil
Cimetidine (Tagamet)
Cyclosporine (Neoral, Sandimmune)
Digoxin (Lanoxin)
Diltiazem (Cardizem)
Disulfiram (Antabuse)
Ergotamine
Fluoxetine (Prozac)
Fluvoxamine (Luvox)

Grapefruit juice
Isoniazid (Rifamate)
Nefazodone (Serzone)
Nicardipine (Cardene)
Nifedipine (Adalat, Procardia)
Oral contraceptives
Other central nervous system depressants such as Valium and Demerol
Paroxetine (Paxil)
Propoxyphene (Darvon)
Sertraline (Zoloft)

Special information about pregnancy and breastfeeding

Xanax should be avoided by patients who are pregnant or plan to become pregnant. There is an increased risk of respiratory problems and muscular weakness in the baby. Infants may also experience withdrawal symptoms.

Xanax may appear in breast milk and could affect a nursing infant. If this medication is essential to the mother's health, the doctor may advise her to stop breastfeeding until treatment is finished.

Recommended dosage

ADULTS

Anxiety disorder

The usual starting dose of Xanax is 0.25 to 0.5 milligram taken 3 times a day. The dose may be increased every 3 to 4 days to a maximum daily dose of 4 milligrams, divided into smaller doses.

Panic disorder

The usual starting dose is 0.5 milligram 3 times a day. This dose can be increased by 1 milligram a day every 3 or 4 days. The daily dose ranges from 1 up to a total of 10 milligrams, according to the patient's needs. A typical dose is 5 to 6 milligrams a day.

The doctor will reassess treatment periodically to be sure the patient is getting the right amount of medication.

CHILDREN

Safety and effectiveness have not been established in children under 18 years of age.

OLDER ADULTS

The usual starting dose for an anxiety disorder is 0.25 milligram, 2 or 3 times daily. This dose may be gradually increased if needed and tolerated.

Overdosage

An overdose of Xanax, alone or after combining it with alcohol, can be fatal. If an overdose is suspected, seek medical attention immediately.

■ *Symptoms of Xanax overdose may include:*
Confusion, coma, impaired coordination, sleepiness, slowed reaction time

Generic name:

Zaleplon

See Sonata, page 191

Generic name:

Ziprasidone

See Geodon, page 80

Brand name:

Zoloft

Pronounced: ZOE-loft
Generic name: Sertraline

Why is this drug prescribed?

Zoloft is prescribed for major depressive disorder and obsessive-compulsive disorder. It is also used for the treatment of panic disorder, premenstrual dysphoric disorder (PMDD), and posttraumatic stress disorder.

Zoloft is a member of the family of drugs called "selective serotonin reuptake inhibitors." Serotonin is one of the chemical messengers believed to govern moods. Ordinarily, it is quickly reabsorbed after its release at the junctures between nerves. Reuptake inhibitors such as Zoloft slow this process, thereby boosting the levels of serotonin available in the brain.

Most important fact about this drug

Zoloft must not be used within 2 weeks of taking any drug classified as an MAO inhibitor, such as the antidepressants Nardil and Parnate. When serotonin boosters such as Zoloft are combined with MAO inhibitors, serious and sometimes fatal reactions can occur.

How should this medication be taken?

Zoloft should be taken exactly as prescribed, once a day in either the morning or the evening.

Zoloft is available in capsule and oral concentrate forms. Zoloft oral concentrate should be prepared with the dropper provided. The amount of concentrate prescribed by the doctor should be mixed with 4 ounces of water, ginger ale, lemon/lime soda, lemonade, or orange juice. (No other type of beverage should be used.) The mixture must be taken immediately; it should not be prepared in advance for later use. At times, a slight haze may appear after mixing, but this is normal.

Improvement with Zoloft may not be seen for several days to a few weeks. Treatment typically lasts for at least several months.

Zoloft may make the mouth dry. Sucking a hard candy, chewing gum, or melting bits of ice in the mouth can provide temporary relief.

■ *Missed dose...*
Generally, the forgotten dose should be taken as soon as remembered. However, if several hours have passed, it should be skipped and the patient should return to the regular schedule. Doses should never be doubled.

■ *Storage instructions...*
Zoloft may be stored at room temperature.

What side effects may occur?
Side effects cannot be predicted. If any develop or change in intensity, patients should inform their doctor as soon as possible.

■ *More common side effects may include:*
Abdominal pain, agitation, anxiety, constipation, decreased sex drive, diarrhea or loose stools, difficulty with ejaculation, dizziness, dry mouth, fatigue, gas, headache, decreased appetite, increased sweating, indigestion, insomnia, nausea, nervousness, rash, sleepiness, tingling or pins and needles, tremor, vision problems, vomiting

■ *Less common or rare side effects may include:*
Acne, allergic reaction, altered taste, back pain, blindness, breast development in males, breast pain or enlargement, breathing difficulties, bruise-like marks on the skin, cataracts, changeable emotions, chest pain, cold, clammy skin, conjunctivitis (pinkeye), coughing, difficulty breathing, difficulty swallowing, double vision, dry eyes, eye pain, fainting, feeling faint upon arising from a sitting or lying position, feeling of illness, female and male sexual problems, fever, fluid retention, flushing, frequent urination, hair loss, heart attack, hemorrhoids, hiccups, high blood pressure, high pressure within the eye (glaucoma), hearing problems, hot flushes, impotence, inability to stay seated, increased appetite, increased salivation, increased sex drive, inflamed nasal passages, inflammation of the penis, intolerance to light, irregular heartbeat, itching, joint pains, kidney failure, lack of coordination, lack of sensation, leg cramps, menstrual problems, low blood pressure, migraine, movement problems, muscle cramps or weakness, need to urinate during the night, nosebleed, pain upon urination, prolonged erection, purplish spots on the skin, racing heartbeat,

rectal hemorrhage, respiratory infection/lung problems, ringing in the ears, rolling eyes, sensitivity to light, sinus inflammation, skin eruptions or inflammation, sleepwalking, sores on tongue, speech problems, stomach and intestinal inflammation, swelling of the face and throat, swollen wrists and ankles, thirst, throbbing heartbeat, twitching, vaginal inflammation, hemorrhage or discharge, yawning

■ *Zoloft may also cause mental or emotional symptoms such as:* Abnormal dreams or thoughts, aggressiveness, exaggerated feeling of well-being, depersonalization ("unreal" feeling), hallucinations, impaired concentration, memory loss, paranoia, rapid mood shifts, suicidal thoughts, tooth-grinding, worsened depression

Many people lose a pound or two of body weight while taking Zoloft. This usually poses no problem but may be a concern if depression has already caused a great deal of weight loss.

In a few people, Zoloft may trigger the grandiose, inappropriate, out-of-control behavior called mania or the similar, but less dramatic, "hyper" state called hypomania.

Why should this drug not be prescribed?
This drug should never be combined with an MAO inhibitor (see "Most important fact about this drug"). Due to its alcohol content, Zoloft oral concentrate cannot be used with the anti-alcohol medication Antabuse.

Special warnings about this medication
Patients with a kidney or liver disorder, and those subject to seizures, need to take Zoloft cautiously and under close medical supervision. The doctor may limit the dosage under these circumstances.

Zoloft has not been found to impair the ability to drive or operate machinery. Nevertheless, the manufacturer recommends caution until patients know how the drug affects them.

People who are sensitive to latex should use caution when handling the dropper provided with the oral concentrate.

Possible food and drug interactions when taking this medication
Although alcohol does not appear to interact with Zoloft, the manufacturer recommends avoiding the combination. Likewise, over-the-counter remedies should be used with caution. Although none is known to interact with Zoloft, interactions remain a possibility.

If Zoloft is taken with certain other drugs, the effects of either could be increased, decreased, or altered. Here is an overview of drugs that may cause a problem:

Cimetidine (Tagamet)
Diazepam (Valium)
Digitoxin (Crystodigin)

Flecainide (Tambocor)
Lithium (Eskalith, Lithobid)
MAO inhibitor drugs such as the antidepressants Nardil and Parnate
Other serotonin-boosting drugs such as Paxil and Prozac
Other antidepressants such as Elavil and Serzone
Propafenone (Rythmol)
Sumatriptan (Imitrex)
Tolbutamide (Orinase)
Warfarin (Coumadin)

Special information about pregnancy and breastfeeding

The effects of Zoloft during pregnancy have not been adequately studied. Patients who are pregnant or plan to become pregnant should inform their doctor immediately. Zoloft should be taken during pregnancy only if it is clearly needed.

It is not known whether Zoloft appears in breast milk. Caution is advised when using Zoloft during breastfeeding.

Recommended dosage

ADULTS

Depressive or Obsessive Compulsive Disorder and PMDD
The usual starting dose is 50 milligrams once a day, taken either in the morning or in the evening. The doctor may increase the dose depending upon the patient's response. The maximum dose for PMDD is 150 milligrams daily. For other disorders, the maximum dose is 200 milligrams a day.

Panic Disorder and Posttraumatic Stress Disorder
During the first week, the usual dose is 25 milligrams once a day. After that, the dose increases to 50 milligrams once a day. Depending on response, the doctor may continue to increase the dose up to a maximum of 200 milligrams a day.

CHILDREN

Obsessive-Compulsive Disorder
The starting dose for children aged 6 to 12 is 25 milligrams and for adolescents aged 13 to 17, 50 milligrams. The doctor will adjust the dose as necessary.

Safety and effectiveness have not been established for children under 6.

Overdosage

An overdose of Zoloft can be fatal. If an overdose is suspected, seek medical attention immediately.

■ *Common symptoms of Zoloft overdose include:*
Agitation, dizziness, nausea, rapid heartbeat, sleepiness, tremor, vomiting

Other possible symptoms include coma, stupor, fainting, convulsions, delirium, hallucinations, mania, high or low blood pressure, and slow, rapid, or irregular heartbeat

Generic name:

Zolpidem

See Ambien, page 4

Brand name:

Zyprexa

Pronounced: Zye-PRECKS-ah
Generic name: Olanzapine

Why is this drug prescribed?

Zyprexa helps manage symptoms of schizophrenia, the manic phase of manic-depression, and other psychotic disorders. It is thought to work by opposing the action of serotonin and dopamine, two of the brain's major chemical messengers. The drug is available as Zyprexa tablets and Zyprexa Zydis, which dissolves rapidly with or without liquid.

Most important fact about this drug

At the start of Zyprexa therapy, the drug can cause extreme low blood pressure, increased heart rate, dizziness, and, in rare cases, a tendency to faint when first standing up. These problems are more likely if the patient is dehydrated, has heart disease, or takes blood pressure medicine. To avoid such problems, the doctor may start with a low dose of Zyprexa and increase the dosage gradually.

How should this medication be taken?

Zyprexa should be taken once a day with or without food. To use Zyprexa Zydis, patients should open the sachet, peel back the foil on the blister pack, remove the tablet, and place the entire tablet in their mouth. The tablet should not be pushed through the foil. The medication can be taken with or without water; saliva will cause the tablet to dissolve.

■ *Missed dose...*

Generally, a forgotten dose should be taken as soon as remembered. However, if it is almost time for the next dose, the missed dose should be skipped and the patient should go back to the regular schedule. Doses should never be doubled.

■ *Storage instructions...*
Zyprexa should be stored at room temperature away from light and moisture.

What side effects may occur?

Side effects cannot be predicted. If any develop or change in intensity, patients should inform their doctor as soon as possible.

■ *More common side effects may include:*
Abdominal pain, abnormal gait, accidental injury, agitation, anxiety, back pain, behavior problems, blood in urine, blurred vision, chest pain, constipation, cough, dehydration, dizziness, drowsiness, dry mouth, extreme low blood pressure, eye problems, feeling of well-being, fever, headache, high blood pressure, hostility, increased appetite, increased cough, indigestion, inflammation of the nasal passages and throat, insomnia, joint pain, movement disorders, muscle rigidity, nausea, nervousness, pain in arms and legs, rapid heartbeat, restlessness, tension, tremor, weakness, weight gain

■ *Less common side effects may include:*
Abnormal dreams, decreased sex drive, dental pain, diabetes, difficulty breathing, emotional instability, eye infection, increased salivation, intentional injury, involuntary movement, joint stiffness, low blood pressure, menstrual irregularities, nasal stuffiness, sleepiness, sore throat, suicide attempts, sweating, swelling of arms and legs, thirst, twitching, urinary problems, vaginal infection, vomiting

■ *Rare side effects may include:*
Abnormal ejaculation, black bowel movements, bleeding, blood clots, bone pain, breast growth in males, breast pain, burping, chills, congestive heart failure, difficulty swallowing, dry eyes, dry skin, ear pain, change in taste sensation, enlarged abdomen, fever, gas, stomach upset, hair loss, hangover feeling, heart attack, inability to control bowel movements, migraine, mouth sores, neck pain, neck rigidity, osteoporosis, pallor, rash, rectal bleeding, rheumatoid arthritis, ringing in the ears, sensitivity to light, stroke, sudden death, swelling of face, swollen gums, yeast infection

Why should this drug not be prescribed?

Anyone who is allergic to Zyprexa cannot use this drug.

Special warnings about this drug

Zyprexa sometimes causes drowsiness and can impair judgment, thinking, and motor skills. Patients should use caution while driving and shouldn't operate dangerous machinery until they know how the drug affects them.

Medicines such as Zyprexa can interfere with regulation of the body's temperature. Patients should avoid getting overheated or becoming dehydrated while taking Zyprexa. They need to stay away from extreme heat and drink plenty of fluids.

People with the following conditions should use Zyprexa with caution: Alzheimer's disease, trouble swallowing, narrow angle glaucoma (high pressure in the eye), an enlarged prostate, heart irregularities, heart disease, heart failure, liver disease, or a history of heart attack, seizures, or intestinal blockage.

Drugs such as Zyprexa sometimes cause a condition called Neuroleptic Malignant Syndrome. Symptoms include high fever, muscle rigidity, irregular pulse or blood pressure, rapid heartbeat, excessive perspiration, and changes in heart rhythm. If these symptoms appear, the doctor will discontinue Zyprexa while the condition is under treatment.

There is also a risk of developing tardive dyskinesia, a condition marked by slow, rhythmical, involuntary movements. This problem is more likely to surface in older adults, especially elderly women. When it does, use of Zyprexa is usually stopped.

Children with phenylketonuria (the inability to process phenylalanine, a condition that quickly leads to mental retardation) should never be given Zyprexa, which contains this substance.

Possible food and drug interactions when taking this medication

Patients should avoid alcohol while taking Zyprexa. The combination can cause a sudden drop in blood pressure.

If Zyprexa is taken with certain other drugs, the effects of either can be increased, decreased, or altered. Patients should check with the doctor before taking any prescription or over-the-counter drugs. Medications of particular concern include the following:

Blood pressure medications
Carbamazepine (Tegretol)
Diazepam (Valium)
Drugs that boost the effect of dopamine, such as the Parkinson's medications Mirapex, Parlodel, Permax, and Requip
Fluvoxamine (Luvox)
Levodopa (Larodopa)
Omeprazole (Prilosec)
Rifampin (Rifadin, Rimactane)

Special information about pregnancy and breastfeeding

Patients who are pregnant or plan to become pregnant should inform their doctor immediately. Zyprexa should be used during pregnancy only if absolutely necessary.

The drug may appear in breast milk; women on Zyprexa therapy should not breastfeed.

Recommended dosage

ADULTS

Schizophrenia

The usual starting dose is 5 to 10 milligrams once a day. If the patient starts at the lower dose, after a few days the doctor will increase it to 10. After that, the dosage will be increased no more than once a week, 5 milligrams at a time, up to a maximum of 20 milligrams a day.

Those most likely to start at 5 milligrams are the debilitated, people prone to low blood pressure, and nonsmoking women over 65 (because they tend to have a slow metabolism).

Manic Episodes in Manic-Depression

The usual starting dose is 10 to 15 milligrams once a day. The drug is typically taken for no more than 3 or 4 weeks at a time.

Overdosage

An overdose of Zyprexa is usually not life-threatening, but fatalities have been reported. If an overdose is suspected, seek medical attention immediately.

Symptoms of Zyprexa overdose may include:
Agitation, drowsiness, rapid or irregular heartbeat, slurred or disrupted speech, stupor

Overdoses of Zyprexa have also led to breathing difficulties, changes in blood pressure, excessive perspiration, fever, muscle rigidity, cardiac arrest, coma, and convulsions.

Section 2

Interactions with Psychotropic Drugs

Listed in this section are over 1,400 possible interactions with the psychotropic medications profiled in Section 1. Entries are organized alphabetically, first by the generic name of the psychotropic drug, then by the generic name of the potentially interactive medication. Each entry includes a brief description of the possible results of concurrent use, plus ratings of the interaction's rapidity of onset, degree of severity, and level of supporting documentation. A key to these ratings follows.

Onset
  - **0 = Unspecified**
  - **1 = Rapid:** Develops within 24 hours
  - **2 = Delayed:** Will not occur during the first 24 hours

Severity
  - **1 = Contraindicated:** The interaction may be life-threatening. Concomitant use of the interacting agents is contraindicated.
  - **2 = Major:** The interaction may be life-threatening and/or require medical intervention to minimize or prevent serious adverse effects.
  - **3 = Moderate:** The interaction may result in an exacerbation of the patient's condition and/or require an alteration in therapy.
  - **4 = Minor:** The interaction would have limited clinical effects. Manifestations may include an increase in the frequency or severity of side effects but generally would not require a major alteration in therapy.

Evidence
  - **1 = Excellent:** Controlled studies have clearly established the existence of the interaction.
  - **2 = Good:** Documentation strongly suggests the interaction exists, but well-controlled studies are lacking.
  - **3 = Fair:** Available documentation is fair, but pharmacologic considerations lead clinicians to suspect the interaction exists; or, documentation is good for a pharmacologically similar drug.
  - **4 = Poor:** Documentation is poor (such as limited case reports), but the interaction is theoretically possible.

The information in this section is extracted from the DRUG-REAX System, a drug therapy screening program produced by *Physicians' Desk Reference*® affiliate Micromedex, Inc., the world leader in specialized information on pharmaceuticals. The entries are based on an independent review of the medical literature by a staff of more than 100 clinicians, and may vary from the summary information presented in Section 1.

Alprazolam

INTERACTION	ONSET	SEVERITY	EVIDENCE
CIMETIDINE Concurrent use of ALPRAZOLAM and CIMETIDINE may result in an increased risk of alprazolam toxicity (central nervous system depression).	1	3	3
CLARITHROMYCIN Concurrent use of ALPRAZOLAM and CLARITHROMYCIN may result in increased alprazolam toxicity (central nervous system depression, poor coordination, lethargy).	2	3	3
ERYTHROMYCIN Concurrent use of ALPRAZOLAM and ERYTHROMYCIN may result in increased alprazolam toxicity (central nervous system depression, poor coordination, lethargy).	2	3	3
ETHANOL Concurrent use of ALPRAZOLAM and ETHANOL may result in increased sedation.	1	3	2
FLUCONAZOLE Concurrent use of ALPRAZOLAM and FLUCONAZOLE may result in increased alprazolam serum concentrations and potential alprazolam toxicity (sedation, slurred speech, central nervous system depression).	1	2	3
FLUOXETINE Concurrent use of ALPRAZOLAM and FLUOXETINE may result in an increased risk of alprazolam toxicity (somnolence, dizziness, poor coordination, slurred speech, low blood pressure, psychomotor impairment).	1	3	2
FLUVOXAMINE Concurrent use of ALPRAZOLAM and FLUVOXAMINE may result in elevated plasma alprazolam levels and an increased risk of side effects (central nervous system depression).	2	3	2
ITRACONAZOLE Concurrent use of ALPRAZOLAM and ITRACONAZOLE may result in increased alprazolam serum concentrations and potential alprazolam toxicity (sedation, slurred speech, central nervous system depression).	1	1	3
JOSAMYCIN Concurrent use of ALPRAZOLAM and JOSAMYCIN may result in increased alprazolam toxicity (central nervous system depression, poor coordination, lethargy).	2	3	3
KETOCONAZOLE Concurrent use of ALPRAZOLAM and KETOCONAZOLE may result in increased alprazolam serum concentrations and potential alprazolam toxicity (sedation, slurred speech, central nervous system depression).	1	1	2

Onset: 0=Unspecified   1=Rapid   2=Delayed
Severity: 1=Contraindicated   2=Major   3=Moderate   4=Minor
Evidence: 1=Excellent   2=Good   3=Fair   4=Poor

INTERACTION	ONSET	SEVERITY	EVIDENCE
NEFAZODONE Concurrent use of ALPRAZOLAM and NEFAZODONE may result in psychomotor impairment and sedation.	1	3	2
OMEPRAZOLE Concurrent use of ALPRAZOLAM and OMEPRAZOLE may result in alprazolam toxicity (central nervous system depression, poor coordination, lethargy).	2	3	3
ORAL CONTRACEPTIVES Concurrent use of ALPRAZOLAM and ORAL CONTRACEPTIVES may result in an increased risk of alprazolam toxicity (central nervous system depression, low blood pressure).	2	3	3
PROPOXYPHENE Concurrent use of ALPRAZOLAM and PROPOXYPHENE may result in an increased risk of alprazolam toxicity (central nervous system depression).	2	3	3
RITONAVIR Concurrent use of ALPRAZOLAM and RITONAVIR may result in increased plasma concentrations of alprazolam and enhanced alprazolam effects.	2	3	3
ROXITHROMYCIN Concurrent use of ALPRAZOLAM and ROXITHROMYCIN may result in increased alprazolam toxicity (central nervous system depression, poor coordination, lethargy).	2	3	3
SERTRALINE Concurrent use of ALPRAZOLAM and SERTRALINE may result in an increased risk of psychomotor impairment and sedation.	1	3	3
THEOPHYLLINE Concurrent use of ALPRAZOLAM and THEOPHYLLINE may result in decreased alprazolam effectiveness.	1	3	2
TROLEANDOMYCIN Concurrent use of ALPRAZOLAM and TROLEANDOMYCIN may result in increased alprazolam toxicity (central nervous system depression, poor coordination, lethargy).	2	3	3

Amitriptyline

INTERACTION	ONSET	SEVERITY	EVIDENCE
ACENOCOUMAROL Concurrent use of AMITRIPTYLINE and ACENOCOUMAROL may result in an increased risk of bleeding.	2	3	3
AMPRENAVIR Concurrent use of AMITRIPTYLINE and AMPRENAVIR may result in increased amitriptyline serum concentrations and potential toxicity (antispasmodic effects, sedation, confusion, cardiac irregularities).	2	2	3

INTERACTION	ONSET	SEVERITY	EVIDENCE
ANISINDIONE Concurrent use of AMITRIPTYLINE and ANISINDIONE may result in an increased risk of bleeding.	2	3	3
BEPRIDIL Concurrent use of AMITRIPTYLINE and BEPRIDIL may result in irregular heartbeat.	1	1	3
BETHANIDINE Concurrent use of AMITRIPTYLINE and BETHANIDINE may result in decreased antihypertensive effectiveness.	1	3	2
CARBAMAZEPINE Concurrent use of AMITRIPTYLINE and CARBAMAZEPINE may result in decreased amitriptyline effectiveness.	2	3	3
CIMETIDINE Concurrent use of AMITRIPTYLINE and CIMETIDINE may result in amitriptyline toxicity (dry mouth, blurred vision, urinary retention).	2	3	2
CISAPRIDE Concurrent use of AMITRIPTYLINE and CISAPRIDE may result in cardiotoxicity (irregular heartbeat, cardiac arrest).	1	1	3
CLONIDINE Concurrent use of AMITRIPTYLINE and CLONIDINE may result in decreased antihypertensive effectiveness.	2	2	3
CLORGYLINE Concurrent use of AMITRIPTYLINE and CLORGYLINE may result in neurotoxicity, seizures, or serotonin syndrome (high blood pressure, high fever, spasms, mental status changes).	2	1	3
DICUMAROL Concurrent use of AMITRIPTYLINE and DICUMAROL may result in an increased risk of bleeding.	2	3	3
DROPERIDOL Concurrent use of AMITRIPTYLINE and DROPERIDOL may result in an increased risk of cardiotoxicity (irregular heartbeat, cardiac arrest).	1	2	3
EPINEPHRINE Concurrent use of AMITRIPTYLINE and EPINEPHRINE may result in high blood pressure, cardiac irregularities, and rapid heartbeat.	1	2	2
ETHANOL Concurrent use of AMITRIPTYLINE and ETHANOL may result in enhanced central nervous system depression and impairment of motor skills.	1	3	1

Onset: 0=Unspecified 1=Rapid 2=Delayed
Severity: 1=Contraindicated 2=Major 3=Moderate 4=Minor
Evidence: 1=Excellent 2=Good 3=Fair 4=Poor

INTERACTION	ONSET	SEVERITY	EVIDENCE
ETILEFRINE Concurrent use of AMITRIPTYLINE and ETILEFRINE may result in high blood pressure, cardiac irregularities, and rapid heartbeat.	1	2	2
FLUCONAZOLE Concurrent use of AMITRIPTYLINE and FLUCONAZOLE may result in an increased risk of amitriptyline toxicity.	2	3	3
FLUOXETINE Concurrent use of AMITRIPTYLINE and FLUOXETINE may result in amitriptyline toxicity (dry mouth, urinary retention, sedation).	2	3	3
FLUVOXAMINE Concurrent use of AMITRIPTYLINE and FLUVOXAMINE may result in amitriptyline toxicity (dry mouth, urinary retention, sedation).	2	3	3
FURAZOLIDONE Concurrent use of AMITRIPTYLINE and FURAZOLIDONE may result in neurotoxicity, seizures, or serotonin syndrome (high blood pressure, high fever, spasms, mental status changes).	2	1	3
GREPAFLOXACIN Concurrent use of AMITRIPTYLINE and GREPAFLOXACIN may result in an increased risk of cardiotoxicity (irregular heartbeat, cardiac arrest).	2	1	3
GUANADREL Concurrent use of AMITRIPTYLINE and GUANADREL may result in decreased antihypertensive effectiveness.	2	3	3
GUANETHIDINE Concurrent use of AMITRIPTYLINE and GUANETHIDINE may result in decreased antihypertensive effectiveness.	2	3	2
GUANFACINE Concurrent use of AMITRIPTYLINE and GUANFACINE may result in decreased antihypertensive effectiveness.	2	3	3
HALOFANTRINE Concurrent use of AMITRIPTYLINE and HALOFANTRINE may result in cardiotoxicity (irregular heartbeat, cardiac arrest).	2	2	3
IBUTILIDE Concurrent use of AMITRIPTYLINE and IBUTILIDE may result in an increased risk of cardiac irregularities.	1	2	3
IPRONIAZID Concurrent use of AMITRIPTYLINE and IPRONIAZID may result in neurotoxicity, seizures, or serotonin syndrome (high blood pressure, high fever, spasms, mental status changes).	2	1	3

INTERACTION	ONSET	SEVERITY	EVIDENCE
ISOCARBOXAZID Concurrent use of AMITRIPTYLINE and ISOCARBOXAZID may result in neurotoxicity, seizures, or serotonin syndrome (high blood pressure, high fever, spasms, mental status changes).	2	1	3
LEVOMETHADYL Concurrent use of AMITRIPTYLINE and LEVOMETHADYL may result in an increased risk of cardiotoxicity (irregular heartbeat, cardiac arrest).	2	1	3
METHOXAMINE Concurrent use of TRICYCLIC ANTIDEPRESSANTS such as amitriptyline and METHOXAMINE may result in high blood pressure, cardiac irregularities, and rapid heartbeat.	1	2	2
MIDODRINE Concurrent use of TRICYCLIC ANTIDEPRESSANTS and MIDODRINE may result in high blood pressure, cardiac irregularities, and rapid heartbeat.	1	2	2
MOCLOBEMIDE Concurrent use of AMITRIPTYLINE and MOCLOBEMIDE may result in neurotoxicity, seizures, or serotonin syndrome (high blood pressure, high fever, spasms, mental status changes).	2	1	3
NEFAZODONE Concurrent use of AMITRIPTYLINE and NEFAZODONE may result in increased risk of serotonin syndrome (high blood pressure, high fever, spasms, mental status changes).	1	2	3
NIALAMIDE Concurrent use of AMITRIPTYLINE and NIALAMIDE may result in neurotoxicity, seizures, or serotonin syndrome (high blood pressure, high fever, spasms, mental status changes).	2	1	3
NOREPINEPHRINE Concurrent use of AMITRIPTYLINE and NOREPINEPHRINE may result in high blood pressure, cardiac irregularities, and rapid heartbeat.	1	2	2
OXILOFRINE Concurrent use of AMITRIPTYLINE and OXILOFRINE may result in high blood pressure, cardiac irregularities, and rapid heartbeat.	1	2	2
PARGYLINE Concurrent use of AMITRIPTYLINE and PARGYLINE may result in neurotoxicity, seizures, or serotonin syndrome (high blood pressure, high fever, spasms, mental status changes).	2	1	3
PHENELZINE Concurrent use of AMITRIPTYLINE and PHENELZINE may result in neurotoxicity, seizures, or serotonin syndrome (high blood pressure, high fever, spasms, mental status changes).	2	1	3

Onset: 0=Unspecified 1=Rapid 2=Delayed
Severity: 1=Contraindicated 2=Major 3=Moderate 4=Minor
Evidence: 1=Excellent 2=Good 3=Fair 4=Poor

INTERACTION	ONSET	SEVERITY	EVIDENCE
PHENINDIONE Concurrent use of AMITRIPTYLINE and PHENINDIONE may result in an increased risk of bleeding.	2	3	3
PHENPROCOUMON Concurrent use of AMITRIPTYLINE and PHENPROCOUMON may result in an increased risk of bleeding.	2	3	3
PHENYLEPHRINE Concurrent use of AMITRIPTYLINE and PHENYLEPHRINE may result in high blood pressure, cardiac irregularities, and rapid heartbeat.	1	2	2
PIMOZIDE Concurrent use of AMITRIPTYLINE and PIMOZIDE may result in an increased risk of cardiotoxicity (irregular heartbeat, cardiac arrest).	1	1	3
PROCARBAZINE Concurrent use of AMITRIPTYLINE and PROCARBAZINE may result in neurotoxicity, seizures.	2	1	3
SELEGILINE Concurrent use of AMITRIPTYLINE and SELEGILINE may result in neurotoxicity, seizures, or serotonin syndrome (high blood pressure, high fever, spasms, mental status changes).	2	1	3
SERTRALINE Concurrent use of AMITRIPTYLINE and SERTRALINE may result in elevated amitriptyline serum levels or possible serotonin syndrome (high blood pressure, high fever, spasms, mental status changes).	2	2	3
SPARFLOXACIN Concurrent use of AMITRIPTYLINE and SPARFLOXACIN may result in irregular heartbeat.	2	1	3
ST JOHN'S WORT Concurrent use of AMITRIPTYLINE and ST JOHN'S WORT may result in decreased effectiveness of amitriptyline and possible increased risk of serotonin syndrome (high blood pressure, high fever, spasms, mental status changes).	2	3	3
TOLOXATONE Concurrent use of AMITRIPTYLINE and TOLOXATONE may result in neurotoxicity, seizures, or serotonin syndrome (high blood pressure, high fever, spasms, mental status changes).	2	1	3
TRAMADOL Concurrent use of AMITRIPTYLINE and TRAMADOL may result in an increased risk of seizures.	1	2	3
TRANYLCYPROMINE Concurrent use of AMITRIPTYLINE and TRANYLCYPROMINE may result in neurotoxicity, seizures, or serotonin syndrome (high blood pressure, high fever, spasms, mental status changes).	2	1	3

INTERACTION	ONSET	SEVERITY	EVIDENCE
WARFARIN Concurrent use of AMITRIPTYLINE and WARFARIN may result in an increased risk of bleeding.	2	3	3

Amoxapine

INTERACTION	ONSET	SEVERITY	EVIDENCE
ACENOCOUMAROL Concurrent use of AMOXAPINE and ACENOCOUMAROL may result in increased risk of bleeding.	2	3	3
AMPRENAVIR Concurrent use of AMOXAPINE and AMPRENAVIR may result in increased amoxapine serum concentrations and potential toxicity (antispasmodic effects, sedation, confusion, cardiac irregularities).	2	2	3
ANISINDIONE Concurrent use of AMOXAPINE and ANISINDIONE may result in increased risk of bleeding.	2	3	3
BEPRIDIL Concurrent use of AMOXAPINE and BEPRIDIL may result in irregular heartbeat.	1	1	3
CIMETIDINE Concurrent use of AMOXAPINE and CIMETIDINE may result in amoxapine toxicity (dry mouth, urinary retention, blurred vision).	2	3	3
CISAPRIDE Concurrent use of AMOXAPINE and CISAPRIDE may result in cardiotoxicity (irregular heartbeat, cardiac arrest).	1	1	3
CLONIDINE Concurrent use of AMOXAPINE and CLONIDINE may result in decreased clonidine effectiveness.	2	2	3
CLORGYLINE Concurrent use of AMOXAPINE and CLORGYLINE may result in neurotoxicity, seizures, or serotonin syndrome (high blood pressure, high fever, spasms, mental status changes).	2	2	3
DICUMAROL Concurrent use of AMOXAPINE and DICUMAROL may result in increased risk of bleeding.	2	3	3
DROPERIDOL Concurrent use of AMOXAPINE and DROPERIDOL may result in an increased risk of cardiotoxicity (irregular heartbeat, cardiac arrest).	1	2	3
EPINEPHRINE Concurrent use of as AMOXAPINE and EPINEPHRINE may result in high blood pressure, cardiac irregularities, and rapid heartbeat.	1	2	2

Onset: 0=Unspecified 1=Rapid 2=Delayed
Severity: 1=Contraindicated 2=Major 3=Moderate 4=Minor
Evidence: 1=Excellent 2=Good 3=Fair 4=Poor

INTERACTION	ONSET	SEVERITY	EVIDENCE
ETILEFRINE Concurrent use of as AMOXAPINE and ETILEFRINE may result in high blood pressure, cardiac irregularities, and rapid heartbeat.	1	2	2
FLUOXETINE Concurrent use of AMOXAPINE and FLUOXETINE may result in increased amoxapine concentration and toxicity (antispasmodic effects, sedation, cardiac effects).	2	3	3
GREPAFLOXACIN Concurrent use of AMOXAPINE and GREPAFLOXACIN may result in an increased risk of cardiotoxicity (irregular heartbeat, cardiac arrest).	2	1	3
GUANADREL Concurrent use of AMOXAPINE and GUANADREL may result in decreased guanadrel effectiveness.	2	3	3
HALOFANTRINE Concurrent use of AMOXAPINE and HALOFANTRINE may result in cardiotoxicity (irregular heartbeat, cardiac arrest).	2	2	3
IBUTILIDE Concurrent use of AMOXAPINE and IBUTILIDE may result in an increased risk of irregular heartbeat.	1	2	3
ISOCARBOXAZID Concurrent use of AMOXAPINE and ISOCARBOXAZID may result in neurotoxicity, seizures, or serotonin syndrome (high blood pressure, high fever, spasms, mental status changes).	2	1	3
LEVOMETHADYL Concurrent use of AMOXAPINE and LEVOMETHADYL may result in an increased risk of cardiotoxicity (irregular heartbeat, cardiac arrest).	2	1	3
METHOXAMINE Concurrent use of as AMOXAPINE and METHOXAMINE may result in high blood pressure, cardiac irregularities, and rapid heartbeat.	1	2	2
MIDODRINE Concurrent use of AMOXAPINE and MIDODRINE may result in high blood pressure, cardiac irregularities, and rapid heartbeat.	1	2	2
MOCLOBEMIDE Concurrent use of AMOXAPINE and MOCLOBEMIDE may result in neurotoxicity, seizures, or serotonin syndrome (high blood pressure, high fever, spasms, mental status changes).	2	2	3
NOREPINEPHRINE Concurrent use of AMOXAPINE and NOREPINEPHRINE may result in high blood pressure, cardiac irregularities, and rapid heartbeat.	1	2	2

INTERACTION	ONSET	SEVERITY	EVIDENCE
OXILOFRINE Concurrent use of AMOXAPINE and OXILOFRINE may result in high blood pressure, cardiac irregularities, and rapid heartbeat.	1	2	2
PHENELZINE Concurrent use of AMOXAPINE and PHENELZINE may result in neurotoxicity, seizures, or serotonin syndrome (high blood pressure, high fever, spasms, mental status changes).	2	2	3
PHENINDIONE Concurrent use of AMOXAPINE and PHENINDIONE may result in increased risk of bleeding.	2	3	3
PHENPROCOUMON Concurrent use of AMOXAPINE and PHENPROCOUMON may result in increased risk of bleeding.	2	3	3
PHENYLEPHRINE Concurrent use of AMOXAPINE and PHENYLEPHRINE may result in high blood pressure, cardiac irregularities, and rapid heartbeat.	1	2	2
PIMOZIDE Concurrent use of AMOXAPINE and PIMOZIDE may result in an increased risk of cardiotoxicity (irregular heartbeat, cardiac arrest).	1	1	3
PROCARBAZINE Concurrent use of AMOXAPINE and PROCARBAZINE may result in neurotoxicity, seizures.	2	2	3
SELEGILINE Concurrent use of AMOXAPINE and SELEGILINE may result in neurotoxicity, seizures, or serotonin syndrome (high blood pressure, high fever, spasms, mental status changes).	2	2	3
SPARFLOXACIN Concurrent use of AMOXAPINE and SPARFLOXACIN may result in irregular heartbeat.	2	1	3
TRAMADOL Concurrent use of AMOXAPINE and TRAMADOL may result in an increased risk of seizures.	1	2	3
TRANYLCYPROMINE Concurrent use of AMOXAPINE and TRANYLCYPROMINE may result in neurotoxicity, seizures, or serotonin syndrome (high blood pressure, high fever, spasms, mental status changes).	2	2	3
WARFARIN Concurrent use of AMOXAPINE and WARFARIN may result in an increased risk of bleeding.	2	3	3

Onset: 0=Unspecified 1=Rapid 2=Delayed
Severity: 1=Contraindicated 2=Major 3=Moderate 4=Minor
Evidence: 1=Excellent 2=Good 3=Fair 4=Poor

Amphetamine

INTERACTION	ONSET	SEVERITY	EVIDENCE
ACETAZOLAMIDE Concurrent use of AMPHETAMINE and ACETAZOLAMIDE may result in amphetamine toxicity (high blood pressure, high fever, seizures).	2	4	3
CLORGYLINE Concurrent use of AMPHETAMINE and CLORGYLINE may result in hypertensive crisis (headache, high fever, high blood pressure).	1	1	3
GUANETHIDINE Concurrent use of AMPHETAMINE and GUANETHIDINE may result in decreased guanethidine effectiveness.	1	3	2
IPRONIAZID Concurrent use of AMPHETAMINE and IPRONIAZID may result in a hypertensive crisis (headache, high fever, high blood pressure).	1	1	3
ISOCARBOXAZID Concurrent use of AMPHETAMINE and ISOCARBOXAZID may result in hypertensive crisis (headache, high fever, high blood pressure).	1	1	3
MOCLOBEMIDE Concurrent use of AMPHETAMINE and MOCLOBEMIDE may result in hypertensive crisis (headache, high fever, high blood pressure).	1	1	3
NIALAMIDE Concurrent use of AMPHETAMINE and NIALAMIDE may result in a hypertensive crisis (headache, high fever, high blood pressure).	1	1	3
PARGYLINE Concurrent use of AMPHETAMINE and PARGYLINE may result in hypertensive crisis (headache, high fever, high blood pressure).	1	1	3
PHENELZINE Concurrent use of AMPHETAMINE and PHENELZINE may result in hypertensive crisis (headache, high fever, high blood pressure).	1	1	2
PROCARBAZINE Concurrent use of AMPHETAMINE and PROCARBAZINE may result in a hypertensive crisis (headache, high fever, high blood pressure).	1	1	3
SELEGILINE Concurrent use of AMPHETAMINE and SELEGILINE may result in hypertensive crisis (headache, high fever, high blood pressure).	1	1	2
SIBUTRAMINE Concurrent use of AMPHETAMINE and SIBUTRAMINE may result in an increased risk of high blood pressure and rapid heartbeat.	1	1	3

INTERACTION	ONSET	SEVERITY	EVIDENCE
SODIUM BICARBONATE Concurrent use of AMPHETAMINE and SODIUM BICARBONATE may result in amphetamine toxicity (high blood pressure, high fever, seizures).	2	3	3
TOLOXATONE Concurrent use of AMPHETAMINE and TOLOXATONE may result in a hypertensive crisis (headache, high fever, high blood pressure).	1	1	3
TRANYLCYPROMINE Concurrent use of AMPHETAMINE and TRANYLCYPROMINE may result in hypertensive crisis (headache, high fever, high blood pressure).	1	1	2

Bupropion

INTERACTION	ONSET	SEVERITY	EVIDENCE
CLORGYLINE Concurrent use of BUPROPION and CLORGYLINE may result in bupropion toxicity.	1	1	3
DROPERIDOL Concurrent use of BUPROPION and DROPERIDOL may result in an increased risk of cardiotoxicity (irregular heartbeat, cardiac arrest).	1	2	3
ETHANOL Concurrent use of BUPROPION and ETHANOL may result in an increased risk of seizures.	2	2	3
IPRONIAZID Concurrent use of BUPROPION and IPRONIAZID may result in bupropion toxicity (seizures, agitation, psychotic changes).	1	1	3
ISOCARBOXAZID Concurrent use of BUPROPION and ISOCARBOXAZID may result in bupropion toxicity (seizures, agitation, psychotic changes).	1	1	3
MOCLOBEMIDE Concurrent use of BUPROPION and MOCLOBEMIDE may result in bupropion toxicity (seizures, agitation, psychotic changes).	1	1	3
NIALAMIDE Concurrent use of BUPROPION and NIALAMIDE may result in bupropion toxicity (seizures, agitation, psychotic changes).	1	1	3
PARGYLINE Concurrent use of BUPROPION and PARGYLINE may result in bupropion toxicity (seizures, agitation, psychotic changes).	1	1	3

Onset: 0=Unspecified 1=Rapid 2=Delayed
Severity: 1=Contraindicated 2=Major 3=Moderate 4=Minor
Evidence: 1=Excellent 2=Good 3=Fair 4=Poor

INTERACTION	ONSET	SEVERITY	EVIDENCE
PHENELZINE Concurrent use of BUPROPION and PHENELZINE may result in bupropion toxicity (seizures, agitation, psychotic changes).	1	1	3
PROCARBAZINE Concurrent use of BUPROPION and PROCARBAZINE may result in bupropion toxicity (seizures, agitation, psychotic changes).	1	1	3
SELEGILINE Concurrent use of BUPROPION and SELEGILINE may result in bupropion toxicity (seizures, agitation, psychotic changes).	1	1	3
TOLOXATONE Concurrent use of BUPROPION and TOLOXATONE may result in bupropion toxicity (seizures, agitation, psychotic changes).	1	1	3
TRANYLCYPROMINE Concurrent use of BUPROPION and TRANYLCYPROMINE may result in bupropion toxicity (seizures, agitation, psychotic changes).	1	1	3

Buspirone

INTERACTION	ONSET	SEVERITY	EVIDENCE
CLORGYLINE Concurrent use of BUSPIRONE and CLORGYLINE may result in hypertensive crisis (headache, high fever, high blood pressure).	1	2	3
DILTIAZEM Concurrent use of BUSPIRONE and DILTIAZEM may result in an increased risk of enhanced buspirone effects.	1	3	3
ERYTHROMYCIN Concurrent use of BUSPIRONE and ERYTHROMYCIN may result in increased buspirone plasma concentrations; increased buspirone side effects (impaired psychomotor performance, sedation).	1	3	3
GRAPEFRUIT JUICE Concurrent use of BUSPIRONE and GRAPEFRUIT JUICE may result in an increased risk of buspirone toxicity (dizziness, sedation).	1	3	3
IPRONIAZID Concurrent use of BUSPIRONE and IPRONIAZID may result in hypertensive crisis (headache, high fever, high blood pressure).	1	2	3
ISOCARBOXAZID Concurrent use of BUSPIRONE and ISOCARBOXAZID may result in hypertensive crisis (headache, high fever, high blood pressure).	1	1	3

INTERACTION	ONSET	SEVERITY	EVIDENCE
ITRACONAZOLE Concurrent use of BUSPIRONE and ITRACONAZOLE may result in increased buspirone plasma concentrations; increased buspirone side effects (impaired psychomotor performance, sedation).	1	3	3
MOCLOBEMIDE Concurrent use of BUSPIRONE and MOCLOBEMIDE may result in hypertensive crisis (headache, high fever, high blood pressure).	1	2	3
NIALAMIDE Concurrent use of BUSPIRONE and NIALAMIDE may result in hypertensive crisis (headache, high fever, high blood pressure).	1	2	3
PARGYLINE Concurrent use of BUSPIRONE and PARGYLINE may result in hypertensive crisis (headache, high fever, high blood pressure).	1	2	3
PHENELZINE Concurrent use of BUSPIRONE and PHENELZINE may result in hypertensive crisis (headache, high fever, high blood pressure).	1	1	3
PROCARBAZINE Concurrent use of BUSPIRONE and PROCARBAZINE may result in hypertensive crisis (headache, high fever, high blood pressure).	1	2	3
RIFAMPIN Concurrent use of BUSPIRONE and RIFAMPIN may result in reduced anxiolytic effects of buspirone.	1	3	3
SELEGILINE Concurrent use of BUSPIRONE and SELEGILINE may result in hypertensive crisis (headache, high fever, high blood pressure).	1	2	3
TOLOXATONE Concurrent use of BUSPIRONE and TOLOXATONE may result in hypertensive crisis (headache, high fever, high blood pressure).	1	2	3
TRANYLCYPROMINE Concurrent use of BUSPIRONE and TRANYLCYPROMINE may result in hypertensive crisis (headache, high fever, high blood pressure).	1	1	3
VERAPAMIL Concurrent use of BUSPIRONE and VERAPAMIL may result in an increased risk of enhanced buspirone effects.	1	3	3

Onset: 0=Unspecified 1=Rapid 2=Delayed
Severity: 1=Contraindicated 2=Major 3=Moderate 4=Minor
Evidence: 1=Excellent 2=Good 3=Fair 4=Poor

Chlordiazepoxide

INTERACTION	ONSET	SEVERITY	EVIDENCE
CIMETIDINE Concurrent use of CHLORDIAZEPOXIDE and CIMETIDINE may result in chlordiazepoxide toxicity (central nervous system depression).	1	4	3
DISULFIRAM Concurrent use of CHLORDIAZEPOXIDE and DISULFIRAM may result in an increased risk of chlordiazepoxide toxicity (central nervous system depression).	2	4	3
ETHANOL Concurrent use of CHLORDIAZEPOXIDE and ETHANOL may result in increased sedation.	1	3	1
KETOCONAZOLE Concurrent use of CHLORDIAZEPOXIDE and KETOCONAZOLE may result in moderate decreases in chlordiazepoxide clearance and possible chlordiazepoxide toxicity (sedation, drowsiness, slurred speech, psychomotor impairment).	1	4	3
THEOPHYLLINE Concurrent use of CHLORDIAZEPOXIDE and THEOPHYLLINE may result in decreased chlordiazepoxide effectiveness.	1	3	2

Chlorpromazine

INTERACTION	ONSET	SEVERITY	EVIDENCE
ANTACIDS Concurrent use of CHLORPROMAZINE and ANTACIDS may result in decreased chlorpromazine effectiveness.	2	4	3
ATENOLOL Concurrent use of CHLORPROMAZINE and ATENOLOL may result in low blood pressure and/or chlorpromazine toxicity.	1	3	2
BELLADONNA Concurrent use of CHLORPROMAZINE and BELLADONNA may result in increased manic, agitated reactions, or enhanced antispasmodic effects resulting in cardiorespiratory failure, especially in cases of belladonna overdose.	1	3	2
BENZTROPINE Concurrent use of CHLORPROMAZINE and BENZTROPINE may result in decreased chlorpromazine serum concentrations, decreased chlorpromazine effectiveness, enhanced antispasmodic effects (intestinal blockage, high fever, sedation, dry mouth).	2	3	3
CABERGOLINE Concurrent use of CHLORPROMAZINE and CABERGOLINE may result in the decreased therapeutic effect of both drugs.	1	3	3

INTERACTION	ONSET	SEVERITY	EVIDENCE
CISAPRIDE Concurrent use of CHLORPROMAZINE and CISAPRIDE may result in cardiotoxicity (irregular heartbeat, cardiac arrest).	1	1	3
DROPERIDOL Concurrent use of CHLORPROMAZINE and DROPERIDOL may result in an increased risk of cardiotoxicity (irregular heartbeat, cardiac arrest).	1	2	3
EPINEPHRINE Concurrent use of CHLORPROMAZINE and EPINEPHRINE may result in low blood pressure and rapid heartbeat.	1	3	3
ETHANOL Concurrent use of CHLORPROMAZINE and ETHANOL may result in increased sedation.	1	3	2
FOSPHENYTOIN Concurrent use of CHLORPROMAZINE and FOSPHENYTOIN may result in increased or decreased phenytoin levels and possibly reduced chlorpromazine levels.	2	4	3
GREPAFLOXACIN Concurrent use of CHLORPROMAZINE and GREPAFLOXACIN may result in an increased risk of cardiotoxicity (irregular heartbeat, cardiac arrest).	2	1	3
GUANETHIDINE Concurrent use of CHLORPROMAZINE and GUANETHIDINE may result in decreased guanethidine effectiveness.	1	3	2
HALOFANTRINE Concurrent use of CHLORPROMAZINE and HALOFANTRINE may result in cardiotoxicity (irregular heartbeat, cardiac arrest).	2	2	3
IBUTILIDE Concurrent use of CHLORPROMAZINE and IBUTILIDE may result in an increased risk of irregularities.	1	2	3
LEVODOPA Concurrent use of CHLORPROMAZINE and LEVODOPA may result in loss of levodopa efficacy.	1	3	2
LEVOMETHADYL Concurrent use of CHLORPROMAZINE and LEVOMETHADYL may result in an increased risk of cardiotoxicity (irregular heartbeat, cardiac arrest).	2	1	3
LITHIUM Concurrent use of CHLORPROMAZINE and LITHIUM may result in weakness, movement disorders, brain disorders, and brain damage.	2	2	1

Onset: 0=Unspecified 1=Rapid 2=Delayed
Severity: 1=Contraindicated 2=Major 3=Moderate 4=Minor
Evidence: 1=Excellent 2=Good 3=Fair 4=Poor

INTERACTION	ONSET	SEVERITY	EVIDENCE
MEPERIDINE Concurrent use of CHLORPROMAZINE and MEPERIDINE may result in an increase in central nervous system and respiratory depression.	1	3	2
METOPROLOL Concurrent use of CHLORPROMAZINE and METOPROLOL may result in low blood pressure and/or chlorpromazine toxicity.	1	3	2
NOREPINEPHRINE Concurrent use of CHLORPROMAZINE and NOREPINEPHRINE may result in decreased norepinephrine effectiveness.	1	3	3
ORPHENADRINE Concurrent use of CHLORPROMAZINE and ORPHENADRINE may result in decreased chlorpromazine serum concentrations, decreased chlorpromazine effectiveness, enhanced antispasmodic effects (intestinal blockage, high fever, sedation, dry mouth).	2	3	3
PHENMETRAZINE Concurrent use of CHLORPROMAZINE and PHENMETRAZINE may result in decreased phenmetrazine effectiveness.	1	3	2
PHENOBARBITAL Concurrent use of CHLORPROMAZINE and PHENOBARBITAL may result in decreased chlorpromazine effectiveness.	1	3	3
PHENYTOIN Concurrent use of CHLORPROMAZINE and PHENYTOIN may result in increased or decreased phenytoin levels and possibly reduced chlorpromazine levels.	2	4	3
PORFIMER Concurrent use of CHLORPROMAZINE and PORFIMER may result in excessive intracellular damage in photosensitized tissues.	2	3	3
PROCYCLIDINE Concurrent use of CHLORPROMAZINE and PROCYCLIDINE may result in decreased chlorpromazine serum concentrations, decreased chlorpromazine effectiveness, enhanced antispasmodic effects (intestinal blockage, high fever, sedation, dry mouth).	2	3	3
PROPRANOLOL Concurrent use of CHLORPROMAZINE and PROPRANOLOL may result in chlorpromazine toxicity (sedation, movement disorders, delirium), seizures.	2	3	3
SPARFLOXACIN Concurrent use of CHLORPROMAZINE and SPARFLOXACIN may result in irregular heartbeat.	2	1	3

INTERACTION	ONSET	SEVERITY	EVIDENCE
TRAMADOL Concurrent use of CHLORPROMAZINE and TRAMADOL may result in an increased risk of seizures.	1	2	3
TRIHEXYPHENIDYL Concurrent use of CHLORPROMAZINE and TRIHEXYPHENIDYL may result in decreased chlorpromazine serum concentrations, decreased chlorpromazine effectiveness, enhanced antispasmodic effects (intestinal blockage, high fever, sedation, dry mouth).	2	3	3
ZIPRASIDONE Concurrent use of CHLORPROMAZINE and ZIPRASIDONE may result in an increased risk of cardiotoxicity (irregular heartbeat, cardiac arrest).	2	1	3

Citalopram

INTERACTION	ONSET	SEVERITY	EVIDENCE
ALMOTRIPTAN Concurrent use of CITALOPRAM and ALMOTRIPTAN may result in weakness, exaggerated reflexes, and incoordination.	0	3	3
CLORGYLINE Concurrent use of CITALOPRAM and CLORGYLINE may result in central nervous system toxicity or serotonin syndrome (high blood pressure, high fever, spasms, mental status changes).	1	1	3
DEXFENFLURAMINE Concurrent use of CITALOPRAM and DEXFENFLURAMINE may result in serotonin syndrome (high blood pressure, high fever, spasms, mental status changes).	1	2	3
DROPERIDOL Concurrent use of CITALOPRAM and DROPERIDOL may result in an increased risk of cardiotoxicity (irregular heartbeat, cardiac arrest).	1	2	3
FENFLURAMINE Concurrent use of CITALOPRAM and FENFLURAMINE may result in serotonin syndrome (high blood pressure, high fever, spasms, mental status changes).	1	2	3
FURAZOLIDONE Concurrent use of CITALOPRAM and FURAZOLIDONE may result in weakness, exaggerated reflexes, and incoordination.	2	1	3
HYDROXYTRYPTOPHAN Concurrent use of CITALOPRAM and HYDROXYTRYPTOPHAN may result in an increased risk of serotonin syndrome (high blood pressure, high fever, spasms, mental status changes).	1	3	3

Onset:　　0=Unspecified　1=Rapid　2=Delayed
Severity:　1=Contraindicated　2=Major　3=Moderate　4=Minor
Evidence:　1=Excellent　2=Good　3=Fair　4=Poor

INTERACTION	ONSET	SEVERITY	EVIDENCE
IPRONIAZID Concurrent use of CITALOPRAM and IPRONIAZID may result in central nervous system toxicity or serotonin syndrome (high blood pressure, high fever, spasms, mental status changes).	1	1	3
ISOCARBOXAZID Concurrent use of CITALOPRAM and ISOCARBOXAZID may result in central nervous system toxicity or serotonin syndrome (high blood pressure, high fever, spasms, mental status changes).	1	1	3
LEVOMETHADYL Concurrent use of CITALOPRAM and LEVOMETHADYL may result in an increased risk of cardiotoxicity (irregular heartbeat, cardiac arrest).	2	1	3
MOCLOBEMIDE Concurrent use of CITALOPRAM and MOCLOBEMIDE may result in serotonin syndrome (high blood pressure, high fever, spasms, mental status changes).	1	1	3
NIALAMIDE Concurrent use of CITALOPRAM and NIALAMIDE may result in central nervous system toxicity or serotonin syndrome (high blood pressure, high fever, spasms, mental status changes).	1	1	3
PARGYLINE Concurrent use of CITALOPRAM and PARGYLINE may result in central nervous system toxicity or serotonin syndrome (high blood pressure, high fever, spasms, mental status changes).	1	1	3
PHENELZINE Concurrent use of CITALOPRAM and PHENELZINE may result in central nervous system toxicity or serotonin syndrome (high blood pressure, high fever, spasms, mental status changes).	1	1	3
PROCARBAZINE Concurrent use of CITALOPRAM and PROCARBAZINE may result in central nervous system toxicity or serotonin syndrome (high blood pressure, high fever, spasms, mental status changes).	1	1	3
SELEGILINE Concurrent use of CITALOPRAM and SELEGILINE may result in central nervous system toxicity or serotonin syndrome (high blood pressure, high fever, spasms, mental status changes).	1	1	3
SIBUTRAMINE Concurrent use of CITALOPRAM and SIBUTRAMINE may result in an increased risk of serotonin syndrome (high blood pressure, high fever, spasms, mental status changes).	1	2	3

INTERACTION	ONSET	SEVERITY	EVIDENCE
TOLOXATONE Concurrent use of CITALOPRAM and TOLOXATONE may result in central nervous system toxicity or serotonin syndrome (high blood pressure, high fever, spasms, mental status changes).	1	1	3
TRAMADOL Concurrent use of CITALOPRAM and TRAMADOL may result in an increased risk of seizures and serotonin syndrome (high blood pressure, high fever, spasms, mental status changes).	1	2	2
TRANYLCYPROMINE Concurrent use of CITALOPRAM and TRANYLCYPROMINE may result in central nervous system toxicity or serotonin syndrome (high blood pressure, high fever, spasms, mental status changes).	1	1	3

Clomipramine

INTERACTION	ONSET	SEVERITY	EVIDENCE
ACENOCOUMAROL Concurrent use of CLOMIPRAMINE and ACENOCOUMAROL may result in increased risk of bleeding.	2	3	3
AMPRENAVIR Concurrent use of CLOMIPRAMINE and AMPRENAVIR may result in increased clomipramine serum concentrations and potential toxicity (antispasmodic effects, sedation, confusion, cardiac irregularities).	2	2	3
ANISINDIONE Concurrent use of CLOMIPRAMINE and ANISINDIONE may result in increased risk of bleeding.	2	3	3
BEPRIDIL Concurrent use of CLOMIPRAMINE and BEPRIDIL may result in irregular heartbeat.	1	1	3
BETHANIDINE Concurrent use of CLOMIPRAMINE and BETHANIDINE may result in decreased antihypertensive effectiveness.	1	3	3
CIMETIDINE Concurrent use of CLOMIPRAMINE and CIMETIDINE may result in clomipramine toxicity (dry mouth, blurred vision, urinary retention).	2	3	3
CISAPRIDE Concurrent use of CLOMIPRAMINE and CISAPRIDE may result in cardiotoxicity (irregular heartbeat, cardiac arrest).	1	1	3
CLONIDINE Concurrent use of CLOMIPRAMINE and CLONIDINE may result in decreased antihypertensive effectiveness.	2	2	3

Onset: 0=Unspecified 1=Rapid 2=Delayed
Severity: 1=Contraindicated 2=Major 3=Moderate 4=Minor
Evidence: 1=Excellent 2=Good 3=Fair 4=Poor

INTERACTION	ONSET	SEVERITY	EVIDENCE
CLORGYLINE Concurrent use of CLOMIPRAMINE and CLORGYLINE may result in neurotoxicity, seizures, or serotonin syndrome (high blood pressure, high fever, spasms, mental status changes).	2	2	3
DICUMAROL Concurrent use of CLOMIPRAMINE and DICUMAROL may result in increased risk of bleeding.	2	3	3
DROPERIDOL Concurrent use of CLOMIPRAMINE and DROPERIDOL may result in an increased risk of cardiotoxicity (irregular heartbeat, cardiac arrest).	1	2	3
EPINEPHRINE Concurrent use of CLOMIPRAMINE and EPINEPHRINE may result in high blood pressure, cardiac irregularities, and rapid heartbeat.	1	2	2
ETILEFRINE Concurrent use of CLOMIPRAMINE and ETILEFRINE may result in high blood pressure, cardiac irregularities, and rapid heartbeat.	1	2	2
FLUOXETINE Concurrent use of CLOMIPRAMINE and FLUOXETINE may result in clomipramine toxicity (dry mouth, urinary retention, sedation).	2	3	3
FLUVOXAMINE Concurrent use of CLOMIPRAMINE and FLUVOXAMINE may result in clomipramine toxicity (dry mouth, urinary retention, sedation).	2	3	3
GREPAFLOXACIN Concurrent use of CLOMIPRAMINE and GREPAFLOXACIN may result in an increased risk of cardiotoxicity (irregular heartbeat, cardiac arrest).	2	1	3
GUANADREL Concurrent use of CLOMIPRAMINE and GUANADREL may result in decreased antihypertensive effectiveness.	2	3	3
HALOFANTRINE Concurrent use of CLOMIPRAMINE and HALOFANTRINE may result in cardiotoxicity (irregular heartbeat, cardiac arrest).	2	2	3
IBUTILIDE Concurrent use of CLOMIPRAMINE and IBUTILIDE may result in an increased risk of cardiac irregularities.	1	2	3
ISOCARBOXAZID Concurrent use of CLOMIPRAMINE and ISOCARBOXAZID may result in neurotoxicity, seizures, or serotonin syndrome (high blood pressure, high fever, spasms, mental status changes).	2	1	3
METHOXAMINE Concurrent use of CLOMIPRAMINE and METHOXAMINE may result in high blood pressure, cardiac irregularities, and rapid heartbeat.	1	2	2

INTERACTION	ONSET	SEVERITY	EVIDENCE
MIDODRINE Concurrent use of CLOMIPRAMINE and MIDODRINE may result in high blood pressure, cardiac irregularities, and rapid heartbeat.	1	2	2
MOCLOBEMIDE Concurrent use of CLOMIPRAMINE and MOCLOBEMIDE may result in neurotoxicity, seizures, or serotonin syndrome (high blood pressure, high fever, spasms, mental status changes).	1	2	3
NOREPINEPHRINE Concurrent use of CLOMIPRAMINE and NOREPINEPHRINE may result in high blood pressure, cardiac irregularities, and rapid heartbeat.	1	2	2
OLANZAPINE Concurrent use of CLOMIPRAMINE and OLANZAPINE may result in an increased risk of seizures.	2	2	2
OXILOFRINE Concurrent use of CLOMIPRAMINE and OXILOFRINE may result in high blood pressure, cardiac irregularities, and rapid heartbeat.	1	2	2
PHENELZINE Concurrent use of CLOMIPRAMINE and PHENELZINE may result in neurotoxicity, seizures, or serotonin syndrome (high blood pressure, high fever, spasms, mental status changes).	2	2	3
PHENINDIONE Concurrent use of CLOMIPRAMINE and PHENINDIONE may result in increased risk of bleeding.	2	3	3
PHENPROCOUMON Concurrent use of CLOMIPRAMINE and PHENPROCOUMON may result in increased risk of bleeding.	2	3	3
PHENYLEPHRINE Concurrent use of CLOMIPRAMINE and PHENYLEPHRINE may result in high blood pressure, cardiac irregularities, and rapid heartbeat.	1	2	2
PIMOZIDE Concurrent use of CLOMIPRAMINE and PIMOZIDE may result in an increased risk of cardiotoxicity (irregular heartbeat, cardiac arrest).	1	1	3
PROCARBAZINE Concurrent use of CLOMIPRAMINE and PROCARBAZINE may result in neurotoxicity, seizures.	2	2	3

Onset: 0=Unspecified 1=Rapid 2=Delayed
Severity: 1=Contraindicated 2=Major 3=Moderate 4=Minor
Evidence: 1=Excellent 2=Good 3=Fair 4=Poor

INTERACTION	ONSET	SEVERITY	EVIDENCE
SELEGILINE Concurrent use of CLOMIPRAMINE and SELEGILINE may result in neurotoxicity, seizures, or serotonin syndrome (high blood pressure, high fever, spasms, mental status changes).	2	2	3
SPARFLOXACIN Concurrent use of CLOMIPRAMINE and SPARFLOXACIN may result in irregular heartbeat.	2	1	3
TRAMADOL Concurrent use of CLOMIPRAMINE and TRAMADOL may result in an increased risk of seizures.	1	2	3
TRANYLCYPROMINE Concurrent use of CLOMIPRAMINE and TRANYLCYPROMINE may result in neurotoxicity, seizures, or serotonin syndrome (high blood pressure, high fever, spasms, mental status changes).	2	2	3
VALPROIC ACID Concurrent use of CLOMIPRAMINE and VALPROIC ACID may result in increased risk of clomipramine toxicity (agitation, confusion, hallucinations, urinary retention, rapid heartbeat, seizures, coma).	2	3	3
WARFARIN Concurrent use of CLOMIPRAMINE and WARFARIN may result in an increased risk of bleeding.	2	3	3

Clonazepam

INTERACTION	ONSET	SEVERITY	EVIDENCE
CARBAMAZEPINE Concurrent use of CLONAZEPAM and CARBAMAZEPINE may result in reduced plasma levels of clonazepam.	2	3	3
CIMETIDINE Concurrent use of CLONAZEPAM and CIMETIDINE may result in clonazepam toxicity (central nervous system depression).	1	4	3
KETOCONAZOLE Concurrent use of CLONAZEPAM and KETOCONAZOLE may result in increased clonazepam serum concentrations and clonazepam adverse effects (sedation, slurred speech, central nervous system depression).	2	4	3
THEOPHYLLINE Concurrent use of CLONAZEPAM and THEOPHYLLINE may result in decreased clonazepam effectiveness.	1	3	2

Clorazepate

INTERACTION	ONSET	SEVERITY	EVIDENCE
CIMETIDINE Concurrent use of CLORAZEPATE and CIMETIDINE may result in clorazepate toxicity (central nervous system depression).	1	4	3
ETHANOL Concurrent use of CLORAZEPATE and ETHANOL may result in increased sedation.	1	3	2
KETOCONAZOLE Concurrent use of CLORAZEPATE and KETOCONAZOLE may result in increased clorazepate serum concentrations and clorazepate adverse effects (sedation, slurred speech, central nervous system depression).	2	4	3
THEOPHYLLINE Concurrent use of CLORAZEPATE and THEOPHYLLINE may result in decreased benzodiazepine effectiveness.	1	3	2

Clozapine

INTERACTION	ONSET	SEVERITY	EVIDENCE
CARBAMAZEPINE Concurrent use of CLOZAPINE and CARBAMAZEPINE may result in an increased risk of bone marrow suppression, involuntary jerking movements, or decreased serum clozapine levels.	2	2	3
DROPERIDOL Concurrent use of CLOZAPINE and DROPERIDOL may result in an increased risk of cardiotoxicity (irregular heartbeat, cardiac arrest).	1	2	3
ERYTHROMYCIN Concurrent use of CLOZAPINE and ERYTHROMYCIN may result in increased clozapine serum concentrations and risk of side effects (sedation, incoordination, slurred speech, seizures, blood abnormalities).	2	3	3
FLUOXETINE Concurrent use of CLOZAPINE and FLUOXETINE may result in an increased risk of clozapine toxicity (sedation, seizures, low blood pressure).	2	3	3
FOSPHENYTOIN Concurrent use of CLOZAPINE and FOSPHENYTOIN may result in decreased clozapine plasma levels associated with marked worsening of psychosis.	2	3	3
GUARANA Concomitant administration of CLOZAPINE and GUARANA may lead to increased clozapine levels, (blood disorders and seizures) or increased guarana levels, (headache, insomnia, restlessness, fluid loss, rapid heartbeat).	2	2	3

Onset: 0=Unspecified 1=Rapid 2=Delayed
Severity: 1=Contraindicated 2=Major 3=Moderate 4=Minor
Evidence: 1=Excellent 2=Good 3=Fair 4=Poor

INTERACTION	ONSET	SEVERITY	EVIDENCE
LITHIUM Concurrent use of CLOZAPINE and LITHIUM may result in weakness, movement disorders, brain disorders, and brain damage.	2	2	1
LORAZEPAM Concurrent use of CLOZAPINE and LORAZEPAM may result in central nervous system depression.	1	4	3
PHENOBARBITAL Concurrent use of CLOZAPINE and PHENOBARBITAL may result in decreased clozapine plasma levels associated with marked worsening of psychosis.	2	3	3
PHENYTOIN Concurrent administration of CLOZAPINE and PHENYTOIN may result in decreased clozapine plasma levels associated with marked worsening of psychosis.	2	3	3
SERTRALINE Concurrent use of CLOZAPINE and SERTRALINE may result in an increased risk of clozapine toxicity (sedation, seizures, low blood pressure).	2	3	3
TRAMADOL Concurrent use of CLOZAPINE and TRAMADOL may result in an increased risk of seizures.	1	2	3

Desipramine

INTERACTION	ONSET	SEVERITY	EVIDENCE
ACENOCOUMAROL Concurrent use of DESIPRAMINE and ACENOCOUMAROL may result in increased risk of bleeding.	2	3	3
AMPRENAVIR Concurrent use of DESIPRAMINE and AMPRENAVIR may result in increased desipramine serum concentrations and potential toxicity (antispasmodic effects, sedation, confusion, cardiac irregularities).	2	2	3
ANISINDIONE Concurrent use of DESIPRAMINE and ANISINDIONE may result in increased risk of bleeding.	2	3	3
BEPRIDIL Concurrent use of DESIPRAMINE and BEPRIDIL may result in cardiac irregularities.	1	1	3
BETHANIDINE Concurrent use of DESIPRAMINE and BETHANIDINE may result in decreased antihypertensive effectiveness.	1	3	2
CIMETIDINE Concurrent use of DESIPRAMINE and CIMETIDINE may result in desipramine toxicity (dry mouth, blurred vision, urinary retention).	2	3	2

INTERACTION	ONSET	SEVERITY	EVIDENCE
CISAPRIDE Concurrent use of DESIPRAMINE and CISAPRIDE may result in cardiotoxicity (irregular heartbeat, cardiac arrest).	1	1	3
CLONIDINE Concurrent use of DESIPRAMINE and CLONIDINE may result in decreased antihypertensive effectiveness.	2	2	2
CLORGYLINE Concurrent use of DESIPRAMINE and CLORGYLINE may result in neurotoxicity, seizures, or serotonin syndrome (high blood pressure, high fever, spasms, mental status changes).	2	2	3
DICUMAROL Concurrent use of DESIPRAMINE and DICUMAROL may result in increased risk of bleeding.	2	3	3
DROPERIDOL Concurrent use of DESIPRAMINE and DROPERIDOL may result in an increased risk of cardiotoxicity (irregular heartbeat, cardiac arrest).	1	2	3
EPINEPHRINE Concurrent use of DESIPRAMINE and EPINEPHRINE may result in high blood pressure, cardiac irregularities, and rapid heartbeat.	1	2	2
ETILEFRINE Concurrent use of DESIPRAMINE and ETILEFRINE may result in high blood pressure, cardiac irregularities, and rapid heartbeat.	1	2	2
FLUOXETINE Concurrent use of DESIPRAMINE and FLUOXETINE may result in desipramine toxicity (dry mouth, urinary retention, sedation).	2	3	2
GREPAFLOXACIN Concurrent use of DESIPRAMINE and GREPAFLOXACIN may result in an increased risk of cardiotoxicity (irregular heartbeat, cardiac arrest).	2	1	3
GUANADREL Concurrent use of DESIPRAMINE and GUANADREL may result in decreased antihypertensive effectiveness.	2	3	3
GUANETHIDINE Concurrent use of DESIPRAMINE and GUANETHIDINE may result in decreased antihypertensive effectiveness.	2	3	1
HALOFANTRINE Concurrent use of DESIPRAMINE and HALOFANTRINE may result in cardiotoxicity (irregular heartbeat, cardiac arrest).	2	2	3
ISOCARBOXAZID Concurrent use of DESIPRAMINE and ISOCARBOXAZID may result in neurotoxicity, seizures, or serotonin syndrome (high blood pressure, high fever, spasms, mental status changes).	2	1	3

Onset: 0=Unspecified 1=Rapid 2=Delayed
Severity: 1=Contraindicated 2=Major 3=Moderate 4=Minor
Evidence: 1=Excellent 2=Good 3=Fair 4=Poor

INTERACTION	ONSET	SEVERITY	EVIDENCE
LEVOMETHADYL Concurrent use of DESIPRAMINE and LEVOMETHADYL may result in an increased risk of cardiotoxicity (irregular heartbeat, cardiac arrest).	2	1	3
METHOXAMINE Concurrent use of DESIPRAMINE and METHOXAMINE may result in high blood pressure, cardiac irregularities, and rapid heartbeat.	1	2	2
MIDODRINE Concurrent use of DESIPRAMINE and MIDODRINE may result in high blood pressure, cardiac irregularities, and rapid heartbeat.	1	2	2
MOCLOBEMIDE Concurrent use of DESIPRAMINE and MOCLOBEMIDE may result in neurotoxicity, seizures, or serotonin syndrome (high blood pressure, high fever, spasms, mental status changes).	2	2	3
NOREPINEPHRINE Concurrent use of DESIPRAMINE and NOREPINEPHRINE may result in high blood pressure, cardiac irregularities, and rapid heartbeat.	1	2	2
OXILOFRINE Concurrent use of DESIPRAMINE and OXILOFRINE may result in high blood pressure, cardiac irregularities, and rapid heartbeat.	1	2	2
PHENELZINE Concurrent use of DESIPRAMINE and PHENELZINE may result in neurotoxicity, seizures, or serotonin syndrome (high blood pressure, high fever, spasms, mental status changes).	2	2	3
PHENINDIONE Concurrent use of DESIPRAMINE and PHENINDIONE may result in increased risk of bleeding.	2	3	3
PHENPROCOUMON Concurrent use of DESIPRAMINE and PHENPRO-COUMON may result in increased risk of bleeding.	2	3	3
PHENYLEPHRINE Concurrent use of DESIPRAMINE and PHENYLEPHRINE may result in high blood pressure, cardiac irregularities, and rapid heartbeat.	1	2	2
PIMOZIDE Concurrent use of DESIPRAMINE and PIMOZIDE may result in an increased risk of cardiotoxicity (irregular heartbeat, cardiac arrest).	1	1	3
PROCARBAZINE Concurrent use of DESIPRAMINE and PROCARBAZINE may result in neurotoxicity, seizures.	2	2	3
QUINIDINE Concurrent use of DESIPRAMINE and QUINIDINE may result in desipramine toxicity (dry mouth, sedation) and an increased risk of cardiotoxicity.	2	3	3

INTERACTION	ONSET	SEVERITY	EVIDENCE
RITONAVIR Concurrent use of DESIPRAMINE and RITONAVIR may result in increased desipramine plasma concentrations and potential desipramine toxicity (dry mouth, urinary retention, sedation, blurred vision).	2	3	3
SELEGILINE Concurrent use of DESIPRAMINE and SELEGILINE may result in neurotoxicity, seizures, or serotonin syndrome (high blood pressure, high fever, spasms, mental status changes).	2	2	3
SPARFLOXACIN Concurrent use of DESIPRAMINE and SPARFLOXACIN may result in irregular heartbeat.	2	1	3
TRAMADOL Concurrent use of DESIPRAMINE and TRAMADOL may result in an increased risk of seizures.	1	2	3
TRANYLCYPROMINE Concurrent use of DESIPRAMINE and TRANYL-CYPROMINE may result in neurotoxicity, seizures, or serotonin syndrome (high blood pressure, high fever, spasms, mental status changes).	2	2	3
WARFARIN Concurrent use of DESIPRAMINE and WARFARIN may result in an increased risk of bleeding.	2	3	3

Dexmethylphenidate

INTERACTION	ONSET	SEVERITY	EVIDENCE
CLORGYLINE Concurrent use of DEXMETHYLPHENIDATE and CLORGYLINE may result in hypertensive crisis (headache, palpitation, neck stiffness).	1	1	3
COUMARIN Concurrent use of DEXMETHYLPHENIDATE and COUMARIN may result in an increased risk of bleeding.	1	3	3
IPRONIAZID Concurrent use of DEXMETHYLPHENIDATE and IPRONIAZID may result in hypertensive crisis (headache, palpitation, neck stiffness).	1	1	3
ISOCARBOXAZID Concurrent use of DEXMETHYLPHENIDATE and ISOCARBOXAZID may result in hypertensive crisis (headache, palpitation, neck stiffness).	1	1	3
LAZABEMIDE Concurrent use of DEXMETHYLPHENIDATE and LAZABEMIDE may result in hypertensive crisis (headache, palpitation, neck stiffness).	1	1	3

Onset: 0=Unspecified 1=Rapid 2=Delayed
Severity: 1=Contraindicated 2=Major 3=Moderate 4=Minor
Evidence: 1=Excellent 2=Good 3=Fair 4=Poor

INTERACTION	ONSET	SEVERITY	EVIDENCE
MOCLOBEMIDE Concurrent use of DEXMETHYLPHENIDATE and MOCLOBEMIDE may result in hypertensive crisis (headache, palpitation, neck stiffness).	1	1	3
NIALAMIDE Concurrent use of DEXMETHYLPHENIDATE and NIALAMIDE may result in hypertensive crisis (headache, palpitation, neck stiffness).	1	1	3
PARGYLINE Concurrent use of DEXMETHYLPHENIDATE and PARGYLINE may result in hypertensive crisis (headache, palpitation, neck stiffness).	1	1	3
PHENELZINE Concurrent use of DEXMETHYLPHENIDATE and PHENELZINE may result in hypertensive crisis (headache, palpitation, neck stiffness).	1	1	3
PHENOBARBITAL Concurrent use of DEXMETHYLPHENIDATE and PHENOBARBITAL may result in an increase in phenobarbital plasma concentrations.	1	3	3
PHENYTOIN Concurrent use of DEXMETHYLPHENIDATE and PHENYTOIN may result in an increase in phenytoin plasma concentrations.	1	3	3
PRIMIDONE Concurrent use of DEXMETHYLPHENIDATE and PRIMIDONE may result in an increase in primidone plasma concentrations.	1	3	3
PROCARBAZINE Concurrent use of DEXMETHYLPHENIDATE and PROCARBAZINE may result in hypertensive crisis (headache, palpitation, neck stiffness).	1	1	3
SELEGILINE Concurrent use of DEXMETHYLPHENIDATE and SELEGILINE may result in hypertensive crisis (headache, palpitation, neck stiffness).	1	1	3
TOLOXATONE Concurrent use of DEXMETHYLPHENIDATE and TOLOXATONE may result in hypertensive crisis (headache, palpitation, neck stiffness).	1	1	3
TRANYLCYPROMINE Concurrent use of DEXMETHYLPHENIDATE and TRANYLCYPROMINE may result in hypertensive crisis (headache, palpitation, neck stiffness).	1	1	3

Dextroamphetamine

INTERACTION	ONSET	SEVERITY	EVIDENCE
ACETAZOLAMIDE Concurrent use of DEXTROAMPHETAMINE and ACETAZOLAMIDE may result in amphetamine toxicity (high blood pressure, high fever, seizures).	1	3	2
ACIDIC FOODS Concurrent use of DEXTROAMPHETAMINE and ACIDIC FOODS may result in altered serum concentrations.	1	4	2
CLORGYLINE Concurrent use of DEXTROAMPHETAMINE and CLORGYLINE may result in a hypertensive crisis (headache, high fever, high blood pressure).	1	1	3
FURAZOLIDONE Concurrent use of DEXTROAMPHETAMINE and FURAZOLIDONE may result in a hypertensive crisis (headache, high fever, high blood pressure).	1	1	3
IPRONIAZID Concurrent use of DEXTROAMPHETAMINE and IPRONIAZID may result in a hypertensive crisis (headache, high fever, high blood pressure).	1	1	3
ISOCARBOXAZID Concurrent use of DEXTROAMPHETAMINE and ISOCARBOXAZID may result in a hypertensive crisis (headache, high fever, high blood pressure).	1	1	3
MOCLOBEMIDE Concurrent use of DEXTROAMPHETAMINE and MOCLOBEMIDE may result in a hypertensive crisis (headache, high fever, high blood pressure).	1	1	3
NIALAMIDE Concurrent use of DEXTROAMPHETAMINE and NIALAMIDE may result in a hypertensive crisis (headache, high fever, high blood pressure).	1	1	3
PARGYLINE Concurrent use of DEXTROAMPHETAMINE and PARGYLINE may result in a hypertensive crisis (headache, high fever, high blood pressure).	1	1	1
PHENELZINE Concurrent use of DEXTROAMPHETAMINE and PHENELZINE may result in a hypertensive crisis (headache, high fever, high blood pressure).	1	1	3
PROCARBAZINE Concurrent use of DEXTROAMPHETAMINE and PROCARBAZINE may result in a hypertensive crisis (headache, high fever, high blood pressure).	1	1	3

Onset: 0=Unspecified 1=Rapid 2=Delayed
Severity: 1=Contraindicated 2=Major 3=Moderate 4=Minor
Evidence: 1=Excellent 2=Good 3=Fair 4=Poor

INTERACTION	ONSET	SEVERITY	EVIDENCE
SELEGILINE Concurrent use of DEXTROAMPHETAMINE and SELEGILINE may result in a hypertensive crisis (headache, high fever, high blood pressure).	1	1	3
SIBUTRAMINE Concurrent use of DEXTROAMPHETAMINE and SIBUTRAMINE may result in an increased risk of high blood pressure and rapid heartbeat.	1	1	3
SODIUM BICARBONATE Concurrent use of DEXTROAMPHETAMINE and SODIUM BICARBONATE may result in amphetamine toxicity (high blood pressure, high fever, seizures).	2	3	3
TOLOXATONE Concurrent use of DEXTROAMPHETAMINE and TOLOXATONE may result in a hypertensive crisis (headache, high fever, high blood pressure).	1	1	3
TRANYLCYPROMINE Concurrent use of DEXTROAMPHETAMINE and TRANYLCYPROMINE may result in a hypertensive crisis (headache, high fever, high blood pressure).	1	1	3

Diazepam

INTERACTION	ONSET	SEVERITY	EVIDENCE
CIMETIDINE Concurrent use of DIAZEPAM and CIMETIDINE may result in diazepam toxicity (central nervous system depression).	1	4	2
CLARITHROMYCIN Concurrent use of DIAZEPAM and CLARITHROMYCIN may result in increased diazepam toxicity (central nervous system depression, poor coordination, lethargy).	2	3	3
DISULFIRAM Concurrent use of DIAZEPAM and DISULFIRAM may result in an increased risk of central nervous system depression.	2	3	3
ERYTHROMYCIN Concurrent use of DIAZEPAM and ERYTHROMYCIN may result in increased diazepam toxicity (central nervous system depression, poor coordination, lethargy).	2	3	3
ETHANOL Concurrent use of DIAZEPAM and ETHANOL may result in increased sedation.	1	3	1
FLUOXETINE Concurrent use of DIAZEPAM and FLUOXETINE may result in higher serum concentrations of diazepam.	2	4	3
FLUVOXAMINE Concurrent use of DIAZEPAM and FLUVOXAMINE may result in diazepam and N-desmethyldiazepam accumulation.	2	3	2

INTERACTION	ONSET	SEVERITY	EVIDENCE
FOOD Concurrent use of DIAZEPAM and FOOD may result in increased diazepam concentrations.	1	4	3
ITRACONAZOLE Concurrent use of DIAZEPAM and ITRACONAZOLE may result in increased diazepam serum concentrations and diazepam adverse effects (sedation, slurred speech, central nervous system depression).	2	3	3
JOSAMYCIN Concurrent use of DIAZEPAM and JOSAMYCIN may result in increased diazepam toxicity (central nervous system depression, poor coordination, lethargy).	2	3	3
KETOCONAZOLE Concurrent use of DIAZEPAM and KETOCONAZOLE may result in increased diazepam serum concentrations and diazepam adverse effects (sedation, slurred speech, central nervous system depression).	2	4	3
RIFAMPIN Concurrent use of DIAZEPAM and RIFAMPIN may result in decreased diazepam effectiveness.	2	3	3
ROXITHROMYCIN Concurrent use of DIAZEPAM and ROXITHROMYCIN may result in increased diazepam toxicity (central nervous system depression, poor coordination, lethargy).	2	3	3
THEOPHYLLINE Concurrent use of DIAZEPAM and THEOPHYLLINE may result in decreased diazepam effectiveness.	1	3	2
TROLEANDOMYCIN Concurrent use of DIAZEPAM and TROLEANDOMYCIN may result in increased diazepam toxicity (central nervous system depression, poor coordination, lethargy).	2	3	3

Donepezil

INTERACTION	ONSET	SEVERITY	EVIDENCE
SUCCINYLCHOLINE Concurrent use of DONEPEZIL and SUCCINYLCHOLINE may result in prolonged neuromuscular blockade (paralysis).	1	2	3

Doxepin

INTERACTION	ONSET	SEVERITY	EVIDENCE
ACENOCOUMAROL Concurrent use of DOXEPIN and ACENOCOUMAROL may result in increased risk of bleeding.	2	3	3

Onset: 0=Unspecified 1=Rapid 2=Delayed
Severity: 1=Contraindicated 2=Major 3=Moderate 4=Minor
Evidence: 1=Excellent 2=Good 3=Fair 4=Poor

INTERACTION	ONSET	SEVERITY	EVIDENCE
AMPRENAVIR Concurrent use of DOXEPIN and AMPRENAVIR may result in increased doxepin serum concentrations and potential toxicity (antispasmodic effects, sedation, confusion, cardiac irregularities).	2	2	3
ANISINDIONE Concurrent use of DOXEPIN and ANISINDIONE may result in increased risk of bleeding.	2	3	3
BEPRIDIL Concurrent use of DOXEPIN and BEPRIDIL may result in cardiac irregularities.	1	1	3
BETHANIDINE Concurrent use of DOXEPIN and BETHANIDINE may result in decreased antihypertensive effectiveness.	1	3	2
CIMETIDINE Concurrent use of DOXEPIN and CIMETIDINE may result in doxepin toxicity (dry mouth, blurred vision, urinary retention).	2	3	2
CISAPRIDE Concurrent use of DOXEPIN and CISAPRIDE may result in cardiotoxicity (irregular heartbeat, cardiac arrest).	1	1	3
CLONIDINE Concurrent use of DOXEPIN and CLONIDINE may result in decreased antihypertensive effectiveness.	2	2	3
CLORGYLINE Concurrent use of DOXEPIN and CLORGYLINE may result in neurotoxicity, seizures, or serotonin syndrome (high blood pressure, high fever, spasms, mental status changes).	2	2	3
DICUMAROL Concurrent use of DOXEPIN and DICUMAROL may result in increased risk of bleeding.	2	3	3
DROPERIDOL Concurrent use of DOXEPIN and DROPERIDOL may result in an increased risk of cardiotoxicity (irregular heartbeat, cardiac arrest).	1	2	3
EPINEPHRINE Concurrent use of DOXEPIN and EPINEPHRINE may result in high blood pressure, cardiac irregularities, and rapid heartbeat.	1	2	2
ETILEFRINE Concurrent use of DOXEPIN and ETILEFRINE may result in high blood pressure, cardiac irregularities, and rapid heartbeat.	1	2	2
FLUOXETINE Concurrent use of DOXEPIN and FLUOXETINE may result in doxepin toxicity (dry mouth, urinary retention, sedation).	2	3	3
GREPAFLOXACIN Concurrent use of DOXEPIN and GREPAFLOXACIN may result in an increased risk of cardiotoxicity (irregular heartbeat, cardiac arrest).	2	1	3

INTERACTION	ONSET	SEVERITY	EVIDENCE
GUANADREL Concurrent use of DOXEPIN and GUANADREL may result in decreased antihypertensive effectiveness.	2	3	3
GUANETHIDINE Concurrent use of DOXEPIN and GUANETHIDINE may result in decreased antihypertensive effectiveness.	2	3	3
HALOFANTRINE Concurrent use of DOXEPIN and HALOFANTRINE may result in cardiotoxicity (irregular heartbeat, cardiac arrest).	2	2	3
IBUTILIDE Concurrent use of DOXEPIN and IBUTILIDE may result in an increased risk of irregularities.	1	2	3
ISOCARBOXAZID Concurrent use of DOXEPIN and ISOCARBOXAZID may result in neurotoxicity, seizures, or serotonin syndrome (high blood pressure, high fever, spasms, mental status changes).	2	1	3
METHOXAMINE Concurrent use of DOXEPIN and METHOXAMINE may result in high blood pressure, cardiac irregularities, and rapid heartbeat.	1	2	2
MIDODRINE Concurrent use of DOXEPIN and MIDODRINE may result in high blood pressure, cardiac irregularities, and rapid heartbeat.	1	2	2
MOCLOBEMIDE Concurrent use of DOXEPIN and MOCLOBEMIDE may result in neurotoxicity, seizures, or serotonin syndrome (high blood pressure, high fever, spasms, mental status changes).	2	2	3
NOREPINEPHRINE Concurrent use of DOXEPIN and NOREPINEPHRINE may result in high blood pressure, cardiac irregularities, and rapid heartbeat.	1	2	2
OXILOFRINE Concurrent use of DOXEPIN and OXILOFRINE may result in high blood pressure, cardiac irregularities, and rapid heartbeat.	1	2	2
PHENELZINE Concurrent use of DOXEPIN and PHENELZINE may result in neurotoxicity, seizures, or serotonin syndrome (high blood pressure, high fever, spasms, mental status changes).	2	2	3
PHENINDIONE Concurrent use of DOXEPIN and PHENINDIONE may result in increased risk of bleeding.	2	3	3
PHENPROCOUMON Concurrent use of DOXEPIN and PHENPROCOUMON may result in increased risk of bleeding.	2	3	3

Onset: 0=Unspecified 1=Rapid 2=Delayed
Severity: 1=Contraindicated 2=Major 3=Moderate 4=Minor
Evidence: 1=Excellent 2=Good 3=Fair 4=Poor

INTERACTION	ONSET	SEVERITY	EVIDENCE
PHENYLEPHRINE Concurrent use of DOXEPIN and PHENYLEPHRINE may result in high blood pressure, cardiac irregularities, and rapid heartbeat.	1	2	2
PIMOZIDE Concurrent use of DOXEPIN and PIMOZIDE may result in an increased risk of cardiotoxicity (irregular heartbeat, cardiac arrest).	1	1	3
PROCARBAZINE Concurrent use of DOXEPIN and PROCARBAZINE may result in neurotoxicity, seizures.	2	2	3
SELEGILINE Concurrent use of DOXEPIN and SELEGILINE may result in neurotoxicity, seizures, or serotonin syndrome (high blood pressure, high fever, spasms, mental status changes).	2	2	3
SPARFLOXACIN Concurrent use of DOXEPIN and SPARFLOXACIN may result in irregular heartbeat.	2	1	3
TRAMADOL Concurrent use of DOXEPIN and TRAMADOL may result in an increased risk of seizures.	1	2	3
TRANYLCYPROMINE Concurrent use of DOXEPIN and TRANYLCYPROMINE may result in neurotoxicity, seizures, or serotonin syndrome (high blood pressure, high fever, spasms, mental status changes).	2	2	3
WARFARIN Concurrent use of DOXEPIN and WARFARIN may result in an increased risk of bleeding.	2	3	3

Estazolam

INTERACTION	ONSET	SEVERITY	EVIDENCE
CIMETIDINE Concurrent use of ESTAZOLAM and CIMETIDINE may result in estazolam toxicity (central nervous system depression).	1	4	3
KETOCONAZOLE Concurrent use of ESTAZOLAM and KETOCONAZOLE may result in increased estazolam serum concentrations and estazolam adverse effects (sedation, slurred speech, central nervous system depression).	2	4	3
THEOPHYLLINE Concurrent use of ESTAZOLAM and THEOPHYLLINE may result in decreased estazolam effectiveness.	1	3	2

Fluoxetine

INTERACTION	ONSET	SEVERITY	EVIDENCE
ALMOTRIPTAN Concurrent use of FLUOXETINE and ALMOTRIPTAN may result in weakness, exaggerated reflexes, and/or incoordination.	0	3	3

INTERACTION	ONSET	SEVERITY	EVIDENCE
ALPRAZOLAM Concurrent use of FLUOXETINE and ALPRAZOLAM may result in an increased risk of alprazolam toxicity (somnolence, dizziness, poor coordination, slurred speech, low blood pressure, psychomotor impairment).	1	3	2
AMITRIPTYLINE Concurrent use of FLUOXETINE and AMITRIPTYLINE may result in amitriptyline toxicity (dry mouth, urinary retention, sedation).	2	3	3
AMOXAPINE Concurrent use of FLUOXETINE and AMOXAPINE may result in increased amoxapine concentration and toxicity (antispasmodic effects, sedation, cardiac effects).	2	3	3
ASTEMIZOLE Concurrent use of FLUOXETINE and ASTEMIZOLE may result in cardiotoxicity (irregular heartbeat, cardiac arrest).	1	2	3
CLOMIPRAMINE Concurrent use of FLUOXETINE and CLOMIPRAMINE may result in clomipramine toxicity (dry mouth, urinary retention, sedation).	2	3	3
CLORGYLINE Concurrent use of FLUOXETINE and CLORGYLINE may result in central nervous system toxicity or serotonin syndrome (high blood pressure, high fever, spasms, mental status changes).	1	1	2
CLOZAPINE Concurrent use of FLUOXETINE and CLOZAPINE may result in an increased risk of clozapine toxicity (sedation, seizures, low blood pressure).	2	3	3
DESIPRAMINE Concurrent use of FLUOXETINE and DESIPRAMINE may result in desipramine toxicity (dry mouth, urinary retention, sedation).	2	3	2
DEXFENFLURAMINE Concurrent use of FLUOXETINE and DEXFENFLURAMINE may result in serotonin syndrome (high blood pressure, high fever, spasms, mental status changes).	1	2	3
DEXTROMETHORPHAN Concurrent use of FLUOXETINE and DEXTROMETHORPHAN may result in possible dextromethorphan toxicity (nausea, vomiting, blurred vision, hallucinations) or serotonin syndrome (high blood pressure, high fever, spasms, mental status changes).	1	2	3
DIAZEPAM Concurrent use of FLUOXETINE and DIAZEPAM may result in higher serum concentrations of diazepam.	2	4	3

Onset: 0=Unspecified 1=Rapid 2=Delayed
Severity: 1=Contraindicated 2=Major 3=Moderate 4=Minor
Evidence: 1=Excellent 2=Good 3=Fair 4=Poor

INTERACTION	ONSET	SEVERITY	EVIDENCE
DOTHIEPIN Concurrent use of FLUOXETINE and DOTHIEPIN may result in dothiepin toxicity (dry mouth, urinary retention, sedation).	2	3	3
DOXEPIN Concurrent use of FLUOXETINE and DOXEPIN may result in doxepin toxicity (dry mouth, urinary retention, sedation).	2	3	3
DROPERIDOL Concurrent use of FLUOXETINE and DROPERIDOL may result in an increased risk of cardiotoxicity (irregular heartbeat, cardiac arrest).	1	2	3
FENFLURAMINE Concurrent use of FLUOXETINE and FENFLURAMINE may result in serotonin syndrome (high blood pressure, high fever, spasms, mental status changes).	1	2	3
FOSPHENYTOIN Concurrent use of FLUOXETINE and FOSPHENYTOIN may result in an increased risk of phenytoin toxicity (poor coordination, exaggerated reflexes, rolling eyes, tremor).	2	3	3
FURAZOLIDONE Concurrent use of FLUOXETINE and FURAZOLIDONE may result in weakness, exaggerated reflexes, and incoordination.	2	1	3
HYDROXYTRYPTOPHAN Concurrent use of FLUOXETINE and HYDROXYTRYPTOPHAN may result in an increased risk of serotonin syndrome (high blood pressure, high fever, spasms, mental status changes).	1	3	3
IMIPRAMINE Concurrent use of FLUOXETINE and IMIPRAMINE may result in imipramine toxicity (dry mouth, urinary retention, sedation).	2	3	3
IPRONIAZID Concurrent use of FLUOXETINE and IPRONIAZID may result in central nervous system toxicity or serotonin syndrome (high blood pressure, high fever, spasms, mental status changes).	1	1	2
ISOCARBOXAZID Concurrent use of FLUOXETINE and ISOCARBOXAZID may result in central nervous system toxicity or serotonin syndrome (high blood pressure, high fever, spasms, mental status changes).	1	1	2
LEVOMETHADYL Concurrent use of FLUOXETINE and LEVOMETHADYL may result in an increased risk of cardiotoxicity (irregular heartbeat, cardiac arrest).	2	1	3

INTERACTION	ONSET	SEVERITY	EVIDENCE
MOCLOBEMIDE Concurrent use of FLUOXETINE and MOCLOBEMIDE may result in central nervous system toxicity or serotonin syndrome (high blood pressure, high fever, spasms, mental status changes).	1	1	3
NIALAMIDE Concurrent use of FLUOXETINE and NIALAMIDE may result in central nervous system toxicity or serotonin syndrome (high blood pressure, high fever, spasms, mental status changes).	1	1	2
NORTRIPTYLINE Concurrent use of FLUOXETINE and NORTRIPTYLINE may result in nortriptyline toxicity (dry mouth, urinary retention, sedation).	2	3	3
PARGYLINE Concurrent use of FLUOXETINE and PARGYLINE may result in central nervous system toxicity or serotonin syndrome (high blood pressure, high fever, spasms, mental status changes).	1	1	2
PHENELZINE Concurrent use of FLUOXETINE and PHENELZINE may result in central nervous system toxicity or serotonin syndrome (high blood pressure, high fever, spasms, mental status changes).	1	1	2
PHENYTOIN Concurrent use of FLUOXETINE and PHENYTOIN may result in an increased risk of phenytoin toxicity (poor coordination, exaggerated reflexes, rolling eyes, tremor).	2	3	3
PROCARBAZINE Concurrent use of FLUOXETINE and PROCARBAZINE may result in central nervous system toxicity or serotonin syndrome (high blood pressure, high fever, spasms, mental status changes).	1	1	2
PROTRIPTYLINE Concurrent use of FLUOXETINE and PROTRIPTYLINE may result in protriptyline toxicity (dry mouth, urinary retention, sedation).	2	3	3
SELEGILINE Concurrent use of FLUOXETINE and SELEGILINE may result in central nervous system toxicity or serotonin syndrome (high blood pressure, high fever, spasms, mental status changes).	1	1	2
SIBUTRAMINE Concurrent use of FLUOXETINE and SIBUTRAMINE may result in an increased risk of serotonin syndrome (high blood pressure, high fever, spasms, mental status changes).	1	2	3

Onset: 0=Unspecified 1=Rapid 2=Delayed
Severity: 1=Contraindicated 2=Major 3=Moderate 4=Minor
Evidence: 1=Excellent 2=Good 3=Fair 4=Poor

INTERACTION	ONSET	SEVERITY	EVIDENCE
THIORIDAZINE Concurrent use of FLUOXETINE and THIORIDAZINE may result in an increased risk of thioridazine toxicity and cardiotoxicity (irregular heartbeat, cardiac arrest).	1	1	3
TOLOXATONE Concurrent use of FLUOXETINE and TOLOXATONE may result in central nervous system toxicity or serotonin syndrome (high blood pressure, high fever, spasms, mental status changes).	1	1	2
TRAMADOL Concurrent use of FLUOXETINE and TRAMADOL may result in an increased risk of seizures and serotonin syndrome (high blood pressure, high fever, spasms, mental status changes).	1	2	2
TRANYLCYPROMINE Concurrent use of FLUOXETINE and TRANYLCYPROMINE may result in central nervous system toxicity or serotonin syndrome (high blood pressure, high fever, spasms, mental status changes).	1	1	2
TRAZODONE Concurrent use of FLUOXETINE and TRAZODONE may result in trazodone toxicity (sedation, dry mouth, urinary retention) or serotonin syndrome (high blood pressure, high fever, spasms, mental status changes).	2	2	3
TRIMIPRAMINE Concurrent use of FLUOXETINE and TRIMIPRAMINE may result in trimipramine toxicity (dry mouth, urinary retention, sedation).	2	3	3
TRYPTOPHAN Concurrent use of FLUOXETINE and TRYPTOPHAN may result in serotonin syndrome (high blood pressure, high fever, spasms, mental status changes).	2	2	3
WARFARIN Concurrent use of FLUOXETINE and WARFARIN may result in an increased risk of bleeding.	2	3	3

Fluphenazine

INTERACTION	ONSET	SEVERITY	EVIDENCE
BELLADONNA Concurrent use of FLUPHENAZINE and BELLADONNA may result in increased manic, agitated reactions, or enhanced antispasmodic effects resulting in cardiorespiratory failure, especially in cases of belladonna overdose.	1	3	2
BENZTROPINE Concurrent use of FLUPHENAZINE and BENZTROPINE may result in decreased fluphenazine serum concentrations, decreased fluphenazine effectiveness, enhanced antispasmodic effects (intestinal blockage, high fever, sedation, dry mouth).	2	3	3

INTERACTION	ONSET	SEVERITY	EVIDENCE
CABERGOLINE Concurrent use of FLUPHENAZINE and CABERGOLINE may result in the decreased therapeutic effect of both drugs.	1	3	3
CISAPRIDE Concurrent use of FLUPHENAZINE and CISAPRIDE may result in cardiotoxicity (irregular heartbeat, cardiac arrest).	1	1	3
ETHANOL Concurrent use of FLUPHENAZINE and ETHANOL may result in increased central nervous system depression and an increased risk of movement disorders.	1	3	2
FOSPHENYTOIN Concurrent use of FLUPHENAZINE and FOSPHENYTOIN may result in increased or decreased phenytoin levels and possibly reduced fluphenazine levels.	2	4	3
GREPAFLOXACIN Concurrent use of FLUPHENAZINE and GREPAFLOXACIN may result in an increased risk of cardiotoxicity (irregular heartbeat, cardiac arrest).	2	1	3
HALOFANTRINE Concurrent use of FLUPHENAZINE and HALOFANTRINE may result in cardiotoxicity (irregular heartbeat, cardiac arrest).	2	2	3
LEVODOPA Concurrent use of FLUPHENAZINE and LEVODOPA may result in loss of levodopa efficacy.	1	3	2
LITHIUM Concurrent use of FLUPHENAZINE and LITHIUM may result in weakness, movement disorders, brain disorders, and brain damage.	2	2	1
MEPERIDINE Concurrent use of FLUPHENAZINE and MEPERIDINE may result in an increase in central nervous system and respiratory depression.	1	3	2
ORPHENADRINE Concurrent use of FLUPHENAZINE and ORPHENADRINE may result in decreased fluphenazine serum concentrations, decreased fluphenazine effectiveness, enhanced antispasmodic effects (intestinal blockage, high fever, sedation, dry mouth).	2	3	3
PHENYTOIN Concurrent use of FLUPHENAZINE and PHENYTOIN may result in increased or decreased phenytoin levels and possibly reduced fluphenazine levels.	2	4	3
PORFIMER Concurrent use of FLUPHENAZINE and PORFIMER may result in excessive intracellular damage in photosensitized tissues.	2	3	3

Onset: 0=Unspecified 1=Rapid 2=Delayed
Severity: 1=Contraindicated 2=Major 3=Moderate 4=Minor
Evidence: 1=Excellent 2=Good 3=Fair 4=Poor

INTERACTION	ONSET	SEVERITY	EVIDENCE
PROCYCLIDINE Concurrent use of FLUPHENAZINE and PROCYCLIDINE may result in decreased fluphenazine serum concentrations, decreased fluphenazine effectiveness, enhanced antispasmodic effects (intestinal blockage, high fever, sedation, dry mouth).	2	3	3
SPARFLOXACIN Concurrent use of FLUPHENAZINE and SPARFLOXACIN may result in irregular heartbeat.	2	1	3
TRAMADOL Concurrent use of FLUPHENAZINE and TRAMADOL may result in an increased risk of seizures.	1	2	3
TRIHEXYPHENIDYL Concurrent use of FLUPHENAZINE and TRIHEXYPHENIDYL may result in decreased fluphenazine serum concentrations, decreased fluphenazine effectiveness, enhanced antispasmodic effects (intestinal blockage, high fever, sedation, dry mouth).	2	3	3

Flurazepam

INTERACTION	ONSET	SEVERITY	EVIDENCE
CIMETIDINE Concurrent use of FLURAZEPAM and CIMETIDINE may result in flurazepam toxicity (central nervous system depression).	2	4	3
KETOCONAZOLE Concurrent use of FLURAZEPAM and KETOCONAZOLE may result in increased flurazepam serum concentrations and flurazepam adverse effects (sedation, slurred speech, central nervous system depression).	2	4	3
THEOPHYLLINE Concurrent use of FLURAZEPAM and THEOPHYLLINE may result in decreased flurazepam effectiveness.	1	3	2

Fluvoxamine

INTERACTION	ONSET	SEVERITY	EVIDENCE
ALMOTRIPTAN Concurrent use of FLUVOXAMINE and ALMOTRIPTAN may result in weakness, exaggerated reflexes, and/or incoordination.	0	3	3
ALPRAZOLAM Concurrent use of FLUVOXAMINE and ALPRAZOLAM may result in elevated plasma alprazolam levels and an increased risk of side effects (central nervous system depression).	2	3	2
AMITRIPTYLINE Concurrent use of FLUVOXAMINE and AMITRIPTYLINE may result in amitriptyline toxicity (dry mouth, urinary retention, sedation).	2	3	3

INTERACTION	ONSET	SEVERITY	EVIDENCE
ASTEMIZOLE Concurrent use of FLUVOXAMINE and ASTEMIZOLE may result in cardiotoxicity (irregular heartbeat, cardiac arrest).	1	1	3
CISAPRIDE Concurrent use of FLUVOXAMINE and CISAPRIDE may result in cardiotoxicity (irregular heartbeat, cardiac arrest).	1	1	3
CLOMIPRAMINE Concurrent use of FLUVOXAMINE and CLOMIPRAMINE may result in clomipramine toxicity (dry mouth, urinary retention, sedation).	2	3	3
CLORGYLINE Concurrent use of FLUVOXAMINE and CLORGYLINE may result in central nervous system toxicity or serotonin syndrome (high blood pressure, high fever, spasms, mental status changes).	1	2	2
DEXFENFLURAMINE Concurrent use of FLUVOXAMINE and DEXFENFLURAMINE may result in serotonin syndrome (high blood pressure, high fever, spasms, mental status changes).	1	2	3
DIAZEPAM Concurrent use of FLUVOXAMINE and DIAZEPAM may result in diazepam and N-desmethyldiazepam accumulation.	2	3	2
DROPERIDOL Concurrent use of FLUVOXAMINE and DROPERIDOL may result in an increased risk of cardiotoxicity (irregular heartbeat, cardiac arrest).	1	2	3
FENFLURAMINE Concurrent use of FLUVOXAMINE and FENFLURAMINE may result in serotonin syndrome (high blood pressure, high fever, spasms, mental status changes).	1	2	3
FOSPHENYTOIN Concurrent use of FLUVOXAMINE and FOSPHENYTOIN may result in an increased risk of phenytoin toxicity (poor coordination, exaggerated reflexes, rolling eyes, tremors).	2	3	3
FURAZOLIDONE Concurrent use of FLUVOXAMINE and FURAZOLIDONE may result in weakness, exaggerated reflexes, and incoordination.	2	1	3
GUARANA Concomitant administration of FLUVOXAMINE and GUARANA may result in symptoms of excessive caffeine (insomnia, headache, restlessness, nervousness, palpitations, and cardiac irregularities).	1	3	3

Onset: 0=Unspecified 1=Rapid 2=Delayed
Severity: 1=Contraindicated 2=Major 3=Moderate 4=Minor
Evidence: 1=Excellent 2=Good 3=Fair 4=Poor

INTERACTION	ONSET	SEVERITY	EVIDENCE
HYDROXYTRYPTOPHAN Concurrent use of FLUVOXAMINE and HYDROXYTRYPTOPHAN may result in an increased risk of serotonin syndrome (high blood pressure, high fever, spasms, mental status changes).	1	3	3
IMIPRAMINE Concurrent use of FLUVOXAMINE and IMIPRAMINE may result in imipramine toxicity (dry mouth, urinary retention, sedation).	2	3	3
IPRONIAZID Concurrent use of FLUVOXAMINE and IPRONIAZID may result in central nervous system toxicity or serotonin syndrome (high blood pressure, high fever, spasms, mental status changes).	1	2	2
ISOCARBOXAZID Concurrent use of FLUVOXAMINE and ISOCARBOXAZID may result in central nervous system toxicity or serotonin syndrome (high blood pressure, high fever, spasms, mental status changes).	1	1	2
LEVOMETHADYL Concurrent use of FLUVOXAMINE and LEVOMETHADYL may result in an increased risk of cardiotoxicity (irregular heartbeat, cardiac arrest).	2	1	3
MELATONIN Concurrent use of FLUVOXAMINE and MELATONIN may result in increased central nervous system depression.	1	4	3
METHADONE Concurrent use of FLUVOXAMINE and METHADONE may result in increased plasma methadone levels.	2	3	3
MIDAZOLAM Concurrent use of FLUVOXAMINE and MIDAZOLAM may result in elevated serum midazolam concentrations.	2	3	3
MOCLOBEMIDE Concurrent use of FLUVOXAMINE and MOCLOBEMIDE may result in central nervous system toxicity or serotonin syndrome (high blood pressure, high fever, spasms, mental status changes).	1	2	2
NIALAMIDE Concurrent use of FLUVOXAMINE and NIALAMIDE may result in central nervous system toxicity or serotonin syndrome (high blood pressure, high fever, spasms, mental status changes).	1	2	2
OLANZAPINE Concurrent use of FLUVOXAMINE and OLANZAPINE may result in an increased risk of olanzapine adverse effects.	2	3	3

INTERACTION	ONSET	SEVERITY	EVIDENCE
PARGYLINE Concurrent use of FLUVOXAMINE and PARGYLINE may result in central nervous system toxicity or serotonin syndrome (high blood pressure, high fever, spasms, mental status changes).	1	2	2
PHENELZINE Concurrent use of FLUVOXAMINE and PHENELZINE may result in central nervous system toxicity or serotonin syndrome (high blood pressure, high fever, spasms, mental status changes).	1	1	2
PHENYTOIN Concurrent use of FLUVOXAMINE and PHENYTOIN may result in an increased risk of phenytoin toxicity (poor coordination, exaggerated reflexes, rolling eyes, tremors).	2	3	3
PROCARBAZINE Concurrent use of FLUVOXAMINE and PROCARBAZINE may result in central nervous system toxicity or serotonin syndrome (high blood pressure, high fever, spasms, mental status changes).	1	2	2
PROPRANOLOL Concurrent use of FLUVOXAMINE and PROPRANOLOL may result in slow heartbeat and low blood pressure.	2	3	3
ROPIVACAINE Concurrent use of FLUVOXAMINE and ROPIVACAINE may result in increased plasma levels of ropivacaine.	1	3	3
SELEGILINE Concurrent use of FLUVOXAMINE and SELEGILINE may result in central nervous system toxicity or serotonin syndrome (high blood pressure, high fever, spasms, mental status changes).	1	2	2
SIBUTRAMINE Concurrent use of FLUVOXAMINE and SIBUTRAMINE may result in an increased risk of serotonin syndrome (high blood pressure, hypothermia, spasms, mental status changes).	1	2	3
TACRINE Concurrent use of FLUVOXAMINE and TACRINE may result in an increase in the plasma concentration of tacrine.	1	3	3
TERFENADINE Concurrent use of FLUVOXAMINE and TERFENADINE may result in cardiotoxicity (irregular heartbeat, cardiac arrest).	1	1	3
THEOPHYLLINE Concurrent use of FLUVOXAMINE and THEOPHYLLINE may result in theophylline toxicity (nausea, vomiting, palpitations, seizures).	2	3	3

Onset: 0=Unspecified 1=Rapid 2=Delayed
Severity: 1=Contraindicated 2=Major 3=Moderate 4=Minor
Evidence: 1=Excellent 2=Good 3=Fair 4=Poor

INTERACTION	ONSET	SEVERITY	EVIDENCE
THIORIDAZINE Concurrent use of FLUVOXAMINE and THIORIDAZINE may result in an increased risk of thioridazine toxicity and cardiotoxicity (irregular heartbeat, cardiac arrest).	1	1	3
TOBACCO Concurrent use of FLUVOXAMINE and TOBACCO may result in increased fluvoxamine metabolism.	2	4	3
TOLOXATONE Concurrent use of FLUVOXAMINE and TOLOXATONE may result in central nervous system toxicity or serotonin syndrome (high blood pressure, high fever, spasms, mental status changes).	1	2	2
TRAMADOL Concurrent use of FLUVOXAMINE and TRAMADOL may result in an increased risk of seizures and serotonin syndrome (high blood pressure, high fever, spasms, mental status changes).	1	2	2
TRANYLCYPROMINE Concurrent use of FLUVOXAMINE and TRANYLCYPROMINE may result in central nervous system toxicity or serotonin syndrome (high blood pressure, high fever, spasms, mental status changes).	1	2	2
TRIAZOLAM Concurrent use of FLUVOXAMINE and TRIAZOLAM may result in elevated serum triazolam concentrations.	2	3	3
WARFARIN Concurrent use of FLUVOXAMINE and WARFARIN may result in an increased risk of bleeding.	2	3	3

Haloperidol

INTERACTION	ONSET	SEVERITY	EVIDENCE
BENZTROPINE Concurrent use of HALOPERIDOL and BENZTROPINE may result in excessive antispasmodic effects (sedation, constipation, dry mouth).	2	3	2
CABERGOLINE Concurrent use of HALOPERIDOL and CABERGOLINE may result in the decreased therapeutic effect of both drugs.	1	3	3
CARBAMAZEPINE Concurrent use of HALOPERIDOL and CARBAMAZEPINE may result in decreased haloperidol effectiveness.	2	3	2
DROPERIDOL Concurrent use of HALOPERIDOL and DROPERIDOL may result in an increased risk of cardiotoxicity (irregular heartbeat, cardiac arrest).	1	2	3

INTERACTION	ONSET	SEVERITY	EVIDENCE
LITHIUM Concurrent use of HALOPERIDOL and LITHIUM may result in weakness, movement disorders, brain disorders, and brain damage.	2	2	1
RIFAMPIN Concurrent use of HALOPERIDOL and RIFAMPIN may result in decreased haloperidol effectiveness.	2	3	3
SPARFLOXACIN Concurrent use of HALOPERIDOL and SPARFLOXACIN may result in irregular heartbeat.	2	1	3
TRAMADOL Concurrent use of HALOPERIDOL and TRAMADOL may result in an increased risk of seizures.	1	2	3
ZOTEPINE Concurrent use of HALOPERIDOL and ZOTEPINE may result in increased risk of seizures.	2	2	3

Imipramine

INTERACTION	ONSET	SEVERITY	EVIDENCE
ACENOCOUMAROL Concurrent use of IMIPRAMINE and ACENOCOUMAROL may result in increased risk of bleeding.	2	3	3
AMPRENAVIR Concurrent use of IMIPRAMINE and AMPRENAVIR may result in increased imipramine serum concentrations and potential toxicity (antispasmodic effects, sedation, confusion, cardiac irregularities).	2	2	3
ANISINDIONE Concurrent use of IMIPRAMINE and ANISINDIONE may result in increased risk of bleeding.	2	3	3
BEPRIDIL Concurrent use of IMIPRAMINE and BEPRIDIL may result in cardiac irregularities.	1	1	3
BETHANIDINE Concurrent use of IMIPRAMINE and BETHANIDINE may result in decreased antihypertensive effectiveness.	1	3	2
CARBAMAZEPINE Concurrent use of IMIPRAMINE and CARBAMAZEPINE may result in decreased imipramine effectiveness.	2	3	3
CIMETIDINE Concurrent use of IMIPRAMINE and CIMETIDINE may result in imipramine toxicity (dry mouth, urinary retention, blurred vision).	2	3	2

Onset: 0=Unspecified 1=Rapid 2=Delayed
Severity: 1=Contraindicated 2=Major 3=Moderate 4=Minor
Evidence: 1=Excellent 2=Good 3=Fair 4=Poor

INTERACTION	ONSET	SEVERITY	EVIDENCE
CISAPRIDE Concurrent use of IMIPRAMINE and CISAPRIDE may result in cardiotoxicity (irregular heartbeat, cardiac arrest).	1	1	3
CLONIDINE Concurrent use of IMIPRAMINE and CLONIDINE may result in decreased antihypertensive effectiveness.	2	2	3
CLORGYLINE Concurrent use of IMIPRAMINE and CLORGYLINE may result in neurotoxicity, seizures, or serotonin syndrome (high blood pressure, high fever, spasms, mental status changes).	2	2	3
DICUMAROL Concurrent use of IMIPRAMINE and DICUMAROL may result in increased risk of bleeding.	2	3	3
DILTIAZEM Concurrent use of IMIPRAMINE and DILTIAZEM may result in imipramine toxicity (dry mouth, sedation).	2	4	3
DROPERIDOL Concurrent use of IMIPRAMINE and DROPERIDOL may result in an increased risk of cardiotoxicity (irregular heartbeat, cardiac arrest).	1	2	3
EPINEPHRINE Concurrent use of IMIPRAMINE and EPINEPHRINE may result in high blood pressure, cardiac irregularities, and rapid heartbeat.	1	2	2
ETILEFRINE Concurrent use of IMIPRAMINE and ETILEFRINE may result in high blood pressure, cardiac irregularities, and rapid heartbeat.	1	2	2
FLUOXETINE Concurrent use of IMIPRAMINE and FLUOXETINE may result in imipramine toxicity (dry mouth, urinary retention, sedation).	2	3	3
FLUVOXAMINE Concurrent use of IMIPRAMINE and FLUVOXAMINE may result in imipramine toxicity (dry mouth, urinary retention, sedation).	2	3	3
GREPAFLOXACIN Concurrent use of IMIPRAMINE and GREPAFLOXACIN may result in an increased risk of cardiotoxicity (irregular heartbeat, cardiac arrest).	2	1	3
GUANADREL Concurrent use of IMIPRAMINE and GUANADREL may result in decreased antihypertensive effectiveness.	2	3	3
GUANETHIDINE Concurrent use of IMIPRAMINE and GUANETHIDINE may result in decreased antihypertensive effectiveness.	2	3	2

INTERACTION	ONSET	SEVERITY	EVIDENCE
GUANFACINE Concurrent use of IMIPRAMINE and GUANFACINE may result in decreased antihypertensive effectiveness.	2	3	3
HALOFANTRINE Concurrent use of IMIPRAMINE and HALOFANTRINE may result in cardiotoxicity (irregular heartbeat, cardiac arrest).	2	2	3
IBUTILIDE Concurrent use of IMIPRAMINE and IBUTILIDE may result in an increased risk of cardiac irregularities.	1	2	3
ISOCARBOXAZID Concurrent use of IMIPRAMINE and ISOCARBOXAZID may result in neurotoxicity, seizures, or serotonin syndrome (high blood pressure, high fever, spasms, mental status changes).	2	1	3
LABETALOL Concurrent use of IMIPRAMINE and LABETALOL may result in imipramine toxicity (dry mouth, urinary retention, sedation).	2	3	3
LEVOMETHADYL Concurrent use of IMIPRAMINE and LEVOMETHADYL may result in an increased risk of cardiotoxicity (irregular heartbeat, cardiac arrest).	2	1	3
METHOXAMINE Concurrent use of IMIPRAMINE and METHOXAMINE may result in high blood pressure, cardiac irregularities, and rapid heartbeat.	1	2	2
MIDODRINE Concurrent use of IMIPRAMINE and MIDODRINE may result in high blood pressure, cardiac irregularities, and rapid heartbeat.	1	2	2
MOCLOBEMIDE Concurrent use of IMIPRAMINE and MOCLOBEMIDE may result in neurotoxicity, seizures, or serotonin syndrome (high blood pressure, high fever, spasms, mental status changes).	2	2	3
NOREPINEPHRINE Concurrent use of IMIPRAMINE and NOREPINEPHRINE may result in high blood pressure, cardiac irregularities, and rapid heartbeat.	1	2	2
OXILOFRINE Concurrent use of IMIPRAMINE and OXILOFRINE may result in high blood pressure, cardiac irregularities, and rapid heartbeat.	1	2	2
PHENELZINE Concurrent use of IMIPRAMINE and PHENELZINE may result in neurotoxicity, seizures, or serotonin syndrome (high blood pressure, high fever, spasms, mental status changes).	2	2	3

Onset: 0=Unspecified 1=Rapid 2=Delayed
Severity: 1=Contraindicated 2=Major 3=Moderate 4=Minor
Evidence: 1=Excellent 2=Good 3=Fair 4=Poor

INTERACTION	ONSET	SEVERITY	EVIDENCE
PHENINDIONE Concurrent use of IMIPRAMINE and PHENINDIONE may result in increased risk of bleeding.	2	3	3
PHENPROCOUMON Concurrent use of IMIPRAMINE and PHENPROCOUMON may result in increased risk of bleeding.	2	3	3
PHENYLEPHRINE Concurrent use of IMIPRAMINE and PHENYLEPHRINE may result in high blood pressure, cardiac irregularities, and rapid heartbeat.	1	2	2
PHENYTOIN Concurrent use of IMIPRAMINE and PHENYTOIN may result in an increased risk of phenytoin toxicity (poor coordination, exaggerated reflexes, rolling eyes, tremors).	2	3	3
PIMOZIDE Concurrent use of IMIPRAMINE and PIMOZIDE may result in an increased risk of cardiotoxicity (irregular heartbeat, cardiac arrest).	1	1	3
PROCARBAZINE Concurrent use of IMIPRAMINE and PROCARBAZINE may result in neurotoxicity, seizures.	2	2	3
PROPAFENONE Concurrent use of IMIPRAMINE and PROPAFENONE may result in imipramine toxicity (dry mouth, sedation).	2	3	3
QUINIDINE Concurrent use of IMIPRAMINE and QUINIDINE may result in imipramine toxicity (dry mouth, sedation) and an increased risk of cardiotoxicity.	2	3	3
SELEGILINE Concurrent use of IMIPRAMINE and SELEGILINE may result in neurotoxicity, seizures, or serotonin syndrome (high blood pressure, high fever, spasms, mental status changes).	2	2	3
SPARFLOXACIN Concurrent use of IMIPRAMINE and SPARFLOXACIN may result in irregular heartbeat.	2	1	3
TOBACCO Concurrent use of IMIPRAMINE and TOBACCO may result in decreased imipramine concentrations.	2	3	3
TRAMADOL Concurrent use of IMIPRAMINE and TRAMADOL may result in an increased risk of seizures.	1	2	3
TRANYLCYPROMINE Concurrent use of IMIPRAMINE and TRANYLCYPROMINE may result in neurotoxicity, seizures, or serotonin syndrome (high blood pressure, high fever, spasms, mental status changes).	2	2	3

INTERACTION	ONSET	SEVERITY	EVIDENCE
VERAPAMIL Concurrent use of IMIPRAMINE and VERAPAMIL may result in imipramine toxicity (dry mouth, sedation, urinary retention).	2	4	2
WARFARIN Concurrent use of IMIPRAMINE and WARFARIN may result in an increased risk of bleeding.	2	3	3

Lithium

INTERACTION	ONSET	SEVERITY	EVIDENCE
ACETAZOLAMIDE Concurrent use of LITHIUM and ACETAZOLAMIDE may result in decreased lithium effectiveness or increased lithium concentrations.	2	3	3
ACETOPHENAZINE Concurrent use of LITHIUM and ACETOPHENAZINE may result in weakness, movement disorders, brain disorders, and brain damage.	2	2	1
AZOSEMIDE Concurrent use of LITHIUM and AZOSEMIDE may result in increased lithium concentrations and lithium toxicity (weakness, tremor, excessive thirst, confusion).	2	2	3
BEMETIZIDE Concurrent use of LITHIUM and BEMETIZIDE may result in lithium toxicity (weakness, tremor, excessive thirst, confusion).	2	2	3
BENDROFLUMETHIAZIDE Concurrent use of LITHIUM and BENDROFLUMETHIAZIDE may result in increased lithium concentrations and lithium toxicity (weakness, tremor, excessive thirst, confusion).	2	2	3
BENZTHIAZIDE Concurrent use of LITHIUM and BENZTHIAZIDE may result in increased lithium concentrations and lithium toxicity (weakness, tremor, excessive thirst, confusion).	2	2	3
BROMPERIDOL Concurrent use of LITHIUM and BROMPERIDOL may result in weakness, movement disorders, brain disorders, and brain damage.	2	2	1
BUMETANIDE Concurrent use of LITHIUM and BUMETANIDE may result in increased lithium concentrations and lithium toxicity (weakness, tremor, excessive thirst, confusion).	2	2	3
BUTHIAZIDE Concurrent use of LITHIUM and BUTHIAZIDE may result in increased lithium concentrations and lithium toxicity (weakness, tremor, excessive thirst, confusion).	2	2	3

Onset: 0=Unspecified 1=Rapid 2=Delayed
Severity: 1=Contraindicated 2=Major 3=Moderate 4=Minor
Evidence: 1=Excellent 2=Good 3=Fair 4=Poor

INTERACTION	ONSET	SEVERITY	EVIDENCE
CANRENOATE Concurrent use of LITHIUM and CANRENOATE may result in increased lithium concentrations and an increased risk of lithium toxicity (weakness, tremor, excessive thirst, confusion).	2	2	3
CHLOROTHIAZIDE Concurrent use of LITHIUM and CHLOROTHIAZIDE may result in increased lithium concentrations and lithium toxicity (weakness, tremor, excessive thirst, confusion).	2	2	3
CHLORPROMAZINE Concurrent use of LITHIUM and CHLORPROMAZINE may result in weakness, movement disorders, brain disorders, and brain damage.	2	2	1
CHLORPROTHIXENE Concurrent use of LITHIUM and CHLORPROTHIXENE may result in weakness, movement disorders, brain disorders, and brain damage.	2	2	1
CHLORTHALIDONE Concurrent use of LITHIUM and CHLORTHALIDONE may result in increased lithium concentrations and lithium toxicity (weakness, tremor, excessive thirst, confusion).	2	2	3
CLOZAPINE Concurrent use of LITHIUM and CLOZAPINE may result in weakness, movement disorders, brain disorders, and brain damage.	2	2	1
CYCLOTHIAZIDE Concurrent use of LITHIUM and CYCLOTHIAZIDE may result in increased lithium concentrations and lithium toxicity (weakness, tremor, excessive thirst, confusion).	2	2	3
DICLOFENAC Concurrent use of LITHIUM and DICLOFENAC may result in lithium toxicity (weakness, tremor, excessive thirst, confusion).	2	3	3
DILTIAZEM Concurrent use of LITHIUM and DILTIAZEM may result in neurotoxicity, psychosis.	2	3	3
DOMPERIDONE Concurrent use of LITHIUM and DOMPERIDONE may result in weakness, movement disorders, brain disorders, and brain damage.	2	2	1
DROPERIDOL Concurrent use of LITHIUM and DROPERIDOL may result in weakness, movement disorders, brain disorders, and brain damage.	2	2	1
ETHACRYNIC ACID Concurrent use of LITHIUM and ETHACRYNIC ACID may result in increased lithium concentrations and lithium toxicity (weakness, tremor, excessive thirst, confusion).	2	2	3

INTERACTION	ONSET	SEVERITY	EVIDENCE
ETHOPROPAZINE Concurrent use of LITHIUM and ETHOPROPAZINE may result in weakness, movement disorders, brain disorders, and brain damage.	2	2	1
FILGRASTIM Concurrent use of LITHIUM and FILGRASTIM may result in a greater than expected increase in white blood cell count.	2	3	3
FLUPENTHIXOL Concurrent use of LITHIUM and FLUPENTHIXOL may result in weakness, movement disorders, brain disorders, and brain damage.	2	2	1
FLUPHENAZINE Concurrent use of LITHIUM and FLUPHENAZINE may result in weakness, movement disorders, brain disorders, and brain damage.	2	2	1
FOOD Concurrent use of LITHIUM and FOOD may result in increased lithium concentrations.	1	3	3
FOSINOPRIL Concurrent use of LITHIUM and FOSINOPRIL may result in lithium toxicity (weakness, tremor, excessive thirst, confusion) and/or kidney damage.	2	3	3
FUROSEMIDE Concurrent use of LITHIUM and FUROSEMIDE may result in increased lithium concentrations and lithium toxicity (weakness, tremor, excessive thirst, confusion).	2	2	3
GUARANA Concomitant administration of LITHIUM and GUARANA may cause alterations in serum lithium levels.	2	3	3
HALOPERIDOL Concurrent use of LITHIUM and HALOPERIDOL may result in weakness, movement disorders, brain disorders, and brain damage.	2	2	1
HYDROCHLOROTHIAZIDE Concurrent use of LITHIUM and HYDROCHLOROTHIAZIDE may result in increased lithium concentrations and lithium toxicity (weakness, tremor, excessive thirst, confusion).	2	2	2
HYDROFLUMETHIAZIDE Concurrent use of LITHIUM and HYDROFLUMETHIAZIDE may result in increased lithium concentrations and lithium toxicity (weakness, tremor, excessive thirst, confusion).	2	2	3
IBUPROFEN Concurrent use of LITHIUM and IBUPROFEN may result in an increased risk of lithium toxicity (weakness, tremor, excessive thirst, confusion).	2	3	3

Onset: 0=Unspecified 1=Rapid 2=Delayed
Severity: 1=Contraindicated 2=Major 3=Moderate 4=Minor
Evidence: 1=Excellent 2=Good 3=Fair 4=Poor

INTERACTION	ONSET	SEVERITY	EVIDENCE
INDAPAMIDE Concurrent use of LITHIUM and INDAPAMIDE may result in increased lithium concentrations and lithium toxicity (weakness, tremor, excessive thirst, confusion).	2	2	3
INDOMETHACIN Concurrent use of LITHIUM and INDOMETHACIN may result in an increased risk of lithium toxicity (weakness, tremor, excessive thirst, confusion).	2	3	3
KETOROLAC Concurrent use of LITHIUM and KETOROLAC may result in lithium toxicity (weakness, tremor, excessive thirst, confusion).	2	3	2
LISINOPRIL Concurrent use of LITHIUM and LISINOPRIL may result in lithium toxicity (weakness, tremor, excessive thirst, confusion) and/or kidney damage.	2	3	3
LOXAPINE Concurrent use of LITHIUM and LOXAPINE may result in weakness, movement disorders, brain disorders, and brain damage.	2	2	1
MEFENAMIC ACID Concurrent use of LITHIUM and MEFENAMIC ACID may result in lithium toxicity (weakness, tremor, excessive thirst, confusion).	2	3	3
MELOXICAM Concurrent use of LITHIUM and MELOXICAM may result in elevation of plasma lithium levels and reduced excretion of lithium by the kidneys.	1	3	3
MELPERONE Concurrent use of LITHIUM and MELPERONE may result in weakness, movement disorders, brain disorders, and brain damage.	2	2	1
MESORIDAZINE Concurrent use of LITHIUM and MESORIDAZINE may result in weakness, movement disorders, brain disorders, and brain damage.	2	2	1
METHOTRIMEPRAZINE Concurrent use of LITHIUM and METHOTRIMEPRAZINE may result in weakness, movement disorders, brain disorders, and brain damage.	2	2	1
METHYCLOTHIAZIDE Concurrent use of LITHIUM and METHYCLOTHIAZIDE may result in increased lithium concentrations and lithium toxicity (weakness, tremor, excessive thirst, confusion).	2	2	3
METHYLDOPA Concurrent use of LITHIUM and METHYLDOPA may result in an increased risk of lithium toxicity (tremor, weakness, excessive thirst, confusion).	2	3	3

INTERACTION	ONSET	SEVERITY	EVIDENCE
METOLAZONE Concurrent use of LITHIUM and METOLAZONE may result in increased lithium concentrations and lithium toxicity (weakness, tremor, excessive thirst, confusion).	2	2	3
METRONIDAZOLE Concurrent use of LITHIUM and METRONIDAZOLE may result in elevated lithium plasma levels and lithium toxicity (weakness, tremor, excessive thirst, confusion).	2	3	3
MOLINDONE Concurrent use of LITHIUM and MOLINDONE may result in weakness, movement disorders, brain disorders, and brain damage.	2	2	1
NAPROXEN Concurrent use of LITHIUM and NAPROXEN may result in elevated lithium plasma levels and lithium toxicity (weakness, tremor, excessive thirst, confusion).	2	3	3
OLANZAPINE Concurrent use of LITHIUM and OLANZAPINE may result in weakness, movement disorders, increased extrapyramidal symptoms, brain disorders, and brain damage.	2	2	1
PEGFILGRASTIM Concurrent use of LITHIUM and PEGFILGRASTIM may result in a greater than expected increase in white blood cell count.	2	3	3
PENFLURIDOL Concurrent use of LITHIUM and PENFLURIDOL may result in weakness, movement disorders, brain disorders, and brain damage.	2	2	1
PERICIAZINE Concurrent use of LITHIUM and PERICIAZINE may result in weakness, movement disorders, brain disorders, and brain damage.	2	2	1
PERPHENAZINE Concurrent use of LITHIUM and PERPHENAZINE may result in weakness, movement disorders, brain disorders, and brain damage.	2	2	1
PHENYLBUTAZONE Concurrent use of LITHIUM and PHENYLBUTAZONE may result in lithium toxicity (weakness, tremor, excessive thirst, confusion).	2	3	3
PIMOZIDE Concurrent use of LITHIUM and PIMOZIDE may result in weakness, movement disorders, brain disorders, and brain damage.	2	2	1

Onset: 0=Unspecified 1=Rapid 2=Delayed
Severity: 1=Contraindicated 2=Major 3=Moderate 4=Minor
Evidence: 1=Excellent 2=Good 3=Fair 4=Poor

INTERACTION	ONSET	SEVERITY	EVIDENCE
PIPAMPERONE Concurrent use of LITHIUM and PIPAMPERONE may result in weakness, movement disorders, brain disorders, and brain damage.	2	2	1
PIPOTIAZINE Concurrent use of LITHIUM and PIPOTIAZINE may result in weakness, movement disorders, brain disorders, and brain damage.	2	2	1
PIRETANIDE Concurrent use of LITHIUM and PIRETANIDE may result in increased lithium concentrations and lithium toxicity (weakness, tremor, excessive thirst, confusion).	2	2	3
PIROXICAM Concurrent use of LITHIUM and PIROXICAM may result in lithium toxicity (weakness, tremor, excessive thirst, confusion).	2	3	3
POLYTHIAZIDE Concurrent use of LITHIUM and POLYTHIAZIDE may result in increased lithium concentrations and lithium toxicity (weakness, tremor, excessive thirst, confusion).	2	2	3
PROCHLORPERAZINE Concurrent use of LITHIUM and PROCHLORPERAZINE may result in weakness, movement disorders, brain disorders, and brain damage.	2	2	1
PROMAZINE Concurrent use of LITHIUM and PROMAZINE may result in weakness, movement disorders, brain disorders, and brain damage.	2	2	1
PROMETHAZINE Concurrent use of LITHIUM and PROMETHAZINE may result in weakness, movement disorders, brain disorders, and brain damage.	2	2	1
QUINETHAZONE Concurrent use of LITHIUM and QUINETHAZONE may result in increased lithium concentrations and lithium toxicity (weakness, tremor, excessive thirst, confusion).	2	2	3
REMOXIPRIDE Concurrent use of LITHIUM and REMOXIPRIDE may result in weakness, movement disorders, brain disorders, and brain damage.	2	2	1
RISPERIDONE Concurrent use of LITHIUM and RISPERIDONE may result in weakness, movement disorders, brain disorders, and brain damage.	2	2	1
SERTINDOLE Concurrent use of LITHIUM and SERTINDOLE may result in weakness, movement disorders, brain disorders, and brain damage.	2	2	1

INTERACTION	ONSET	SEVERITY	EVIDENCE
SIBUTRAMINE Concurrent use of LITHIUM and SIBUTRAMINE may result in an increased risk of serotonin syndrome (high blood pressure, high fever, spasms, mental status changes).	1	2	3
SODIUM BICARBONATE Concurrent use of LITHIUM and SODIUM BICARBONATE may result in decreased lithium effectiveness.	2	3	3
SPIRONOLACTONE Concurrent use of LITHIUM and SPIRONOLACTONE may result in increased lithium concentrations and lithium toxicity (weakness, tremor, excessive thirst, confusion).	2	2	3
SULPIRIDE Concurrent use of LITHIUM and SULPIRIDE may result in weakness, movement disorders, brain disorders, and brain damage.	2	2	1
TENIDAP Concurrent use of LITHIUM and TENIDAP may result in increased lithium serum levels and possible lithium toxicity (weakness, tremor, excessive thirst, confusion).	2	3	3
THEOPHYLLINE Concurrent use of LITHIUM and THEOPHYLLINE may result in decreased lithium effectiveness.	2	3	2
THIOPROPAZATE Concurrent use of LITHIUM and THIOPROPAZATE may result in weakness, movement disorders, brain disorders, and brain damage.	2	2	1
THIOPROPERAZINE Concurrent use of LITHIUM and THIOPROPERAZINE may result in weakness, movement disorders, brain disorders, and brain damage.	2	2	1
THIORIDAZINE Concurrent use of LITHIUM and THIORIDAZINE may result in weakness, movement disorders, brain disorders, and brain damage.	2	2	1
THIOTHIXENE Concurrent use of LITHIUM and THIOTHIXENE may result in weakness, movement disorders, brain disorders, and brain damage.	2	2	1
TIAPRIDE Concurrent use of LITHIUM and TIAPRIDE may result in weakness, movement disorders, brain disorders, and brain damage.	2	2	1
TRICHLORMETHIAZIDE Concurrent use of LITHIUM and TRICHLORMETHIAZIDE may result in increased lithium concentrations and lithium toxicity (weakness, tremor, excessive thirst, confusion).	2	2	3

Onset: 0=Unspecified 1=Rapid 2=Delayed
Severity: 1=Contraindicated 2=Major 3=Moderate 4=Minor
Evidence: 1=Excellent 2=Good 3=Fair 4=Poor

INTERACTION	ONSET	SEVERITY	EVIDENCE
TRIFLUOPERAZINE Concurrent use of LITHIUM and TRIFLUOPERAZINE may result in weakness, movement disorders, brain disorders, and brain damage.	2	2	1
TRIFLUPROMAZINE Concurrent use of LITHIUM and TRIFLUPROMAZINE may result in weakness, movement disorders, brain disorders, and brain damage.	2	2	1
TRIMEPRAZINE Concurrent use of LITHIUM and TRIMEPRAZINE may result in weakness, movement disorders, brain disorders, and brain damage.	2	2	1
VALDECOXIB Concurrent use of LITHIUM and VALDECOXIB may result in increased lithium plasma concentrations and an increased risk of lithium toxicity (weakness, tremor, excessive thirst, confusion).	2	3	3
XIPAMIDE Concurrent use of LITHIUM and XIPAMIDE may result in increased lithium concentrations and lithium toxicity (weakness, tremor, excessive thirst, confusion).	2	2	3
ZOTEPINE Concurrent use of LITHIUM and ZOTEPINE may result in weakness, movement disorders, brain disorders, and brain damage.	2	2	1
ZUCLOPENTHIXOL Concurrent use of LITHIUM and ZUCLOPENTHIXOL may result in weakness, movement disorders, brain disorders, and brain damage.	2	2	1

Lorazepam

INTERACTION	ONSET	SEVERITY	EVIDENCE
CLOZAPINE Concurrent use of LORAZEPAM and CLOZAPINE may result in central nervous system depression.	1	4	3
ETHANOL Concurrent use of LORAZEPAM and ETHANOL may result in increased sedation.	1	3	1
ORAL CONTRACEPTIVES Concurrent use of LORAZEPAM and ORAL CONTRACEPTIVES may result in decreased lorazepam effectiveness.	2	4	3
THEOPHYLLINE Concurrent use of LORAZEPAM and THEOPHYLLINE may result in decreased lorazepam effectiveness.	1	3	2

Maprotiline

INTERACTION	ONSET	SEVERITY	EVIDENCE
CISAPRIDE Concurrent use of MAPROTILINE and CISAPRIDE may result in cardiotoxicity (irregular heartbeat, cardiac arrest).	1	1	3
CLORGYLINE Concurrent use of MAPROTILINE and CLORGYLINE may result in neurotoxicity, seizures.	2	1	3
IBUTILIDE Concurrent use of MAPROTILINE and IBUTILIDE may result in an increased risk of irregularities.	1	2	3
IPRONIAZID Concurrent use of MAPROTILINE and IPRONIAZID may result in neurotoxicity, seizures.	2	1	3
ISOCARBOXAZID Concurrent use of MAPROTILINE and ISOCARBOXAZID may result in neurotoxicity, seizures.	2	1	3
MOCLOBEMIDE Concurrent use of MAPROTILINE and MOCLOBEMIDE may result in neurotoxicity, seizures.	2	1	3
NIALAMIDE Concurrent use of MAPROTILINE and NIALAMIDE may result in neurotoxicity, seizures.	2	1	3
PARGYLINE Concurrent use of MAPROTILINE and PARGYLINE may result in neurotoxicity, seizures.	2	1	3
PHENELZINE Concurrent use of MAPROTILINE and PHENELZINE may result in neurotoxicity, seizures.	2	1	3
PROCARBAZINE Concurrent use of MAPROTILINE and PROCARBAZINE may result in neurotoxicity, seizures.	2	1	3
SELEGILINE Concurrent use of MAPROTILINE and SELEGILINE may result in neurotoxicity, seizures.	2	1	3
TOLOXATONE Concurrent use of MAPROTILINE and TOLOXATONE may result in neurotoxicity, seizures.	2	1	3
TRANYLCYPROMINE Concurrent use of MAPROTILINE and TRANYLCYPROMINE may result in neurotoxicity, seizures.	2	1	3

Onset: 0=Unspecified 1=Rapid 2=Delayed
Severity: 1=Contraindicated 2=Major 3=Moderate 4=Minor
Evidence: 1=Excellent 2=Good 3=Fair 4=Poor

Meprobamate

INTERACTION	ONSET	SEVERITY	EVIDENCE
ETHANOL Concurrent use of MEPROAMATE and ETHANOLmay result in increased sedation.	1	3	1

Mesoridazine

INTERACTION	ONSET	SEVERITY	EVIDENCE
BELLADONNA Concurrent use of MESORIDAZINE and BELLADONNA may result in increased manic, agitated reactions, or enhanced antispasmodic effects resulting in cardiorespiratory failure, especially in cases of belladonna overdose.	1	3	2
BENZTROPINE Concurrent use of MESORIDAZINE and BENZTROPINE may result in decreased mesoridazine serum concentrations, decreased mesoridazine effectiveness, enhanced antispasmodic effects (intestinal blockage, high fever, sedation, dry mouth).	2	3	3
CABERGOLINE Concurrent use of MESORIDAZINE and CABERGOLINE may result in the decreased therapeutic effect of both drugs.	1	3	3
CISAPRIDE Concurrent use of MESORIDAZINE and CISAPRIDE may result in cardiotoxicity (irregular heartbeat, cardiac arrest).	1	1	3
DISOPYRAMIDE Concurrent use of MESORIDAZINE and DISOPYRAMIDE may result in cardiac irregularities (ventricular rapid heartbeat).	2	1	2
DROPERIDOL Concurrent use of MESORIDAZINE and DROPERIDOL may result in an increased risk of cardiotoxicity (irregular heartbeat, cardiac arrest).	1	2	3
ETHANOL Concurrent use of MESORIDAZINE and ETHANOL may result in increased central nervous system depression and an increased risk of movement disorders.	1	3	2
FOSPHENYTOIN Concurrent use of MESORIDAZINE and FOSPHENYTOIN may result in increased or decreased phenytoin levels and possibly reduced mesoridazine levels.	2	4	3
GREPAFLOXACIN Concurrent use of MESORIDAZINE and GREPAFLOXACIN may result in an increased risk of cardiotoxicity (irregular heartbeat, cardiac arrest).	2	1	3
HALOFANTRINE Concurrent use of MESORIDAZINE and HALOFANTRINE may result in cardiotoxicity (irregular heartbeat, cardiac arrest).	2	2	3

INTERACTION	ONSET	SEVERITY	EVIDENCE
IBUTILIDE Concurrent use of MESORIDAZINE and IBUTILIDE may result in an increased risk of cardiac irregularities.	1	2	3
LEVODOPA Concurrent use of MESORIDAZINE and LEVODOPA may result in loss of levodopa efficacy.	1	3	2
LEVOMETHADYL Concurrent use of MESORIDAZINE and LEVOMETHADYL may result in an increased risk of cardiotoxicity (irregular heartbeat, cardiac arrest).	2	1	3
LITHIUM Concurrent use of MESORIDAZINE and LITHIUM may result in weakness, movement disorders, brain disorders, and brain damage.	2	2	1
MEPERIDINE Concurrent use of MESORIDAZINE and MEPERIDINE may result in an increase in central nervous system and respiratory depression.	1	3	2
ORPHENADRINE Concurrent use of MESORIDAZINE and ORPHENADRINE may result in decreased mesoridazine serum concentrations, decreased mesoridazine effectiveness, enhanced antispasmodic effects (intestinal blockage, high fever, sedation, dry mouth).	2	3	3
PHENYTOIN Concurrent use of MESORIDAZINE and PHENYTOIN may result in increased or decreased phenytoin levels and possibly reduced mesoridazine levels.	2	4	3
PORFIMER Concurrent use of MESORIDAZINE and PORFIMER may result in excessive intracellular damage in photosensitized tissues.	2	3	3
PROCAINAMIDE Concurrent use of MESORIDAZINE and PROCAINAMIDE may result in cardiac irregularities (ventricular rapid heartbeat).	2	1	2
PROCYCLIDINE Concurrent use of MESORIDAZINE and PROCYCLIDINE may result in decreased mesoridazine serum concentrations, decreased mesoridazine effectiveness, enhanced antispasmodic effects (intestinal blockage, high fever, sedation, dry mouth).	2	3	3
QUINIDINE Concurrent use of MESORIDAZINE and QUINIDINE may result in cardiac irregularities (ventricular rapid heartbeat).	2	1	2
SPARFLOXACIN Concurrent use of MESORIDAZINE and SPARFLOXACIN may result in irregular heartbeat.	2	1	3

Onset: 0=Unspecified 1=Rapid 2=Delayed
Severity: 1=Contraindicated 2=Major 3=Moderate 4=Minor
Evidence: 1=Excellent 2=Good 3=Fair 4=Poor

INTERACTION	ONSET	SEVERITY	EVIDENCE
THIORIDAZINE Concurrent use of MESORIDAZINE and THIORIDAZINE may result in an increased risk of cardiotoxicity (irregular heartbeat, cardiac arrest).	2	1	3
TRAMADOL Concurrent use of MESORIDAZINE and TRAMADOL may result in an increased risk of seizures.	1	2	3
TRIHEXYPHENIDYL Concurrent use of MESORIDAZINE and TRIHEXYPHENIDYL may result in decreased mesoridazine serum concentrations, decreased mesoridazine effectiveness, enhanced antispasmodic effects (intestinal blockage, high fever, sedation, dry mouth).	2	3	3
ZIPRASIDONE Concurrent use of MESORIDAZINE and ZIPRASIDONE may result in an increased risk of cardiotoxicity (irregular heartbeat, cardiac arrest).	2	1	3
ZOTEPINE Concurrent use of MESORIDAZINE and ZOTEPINE may result in increased risk of seizures.	2	2	3

Methamphetamine

INTERACTION	ONSET	SEVERITY	EVIDENCE
CLORGYLINE Concurrent use of METHAMPHETAMINE and CLORGYLINE may result in hypertensive crisis (headache, palpitation, neck stiffness).	1	1	3
GUANETHIDINE Concurrent use of METHAMPHETAMINE and GUANETHIDINE may result in decreased guanethidine effectiveness.	1	3	2
IPRONIAZID Concurrent use of METHAMPHETAMINE and IPRONIAZID may result in hypertensive crisis (headache, palpitation, neck stiffness).	1	1	3
ISOCARBOXAZID Concurrent use of METHAMPHETAMINE and ISOCARBOXAZID may result in hypertensive crisis (headache, palpitation, neck stiffness).	1	1	3
MOCLOBEMIDE Concurrent use of METHAMPHETAMINE and MOCLOBEMIDE may result in hypertensive crisis (headache, palpitation, neck stiffness).	1	1	3
NIALAMIDE Concurrent use of METHAMPHETAMINE and NIALAMIDE may result in hypertensive crisis (headache, palpitation, neck stiffness).	1	1	3

INTERACTION	ONSET	SEVERITY	EVIDENCE
PARGYLINE Concurrent use of METHAMPHETAMINE and PARGYLINE may result in hypertensive crisis (headache, palpitation, neck stiffness).	1	1	3
PHENELZINE Concurrent use of METHAMPHETAMINE and PHENELZINE may result in hypertensive crisis (headache, palpitation, neck stiffness).	1	1	3
PROCARBAZINE Concurrent use of METHAMPHETAMINE and PROCARBAZINE may result in hypertensive crisis (headache, palpitation, neck stiffness).	1	1	3
SELEGILINE Concurrent use of METHAMPHETAMINE and SELEGILINE may result in hypertensive crisis (headache, palpitation, neck stiffness).	1	1	3
TOLOXATONE Concurrent use of METHAMPHETAMINE and TOLOXATONE may result in hypertensive crisis (headache, palpitation, neck stiffness).	1	1	3
TRANYLCYPROMINE Concurrent use of METHAMPHETAMINE and TRANYLCYPROMINE may result in hypertensive crisis (headache, palpitation, neck stiffness).	1	1	3

Methylphenidate

INTERACTION	ONSET	SEVERITY	EVIDENCE
CARBAMAZEPINE Concurrent use of METHYLPHENIDATE and CARBAMAZEPINE may result in loss of methylphenidate efficacy.	2	3	3
CLORGYLINE Concurrent use of METHYLPHENIDATE and CLORGYLINE may result in hypertensive crisis (headache, palpitation, neck stiffness).	1	1	3
GUANETHIDINE Concurrent use of METHYLPHENIDATE and GUANETHIDINE may result in decreased guanethidine effectiveness.	1	3	3
IPRONIAZID Concurrent use of METHYLPHENIDATE and IPRONIAZID may result in hypertensive crisis (headache, palpitation, neck stiffness).	1	1	3
ISOCARBOXAZID Concurrent use of METHYLPHENIDATE and ISOCARBOXAZID may result in hypertensive crisis (headache, palpitation, neck stiffness).	1	1	3

Onset: 0=Unspecified 1=Rapid 2=Delayed
Severity: 1=Contraindicated 2=Major 3=Moderate 4=Minor
Evidence: 1=Excellent 2=Good 3=Fair 4=Poor

INTERACTION	ONSET	SEVERITY	EVIDENCE
LAZABEMIDE Concurrent use of METHYLPHENIDATE and LAZABEMIDE may result in hypertensive crisis (headache, palpitation, neck stiffness).	1	1	3
MOCLOBEMIDE Concurrent use of METHYLPHENIDATE and MOCLOBEMIDE may result in hypertensive crisis (headache, palpitation, neck stiffness).	1	1	3
NIALAMIDE Concurrent use of METHYLPHENIDATE and NIALAMIDE may result in hypertensive crisis (headache, palpitation, neck stiffness).	1	1	3
PARGYLINE Concurrent use of METHYLPHENIDATE and PARGYLINE may result in hypertensive crisis (headache, palpitation, neck stiffness).	1	1	3
PHENELZINE Concurrent use of METHYLPHENIDATE and PHENELZINE may result in hypertensive crisis (headache, palpitation, neck stiffness).	1	1	3
PROCARBAZINE Concurrent use of METHYLPHENIDATE and PROCARBAZINE may result in hypertensive crisis (headache, palpitation, neck stiffness).	1	1	3
SELEGILINE Concurrent use of METHYLPHENIDATE and SELEGILINE may result in hypertensive crisis (headache, palpitation, neck stiffness).	1	1	3
TOLOXATONE Concurrent use of METHYLPHENIDATE and TOLOXATONE may result in hypertensive crisis (headache, palpitation, neck stiffness).	1	1	3
TRANYLCYPROMINE Concurrent use of METHYLPHENIDATE and TRANYLCYPROMINE may result in hypertensive crisis (headache, palpitation, neck stiffness).	1	1	3

Mirtazapine

INTERACTION	ONSET	SEVERITY	EVIDENCE
CLONIDINE Concurrent use of MIRTAZAPINE and CLONIDINE may result in high blood pressure, decreased antihypertensive effectiveness.	2	2	3
CLORGYLINE Concurrent use of MIRTAZAPINE and CLORGYLINE may result in neurotoxicity, seizures.	2	1	3
IPRONIAZID Concurrent use of MIRTAZAPINE and IPRONIAZID may result in neurotoxicity, seizures.	2	1	3

INTERACTION	ONSET	SEVERITY	EVIDENCE
ISOCARBOXAZID Concurrent use of MIRTAZAPINE and ISOCARBOXAZID may result in neurotoxicity, seizures.	2	1	3
MOCLOBEMIDE Concurrent use of MIRTAZAPINE and MOCLOBEMIDE may result in neurotoxicity, seizures.	2	1	3
NIALAMIDE Concurrent use of MIRTAZAPINE and NIALAMIDE may result in neurotoxicity, seizures.	2	1	3
PARGYLINE Concurrent use of MIRTAZAPINE and PARGYLINE may result in neurotoxicity, seizures.	2	1	3
PHENELZINE Concurrent use of MIRTAZAPINE and PHENELZINE may result in neurotoxicity, seizures.	2	1	3
PROCARBAZINE Concurrent use of MIRTAZAPINE and PROCARBAZINE may result in neurotoxicity, seizures.	2	1	3
SELEGILINE Concurrent use of MIRTAZAPINE and SELEGILINE may result in neurotoxicity, seizures.	2	1	3
TOLOXATONE Concurrent use of MIRTAZAPINE and TOLOXATONE may result in neurotoxicity, seizures.	2	1	3
TRANYLCYPROMINE Concurrent use of MIRTAZAPINE and TRANYLCYPROMINE may result in neurotoxicity, seizures.	2	1	3

Molindone

INTERACTION	ONSET	SEVERITY	EVIDENCE
DROPERIDOL Concurrent use of MOLINDONE and DROPERIDOL may result in an increased risk of cardiotoxicity (irregular heartbeat, cardiac arrest).	1	2	3
LITHIUM Concurrent use of MOLINDONE and LITHIUM may result in weakness, movement disorders, brain disorders, and brain damage.	2	2	1
TRAMADOL Concurrent use of MOLINDONE and TRAMADOL may result in an increased risk of seizures.	1	2	3

Onset: 0=Unspecified 1=Rapid 2=Delayed
Severity: 1=Contraindicated 2=Major 3=Moderate 4=Minor
Evidence: 1=Excellent 2=Good 3=Fair 4=Poor

Nefazodone

INTERACTION	ONSET	SEVERITY	EVIDENCE
ALMOTRIPTAN Concurrent use of NEFAZODONE and ALMOTRIPTAN may result in weakness, exaggerated reflexes, and/or incoordination.	0	3	3
ALPRAZOLAM Concurrent use of NEFAZODONE and ALPRAZOLAM may result in psychomotor impairment and sedation.	1	3	2
AMITRIPTYLINE Concurrent use of NEFAZODONE and AMITRIPTYLINE may result in increased risk of serotonin syndrome (high blood pressure, high fever, spasms, mental status changes).	1	2	3
ASTEMIZOLE Concurrent use of NEFAZODONE and ASTEMIZOLE may result in cardiotoxicity (irregular heartbeat, cardiac arrest).	1	1	3
ATORVASTATIN Concurrent use of NEFAZODONE and ATORVASTATIN may result in an increased risk of muscle disorders or severe muscle wasting.	2	2	3
CARBAMAZEPINE Concurrent use of NEFAZODONE and CARBAMAZEPINE may result in an increased risk of carbamazepine toxicity (poor coordination, rolling eyes, double vision, headache, vomiting, disrupted breathing, seizures, coma).	2	3	3
CISAPRIDE Concurrent use of NEFAZODONE and CISAPRIDE may result in an increased risk of cardiotoxicity (irregular heartbeat, cardiac arrest).	1	1	2
CLORGYLINE Concurrent use of NEFAZODONE and CLORGYLINE may result in high fever, rigidity, spasms, seizures, fluctuations of vital signs, or mental status changes.	1	2	2
CYCLOSPORINE Concurrent use of NEFAZODONE and CYCLOSPORINE may result in an increased risk of cyclosporine toxicity (kidney dysfunction, diminished flow of bile, tingling sensation).	2	3	3
DIGOXIN Concurrent use of NEFAZODONE and DIGOXIN may result in an increase in digoxin serum concentrations and possibly increase the risk of digoxin toxicity (nausea, vomiting, cardiac irregularities).	2	3	3
DROPERIDOL Concurrent use of NEFAZODONE and DROPERIDOL may result in an increased risk of cardiotoxicity (irregular heartbeat, cardiac arrest).	1	2	3

INTERACTION	ONSET	SEVERITY	EVIDENCE
ETHANOL Concurrent use of NEFAZODONE and ETHANOL may result in an increased risk of central nervous system side effects.	1	4	3
FURAZOLIDONE Concurrent use of NEFAZODONE and FURAZOLIDONE may result in weakness, exaggerated reflexes, and incoordination.	2	1	3
IPRONIAZID Concurrent use of NEFAZODONE and IPRONIAZID may result in central nervous system toxicity or serotonin syndrome (high blood pressure, high fever, spasms, mental status changes).	1	2	2
ISOCARBOXAZID Concurrent use of NEFAZODONE and ISOCARBOXAZID may result in high fever, rigidity, spasms, seizures, fluctuations of vital signs, or mental status changes.	1	1	2
LOVASTATIN Concurrent use of NEFAZODONE and LOVASTATIN may result in an increased risk of muscle disorders or severe muscle wasting.	2	2	3
MOCLOBEMIDE Concurrent use of NEFAZODONE and MOCLOBEMIDE may result in central nervous system toxicity or serotonin syndrome (high blood pressure, high fever, spasms, mental status changes).	1	2	2
NIALAMIDE Concurrent use of NEFAZODONE and NIALAMIDE may result in central nervous system toxicity or serotonin syndrome (high blood pressure, high fever, spasms, mental status changes).	1	2	2
PARGYLINE Concurrent use of NEFAZODONE and PARGYLINE may result in central nervous system toxicity or serotonin syndrome (high blood pressure, high fever, spasms, mental status changes).	1	2	2
PHENELZINE Concurrent use of NEFAZODONE and PHENELZINE may result in high fever, rigidity, spasms, seizures, fluctuations of vital signs, or mental status changes.	1	1	2
PIMOZIDE Concurrent use of NEFAZODONE and PIMOZIDE may result in an increased risk of cardiotoxicity (irregular heartbeat, cardiac arrest).	1	1	3

Onset: 0=Unspecified 1=Rapid 2=Delayed
Severity: 1=Contraindicated 2=Major 3=Moderate 4=Minor
Evidence: 1=Excellent 2=Good 3=Fair 4=Poor

INTERACTION	ONSET	SEVERITY	EVIDENCE
PROCARBAZINE Concurrent use of NEFAZODONE and PROCARBAZINE may result in central nervous system toxicity or serotonin syndrome (high blood pressure, high fever, spasms, mental status changes).	1	2	2
PROPRANOLOL Concurrent use of NEFAZODONE and PROPRANOLOL may result in decreased propranolol efficacy.	1	4	3
SELEGILINE Concurrent use of NEFAZODONE and SELEGILINE may result in high fever, rigidity, spasms, seizures, fluctuations of vital signs, or mental status changes.	1	2	2
SIBUTRAMINE Concurrent use of NEFAZODONE and SIBUTRAMINE may result in an increased risk of serotonin syndrome (high blood pressure, hypothermia, spasms, mental status changes).	1	2	3
SIMVASTATIN Concurrent use of NEFAZODONE and SIMVASTATIN may result in an increased risk of muscle disorders or severe muscle wasting.	2	2	1
TERFENADINE Concurrent use of NEFAZODONE and TERFENADINE may result in serious, even fatal, cardiovascular events (irregular heartbeat, or cardiac arrest).	1	1	2
TOLOXATONE Concurrent use of NEFAZODONE and TOLOXATONE may result in central nervous system toxicity or serotonin syndrome (high blood pressure, high fever, spasms, mental status changes).	1	2	2
TRANYLCYPROMINE Concurrent use of NEFAZODONE and TRANYLCYPROMINE may result in high fever, rigidity, spasms, seizures, fluctuations of vital signs, or mental status changes.	1	2	2
TRIAZOLAM Concurrent use of NEFAZODONE and TRIAZOLAM may result in psychomotor impairment and excessive sedation.	1	3	2

Nortriptyline

INTERACTION	ONSET	SEVERITY	EVIDENCE
ACENOCOUMAROL Concurrent use of NORTRIPTYLINE and ACENOCOUMAROL may result in an increased risk of bleeding.	2	3	3
AMPRENAVIR Concurrent use of NORTRIPTYLINE and AMPRENAVIR may result in increased nortriptyline serum concentrations and potential toxicity (antispasmodic effects, sedation, confusion, cardiac irregularities).	2	2	3

INTERACTION	ONSET	SEVERITY	EVIDENCE
ANISINDIONE Concurrent use of NORTRIPTYLINE and ANISINDIONE may result in an increased risk of bleeding.	2	3	3
BEPRIDIL Concurrent use of NORTRIPTYLINE and BEPRIDIL may result in cardiac irregularities.	1	1	3
BETHANIDINE Concurrent use of NORTRIPTYLINE and BETHANIDINE may result in decreased antihypertensive effectiveness.	1	3	3
CIMETIDINE Concurrent use of NORTRIPTYLINE and CIMETIDINE may result in nortriptyline toxicity (dry mouth, blurred vision, urinary retention).	2	3	2
CISAPRIDE Concurrent use of NORTRIPTYLINE and CISAPRIDE may result in cardiotoxicity (irregular heartbeat, cardiac arrest).	1	1	3
CLONIDINE Concurrent use of NORTRIPTYLINE and CLONIDINE may result in decreased antihypertensive effectiveness.	2	2	3
CLORGYLINE Concurrent use of NORTRIPTYLINE and CLORGYLINE may result in neurotoxicity, seizures, or serotonin syndrome (high blood pressure, high fever, spasms, mental status changes).	2	2	3
DICUMAROL Concurrent use of NORTRIPTYLINE and DICUMAROL may result in an increased risk of bleeding.	2	3	3
DROPERIDOL Concurrent use of NORTRIPTYLINE and DROPERIDOL may result in an increased risk of cardiotoxicity (irregular heartbeat, cardiac arrest).	1	2	3
EPINEPHRINE Concurrent use of NORTRIPTYLINE and EPINEPHRINE may result in high blood pressure, cardiac irregularities, and rapid heartbeat.	1	2	2
ETILEFRINE Concurrent use of NORTRIPTYLINE and ETILEFRINE may result in high blood pressure, cardiac irregularities, and rapid heartbeat.	1	2	2
FLUOXETINE Concurrent use of NORTRIPTYLINE and FLUOXETINE may result in nortriptyline toxicity (dry mouth, urinary retention, sedation).	2	3	3

Onset: 0=Unspecified 1=Rapid 2=Delayed
Severity: 1=Contraindicated 2=Major 3=Moderate 4=Minor
Evidence: 1=Excellent 2=Good 3=Fair 4=Poor

INTERACTION	ONSET	SEVERITY	EVIDENCE
GREPAFLOXACIN Concurrent use of NORTRIPTYLINE and GREPAFLOXACIN may result in an increased risk of cardiotoxicity (irregular heartbeat, cardiac arrest).	2	1	3
GUANADREL Concurrent use of NORTRIPTYLINE and GUANADREL may result in decreased antihypertensive effectiveness.	2	3	3
GUANETHIDINE Concurrent use of NORTRIPTYLINE and GUANETHIDINE may result in decreased antihypertensive effectiveness.	2	3	2
HALOFANTRINE Concurrent use of NORTRIPTYLINE and HALOFANTRINE may result in cardiotoxicity (irregular heartbeat, cardiac arrest).	2	2	3
IBUTILIDE Concurrent use of NORTRIPTYLINE and IBUTILIDE may result in an increased risk of cardiac irregularities.	1	2	3
ISOCARBOXAZID Concurrent use of NORTRIPTYLINE and ISOCARBOXAZID may result in neurotoxicity, seizures, or serotonin syndrome (high blood pressure, high fever, spasms, mental status changes).	2	1	3
LEVOMETHADYL Concurrent use of NORTRIPTYLINE and LEVOMETHADYL may result in an increased risk of cardiotoxicity (irregular heartbeat, cardiac arrest).	2	1	3
METHOXAMINE Concurrent use of NORTRIPTYLINE and METHOXAMINE may result in high blood pressure, cardiac irregularities, and rapid heartbeat.	1	2	2
MIDODRINE Concurrent use of NORTRIPTYLINE and MIDODRINE may result in high blood pressure, cardiac irregularities, and rapid heartbeat.	1	2	2
MOCLOBEMIDE Concurrent use of NORTRIPTYLINE and MOCLOBEMIDE may result in neurotoxicity, seizures, or serotonin syndrome (high blood pressure, high fever, spasms, mental status changes).	2	2	3
NOREPINEPHRINE Concurrent use of NORTRIPTYLINE and NOREPINEPHRINE may result in high blood pressure, cardiac irregularities, and rapid heartbeat.	1	2	2
OXILOFRINE Concurrent use of NORTRIPTYLINE and OXILOFRINE may result in high blood pressure, cardiac irregularities, and rapid heartbeat.	1	2	2

INTERACTION	ONSET	SEVERITY	EVIDENCE
PHENELZINE Concurrent use of NORTRIPTYLINE and PHENELZINE may result in neurotoxicity, seizures, or serotonin syndrome (high blood pressure, high fever, spasms, mental status changes).	2	2	3
PHENINDIONE Concurrent use of NORTRIPTYLINE and PHENINDIONE may result in an increased risk of bleeding.	2	3	3
PHENPROCOUMON Concurrent use of NORTRIPTYLINE and PHENPROCOUMON may result in an increased risk of bleeding.	2	3	3
PHENYLEPHRINE Concurrent use of NORTRIPTYLINE and PHENYLEPHRINE may result in high blood pressure, cardiac irregularities, and rapid heartbeat.	1	2	2
PIMOZIDE Concurrent use of NORTRIPTYLINE and PIMOZIDE may result in an increased risk of cardiotoxicity (irregular heartbeat, cardiac arrest).	1	1	3
PROCARBAZINE Concurrent use of NORTRIPTYLINE and PROCARBAZINE may result in neurotoxicity, seizures.	2	2	3
SELEGILINE Concurrent use of NORTRIPTYLINE and SELEGILINE may result in neurotoxicity, seizures, or serotonin syndrome (high blood pressure, high fever, spasms, mental status changes).	2	2	3
SERTRALINE Concurrent use of NORTRIPTYLINE and SERTRALINE may result in elevated nortriptyline serum levels or possible serotonin syndrome (high blood pressure, high fever, spasms, mental status changes).	2	2	3
SPARFLOXACIN Concurrent use of NORTRIPTYLINE and SPARFLOXACIN may result in irregular heartbeat.	2	1	3
ST JOHN'S WORT Concurrent use of NORTRIPTYLINE and ST. JOHN'S WORT may result in decreased effectiveness of nortriptyline and possible increased risk of serotonin syndrome (high blood pressure, high fever, spasms, mental status changes).	2	3	3
TOBACCO Concurrent use of NORTRIPTYLINE and TOBACCO may result in decreased nortriptyline concentrations.	2	3	3

Onset: 0=Unspecified 1=Rapid 2=Delayed
Severity: 1=Contraindicated 2=Major 3=Moderate 4=Minor
Evidence: 1=Excellent 2=Good 3=Fair 4=Poor

INTERACTION	ONSET	SEVERITY	EVIDENCE
TRAMADOL Concurrent use of NORTRIPTYLINE and TRAMADOL may result in an increased risk of seizures.	1	2	3
TRANYLCYPROMINE Concurrent use of NORTRIPTYLINE and TRANYLCYPROMINE may result in neurotoxicity, seizures, or serotonin syndrome (high blood pressure, high fever, spasms, mental status changes).	2	2	3
WARFARIN Concurrent use of NORTRIPTYLINE and WARFARIN may result in an increased risk of bleeding.	2	3	3

Olanzapine

INTERACTION	ONSET	SEVERITY	EVIDENCE
CIPROFLOXACIN Concurrent use of OLANZAPINE and CIPROFLOXACIN may result in an increased risk of olanzapine toxicity (increased sedation, low blood pressure and dizziness upon standing up).	2	3	3
CLOMIPRAMINE Concurrent use of OLANZAPINE and CLOMIPRAMINE may result in an increased risk of seizures.	2	2	2
DROPERIDOL Concurrent use of OLANZAPINE and DROPERIDOL may result in an increased risk of cardiotoxicity (irregular heartbeat, cardiac arrest).	1	2	3
ETHANOL Concurrent use of OLANZAPINE and ETHANOL may result in excessive central nervous system depression.	1	3	3
FLUVOXAMINE Concurrent use of OLANZAPINE and FLUVOXAMINE may result in an increased risk of olanzapine adverse effects.	2	3	3
LEVOMETHADYL Concurrent use of OLANZAPINE and LEVOMETHADYL may result in an increased risk of cardiotoxicity (irregular heartbeat, cardiac arrest).	2	1	3
LITHIUM Concurrent use of OLANZAPINE and LITHIUM may result in weakness, movement disorders, brain disorders, and brain damage.	2	2	1

Oxazepam

INTERACTION	ONSET	SEVERITY	EVIDENCE
FOSPHENYTOIN Concurrent use of OXAZEPAM and FOSPHENYTOIN may result in loss of oxazepam efficacy.	2	4	3
PHENYTOIN Concurrent use of OXAZEPAM and PHENYTOIN may result in loss of oxazepam efficacy.	2	4	3

INTERACTION	ONSET	SEVERITY	EVIDENCE
THEOPHYLLINE Concurrent use of OXAZEPAM and THEOPHYLLINE may result in decreased oxazepam effectiveness.	1	3	2

Paroxetine

INTERACTION	ONSET	SEVERITY	EVIDENCE
ALMOTRIPTAN Concurrent use of PAROXETINE and ALMOTRIPTAN may result in weakness, exaggerated reflexes, and/or incoordination.	0	3	3
ASTEMIZOLE Concurrent use of PAROXETINE and ASTEMIZOLE may result in cardiotoxicity (irregular heartbeat, cardiac arrest).	1	2	3
CIMETIDINE Concurrent use of PAROXETINE and CIMETIDINE may result in increased paroxetine serum concentrations and possibly paroxetine toxicity (dizziness, somnolence, nausea, headache).	2	4	3
CLORGYLINE Concurrent use of PAROXETINE and CLORGYLINE may result in central nervous system toxicity or serotonin syndrome (high blood pressure, high fever, spasms, mental status changes).	1	1	2
DEXFENFLURAMINE Concurrent use of PAROXETINE and DEXFENFLURAMINE may result in serotonin syndrome (high blood pressure, high fever, spasms, mental status changes).	1	2	3
DEXTROMETHORPHAN Concurrent use of PAROXETINE and DEXTROMETHORPHAN may result in possible dextromethorphan toxicity (nausea, vomiting, blurred vision, hallucinations) or serotonin syndrome (high blood pressure, high fever, spasms, mental status changes).	1	2	3
DROPERIDOL Concurrent use of PAROXETINE and DROPERIDOL may result in an increased risk of cardiotoxicity (irregular heartbeat, cardiac arrest).	1	2	3
ENCAINIDE Concurrent use of PAROXETINE and ENCAINIDE may result in an increased risk of encainide toxicity (cardiac irregularities).	1	3	3
ETHANOL Concurrent use of PAROXETINE and ETHANOL may result in an increased risk of impairment of mental and motor skills.	1	4	3

Onset: 0=Unspecified 1=Rapid 2=Delayed
Severity: 1=Contraindicated 2=Major 3=Moderate 4=Minor
Evidence: 1=Excellent 2=Good 3=Fair 4=Poor

INTERACTION	ONSET	SEVERITY	EVIDENCE
FENFLURAMINE Concurrent use of PAROXETINE and FENFLURAMINE may result in serotonin syndrome (high blood pressure, high fever, spasms, mental status changes).	1	2	3
FOSPHENYTOIN Concurrent use of PAROXETINE and FOSPHENYTOIN may result in reduced paroxetine efficacy.	2	3	3
FURAZOLIDONE Concurrent use of PAROXETINE and FURAZOLIDONE may result in weakness, exaggerated reflexes, and incoordination.	2	1	3
HYDROXYTRYPTOPHAN Concurrent use of PAROXETINE and HYDROXYTRYPTOPHAN may result in an increased risk of serotonin syndrome (high blood pressure, high fever, spasms, mental status changes).	1	3	3
IPRONIAZID Concurrent use of PAROXETINE and IPRONIAZID may result in central nervous system toxicity or serotonin syndrome (high blood pressure, high fever, spasms, mental status changes).	1	1	2
ISOCARBOXAZID Concurrent use of PAROXETINE and ISOCARBOXAZID may result in central nervous system toxicity or serotonin syndrome (high blood pressure, high fever, spasms, mental status changes).	1	1	2
MOCLOBEMIDE Concurrent use of PAROXETINE and MOCLOBEMIDE may result in central nervous system toxicity or serotonin syndrome (high blood pressure, high fever, spasms, mental status changes).	1	1	2
NIALAMIDE Concurrent use of PAROXETINE and NIALAMIDE may result in central nervous system toxicity or serotonin syndrome (high blood pressure, high fever, spasms, mental status changes).	1	1	2
PARGYLINE Concurrent use of PAROXETINE and PARGYLINE may result in central nervous system toxicity or serotonin syndrome (high blood pressure, high fever, spasms, mental status changes).	1	1	2
PERPHENAZINE Concurrent use of PAROXETINE and PERPHENAZINE may result in increased plasma concentrations and side effects of perphenazine.	1	3	3
PHENELZINE Concurrent use of PAROXETINE and PHENELZINE may result in central nervous system toxicity or serotonin syndrome (high blood pressure, high fever, spasms, mental status changes).	1	1	2

INTERACTION	ONSET	SEVERITY	EVIDENCE
PHENOBARBITAL Concurrent use of PAROXETINE and PHENOBARBITAL may result in reduced paroxetine effectiveness.	1	4	3
PHENYTOIN Concurrent use of PAROXETINE and PHENYTOIN may result in reduced paroxetine efficacy.	2	3	3
PROCARBAZINE Concurrent use of PAROXETINE and PROCARBAZINE may result in central nervous system toxicity or serotonin syndrome (high blood pressure, high fever, spasms, mental status changes).	1	1	2
PROCYCLIDINE Concurrent use of PAROXETINE and PROCYCLIDINE may result in an increased risk of antispasmodic effects (dry mouth, sedation, dilated pupils).	1	4	3
PROPAFENONE Concurrent use of PAROXETINE and PROPAFENONE may result in an increased risk of propafenone toxicity (cardiac irregularities).	1	3	3
RISPERIDONE Concurrent use of PAROXETINE and RISPERIDONE may result in an increased risk for serotonin syndrome (high blood pressure, high fever, spasms, mental status changes).	2	2	2
SELEGILINE Concurrent use of PAROXETINE and SELEGILINE may result in central nervous system toxicity or serotonin syndrome (high blood pressure, high fever, spasms, mental status changes).	1	1	2
SIBUTRAMINE Concurrent use of PAROXETINE and SIBUTRAMINE may result in an increased risk of serotonin syndrome (high blood pressure, high fever, spasms, mental status changes).	1	2	3
THEOPHYLLINE Concurrent use of PAROXETINE and THEOPHYLLINE may result in an increased risk of theophylline toxicity.	2	3	3
THIORIDAZINE Concurrent use of PAROXETINE and THIORIDAZINE may result in an increased risk of thioridazine toxicity, cardiotoxicity (irregular heartbeat, cardiac arrest).	1	1	3
TOLOXATONE Concurrent use of PAROXETINE and TOLOXATONE may result in central nervous system toxicity or serotonin syndrome (high blood pressure, high fever, spasms, mental status changes).	1	1	2

Onset: 0=Unspecified 1=Rapid 2=Delayed
Severity: 1=Contraindicated 2=Major 3=Moderate 4=Minor
Evidence: 1=Excellent 2=Good 3=Fair 4=Poor

INTERACTION	ONSET	SEVERITY	EVIDENCE
TRAMADOL Concurrent use of PAROXETINE and TRAMADOL may result in an increased risk of seizures and serotonin syndrome (high blood pressure, high fever, spasms, mental status changes).	1	2	2
TRANYLCYPROMINE Concurrent use of PAROXETINE and TRANYLCYPROMINE may result in central nervous system toxicity or serotonin syndrome (high blood pressure, high fever, spasms, mental status changes).	1	1	2
TRYPTOPHAN Concurrent use of PAROXETINE and TRYPTOPHAN may result in serotonin syndrome (high blood pressure, high fever, spasms, mental status changes).	2	2	3
VENLAFAXINE Concurrent use of PAROXETINE and VENLAFAXINE may result in an increased risk of serotonin syndrome (high blood pressure, high fever, spasms, mental status changes).	1	2	3

Pentobarbital

INTERACTION	ONSET	SEVERITY	EVIDENCE
ALPRENOLOL Concurrent use of PENTOBARBITAL and ALPRENOLOL may result in decreased alprenolol effectiveness.	2	3	2
DICUMAROL Concurrent use of PENTOBARBITAL and DICUMAROL may result in decreased dicumarol effectiveness.	2	2	2
ETHANOL Concurrent use of PENTOBARBITAL and ETHANOL may result in excessive central nervous system depression.	1	3	1
METOPROLOL Concurrent use of PENTOBARBITAL and METOPROLOL may result in decreased metoprolol effectiveness.	2	3	3
PREDNISOLONE Concurrent use of PENTOBARBITAL and PREDNISOLONE may result in decreased therapeutic effect of prednisolone.	2	3	2
PREDNISONE Concurrent use of PENTOBARBITAL and PREDNISONE may result in decreased therapeutic effect of prednisone.	2	3	2
THEOPHYLLINE Concurrent use of PENTOBARBITAL and THEOPHYLLINE may result in decreased theophylline effectiveness.	2	3	3
VALERIAN Concurrent use of PENTOBARBITAL and VALERIAN may result in increased central nervous system depression.	1	3	3

Perphenazine

INTERACTION	ONSET	SEVERITY	EVIDENCE
BELLADONNA Concurrent use of PERPHENAZINE and BELLADONNA may result in increased manic, agitated reactions, or enhanced antispasmodic effects resulting in cardiorespiratory failure, especially in cases of belladonna overdose.	1	3	2
BENZTROPINE Concurrent use of PERPHENAZINE and BENZTROPINE may result in decreased perphenazine serum concentrations, decreased perphenazine effectiveness, enhanced antispasmodic effects (intestinal blockage, high fever, sedation, dry mouth).	2	3	3
CABERGOLINE Concurrent use of PERPHENAZINE and CABERGOLINE may result in the decreased therapeutic effect of both drugs.	1	3	3
CISAPRIDE Concurrent use of PERPHENAZINE and CISAPRIDE may result in cardiotoxicity (irregular heartbeat, cardiac arrest).	1	1	3
DROPERIDOL Concurrent use of PERPHENAZINE and DROPERIDOL may result in an increased risk of cardiotoxicity (irregular heartbeat, cardiac arrest).	1	2	3
ETHANOL Concurrent use of PERPHENAZINE and ETHANOL may result in increased central nervous system depression and an increased risk of movement disorders.	1	3	2
FOSPHENYTOIN Concurrent use of PERPHENAZINE and FOSPHENYTOIN may result in increased or decreased phenytoin levels and possibly reduced perphenazine levels.	2	4	3
GREPAFLOXACIN Concurrent use of PERPHENAZINE and GREPAFLOXACIN may result in an increased risk of cardiotoxicity (irregular heartbeat, cardiac arrest).	2	1	3
HALOFANTRINE Concurrent use of PERPHENAZINE and HALOFANTRINE may result in cardiotoxicity (irregular heartbeat, cardiac arrest).	2	2	3
LEVODOPA Concurrent use of PERPHENAZINE and LEVODOPA may result in loss of levodopa efficacy.	1	3	2
LITHIUM Concurrent use of PERPHENAZINE and LITHIUM may result in weakness, movement disorders, brain disorders, and brain damage.	2	2	1

Onset: 0=Unspecified 1=Rapid 2=Delayed
Severity: 1=Contraindicated 2=Major 3=Moderate 4=Minor
Evidence: 1=Excellent 2=Good 3=Fair 4=Poor

INTERACTION	ONSET	SEVERITY	EVIDENCE
MEPERIDINE Concurrent use of PERPHENAZINE and MEPERIDINE may result in an increase in central nervous system and respiratory depression.	1	3	2
ORPHENADRINE Concurrent use of PERPHENAZINE and ORPHENADRINE may result in decreased perphenazine serum concentrations, decreased perphenazine effectiveness, enhanced antispasmodic effects (intestinal blockage, high fever, sedation, dry mouth).	2	3	3
PAROXETINE Concurrent use of PERPHENAZINE and PAROXETINE may result in increased plasma concentrations and side effects of perphenazine.	1	3	3
PHENYTOIN Concurrent use of PERPHENAZINE and PHENYTOIN may result in increased or decreased phenytoin levels and possibly reduced perphenazine levels.	2	4	3
PORFIMER Concurrent use of PERPHENAZINE and PORFIMER may result in excessive intracellular damage in photosensitized tissues.	2	3	3
PROCYCLIDINE Concurrent use of PERPHENAZINE and PROCYCLIDINE may result in decreased perphenazine serum concentrations, decreased perphenazine effectiveness, enhanced antispasmodic effects (intestinal blockage, high fever, sedation, dry mouth).	2	3	3
SPARFLOXACIN Concurrent use of PERPHENAZINE and SPARFLOXACIN may result in irregular heartbeat.	2	1	3
TRAMADOL Concurrent use of PERPHENAZINE and TRAMADOL may result in an increased risk of seizures.	1	2	3
TRIHEXYPHENIDYL Concurrent use of PERPHENAZINE and TRIHEXYPHENIDYL may result in decreased perphenazine serum concentrations, decreased perphenazine effectiveness, enhanced antispasmodic effects (intestinal blockage, high fever, sedation, dry mouth).	2	3	3

Phenelzine

INTERACTION	ONSET	SEVERITY	EVIDENCE
ACARBOSE Concurrent use of PHENELZINE and ACARBOSE may result in excessive reductions in blood sugar, central nervous system depression, and seizures.	1	3	2
ACETOHEXAMIDE Concurrent use of PHENELZINE and ACETOHEXAMIDE may result in excessive reductions in blood sugar, central nervous system depression, and seizures.	1	3	2

INTERACTION	ONSET	SEVERITY	EVIDENCE
ALBUTEROL Concurrent use of PHENELZINE and ALBUTEROL may result in an increased risk of rapid heartbeat, agitation, or mild mania.	2	2	2
AMITRIPTYLINE Concurrent use of PHENELZINE and AMITRIPTYLINE may result in neurotoxicity, seizures, or serotonin syndrome (high blood pressure, high fever, spasms, mental status changes).	2	1	3
AMOXAPINE Concurrent use of PHENELZINE and AMOXAPINE may result in neurotoxicity, seizures, or serotonin syndrome (high blood pressure, high fever, spasms, mental status changes).	2	2	3
AMPHETAMINE Concurrent use of PHENELZINE and AMPHETAMINE may result in hypertensive crisis (headache, high fever, high blood pressure).	1	1	2
APRACLONIDINE Concurrent use of PHENELZINE and APRACLONIDINE may result in potentiation of phenelzine effects.	1	1	3
BAMBUTEROL Concurrent use of PHENELZINE and BAMBUTEROL may result in an increased risk of rapid heartbeat, agitation, or mild mania.	2	2	2
BENFLUOREX Concurrent use of PHENELZINE and BENFLUOREX may result in excessive reductions in blood sugar, central nervous system depression, and seizures.	1	3	2
BENZPHETAMINE Concurrent use of PHENELZINE and BENZPHETAMINE may result in hypertensive crisis (headache, high fever, high blood pressure).	1	1	2
BITOLTEROL Concurrent use of PHENELZINE and BITOLTEROL may result in an increased risk of rapid heartbeat, agitation, or mild mania.	2	2	2
BROXATEROL Concurrent use of PHENELZINE and BROXATEROL may result in an increased risk of rapid heartbeat, agitation, or mild mania.	2	2	2
BUPROPION Concurrent use of PHENELZINE and BUPROPION may result in bupropion toxicity (seizures, agitation, psychotic changes).	1	1	3
BUSPIRONE Concurrent use of PHENELZINE and BUSPIRONE may result in hypertensive crisis.	1	1	3

Onset: 0=Unspecified 1=Rapid 2=Delayed
Severity: 1=Contraindicated 2=Major 3=Moderate 4=Minor
Evidence: 1=Excellent 2=Good 3=Fair 4=Poor

INTERACTION	ONSET	SEVERITY	EVIDENCE
CARBAMAZEPINE Concurrent use of PHENELZINE and CARBAMAZEPINE may result in high blood pressure, high fever, and seizures.	1	1	3
CHLORPROPAMIDE Concurrent use of PHENELZINE and CHLORPROPAMIDE may result in excessive reductions in blood sugar, central nervous system depression, and seizures.	1	3	2
CITALOPRAM Concurrent use of PHENELZINE and CITALOPRAM may result in central nervous system toxicity or serotonin syndrome (high blood pressure, high fever, spasms, mental status changes).	1	1	3
CLENBUTEROL Concurrent use of PHENELZINE and CLENBUTEROL may result in an increased risk of rapid heartbeat, agitation, or mild mania.	2	2	2
CLOMIPRAMINE Concurrent use of PHENELZINE and CLOMIPRAMINE may result in neurotoxicity, seizures, or serotonin syndrome (high blood pressure, high fever, spasms, mental status changes).	2	2	3
CLORGYLINE Concurrent use of PHENELZINE and CLORGYLINE may result in hypertensive crisis (headache, palpitation, neck stiffness).	1	1	3
CLOVOXAMINE Concurrent use of PHENELZINE and CLOVOXAMINE may result in central nervous system toxicity or serotonin syndrome (high blood pressure, high fever, spasms, mental status changes).	1	1	3
COCAINE Concurrent use of PHENELZINE and COCAINE may result in hypertensive crisis (headache, high fever, high blood pressure).	1	1	3
CYCLOBENZAPRINE Concurrent use of PHENELZINE and CYCLOBENZAPRINE may result in hypertensive crises (headache, high fever, high blood pressure) or severe convulsive seizures.	1	1	3
CYPROHEPTADINE Concurrent use of PHENELZINE and CYPROHEPTADINE may result in prolonged and intensified effects of cyproheptadine.	2	1	3
DESIPRAMINE Concurrent use of PHENELZINE and DESIPRAMINE may result in neurotoxicity, seizures, or serotonin syndrome (high blood pressure, high fever, spasms, mental status changes).	2	2	3

INTERACTION	ONSET	SEVERITY	EVIDENCE
DEXFENFLURAMINE Concurrent use of PHENELZINE and DEXFENFLURAMINE may result in central nervous system toxicity or serotonin syndrome (high blood pressure, high fever, spasms, mental status changes).	1	1	3
DEXMETHYLPHENIDATE Concurrent use of PHENELZINE and DEXMETHYLPHENIDATE may result in hypertensive crisis (headache, palpitation, neck stiffness).	1	1	3
DEXTROAMPHETAMINE Concurrent use of PHENELZINE and DEXTROAMPHETAMINE may result in a hypertensive crisis (headache, high fever, high blood pressure).	1	1	3
DEXTROMETHORPHAN Concurrent use of PHENELZINE and DEXTROMETHORPHAN may result in an increased risk of serotonin syndrome (high blood pressure, high fever, spasms, mental status changes).	1	1	3
DIETHYLPROPION Concurrent use of PHENELZINE and DIETHYLPROPION may result in hypertensive crisis (headache, high fever, high blood pressure).	1	1	2
DOPAMINE Concurrent use of PHENELZINE and DOPAMINE may result in hypertensive crisis (headache, high fever, high blood pressure).	1	1	1
DOTHIEPIN Concurrent use of PHENELZINE and DOTHIEPIN may result in neurotoxicity, seizures, or serotonin syndrome (high blood pressure, high fever, spasms, mental status changes).	2	2	3
DOXEPIN Concurrent use of PHENELZINE and DOXEPIN may result in neurotoxicity, seizures, or serotonin syndrome (high blood pressure, high fever, spasms, mental status changes).	2	2	3
DROPERIDOL Concurrent use of PHENELZINE and DROPERIDOL may result in an increased risk of cardiotoxicity (irregular heartbeat, cardiac arrest).	1	2	3
EPHEDRINE Concurrent use of PHENELZINE and EPHEDRINE may result in hypertensive crisis (headache, high fever, high blood pressure).	1	2	3
EPINEPHRINE Concurrent use of PHENELZINE and EPINEPHRINE may result in increased hypertensive effects.	1	1	3

Onset: **0**=Unspecified **1**=Rapid **2**=Delayed
Severity: **1**=Contraindicated **2**=Major **3**=Moderate **4**=Minor
Evidence: **1**=Excellent **2**=Good **3**=Fair **4**=Poor

INTERACTION	ONSET	SEVERITY	EVIDENCE
FEMOXETINE Concurrent use of PHENELZINE and FEMOXETINE may result in central nervous system toxicity or serotonin syndrome (high blood pressure, high fever, spasms, mental status changes).	1	1	3
FENFLURAMINE Concurrent use of PHENELZINE and FENFLURAMINE may result in serotonin syndrome (high blood pressure, high fever, spasms, mental status changes).	1	1	3
FENOTEROL Concurrent use of PHENELZINE and FENOTEROL may result in an increased risk of rapid heartbeat, agitation, or mild mania.	2	2	2
FLUOXETINE Concurrent use of PHENELZINE and FLUOXETINE may result in central nervous system toxicity or serotonin syndrome (high blood pressure, high fever, spasms, mental status changes).	1	1	2
FLUVOXAMINE Concurrent use of PHENELZINE and FLUVOXAMINE may result in central nervous system toxicity or serotonin syndrome (high blood pressure, high fever, spasms, mental status changes).	1	1	2
FORMOTEROL Concurrent use of PHENELZINE and FORMOTEROL may result in an increased risk of rapid heartbeat, agitation, or mild mania.	2	2	2
FURAZOLIDONE Concurrent use of PHENELZINE and FURAZOLIDONE may result in hypertensive crisis (headache, palpitation, neck stiffness).	1	1	3
GLICLAZIDE Concurrent use of PHENELZINE and GLICLAZIDE may result in excessive reductions in blood sugar, central nervous system depression, and seizures.	1	3	2
GLIMEPIRIDE Concurrent use of PHENELZINE and GLIMEPIRIDE may result in excessive reductions in blood sugar, central nervous system depression, and seizures.	1	3	2
GLIPIZIDE Concurrent use of PHENELZINE and GLIPIZIDE may result in excessive reductions in blood sugar, central nervous system depression, and seizures.	1	3	2
GLIQUIDONE Concurrent use of PHENELZINE and GLIQUIDONE may result in excessive reductions in blood sugar, central nervous system depression, and seizures.	1	3	2

INTERACTION	ONSET	SEVERITY	EVIDENCE
GLYBURIDE Concurrent use of PHENELZINE and GLYBURIDE may result in excessive reductions in blood sugar, central nervous system depression, and seizures.	1	3	2
GUANADREL Concurrent use of PHENELZINE and GUANADREL may result in decreased antihypertensive response to guanadrel or hypertensive crisis when guanadrel is initiated in a patient already receiving phenelzine.	1	1	3
GUAR GUM Concurrent use of PHENELZINE and GUAR GUM may result in excessive reductions in blood sugar, central nervous system depression, and seizures.	1	3	2
HEXOPRENALINE Concurrent use of PHENELZINE and HEXOPRENALINE may result in an increased risk of rapid heartbeat, agitation, or mild mania.	2	2	2
IMIPRAMINE Concurrent use of PHENELZINE and IMIPRAMINE may result in neurotoxicity, seizures, or serotonin syndrome (high blood pressure, high fever, spasms, mental status changes).	2	2	3
INSULIN Concurrent use of PHENELZINE and INSULIN may result in excessive reductions in blood sugar, central nervous system depression, and seizures.	1	3	2
IPRONIAZID Concurrent use of PHENELZINE and IPRONIAZID may result in hypertensive crisis (headache, palpitation, neck stiffness).	1	1	3
ISOCARBOXAZID Concurrent use of PHENELZINE and ISOCARBOXAZID may result in hypertensive crisis (headache, palpitation, neck stiffness).	1	1	3
ISOETHARINE Concurrent use of PHENELZINE and ISOETHARINE may result in an increased risk of rapid heartbeat, agitation, or mild mania.	2	2	2
ISOMETHEPTENE Concurrent use of PHENELZINE and ISOMETHEPTENE may result in severe headache, hypertensive crisis, cardiac irregularities.	1	1	1
ISOPROTERENOL Concurrent use of PHENELZINE and ISOPROTERENOL may result in increased blood pressure.	1	3	3

Onset: 0=Unspecified 1=Rapid 2=Delayed
Severity: 1=Contraindicated 2=Major 3=Moderate 4=Minor
Evidence: 1=Excellent 2=Good 3=Fair 4=Poor

INTERACTION	ONSET	SEVERITY	EVIDENCE
LAZABEMIDE Concurrent use of PHENELZINE and LAZABEMIDE may result in hypertensive crisis (headache, palpitation, neck stiffness).	1	1	3
LEVALBUTEROL Concurrent use of PHENELZINE and LEVALBUTEROL may result in an increased risk of rapid heartbeat, agitation, or mild mania.	2	2	2
LEVODOPA Concurrent use of PHENELZINE and LEVODOPA may result in high blood pressure.	1	1	3
LEVOMETHADYL Concurrent use of PHENELZINE and LEVOMETHADYL may result in increased levels of levomethadyl or its active metabolites.	2	1	3
LOFEPRAMINE Concurrent use of PHENELZINE and LOFEPRAMINE may result in neurotoxicity, seizures, or serotonin syndrome (high blood pressure, high fever, spasms, mental status changes).	2	2	3
MA HUANG Concurrent use of PHENELZINE and MA HUANG may result in increased risk for excessive phenelzine activity including headache, high fever, cardiac irregularities, and hypertensive crisis.	1	2	3
MAPROTILINE Concurrent use of PHENELZINE and MAPROTILINE may result in neurotoxicity, seizures.	2	1	3
MAZINDOL Concurrent use of PHENELZINE and MAZINDOL may result in hypertensive crisis (headache, high fever, high blood pressure).	1	1	3
MEPERIDINE Concurrent use of PHENELZINE and MEPERIDINE may result in cardiovascular instability, high fever, coma, or death.	1	1	2
METARAMINOL Concurrent use of PHENELZINE and METARAMINOL may result in hypertensive crisis (headache, high fever, high blood pressure).	1	2	3
METFORMIN Concurrent use of PHENELZINE and METFORMIN may result in excessive reductions in blood sugar, central nervous system depression, and seizures.	1	3	2

INTERACTION	ONSET	SEVERITY	EVIDENCE
METHAMPHETAMINE Concurrent use of PHENELZINE and METHAMPHETAMINE may result in hypertensive crisis (headache, high fever, high blood pressure).	1	1	3
METHOTRIMEPRAZINE Concurrent use of PHENELZINE and METHOTRIMEPRAZINE may result in possibly prolonged effect of methotrimeprazine, with potentially increased side effects.	2	1	3
METHYLDOPA Concurrent use of PHENELZINE and METHYLDOPA may result in hypertensive crisis (headache, palpitation, neck stiffness).	1	1	3
METHYLPHENIDATE Concurrent use of PHENELZINE and METHYLPHENIDATE may result in hypertensive crisis (headache, palpitation, neck stiffness).	1	1	3
MIGLITOL Concurrent use of PHENELZINE and MIGLITOL may result in excessive reductions in blood sugar, central nervous system depression, and seizures.	1	3	2
MIRTAZAPINE Concurrent use of PHENELZINE and MIRTAZAPINE may result in neurotoxicity, seizures.	2	1	3
MOCLOBEMIDE Concurrent use of PHENELZINE and MOCLOBEMIDE may result in hypertensive crisis (headache, palpitation, neck stiffness).	1	1	3
MORPHINE Concurrent use of PHENELZINE and MORPHINE may result in low blood pressure and exaggeration of central nervous system and respiratory depressant effects.	1	1	3
NEFAZODONE Concurrent use of PHENELZINE and NEFAZODONE may result in high fever, rigidity, spasms, seizures, fluctuations of vital signs, or mental status changes.	1	1	2
NIALAMIDE Concurrent use of PHENELZINE and NIALAMIDE may result in hypertensive crisis (headache, palpitation, neck stiffness).	1	1	3
NOREPINEPHRINE Concurrent use of PHENELZINE and NOREPINEPHRINE may result in increased blood pressure.	1	1	3

Onset: 0=Unspecified 1=Rapid 2=Delayed
Severity: 1=Contraindicated 2=Major 3=Moderate 4=Minor
Evidence: 1=Excellent 2=Good 3=Fair 4=Poor

INTERACTION	ONSET	SEVERITY	EVIDENCE
NORTRIPTYLINE Concurrent use of PHENELZINE and NORTRIPTYLINE may result in neurotoxicity, seizures, or serotonin syndrome (high blood pressure, high fever, spasms, mental status changes).	2	2	3
OPIPRAMOL Concurrent use of PHENELZINE and OPIPRAMOL may result in neurotoxicity, seizures, or serotonin syndrome (high blood pressure, high fever, spasms, mental status changes).	2	1	3
OXYCODONE Concurrent use of PHENELZINE and OXYCODONE may result in anxiety, confusion and significant respiratory depressant effects or coma.	2	2	3
PARGYLINE Concurrent use of PHENELZINE and PARGYLINE may result in hypertensive crisis (headache, palpitation, neck stiffness).	1	1	3
PAROXETINE Concurrent use of PHENELZINE and PAROXETINE may result in central nervous system toxicity or serotonin syndrome (high blood pressure, high fever, spasms, mental status changes).	1	1	2
PHENDIMETRAZINE Concurrent use of PHENELZINE and PHENDIMETRIZINE may result in hypertensive crisis (headache, high fever, high blood pressure).	1	1	2
PHENMETRAZINE Concurrent use of PHENELZINE and PHENMETRAZINE may result in hypertensive crisis (headache, high fever, high blood pressure).	1	1	2
PHENTERMINE Concurrent use of PHENELZINE and PHENTERMINE may result in hypertensive crisis (headache, high fever, high blood pressure).	1	1	1
PHENYLALANINE Concurrent use of PHENELZINE and PHENYLALANINE may result in hypertensive crisis (headache, palpitation, neck stiffness).	1	1	3
PHENYLEPHRINE Concurrent use of PHENELZINE and PHENYLEPHRINE may result in hypertensive crisis (headache, high fever, high blood pressure).	1	1	2
PHENYLPROPANOLAMINE Concurrent use of PHENELZINE and PHENYLPROPANOLAMINE may result in hypertensive crisis (headache, high fever, high blood pressure).	1	1	1

INTERACTION	ONSET	SEVERITY	EVIDENCE
PIRBUTEROL Concurrent use of PHENELZINE and PIRBUTEROL may result in an increased risk of rapid heartbeat, agitation, or mild mania.	2	2	2
PROCARBAZINE Concurrent use of PHENELZINE and PROCARBAZINE may result in hypertensive crisis (headache, palpitation, neck stiffness).	1	1	3
PROCATEROL Concurrent use of PHENELZINE and PROCATEROL may result in an increased risk of rapid heartbeat, agitation, or mild mania.	2	2	2
PROTRIPTYLINE Concurrent use of PHENELZINE and PROTRIPTYLINE may result in neurotoxicity, seizures, or serotonin syndrome (high blood pressure, high fever, spasms, mental status changes).	2	2	3
PSEUDOEPHEDRINE Concurrent use of PHENELZINE and PSEUDOEPHEDRINE may result in hypertensive crisis (headache, high fever, high blood pressure).	1	1	3
REBOXETINE Concurrent use of PHENELZINE and REBOXETINE may result in high fever, rigidity, spasms, seizures, fluctuations of vital signs, or mental status changes.	1	2	3
RESERPINE Concurrent use of PHENELZINE and RESERPINE may result in elevated levels of several chemical messengers in the brain.	1	1	3
RIMITEROL Concurrent use of PHENELZINE and RIMITEROL may result in an increased risk of rapid heartbeat, agitation, or mild mania.	2	2	2
RITODRINE Concurrent use of PHENELZINE and RITODRINE may result in an increased risk of rapid heartbeat, agitation, or mild mania.	2	2	2
SALMETEROL Concurrent use of PHENELZINE and SALMETEROL may result in an increased risk of rapid heartbeat, agitation, or mild mania.	2	2	2
SELEGILINE Concurrent use of PHENELZINE and SELEGILINE may result in hypertensive crisis (headache, palpitation, neck stiffness).	1	1	3

Onset: 0=Unspecified 1=Rapid 2=Delayed
Severity: 1=Contraindicated 2=Major 3=Moderate 4=Minor
Evidence: 1=Excellent 2=Good 3=Fair 4=Poor

INTERACTION	ONSET	SEVERITY	EVIDENCE
SERTRALINE Concurrent use of PHENELZINE and SERTRALINE may result in central nervous system toxicity or serotonin syndrome (high blood pressure, high fever, spasms, mental status changes).	1	1	2
SIBUTRAMINE Concurrent use of PHENELZINE and SIBUTRAMINE may result in central nervous system toxicity or serotonin syndrome (high blood pressure, high fever, spasms, mental status changes).	1	1	3
ST JOHN'S WORT Concurrent use of PHENELZINE and ST. JOHN'S WORT may result in an increased risk of serotonin syndrome (high blood pressure, high fever, spasms, mental status changes) and/or an increased risk of hypertensive crisis.	2	2	3
SUMATRIPTAN Concurrent use of PHENELZINE and SUMATRIPTAN may result in an increased risk of serotonin syndrome (high blood pressure, high fever, spasms, mental status changes).	1	1	3
TERBUTALINE Concurrent use of PHENELZINE and TERBUTALINE may result in an increased risk of rapid heartbeat, agitation, or mild mania.	2	2	2
TOLAZAMIDE Concurrent use of PHENELZINE and TOLAZAMIDE may result in excessive reductions in blood sugar, central nervous system depression, and seizures.	1	3	2
TOLBUTAMIDE Concurrent use of PHENELZINE and TOLBUTAMIDE may result in excessive reductions in blood sugar, central nervous system depression, and seizures.	1	3	2
TOLCAPONE Concurrent use of PHENELZINE and TOLCAPONE may result in decreased metabolism of certain chemical messengers in the brain.	1	2	3
TOLOXATONE Concurrent use of PHENELZINE and TOLOXATONE may result in hypertensive crisis (headache, palpitation, neck stiffness).	1	1	3
TRAMADOL Concurrent use of PHENELZINE and TRAMADOL may result in nausea, vomiting, cardiovascular collapse, respiratory depression, seizures.	1	2	3
TRANYLCYPROMINE Concurrent use of PHENELZINE and TRANYLCYPROMINE may result in hypertensive crisis (headache, palpitation, neck stiffness).	1	1	3

INTERACTION	ONSET	SEVERITY	EVIDENCE
TRIMIPRAMINE Concurrent use of PHENELZINE and TRIMIPRAMINE may result in neurotoxicity, seizures, or serotonin syndrome (high blood pressure, high fever, spasms, mental status changes).	2	2	3
TROGLITAZONE Concurrent use of PHENELZINE and TROGLITAZONE may result in excessive reductions in blood sugar, central nervous system depression, and seizures.	1	3	2
TRYPTOPHAN Concurrent use of PHENELZINE and TRYPTOPHAN may result in delirium and serotonin syndrome (high blood pressure, high fever, spasms, mental status changes).	1	1	3
TULOBUTEROL Concurrent use of PHENELZINE and TULOBUTEROL may result in an increased risk of rapid heartbeat, agitation, or mild mania.	2	2	2
TYRAMINE FOODS Concurrent use of PHENELZINE and TYRAMINE FOODS may result in increased blood pressure.	1	1	1
VENLAFAXINE Concurrent use of PHENELZINE and VENLAFAXINE may result in central nervous system toxicity or serotonin syndrome (high blood pressure, high fever, spasms, mental status changes).	1	1	2

Phenobarbital

INTERACTION	ONSET	SEVERITY	EVIDENCE
ACENOCOUMAROL Concurrent use of PHENOBARBITAL and ACENOCOUMAROL may result in decreased acenocoumarol effectiveness.	2	2	2
ALPRENOLOL Concurrent use of PHENOBARBITAL and ALPRENOLOL may result in decreased alprenolol effectiveness.	2	3	3
ANISINDIONE Concurrent use of PHENOBARBITAL and ANISINDIONE may result in decreased anisindione effectiveness.	2	2	2
BETAMETHASONE Concurrent use of PHENOBARBITAL and BETAMETHASONE may result in decreased betamethasone effectiveness.	2	3	3
CHLORPROMAZINE Concurrent use of PHENOBARBITAL and CHLORPROMAZINE may result in decreased chlorpromazine effectiveness.	1	3	3

Onset: 0=Unspecified 1=Rapid 2=Delayed
Severity: 1=Contraindicated 2=Major 3=Moderate 4=Minor
Evidence: 1=Excellent 2=Good 3=Fair 4=Poor

INTERACTION	ONSET	SEVERITY	EVIDENCE
CLOZAPINE Concurrent use of PHENOBARBITAL and CLOZAPINE may result in decreased clozapine plasma levels associated with marked worsening of psychosis.	2	3	3
CORTISONE Concurrent use of PHENOBARBITAL and CORTISONE may result in decreased cortisone effectiveness.	2	3	3
CYCLOSPORINE Concurrent use of PHENOBARBITAL and CYCLOSPORINE may result in decreased cyclosporine effectiveness.	2	3	3
DEFLAZACORT Concurrent use of PHENOBARBITAL and DEFLAZACORT may result in decreased corticosteroid effectiveness.	2	3	2
DEXAMETHASONE Concurrent use of PHENOBARBITAL and DEXAMETHASONE may result in decreased dexamethasone effectiveness.	2	3	2
DEXMETHYLPHENIDATE Concurrent use of PHENOBARBITAL and DEXMETHYLPHENIDATE may result in an increase in phenobarbital plasma concentrations.	1	3	3
DICUMAROL Concurrent use of PHENOBARBITAL and DICUMAROL may result in decreased dicumarol effectiveness.	2	2	2
DIGITOXIN Concurrent use of PHENOBARBITAL and DIGITOXIN may result in decreased digitoxin levels.	2	3	3
DISOPYRAMIDE Concurrent use of PHENOBARBITAL and DISOPYRAMIDE may result in decreased disopyramide effectiveness.	2	3	3
ETHANOL Concurrent use of PHENOBARBITAL and ETHANOL may result in excessive central nervous system depression.	1	3	1
ETHOSUXIMIDE Concurrent use of PHENOBARBITAL and ETHOSUXIMIDE may result in decreased ethosuximide serum concentrations.	2	3	3
FELODIPINE Concurrent use of PHENOBARBITAL and FELODIPINE may result in decreased felodipine effectiveness.	2	3	3
FLUDROCORTISONE Concurrent use of PHENOBARBITAL and FLUDROCORTISONE may result in decreased fludrocortisone effectiveness.	2	3	2

INTERACTION	ONSET	SEVERITY	EVIDENCE
FOSPHENYTOIN Concurrent use of PHENOBARBITAL and FOSPHENYTOIN may result in increased or decreased phenytoin levels.	2	4	3
GRISEOFULVIN Concurrent use of PHENOBARBITAL and GRISEOFULVIN may result in decreased effectiveness of griseofulvin.	1	3	3
GUANFACINE Concurrent use of PHENOBARBITAL and GUANFACINE may result in decreased guanfacine effectiveness.	2	3	3
HYDROCORTISONE Concurrent use of PHENOBARBITAL and HYDROCORTISONE may result in decreased hydrocortisone effectiveness.	2	3	2
ITRACONAZOLE Concurrent use of PHENOBARBITAL and ITRACONAZOLE may result in loss of itraconazole efficacy.	2	3	3
LAMOTRIGINE Concurrent use of PHENOBARBITAL and LAMOTRIGINE may result in reduced lamotrigine efficacy, loss of seizure control.	2	3	2
LEVOMETHADYL Concurrent use of PHENOBARBITAL and LEVOMETHADYL may result in an increased risk of cardiotoxicity (irregular heartbeat).	2	3	3
METHOXYFLURANE Concurrent use of PHENOBARBITAL and METHOXYFLURANE may result in kidney damage.	1	2	3
METHYLPREDNISOLONE Concurrent use of PHENOBARBITAL and METHYLPREDNISOLONE may result in decreased methylprednisolone effectiveness.	2	3	2
METOPROLOL Concurrent use of PHENOBARBITAL and METOPROLOL may result in decreased metoprolol effectiveness.	2	3	3
METRONIDAZOLE Concurrent use of PHENOBARBITAL and METRONIDAZOLE may result in decreased metronidazole effectiveness.	2	4	3
ORAL CONTRACEPTIVES Concurrent use of PHENOBARBITAL and ORAL CONTRACEPTIVES may result in decreased contraceptive effectiveness.	2	2	2
PARAMETHASONE Concurrent use of PHENOBARBITAL and PARAMETHASONE may result in decreased paramethasone effectiveness.	2	3	2

Onset: 0=Unspecified   1=Rapid   2=Delayed
Severity: 1=Contraindicated   2=Major   3=Moderate   4=Minor
Evidence: 1=Excellent   2=Good   3=Fair   4=Poor

INTERACTION	ONSET	SEVERITY	EVIDENCE
PAROXETINE Concurrent use of PHENOBARBITAL and PAROXETINE may result in reduced paroxetine effectiveness.	1	4	3
PHENINDIONE Concurrent use of PHENOBARBITAL and PHENINDIONE may result in decreased phenindione effectiveness.	2	2	2
PHENPROCOUMON Concurrent use of PHENOBARBITAL and PHENPROCOUMON may result in decreased phenprocoumon effectiveness.	2	2	2
PHENYTOIN Concurrent use of PHENOBARBITAL and PHENYTOIN may result in increased or decreased phenytoin levels.	2	4	3
PREDNISOLONE Concurrent use of PHENOBARBITAL and PREDNISOLONE may result in decreased prednisolone effectiveness.	2	3	2
PREDNISONE Concurrent use of PHENOBARBITAL and PREDNISONE may result in decreased therapeutic effect of prednisone.	2	3	2
PROPRANOLOL Concurrent use of PHENOBARBITAL and PROPRANOLOL may result in decreased propranolol effectiveness.	2	3	3
QUINIDINE Concurrent use of PHENOBARBITAL and QUINIDINE may result in decreased quinidine effectiveness.	2	3	2
TACROLIMUS Concurrent use of PHENOBARBITAL and TACROLIMUS may result in decreased tacrolimus efficacy.	2	3	3
TENIPOSIDE Concurrent use of PHENOBARBITAL and TENIPOSIDE may result in increased teniposide clearance.	2	3	3
THEOPHYLLINE Concurrent use of PHENOBARBITAL and THEOPHYLLINE may result in decreased theophylline effectiveness.	2	3	2
TOPIRAMATE Concurrent use of PHENOBARBITAL and TOPIRAMATE may result in a decrease in serum concentrations of topiramate.	2	3	3
TRIAMCINOLONE Concurrent use of PHENOBARBITAL and TRIAMCINOLONE may result in decreased triamcinolone effectiveness.	2	3	2
VALERIAN Concurrent use of PHENOBARBITAL and VALERIAN may result in increased central nervous system depression.	1	3	3
VALPROIC ACID Concurrent use of PHENOBARBITAL and VALPROIC ACID may result in phenobarbital toxicity or decreased valproic acid effectiveness.	2	3	1

INTERACTION	ONSET	SEVERITY	EVIDENCE
VERAPAMIL Concurrent use of PHENOBARBITAL and VERAPAMIL may result in decreased verapamil effectiveness.	2	3	3
WARFARIN Concurrent use of PHENOBARBITAL and WARFARIN may result in decreased warfarin effectiveness.	2	3	1

Prochlorperazine

INTERACTION	ONSET	SEVERITY	EVIDENCE
BELLADONNA Concurrent use of PROCHLORPERAZINE and BELLADONNA may result in increased manic, agitated reactions, or enhanced antispasmodic effects resulting in cardiorespiratory failure, especially in cases of belladonna overdose.	1	3	2
BENZTROPINE Concurrent use of PROCHLORPERAZINE and BENZTROPINE may result in decreased prochlorperazine serum concentrations, decreased prochlorperazine effectiveness, and enhanced antispasmodic effects (intestinal blockage, high fever, sedation, dry mouth).	2	3	3
CABERGOLINE Concurrent use of PROCHLORPERAZINE and CABERGOLINE may result in the decreased therapeutic effect of both drugs.	1	3	3
CISAPRIDE Concurrent use of PROCHLORPERAZINE and CISAPRIDE may result in cardiotoxicity (irregular heartbeat, cardiac arrest).	1	1	3
ETHANOL Concurrent use of PROCHLORPERAZINE and ETHANOL may result in increased central nervous system depression and an increased risk of movement disorders.	1	3	2
FOSPHENYTOIN Concurrent use of PROCHLORPERAZINE and FOSPHENYTOIN may result in increased or decreased phenytoin levels and possibly reduced prochlorperazine levels.	2	4	3
GREPAFLOXACIN Concurrent use of PROCHLORPERAZINE and GREPAFLOXACIN may result in an increased risk of cardiotoxicity (irregular heartbeat, cardiac arrest).	2	1	3
GUANETHIDINE Concurrent use of PROCHLORPERAZINE and GUANETHIDINE may result in decreased guanethidine effectiveness.	1	3	2

Onset: 0=Unspecified 1=Rapid 2=Delayed
Severity: 1=Contraindicated 2=Major 3=Moderate 4=Minor
Evidence: 1=Excellent 2=Good 3=Fair 4=Poor

INTERACTION	ONSET	SEVERITY	EVIDENCE
HALOFANTRINE Concurrent use of PROCHLORPERAZINE and HALOFANTRINE may result in cardiotoxicity (irregular heartbeat, cardiac arrest).	2	2	3
IBUTILIDE Concurrent use of PROCHLORPERAZINE and IBUTILIDE may result in an increased risk of cardiac irregularities.	1	2	3
LEVODOPA Concurrent use of PROCHLORPERAZINE and LEVODOPA may result in loss of levodopa efficacy.	1	3	2
LITHIUM Concurrent use of PROCHLORPERAZINE and LITHIUM may result in weakness, movement disorders, brain disorders, and brain damage.	2	2	1
MEPERIDINE Concurrent use of PROCHLORPERAZINE and MEPERIDINE may result in an increase in central nervous system and respiratory depression.	1	3	2
ORPHENADRINE Concurrent use of PROCHLORPERAZINE and ORPHENADRINE may result in decreased prochlorperazine serum concentrations, decreased prochlorperazine effectiveness, and enhanced antispasmodic effects (intestinal blockage, high fever, sedation, dry mouth).	2	3	3
PHENYTOIN Concurrent use of PROCHLORPERAZINE and PHENYTOIN may result in increased or decreased phenytoin levels and possibly reduced prochlorperazine levels.	2	4	3
PORFIMER Concurrent use of PROCHLORPERAZINE and PORFIMER may result in excessive intracellular damage in photosensitized tissues.	2	3	3
PROCYCLIDINE Concurrent use of PROCHLORPERAZINE and PROCYCLIDINE may result in decreased prochlorperazine serum concentrations, decreased prochlorperazine effectiveness, enhanced antispasmodic effects (intestinal blockage, high fever, sedation, dry mouth).	2	3	3
SPARFLOXACIN Concurrent use of PROCHLORPERAZINE and SPARFLOXACIN may result in irregular heartbeat.	2	1	3
TRIHEXYPHENIDYL Concurrent use of PROCHLORPERAZINE and TRIHEXYPHENIDYL may result in decreased prochlorperazine serum concentrations, decreased prochlorperazine effectiveness, and enhanced antispasmodic effects (intestinal blockage, high fever, sedation, dry mouth).	2	3	3

Promethazine

INTERACTION	ONSET	SEVERITY	EVIDENCE
BELLADONNA Concurrent use of PROMETHAZINE and BELLADONNA may result in increased manic, agitated reactions, or enhanced antispasmodic effects resulting in cardiorespiratory failure, especially in cases of belladonna overdose.	1	3	2
BENZTROPINE Concurrent use of PROMETHAZINE and BENZTROPINE may result in decreased promethazine serum concentrations, decreased promethazine effectiveness, and enhanced antispasmodic effects (intestinal blockage, high fever, sedation, dry mouth).	2	3	3
CABERGOLINE Concurrent use of PROMETHAZINE and CABERGOLINE may result in the decreased therapeutic effect of both drugs.	1	3	3
CISAPRIDE Concurrent use of PROMETHAZINE and CISAPRIDE may result in cardiotoxicity (irregular heartbeat, cardiac arrest).	1	1	3
FOSPHENYTOIN Concurrent use of PROMETHAZINE and FOSPHENYTOIN may result in increased or decreased phenytoin levels and possibly reduced promethazine levels.	2	4	3
GREPAFLOXACIN Concurrent use of PROMETHAZINE and GREPAFLOXACIN may result in an increased risk of cardiotoxicity (irregular heartbeat, cardiac arrest).	2	1	3
HALOFANTRINE Concurrent use of PROMETHAZINE and HALOFANTRINE may result in cardiotoxicity (irregular heartbeat, cardiac arrest).	2	2	3
LITHIUM Concurrent use of PROMETHAZINE and LITHIUM may result in weakness, movement disorders, brain disorders, and brain damage.	2	2	1
MEPERIDINE Concurrent use of PROMETHAZINE and MEPERIDINE may result in an increase in central nervous system and respiratory depression.	1	3	2
ORPHENADRINE Concurrent use of PROMETHAZINE and ORPHENADRINE may result in decreased promethazine serum concentrations, decreased promethazine effectiveness, and enhanced antispasmodic effects (intestinal blockage, high fever, sedation, dry mouth).	2	3	3

Onset: 0=Unspecified 1=Rapid 2=Delayed
Severity: 1=Contraindicated 2=Major 3=Moderate 4=Minor
Evidence: 1=Excellent 2=Good 3=Fair 4=Poor

INTERACTION	ONSET	SEVERITY	EVIDENCE
PHENYTOIN Concurrent use of PROMETHAZINE and PHENYTOIN may result in increased or decreased phenytoin levels and possibly reduced promethazine levels.	2	4	3
PORFIMER Concurrent use of PROMETHAZINE and PORFIMER may result in excessive intracellular damage in photosensitized tissues.	2	3	3
PROCYCLIDINE Concurrent use of PROMETHAZINE and PROCYCLIDINE may result in decreased promethazine serum concentrations, decreased promethazine effectiveness, and enhanced antispasmodic effects (intestinal blockage, high fever, sedation, dry mouth).	2	3	3
SPARFLOXACIN Concurrent use of PROMETHAZINE and SPARFLOXACIN may result in irregular heartbeat.	2	1	3
TRAMADOL Concurrent use of PROMETHAZINE and TRAMADOL may result in an increased risk of seizures.	1	2	3
TRIHEXYPHENIDYL Concurrent use of PROMETHAZINE and TRIHEXYPHENIDYL may result in decreased promethazine serum concentrations, decreased promethazine effectiveness, and enhanced antispasmodic effects (intestinal blockage, high fever, sedation, dry mouth).	2	3	3

Protriptyline

INTERACTION	ONSET	SEVERITY	EVIDENCE
ACENOCOUMAROL Concurrent use of PROTRIPTYLINE and ACENOCOUMAROL may result in increased risk of bleeding.	2	3	3
AMPRENAVIR Concurrent use of PROTRIPTYLINE and AMPRENAVIR may result in increased protriptyline serum concentrations and potential toxicity (antispasmodic effects, sedation, confusion, cardiac irregularities).	2	2	3
ANISINDIONE Concurrent use of PROTRIPTYLINE and ANISINDIONE may result in increased risk of bleeding.	2	3	3
BEPRIDIL Concurrent use of PROTRIPTYLINE and BEPRIDIL may result in cardiac irregularities.	1	1	3
BETHANIDINE Concurrent use of PROTRIPTYLINE and BETHANIDINE may result in decreased bethanidine effectiveness.	1	3	2

INTERACTION	ONSET	SEVERITY	EVIDENCE
CARBAMAZEPINE Concurrent use of PROTRIPTYLINE and CARBAMAZEPINE may result in decreased protriptyline plasma concentrations and increased carbamazepine plasma concentrations and possible toxicity (poor coordination, rolling eyes, disrupted breathing, seizures, coma).	2	3	3
CIMETIDINE Concurrent use of PROTRIPTYLINE and CIMETIDINE may result in protriptyline toxicity (dry mouth, blurred vision, urinary retention).	2	3	3
CISAPRIDE Concurrent use of PROTRIPTYLINE and CISAPRIDE may result in cardiotoxicity (irregular heartbeat, cardiac arrest).	1	1	3
CLONIDINE Concurrent use of PROTRIPTYLINE and CLONIDINE may result in decreased clonidine effectiveness.	2	2	3
CLORGYLINE Concurrent use of PROTRIPTYLINE and CLORGYLINE may result in neurotoxicity, seizures, or serotonin syndrome (high blood pressure, high fever, spasms, mental status changes).	2	2	3
DICUMAROL Concurrent use of PROTRIPTYLINE and DICUMAROL may result in increased risk of bleeding.	2	3	3
EPINEPHRINE Concurrent use of PROTRIPTYLINE and EPINEPHRINE may result in high blood pressure, cardiac irregularities, and rapid heartbeat.	1	2	2
ETILEFRINE Concurrent use of PROTRIPTYLINE and ETILEFRINE may result in high blood pressure, cardiac irregularities, and rapid heartbeat.	1	2	2
FLUOXETINE Concurrent use of PROTRIPTYLINE and FLUOXETINE may result in protriptyline toxicity (dry mouth, urinary retention, sedation).	2	3	3
GREPAFLOXACIN Concurrent use of PROTRIPTYLINE and GREPAFLOXACIN may result in an increased risk of cardiotoxicity (irregular heartbeat, cardiac arrest).	2	1	3
GUANADREL Concurrent use of PROTRIPTYLINE and GUANADREL may result in decreased guanadrel effectiveness.	2	3	3
GUANETHIDINE Concurrent use of PROTRIPTYLINE and GUANETHIDINE may result in decreased guanethidine effectiveness.	2	3	1

Onset: 0=Unspecified 1=Rapid 2=Delayed
Severity: 1=Contraindicated 2=Major 3=Moderate 4=Minor
Evidence: 1=Excellent 2=Good 3=Fair 4=Poor

INTERACTION	ONSET	SEVERITY	EVIDENCE
HALOFANTRINE Concurrent use of PROTRIPTYLINE and HALOFANTRINE may result in cardiotoxicity (irregular heartbeat, cardiac arrest).	2	2	3
ISOCARBOXAZID Concurrent use of PROTRIPTYLINE and ISOCARBOXAZID may result in neurotoxicity, seizures, or serotonin syndrome (high blood pressure, high fever, spasms, mental status changes).	2	1	3
METHOXAMINE Concurrent use of PROTRIPTYLINE and METHOXAMINE may result in high blood pressure, cardiac irregularities, and rapid heartbeat.	1	2	2
MIDODRINE Concurrent use of PROTRIPTYLINE and MIDODRINE may result in high blood pressure, cardiac irregularities, and rapid heartbeat.	1	2	2
MOCLOBEMIDE Concurrent use of PROTRIPTYLINE and MOCLOBEMIDE may result in neurotoxicity, seizures, or serotonin syndrome (high blood pressure, high fever, spasms, mental status changes).	2	2	3
NOREPINEPHRINE Concurrent use of PROTRIPTYLINE and NOREPINEPHRINE may result in high blood pressure, cardiac irregularities, and rapid heartbeat.	1	2	2
OXILOFRINE Concurrent use of PROTRIPTYLINE and OXILOFRINE may result in high blood pressure, cardiac irregularities, and rapid heartbeat.	1	2	2
PHENELZINE Concurrent use of PROTRIPTYLINE and PHENELZINE may result in neurotoxicity, seizures, or serotonin syndrome (high blood pressure, high fever, spasms, mental status changes).	2	2	3
PHENINDIONE Concurrent use of PROTRIPTYLINE and PHENINDIONE may result in increased risk of bleeding.	2	3	3
PHENPROCOUMON Concurrent use of PROTRIPTYLINE and PHENPROCOUMON may result in increased risk of bleeding.	2	3	3
PHENYLEPHRINE Concurrent use of PROTRIPTYLINE and PHENYLEPHRINE may result in high blood pressure, cardiac irregularities, and rapid heartbeat.	1	2	2
PIMOZIDE Concurrent use of PROTRIPTYLINE and PIMOZIDE may result in an increased risk of cardiotoxicity (irregular heartbeat, cardiac arrest).	1	1	3

INTERACTION	ONSET	SEVERITY	EVIDENCE
PROCARBAZINE Concurrent use of PROTRIPTYLINE and PROCARBAZINE may result in neurotoxicity, seizures.	2	2	3
SELEGILINE Concurrent use of PROTRIPTYLINE and SELEGILINE may result in neurotoxicity, seizures, or serotonin syndrome (high blood pressure, high fever, spasms, mental status changes).	2	2	3
SPARFLOXACIN Concurrent use of PROTRIPTYLINE and SPARFLOXACIN may result in irregular heartbeat.	2	1	3
TRAMADOL Concurrent use of PROTRIPTYLINE and TRAMADOL may result in an increased risk of seizures.	1	2	3
TRANYLCYPROMINE Concurrent use of PROTRIPTYLINE and TRANYLCYPROMINE may result in neurotoxicity, seizures, or serotonin syndrome (high blood pressure, high fever, spasms, mental status changes).	2	2	3
WARFARIN Concurrent use of PROTRIPTYLINE and WARFARIN may result in an increased risk of bleeding.	2	3	3

Quazepam

INTERACTION	ONSET	SEVERITY	EVIDENCE
CIMETIDINE Concurrent use of QUAZEPAM and CIMETIDINE may result in quazepam toxicity (central nervous system depression).	1	4	3
KETOCONAZOLE Concurrent use of QUAZEPAM and KETOCONAZOLE may result in increased quazepam serum concentrations and quazepam adverse effects (sedation, slurred speech, central nervous system depression).	2	4	3
THEOPHYLLINE Concurrent use of QUAZEPAM and THEOPHYLLINE may result in decreased quazepam effectiveness.	1	3	2

Quetiapine

INTERACTION	ONSET	SEVERITY	EVIDENCE
ETHANOL Concurrent use of QUETIAPINE and ETHANOL may result in potentiation of the cognitive and motor effects of alcohol.	1	3	3

Onset: 0=Unspecified 1=Rapid 2=Delayed
Severity: 1=Contraindicated 2=Major 3=Moderate 4=Minor
Evidence: 1=Excellent 2=Good 3=Fair 4=Poor

Risperidone

INTERACTION	ONSET	SEVERITY	EVIDENCE
DROPERIDOL Concurrent use of RISPERIDONE and DROPERIDOL may result in an increased risk of cardiotoxicity (irregular heartbeat, cardiac arrest).	1	2	3
LEVOMETHADYL Concurrent use of RISPERIDONE and LEVOMETHADYL may result in an increased risk of cardiotoxicity (irregular heartbeat, cardiac arrest).	2	1	3
LITHIUM Concurrent use of RISPERIDONE and LITHIUM may result in weakness, movement disorders, brain disorders, and brain damage.	2	2	1
PAROXETINE Concurrent use of RISPERIDONE and PAROXETINE may result in an increased risk for serotonin syndrome (high blood pressure, high fever, spasms, mental status changes).	2	2	2
TRAMADOL Concurrent use of RISPERIDONE and TRAMADOL may result in an increased risk of seizures.	1	2	3
ZOTEPINE Concurrent use of RISPERIDONE and ZOTEPINE may result in increased risk of seizures.	2	2	3

Secobarbital

INTERACTION	ONSET	SEVERITY	EVIDENCE
DICUMAROL Concurrent use of SECOBARBITAL and DICUMAROL may result in decreased dicumarol effectiveness.	2	2	2
ETHANOL Concurrent use of SECOBARBITAL and ETHANOL may result in excessive central nervous system depression.	1	3	1
FOSPHENYTOIN Concurrent use of SECOBARBITAL and FOSPHENYTOIN may result in increased or decreased phenytoin levels.	2	3	3
METHOXYFLURANE Concurrent use of SECOBARBITAL and METHOXYFLURANE may result in kidney damage.	1	3	3
ORAL CONTRACEPTIVES Concurrent use of SECOBARBITAL and ORAL CONTRACEPTIVES may result in decreased contraceptive effectiveness.	2	2	2
PHENYTOIN Concurrent use of SECOBARBITAL and PHENYTOIN may result in increased or decreased phenytoin levels.	2	4	3
PREDNISOLONE Concurrent use of SECOBARBITAL and PREDNISOLONE may result in decreased therapeutic effect of prednisolone.	2	3	2

INTERACTION	ONSET	SEVERITY	EVIDENCE
PREDNISONE Concurrent use of SECOBARBITAL and PREDNISONE may result in decreased therapeutic effect of prednisone.	2	3	2
THEOPHYLLINE Concurrent use of SECOBARBITAL and THEOPHYLLINE may result in decreased theophylline effectiveness.	2	3	3
VALERIAN Concurrent use of SECOBARBITAL and VALERIAN may result in increased central nervous system depression.	1	3	3
WARFARIN Concurrent use of SECOBARBITAL and WARFARIN may result in decreased warfarin effectiveness.	2	3	1

Sertraline

INTERACTION	ONSET	SEVERITY	EVIDENCE
ALMOTRIPTAN Concurrent use SERTRALINE and ALMOTRIPTAN may result in weakness, exaggerated reflexes, and/or incoordination.	0	3	3
ALPRAZOLAM Concurrent use of SERTRALINE and ALPRAZOLAM may result in an increased risk of psychomotor impairment and sedation.	1	3	3
AMITRIPTYLINE Concurrent use of SERTRALINE and AMITRIPTYLINE may result in elevated amitriptyline serum levels or possible serotonin syndrome (high blood pressure, high fever, spasms, mental status changes).	2	2	3
CARBAMAZEPINE Concurrent use of SERTRALINE and CARBAMAZEPINE may result in an increased risk of carbamazepine toxicity (poor coordination, rolling eyes, double vision, headache, vomiting, disrupted breathing, seizures, coma) and decreased sertraline efficacy.	2	3	3
CIMETIDINE Concurrent use of SERTRALINE and CIMETIDINE may result in elevated sertraline serum concentrations and increased risk of adverse side effects.	1	3	3
CLORGYLINE Concurrent use of SERTRALINE and CLORGYLINE may result in central nervous system toxicity or serotonin syndrome (high blood pressure, high fever, spasms, mental status changes).	1	1	2
CLOZAPINE Concurrent use of SERTRALINE and CLOZAPINE may result in an increased risk of clozapine toxicity (sedation, seizures, low blood pressure).	2	3	3

Onset: 0=Unspecified 1=Rapid 2=Delayed
Severity: 1=Contraindicated 2=Major 3=Moderate 4=Minor
Evidence: 1=Excellent 2=Good 3=Fair 4=Poor

INTERACTION	ONSET	SEVERITY	EVIDENCE
DEXFENFLURAMINE Concurrent use of SERTRALINE and DEXFENFLURAMINE may result in serotonin syndrome (high blood pressure, high fever, spasms, mental status changes).	1	2	3
DROPERIDOL Concurrent use of SERTRALINE and DROPERIDOL may result in an increased risk of cardiotoxicity (irregular heartbeat, cardiac arrest).	1	2	3
FENFLURAMINE Concurrent use of SERTRALINE and FENFLURAMINE may result in serotonin syndrome (high blood pressure, high fever, spasms, mental status changes).	1	2	3
FURAZOLIDONE Concurrent use of SERTRALINE and FURAZOLIDONE may result in weakness, exaggerated reflexes, and incoordination.	2	1	3
HYDROXYTRYPTOPHAN Concurrent use of SERTRALINE and HYDROXYTRYPTOPHAN may result in an increased risk of serotonin syndrome (high blood pressure, high fever, spasms, mental status changes).	1	3	3
IPRONIAZID Concurrent use of SERTRALINE and IPRONIAZID may result in central nervous system toxicity or serotonin syndrome (high blood pressure, high fever, spasms, mental status changes).	1	1	2
ISOCARBOXAZID Concurrent use of SERTRALINE and ISOCARBOXAZID may result in central nervous system toxicity or serotonin syndrome (high blood pressure, high fever, spasms, mental status changes).	1	1	2
LEVOMETHADYL Concurrent use of SERTRALINE and LEVOMETHADYL may result in an increased risk of cardiotoxicity (irregular heartbeat, cardiac arrest).	2	1	3
MOCLOBEMIDE Concurrent use of SERTRALINE and MOCLOBEMIDE may result in central nervous system toxicity or serotonin syndrome (high blood pressure, high fever, spasms, mental status changes).	1	1	2
NIALAMIDE Concurrent use of SERTRALINE and NIALAMIDE may result in central nervous system toxicity or serotonin syndrome (high blood pressure, high fever, spasms, mental status changes).	1	1	2
NORTRIPTYLINE Concurrent use of SERTRALINE and NORTRIPTYLINE may result in elevated nortriptyline serum levels or possible serotonin syndrome (high blood pressure, high fever, spasms, mental status changes).	2	2	3

INTERACTION	ONSET	SEVERITY	EVIDENCE
PARGYLINE Concurrent use of SERTRALINE and PARGYLINE may result in central nervous system toxicity or serotonin syndrome (high blood pressure, high fever, spasms, mental status changes).	1	1	2
PHENELZINE Concurrent use of SERTRALINE and PHENELZINE may result in central nervous system toxicity or serotonin syndrome (high blood pressure, high fever, spasms, mental status changes).	1	1	2
PROCARBAZINE Concurrent use of SERTRALINE and PROCARBAZINE may result in central nervous system toxicity or serotonin syndrome (high blood pressure, high fever, spasms, mental status changes).	1	1	2
SELEGILINE Concurrent use of SERTRALINE and SELEGILINE may result in central nervous system toxicity or serotonin syndrome (high blood pressure, high fever, spasms, mental status changes).	1	1	2
SIBUTRAMINE Concurrent use of SERTRALINE and SIBUTRAMINE may result in an increased risk of serotonin syndrome (high blood pressure, hypothermia, spasms, mental status changes).	1	2	3
TERFENADINE Concurrent use of SERTRALINE and TERFENADINE may result in cardiotoxicity (irregular heartbeat, cardiac arrest).	1	2	3
TOLOXATONE Concurrent use of SERTRALINE and TOLOXATONE may result in central nervous system toxicity or serotonin syndrome (high blood pressure, high fever, spasms, mental status changes).	1	1	2
TRAMADOL Concurrent use of SERTRALINE and TRAMADOL may result in an increased risk of seizures and serotonin syndrome (high blood pressure, high fever, spasms, mental status changes).	1	2	2
TRANYLCYPROMINE Concurrent use of SERTRALINE and TRANYLCYPROMINE may result in central nervous system toxicity or serotonin syndrome (high blood pressure, high fever, spasms, mental status changes).	1	1	2

Tacrine

INTERACTION	ONSET	SEVERITY	EVIDENCE
CIMETIDINE Concurrent use of TACRINE and CIMETIDINE may result in tacrine toxicity (nausea, vomiting, loss of appetite).	1	4	2

Onset: **0**=Unspecified **1**=Rapid **2**=Delayed
Severity: **1**=Contraindicated **2**=Major **3**=Moderate **4**=Minor
Evidence: **1**=Excellent **2**=Good **3**=Fair **4**=Poor

INTERACTION	ONSET	SEVERITY	EVIDENCE
FLUVOXAMINE Concurrent use of TACRINE and FLUVOXAMINE may result in an increase in the plasma concentration of tacrine.	1	3	3
THEOPHYLLINE Concurrent use of TACRINE and THEOPHYLLINE may result in theophylline toxicity (nausea, vomiting, palpitations, seizures).	2	3	3

Temazepam

INTERACTION	ONSET	SEVERITY	EVIDENCE
ETHANOL Concurrent use of TEMAZEPAM and ETHANOL may result in impaired psychomotor functions.	1	3	2
THEOPHYLLINE Concurrent use of TEMAZEPAM and THEOPHYLLINE may result in decreased temazepam effectiveness.	1	3	2

Thioridazine

INTERACTION	ONSET	SEVERITY	EVIDENCE
ACETYLCHOLINE Concurrent use of THIORIDAZINE and ACETYLCHOLINE may result in an increased risk of cardiotoxicity (irregular heartbeat, cardiac arrest).	2	1	3
AJMALINE Concurrent use of THIORIDAZINE and AJMALINE may result in an increased risk of cardiotoxicity (irregular heartbeat, cardiac arrest).	2	1	3
AMIODARONE Concurrent use of THIORIDAZINE and AMIODARONE may result in an increased risk of cardiotoxicity (irregular heartbeat, cardiac arrest).	2	1	3
APRINDINE Concurrent use of THIORIDAZINE and APRINDINE may result in an increased risk of cardiotoxicity (irregular heartbeat, cardiac arrest).	2	1	3
ARSENIC TRIOXIDE Concurrent use of THIORIDAZINE and ARSENIC TRIOXIDE may result in an increased risk of cardiotoxicity (irregular heartbeat, cardiac arrest).	2	1	3
ASTEMIZOLE Concurrent use of THIORIDAZINE and ASTEMIZOLE may result in an increased risk of cardiotoxicity (irregular heartbeat, cardiac arrest).	2	1	3
BELLADONNA Concurrent use of THIORIDAZINE and BELLADONNA may result in increased manic, agitated reactions, or enhanced antispasmodic effects resulting in cardiorespiratory failure, especially in cases of belladonna overdose.	1	3	2

INTERACTION	ONSET	SEVERITY	EVIDENCE
BENZTROPINE Concurrent use of THIORIDAZINE and BENZTROPINE may result in decreased thioridazine serum concentrations, decreased thioridazine effectiveness, enhanced antispasmodic effects (intestinal blockage, high fever, sedation, dry mouth).	2	3	3
CABERGOLINE Concurrent use of THIORIDAZINE and CABERGOLINE may result in the decreased therapeutic effect of both drugs.	1	3	3
CISAPRIDE Concurrent use of THIORIDAZINE and CISAPRIDE may result in cardiotoxicity (irregular heartbeat, cardiac arrest).	1	1	3
CLINDAMYCIN Concurrent use of THIORIDAZINE and CLINDAMYCIN may result in an increased risk of cardiotoxicity (irregular heartbeat, cardiac arrest).	2	1	3
DIETHYLPROPION Concurrent use of THIORIDAZINE and DIETHYLPROPION may result in an increased risk of cardiotoxicity (irregular heartbeat, cardiac arrest).	2	1	3
DROPERIDOL Concurrent use of THIORIDAZINE and DROPERIDOL may result in an increased risk of cardiotoxicity (irregular heartbeat, cardiac arrest).	2	1	3
ETHANOL Concurrent use of THIORIDAZINE and ETHANOL may result in increased central nervous system depression and an increased risk of movement disorders.	1	3	2
FLUOXETINE Concurrent use of THIORIDAZINE and FLUOXETINE may result in an increased risk of thioridazine toxicity, cardiotoxicity (irregular heartbeat, cardiac arrest).	1	1	3
FLUVOXAMINE Concurrent use of THIORIDAZINE and FLUVOXAMINE may result in an increased risk of thioridazine toxicity, cardiotoxicity (irregular heartbeat, cardiac arrest).	1	1	3
FOSPHENYTOIN Concurrent use of THIORIDAZINE and FOSPHENYTOIN may result in increased or decreased phenytoin levels and possibly reduced thioridazine levels.	2	4	3
GREPAFLOXACIN Concurrent use of THIORIDAZINE and GREPAFLOXACIN may result in an increased risk of cardiotoxicity (irregular heartbeat, cardiac arrest).	2	1	3
HALOFANTRINE Concurrent use of THIORIDAZINE and HALOFANTRINE may result in cardiotoxicity (irregular heartbeat, cardiac arrest).	2	2	3

Onset: 0=Unspecified 1=Rapid 2=Delayed
Severity: 1=Contraindicated 2=Major 3=Moderate 4=Minor
Evidence: 1=Excellent 2=Good 3=Fair 4=Poor

INTERACTION	ONSET	SEVERITY	EVIDENCE
IOPAMIDOL Concurrent use of THIORIDAZINE and IOPAMIDOL may result in an increased risk of cardiotoxicity (irregular heartbeat, cardiac arrest).	2	1	3
KETANSERIN Concurrent use of THIORIDAZINE and KETANSERIN may result in an increased risk of cardiotoxicity (irregular heartbeat, cardiac arrest).	2	1	3
LEVODOPA Concurrent use of THIORIDAZINE and LEVODOPA may result in loss of levodopa efficacy.	1	3	2
LEVOMETHADYL Concurrent use of THIORIDAZINE and LEVOMETHADYL may result in an increased risk of cardiotoxicity (irregular heartbeat, cardiac arrest).	2	1	3
LITHIUM Concurrent use of THIORIDAZINE and LITHIUM may result in weakness, movement disorders, brain disorders, and brain damage.	2	2	1
LUBELUZOLE Concurrent use of THIORIDAZINE and LUBELUZOLE may result in an increased risk of cardiotoxicity (irregular heartbeat, cardiac arrest).	2	1	3
MEPERIDINE Concurrent use of THIORIDAZINE and MEPERIDINE may result in an increase in central nervous system and respiratory depression.	1	3	2
MESORIDAZINE Concurrent use of THIORIDAZINE and MESORIDAZINE may result in an increased risk of cardiotoxicity (irregular heartbeat, cardiac arrest).	2	1	3
ORPHENADRINE Concurrent use of THIORIDAZINE and ORPHENADRINE may result in decreased thioridazine serum concentrations, decreased thioridazine effectiveness, enhanced antispasmodic effects (intestinal blockage, high fever, sedation, dry mouth).	2	3	3
PAROXETINE Concurrent use of THIORIDAZINE and PAROXETINE may result in an increased risk of thioridazine toxicity, cardiotoxicity (irregular heartbeat, cardiac arrest).	1	1	3
PENTAMIDINE Concurrent use of THIORIDAZINE and PENTAMIDINE may result in an increased risk of cardiotoxicity (irregular heartbeat, cardiac arrest).	2	1	3
PHENYTOIN Concurrent use of THIORIDAZINE and PHENYTOIN may result in increased or decreased phenytoin levels and possibly reduced thioridazine levels.	2	4	3

INTERACTION	ONSET	SEVERITY	EVIDENCE
PORFIMER Concurrent use of THIORIDAZINE and PORFIMER may result in excessive intracellular damage in photosensitized tissues.	2	3	3
PROBUCOL Concurrent use of THIORIDAZINE and PROBUCOL may result in an increased risk of cardiotoxicity (irregular heartbeat, cardiac arrest).	2	1	3
PROCATEROL Concurrent use of THIORIDAZINE and PROCATEROL may result in an increased risk of cardiotoxicity (irregular heartbeat, cardiac arrest).	2	1	3
PROCYCLIDINE Concurrent use of THIORIDAZINE and PROCYCLIDINE may result in decreased thioridazine serum concentrations, decreased thioridazine effectiveness, enhanced antispasmodic effects (intestinal blockage, high fever, sedation, dry mouth).	2	3	3
PROPRANOLOL Concurrent use of THIORIDAZINE and PROPRANOLOL may result in an increased risk of thioridazine toxicity, cardiotoxicity (irregular heartbeat, cardiac arrest).	2	1	3
PROTIRELIN Concurrent use of THIORIDAZINE and PROTIRELIN may result in decreased thyroid test response.	2	3	3
ROXITHROMYCIN Concurrent use of THIORIDAZINE and ROXITHROMYCIN may result in an increased risk of cardiotoxicity (irregular heartbeat, cardiac arrest).	2	1	3
SEMATILIDE Concurrent use of THIORIDAZINE and SEMATILIDE may result in an increased risk of cardiotoxicity (irregular heartbeat, cardiac arrest).	2	1	3
SPARFLOXACIN Concurrent use of THIORIDAZINE and SPARFLOXACIN may result in irregular heartbeat.	2	1	3
SPIRAMYCIN Concurrent use of THIORIDAZINE and SPIRAMYCIN may result in an increased risk of cardiotoxicity (irregular heartbeat, cardiac arrest).	2	1	3
TERFENADINE Concurrent use of THIORIDAZINE and TERFENADINE may result in an increased risk of cardiotoxicity (irregular heartbeat, cardiac arrest).	2	1	3
TRAMADOL Concurrent use of THIORIDAZINE and TRAMADOL may result in an increased risk of seizures.	1	2	3

Onset: 0=Unspecified 1=Rapid 2=Delayed
Severity: 1=Contraindicated 2=Major 3=Moderate 4=Minor
Evidence: 1=Excellent 2=Good 3=Fair 4=Poor

INTERACTION	ONSET	SEVERITY	EVIDENCE
TRIHEXYPHENIDYL Concurrent use of THIORIDAZINE and TRIHEXYPHENIDYL may result in decreased thioridazine serum concentrations, decreased thioridazine effectiveness, enhanced antispasmodic effects (intestinal blockage, high fever, sedation, dry mouth).	2	3	3
ZIPRASIDONE Concurrent use of THIORIDAZINE and ZIPRASIDONE may result in an increased risk of cardiotoxicity (irregular heartbeat, cardiac arrest).	2	1	3
ZOLMITRIPTAN Concurrent use of THIORIDAZINE and ZOLMITRIPTAN may result in an increased risk of cardiotoxicity (irregular heartbeat, cardiac arrest).	2	1	3

Thiothixene

INTERACTION	ONSET	SEVERITY	EVIDENCE
CABERGOLINE Concurrent use of THIOTHIXENE and CABERGOLINE may result in the decreased therapeutic effect of both drugs.	1	3	3
LITHIUM Concurrent use of THIOTHIXENE and LITHIUM may result in weakness, movement disorders, brain disorders, and brain damage.	2	2	1
TRAMADOL Concurrent use of THIOTHIXENE and TRAMADOL may result in an increased risk of seizures.	1	2	3

Tranylcypromine

INTERACTION	ONSET	SEVERITY	EVIDENCE
ACARBOSE Concurrent use of TRANYLCYPROMINE and ACARBOSE may result in excessive reductions in blood sugar, central nervous system depression, and seizures.	1	3	2
ACETOHEXAMIDE Concurrent use of TRANYLCYPROMINE and ACETOHEXAMIDE may result in excessive reductions in blood sugar, central nervous system depression, and seizures.	1	3	2
ALBUTEROL Concurrent use of TRANYLCYPROMINE and ALBUTEROL may result in an increased risk of rapid heartbeat, agitation, or mild mania.	2	2	2
AMITRIPTYLINE Concurrent use of TRANYLCYPROMINE and AMITRIPTYLINE may result in neurotoxicity, seizures, or serotonin syndrome (high blood pressure, high fever, spasms, mental status changes).	2	1	3

INTERACTION	ONSET	SEVERITY	EVIDENCE
AMOXAPINE Concurrent use of TRANYLCYPROMINE and AMOXAPINE may result in neurotoxicity, seizures, or serotonin syndrome (high blood pressure, high fever, spasms, mental status changes).	2	2	3
AMPHETAMINE Concurrent use of TRANYLCYPROMINE and AMPHETAMINE may result in hypertensive crisis (headache, high fever, high blood pressure).	1	1	2
APRACLONIDINE Concurrent use of TRANYLCYPROMINE and APRACLONIDINE may result in potentiation of tranylcypromine effects.	1	1	3
BAMBUTEROL Concurrent use of TRANYLCYPROMINE and BAMBUTEROL may result in an increased risk of rapid heartbeat, agitation, or mild mania.	2	2	2
BENFLUOREX Concurrent use of TRANYLCYPROMINE and BENFLUOREX may result in excessive reductions in blood sugar, central nervous system depression, and seizures.	1	3	2
BENZPHETAMINE Concurrent use of TRANYLCYPROMINE and BENZPHETAMINE may result in hypertensive crisis (headache, high fever, high blood pressure).	1	1	2
BITOLTEROL Concurrent use of TRANYLCYPROMINE and BITOLTEROL may result in an increased risk of rapid heartbeat, agitation, or mild mania.	2	2	2
BROXATEROL Concurrent use of TRANYLCYPROMINE and BROXATEROL may result in an increased risk of rapid heartbeat, agitation, or mild mania.	2	2	2
BUPROPION Concurrent use of TRANYLCYPROMINE and BUPROPION may result in bupropion toxicity (seizures, agitation, psychotic changes).	1	1	3
BUSPIRONE Concurrent use of TRANYLCYPROMINE and BUSPIRONE may result in hypertensive crisis.	1	1	3
CARBAMAZEPINE Concurrent use of TRANYLCYPROMINE and CARBAMAZEPINE may result in high blood pressure, high fever, and seizures.	1	1	3

Onset: 0=Unspecified 1=Rapid 2=Delayed
Severity: 1=Contraindicated 2=Major 3=Moderate 4=Minor
Evidence: 1=Excellent 2=Good 3=Fair 4=Poor

INTERACTION	ONSET	SEVERITY	EVIDENCE
CHLORPROPAMIDE Concurrent use of TRANYLCYPROMINE and CHLORPROPAMIDE may result in excessive reductions in blood sugar, central nervous system depression, and seizures.	1	3	2
CITALOPRAM Concurrent use of TRANYLCYPROMINE and CITALOPRAM may result in central nervous system toxicity or serotonin syndrome (high blood pressure, high fever, spasms, mental status changes).	1	1	3
CLENBUTEROL Concurrent use of TRANYLCYPROMINE and CLENBUTEROL may result in an increased risk of rapid heartbeat, agitation, or mild mania.	2	2	2
CLOMIPRAMINE Concurrent use of TRANYLCYPROMINE and CLOMIPRAMINE may result in neurotoxicity, seizures, or serotonin syndrome (high blood pressure, high fever, spasms, mental status changes).	2	2	3
CLOVOXAMINE Concurrent use of TRANYLCYPROMINE and CLOVOXAMINE may result in central nervous system toxicity or serotonin syndrome (high blood pressure, high fever, spasms, mental status changes).	1	1	3
CYCLOBENZAPRINE Concurrent use of TRANYLCYPROMINE and CYCLOBENZAPRINE may result in hypertensive crises (headache, high fever, high blood pressure) or severe convulsive seizures.	1	1	3
CYPROHEPTADINE Concurrent use of TRANYLCYPROMINE and CYPROHEPTADINE may result in prolonged and intensified antispasmodic effects.	2	1	3
DESIPRAMINE Concurrent use of TRANYLCYPROMINE and DESIPRAMINE may result in neurotoxicity, seizures, or serotonin syndrome (high blood pressure, high fever, spasms, mental status changes).	2	2	3
DEXFENFLURAMINE Concurrent use of TRANYLCYPROMINE and DEXFENFLURAMINE may result in central nervous system toxicity or serotonin syndrome (high blood pressure, high fever, spasms, mental status changes).	1	1	3
DEXMETHYLPHENIDATE Concurrent use of TRANYLCYPROMINE and DEXMETHYLPHENIDATE may result in hypertensive crisis (headache, palpitation, neck stiffness).	1	1	3

INTERACTION	ONSET	SEVERITY	EVIDENCE
DEXTROAMPHETAMINE Concurrent use of TRANYLCYPROMINE and DEXTROAMPHETAMINE may result in a hypertensive crisis (headache, high fever, high blood pressure).	1	1	3
DEXTROMETHORPHAN Concurrent use of TRANYLCYPROMINE and DEXTROMETHORPHAN may result in an increased risk of serotonin syndrome (high blood pressure, high fever, spasms, mental status changes).	1	1	3
DIETHYLPROPION Concurrent use of TRANYLCYPROMINE and DIETHYLPROPION may result in hypertensive crisis (headache, high fever, high blood pressure).	1	1	2
DOPAMINE Concurrent use of TRANYLCYPROMINE and DOPAMINE may result in hypertensive crisis (headache, high fever, high blood pressure).	1	1	1
DOTHIEPIN Concurrent use of TRANYLCYPROMINE and DOTHIEPIN may result in neurotoxicity, seizures, or serotonin syndrome (high blood pressure, high fever, spasms, mental status changes).	2	2	3
DOXEPIN Concurrent use of TRANYLCYPROMINE and DOXEPIN may result in neurotoxicity, seizures, or serotonin syndrome (high blood pressure, high fever, spasms, mental status changes).	2	2	3
DROPERIDOL Concurrent use of TRANYLCYPROMINE and DROPERIDOL may result in an increased risk of cardiotoxicity (irregular heartbeat, cardiac arrest).	1	2	3
EPHEDRINE Concurrent use of TRANYLCYPROMINE and EPHEDRINE may result in hypertensive crisis (headache, high fever, high blood pressure).	1	2	3
EPINEPHRINE Concurrent use of TRANYLCYPROMINE and EPINEPHRINE may result in increased blood pressure.	1	3	3
FEMOXETINE Concurrent use of TRANYLCYPROMINE and FEMOXETINE may result in central nervous system toxicity or serotonin syndrome (high blood pressure, high fever, spasms, mental status changes).	1	1	3

Onset: 0=Unspecified 1=Rapid 2=Delayed
Severity: 1=Contraindicated 2=Major 3=Moderate 4=Minor
Evidence: 1=Excellent 2=Good 3=Fair 4=Poor

INTERACTION	ONSET	SEVERITY	EVIDENCE
FENFLURAMINE Concurrent use of TRANYLCYPROMINE and FENFLURAMINE may result in serotonin syndrome (high blood pressure, high fever, spasms, mental status changes).	1	1	3
FENOTEROL Concurrent use of TRANYLCYPROMINE and FENOTEROL may result in an increased risk of rapid heartbeat, agitation, or mild mania.	2	2	2
FLUOXETINE Concurrent use of TRANYLCYPROMINE and FLUOXETINE may result in central nervous system toxicity or serotonin syndrome (high blood pressure, high fever, spasms, mental status changes).	1	1	2
FLUVOXAMINE Concurrent use of TRANYLCYPROMINE and FLUVOXAMINE may result in central nervous system toxicity or serotonin syndrome (high blood pressure, high fever, spasms, mental status changes).	1	2	2
FORMOTEROL Concurrent use of TRANYLCYPROMINE and FORMOTEROL may result in an increased risk of rapid heartbeat, agitation, or mild mania.	2	2	2
FURAZOLIDONE Concurrent use of TRANYLCYPROMINE and FURAZOLIDONE may result in an increased risk of a hypertensive crisis or convulsive seizures.	1	1	3
GLICLAZIDE Concurrent use of TRANYLCYPROMINE and GLICLAZIDE may result in excessive reductions in blood sugar, central nervous system depression, and seizures.	1	3	2
GLIMEPIRIDE Concurrent use of TRANYLCYPROMINE and GLIMEPIRIDE may result in excessive reductions in blood sugar, central nervous system depression, and seizures.	1	3	2
GLIPIZIDE Concurrent use of TRANYLCYPROMINE and GLIPIZIDE may result in excessive reductions in blood sugar, central nervous system depression, and seizures.	1	3	2
GLIQUIDONE Concurrent use of TRANYLCYPROMINE and GLIQUIDONE may result in excessive reductions in blood sugar, central nervous system depression, and seizures.	1	3	2
GLYBURIDE Concurrent use of TRANYLCYPROMINE and GLYBURIDE may result in excessive reductions in blood sugar, central nervous system depression, and seizures.	1	3	2

INTERACTION	ONSET	SEVERITY	EVIDENCE
GUANADREL Concurrent use of TRANYLCYPROMINE and GUANADREL may result in decreased response to guanadrel or hypertensive crisis when guanadrel is initiated in a patient already receiving tranylcypromine.	1	1	3
GUAR GUM Concurrent use of TRANYLCYPROMINE and GUAR GUM may result in excessive reductions in blood sugar, central nervous system depression, and seizures.	1	3	2
HEXOPRENALINE Concurrent use of TRANYLCYPROMINE and HEXOPRENALINE may result in an increased risk of rapid heartbeat, agitation, or mild mania.	2	2	2
IMIPRAMINE Concurrent use of TRANYLCYPROMINE and IMIPRAMINE may result in neurotoxicity, seizures, or serotonin syndrome (high blood pressure, high fever, spasms, mental status changes).	2	2	3
INSULIN Concurrent use of TRANYLCYPROMINE and INSULIN may result in excessive reductions in blood sugar, central nervous system depression, and seizures.	1	3	2
ISOCARBOXAZID Concurrent use of TRANYLCYPROMINE and ISOCARBOXAZID may result in an increased risk of a hypertensive crisis or convulsive seizures.	1	1	3
ISOETHARINE Concurrent use of TRANYLCYPROMINE and ISOETHARINE may result in an increased risk of rapid heartbeat, agitation, or mild mania.	2	2	2
ISOMETHEPTENE Concurrent use of TRANYLCYPROMINE and ISOMETHEPTENE may result in severe headache, hypertensive crisis, cardiac irregularities.	1	1	1
ISOPROTERENOL Concurrent use of TRANYLCYPROMINE and ISOPROTERENOL may result in increased blood pressure.	1	3	3
LEVALBUTEROL Concurrent use of TRANYLCYPROMINE and LEVALBUTEROL may result in an increased risk of rapid heartbeat, agitation, or mild mania.	2	2	2
LEVODOPA Concurrent use of TRANYLCYPROMINE and LEVODOPA may result in hypertensive crisis (headache, high fever, high blood pressure).	1	1	3

Onset: 0=Unspecified 1=Rapid 2=Delayed
Severity: 1=Contraindicated 2=Major 3=Moderate 4=Minor
Evidence: 1=Excellent 2=Good 3=Fair 4=Poor

INTERACTION	ONSET	SEVERITY	EVIDENCE
LEVOMETHADYL Concurrent use of TRANYLCYPROMINE and LEVOMETHADYL may result in increased levels of levomethadyl or its active metabolites.	2	1	3
LOFEPRAMINE Concurrent use of TRANYLCYPROMINE and LOFEPRAMINE may result in neurotoxicity, seizures, or serotonin syndrome (high blood pressure, high fever, spasms, mental status changes).	2	2	3
MA HUANG Concurrent use of TRANYLCYPROMINE and MA HUANG may result in increased risk for headache, high fever, cardiac irregularities, and hypertensive crisis (headache, high fever, high blood pressure).	1	2	3
MAPROTILINE Concurrent use of TRANYLCYPROMINE and MAPROTILINE may result in neurotoxicity, seizures.	2	1	3
MAZINDOL Concurrent use of TRANYLCYPROMINE and MAZINDOL may result in hypertensive crisis.	1	1	3
MEPERIDINE Concurrent use of TRANYLCYPROMINE and MEPERIDINE may result in cardiovascular instability, high fever, coma.	1	1	2
METARAMINOL Concurrent use of TRANYLCYPROMINE and METARAMINOL may result in hypertensive crisis (headache, high fever, high blood pressure).	1	2	3
METFORMIN Concurrent use of TRANYLCYPROMINE and METFORMIN may result in excessive reductions in blood sugar, central nervous system depression, and seizures.	1	3	2
METHAMPHETAMINE Concurrent use of TRANYLCYPROMINE and METHAMPHETAMINE may result in hypertensive crisis (headache, high fever, high blood pressure).	1	1	3
METHOTRIMEPRAZINE Concurrent use of TRANYLCYPROMINE and METHOTRIMEPRAZINE may result in possibly prolonged effect of methotrimeprazine, with potentially increased side effects.	2	1	3
METHOXAMINE Concurrent use of TRANYLCYPROMINE and METHOXAMINE may result in hypertensive crisis (headache, high fever, high blood pressure).	1	2	3
METHYLDOPA Concurrent use of TRANYLCYPROMINE and METHYLDOPA may result in hypertensive crisis (headache, palpitation, neck stiffness).	1	1	3

INTERACTION	ONSET	SEVERITY	EVIDENCE
METHYLPHENIDATE Concurrent use of TRANYLCYPROMINE and METHYLPHENIDATE may result in hypertensive crisis (headache, palpitation, neck stiffness).	1	1	3
MIGLITOL Concurrent use of TRANYLCYPROMINE and MIGLITOL may result in excessive reductions in blood sugar, central nervous system depression, and seizures.	1	3	2
MIRTAZAPINE Concurrent use of TRANYLCYPROMINE and MIRTAZAPINE may result in neurotoxicity, seizures.	2	1	3
MORPHINE Concurrent use of TRANYLCYPROMINE and MORPHINE may result in low blood pressure and exaggeration of central nervous system and respiratory depressant effects.	1	1	3
NEFAZODONE Concurrent use of TRANYLCYPROMINE and NEFAZODONE may result in high fever, rigidity, spasms, seizures, fluctuations of vital signs, or mental status changes.	1	2	2
NOREPINEPHRINE Concurrent use of TRANYLCYPROMINE and NOREPINEPHRINE may result in increased blood pressure.	1	3	3
NORTRIPTYLINE Concurrent use of TRANYLCYPROMINE and NORTRIPTYLINE may result in neurotoxicity, seizures, or serotonin syndrome (high blood pressure, high fever, spasms, mental status changes).	2	2	3
OPIPRAMOL Concurrent use of TRANYLCYPROMINE and OPIPRAMOL may result in neurotoxicity, seizures, or serotonin syndrome (high blood pressure, high fever, spasms, mental status changes).	2	1	3
OXYCODONE Concurrent use of TRANYLCYPROMINE and OXYCODONE may result in anxiety, confusion and significant respiratory depressant effects or coma.	2	2	3
PAROXETINE Concurrent use of TRANYLCYPROMINE and PAROXETINE may result in central nervous system toxicity or serotonin syndrome (high blood pressure, high fever, spasms, mental status changes).	1	1	2
PHENDIMETRAZINE Concurrent use of TRANYLCYPROMINE and PHENDIMETRAZINE may result in hypertensive crisis (headache, high fever, high blood pressure).	1	1	2

Onset: 0=Unspecified 1=Rapid 2=Delayed
Severity: 1=Contraindicated 2=Major 3=Moderate 4=Minor
Evidence: 1=Excellent 2=Good 3=Fair 4=Poor

INTERACTION	ONSET	SEVERITY	EVIDENCE
PHENELZINE Concurrent use of TRANYLCYPROMINE and PHENELZINE may result in hypertensive crisis (headache, palpitation, neck stiffness).	1	1	3
PHENMETRAZINE Concurrent use of TRANYLCYPROMINE and PHENMETRAZINE may result in hypertensive crisis (headache, high fever, high blood pressure).	1	1	2
PHENTERMINE Concurrent use of TRANYLCYPROMINE and PHENTERMINE may result in hypertensive crisis (headache, high fever, high blood pressure).	1	1	1
PHENYLEPHRINE Concurrent use of TRANYLCYPROMINE and PHENYLEPHRINE may result in hypertensive crisis (headache, high fever, high blood pressure).	1	1	3
PHENYLPROPANOLAMINE Concurrent use of TRANYLCYPROMINE and PHENYLPROPANOLAMINE may result in hypertensive crisis (headache, high fever, high blood pressure).	1	1	3
PIRBUTEROL Concurrent use of TRANYLCYPROMINE and PIRBUTEROL may result in an increased risk of rapid heartbeat, agitation, or mild mania.	2	2	2
PROCARBAZINE Concurrent use of TRANYLCYPROMINE and PROCARBAZINE may result in an increased risk of a hypertensive crisis or convulsive seizures.	1	1	3
PROCATEROL Concurrent use of TRANYLCYPROMINE and PROCATEROL may result in an increased risk of rapid heartbeat, agitation, or mild mania.	2	2	2
PROTRIPTYLINE Concurrent use of TRANYLCYPROMINE and PROTRIPTYLINE may result in neurotoxicity, seizures, or serotonin syndrome (high blood pressure, high fever, spasms, mental status changes).	2	2	3
PSEUDOEPHEDRINE Concurrent use of TRANYLCYPROMINE and PSEUDOEPHEDRINE may result in severe high blood pressure, high fever, headache.	1	1	3
REBOXETINE Concurrent use of TRANYLCYPROMINE and REBOXETINE may result in high fever, rigidity, spasms, seizures, fluctuations of vital signs, or mental status changes.	1	2	3

INTERACTION	ONSET	SEVERITY	EVIDENCE
RESERPINE Concurrent use of TRANYLCYPROMINE and RESERPINE may result in elevated levels of certain chemical messengers in the brain.	1	1	3
RIMITEROL Concurrent use of TRANYLCYPROMINE and RIMITEROL may result in an increased risk of rapid heartbeat, agitation, or mild mania.	2	2	2
RITODRINE Concurrent use of TRANYLCYPROMINE and RITODRINE may result in an increased risk of rapid heartbeat, agitation, or mild mania.	2	2	2
SALMETEROL Concurrent use of TRANYLCYPROMINE and SALMETEROL may result in an increased risk of rapid heartbeat, agitation, or mild mania.	2	2	2
SERTRALINE Concurrent use of TRANYLCYPROMINE and SERTRALINE may result in central nervous system toxicity or serotonin syndrome (high blood pressure, high fever, spasms, mental status changes).	1	1	2
SIBUTRAMINE Concurrent use of TRANYLCYPROMINE and SIBUTRAMINE may result in central nervous system toxicity or serotonin syndrome (high blood pressure, high fever, spasms, mental status changes).	1	1	3
ST JOHN'S WORT Concurrent use of TRANYLCYPROMINE and ST. JOHN'S WORT may result in an increased risk of serotonin syndrome (high blood pressure, high fever, spasms, mental status changes) and/or an increased risk of hypertensive crisis.	2	2	3
SUMATRIPTAN Concurrent use of TRANYLCYPROMINE and SUMATRIPTAN may result in serotonin syndrome (high blood pressure, high fever, spasms, mental status changes).	1	2	2
TERBUTALINE Concurrent use of TRANYLCYPROMINE and TERBUTALINE may result in an increased risk of rapid heartbeat, agitation, or mild mania.	2	2	2
TOLAZAMIDE Concurrent use of TRANYLCYPROMINE and TOLAZAMIDE may result in excessive reductions in blood sugar, central nervous system depression, and seizures.	1	3	2

Onset: 0=Unspecified 1=Rapid 2=Delayed
Severity: 1=Contraindicated 2=Major 3=Moderate 4=Minor
Evidence: 1=Excellent 2=Good 3=Fair 4=Poor

INTERACTION	ONSET	SEVERITY	EVIDENCE
TOLBUTAMIDE Concurrent use of TRANYLCYPROMINE and TOLBUTAMIDE may result in excessive reductions in blood sugar, central nervous system depression, and seizures.	1	3	2
TOLCAPONE Concurrent use of TRANYLCYPROMINE and TOLCAPONE may result in decreased metabolism of certain chemical messengers in the brain.	1	2	3
TRAMADOL Concurrent use of TRANYLCYPROMINE and TRAMADOL may result in nausea, vomiting, cardiovascular collapse, respiratory depression, seizures.	1	2	3
TRIMIPRAMINE Concurrent use of TRANYLCYPROMINE and TRIMIPRAMINE may result in neurotoxicity, seizures, or serotonin syndrome (high blood pressure, high fever, spasms, mental status changes).	2	2	3
TROGLITAZONE Concurrent use of TRANYLCYPROMINE and TROGLITAZONE may result in excessive reductions in blood sugar, central nervous system depression, and seizures.	1	3	2
TRYPTOPHAN Concurrent use of TRANYLCYPROMINE and TRYPTOPHAN may result in an increased risk of high blood pressure, memory impairment, and disorientation.	1	1	3
TULOBUTEROL Concurrent use of TRANYLCYPROMINE and TULOBUTEROL may result in an increased risk of rapid heartbeat, agitation, or mild mania.	2	2	2
TYRAMINE FOODS Concurrent use of TRANYLCYPROMINE and TYRAMINE FOODS may result in increased blood pressure.	1	1	1
VENLAFAXINE Concurrent use of TRANYLCYPROMINE and VENLAFAXINE may result in central nervous system toxicity or serotonin syndrome (high blood pressure, high fever, spasms, mental status changes).	1	1	2

Trazodone

INTERACTION	ONSET	SEVERITY	EVIDENCE
DROPERIDOL Concurrent use of TRAZODONE and DROPERIDOL may result in an increased risk of cardiotoxicity (irregular heartbeat, cardiac arrest).	1	2	3
FLUOXETINE Concurrent use of TRAZODONE and FLUOXETINE may result in trazodone toxicity (sedation, dry mouth, urinary retention) or serotonin syndrome (high blood pressure, high fever, spasms, mental status changes).	2	2	3

INTERACTION	ONSET	SEVERITY	EVIDENCE
FOOD Concurrent use of TRAZODONE and FOOD may result in increased time to peak levels.	1	4	2
ST JOHN'S WORT Concurrent use of TRAZODONE and ST. JOHN'S WORT may result in an increased risk of serotonin syndrome (high blood pressure, high fever, spasms, mental status changes).	2	2	3

Triazolam

INTERACTION	ONSET	SEVERITY	EVIDENCE
AMPRENAVIR Concurrent use of TRIAZOLAM and AMPRENAVIR may result in an increased risk of triazolam toxicity (excessive sedation, confusion).	1	1	3
AZITHROMYCIN Concurrent use of TRIAZOLAM and AZITHROMYCIN may result in decreased clearance of triazolam and increased pharmacologic effect of triazolam.	0	4	3
CIMETIDINE Concurrent use of TRIAZOLAM and CIMETIDINE may result in triazolam toxicity (excessive sedation, confusion).	1	4	3
CLARITHROMYCIN Concurrent use of TRIAZOLAM and CLARITHROMYCIN may result in increased triazolam toxicity (central nervous system depression, poor coordination, lethargy).	2	3	3
DEHYDROEPIANDROSTERONE Concurrent use of TRIAZOLAM and DEHYDROEPIANDROSTERONE may result in increased central nervous system depression.	1	3	2
EFAVIRENZ Concurrent use of TRIAZOLAM and EFAVIRENZ may result in an increased risk of triazolam toxicity (excessive sedation, confusion).	2	1	3
ETHANOL Concurrent use of TRIAZOLAM and ETHANOL may result in increased sedation.	1	3	1
FLUCONAZOLE Concurrent use of TRIAZOLAM and FLUCONAZOLE may result in increased triazolam serum concentrations.	1	3	3
FLUVOXAMINE Concurrent use of TRIAZOLAM and FLUVOXAMINE may result in elevated serum triazolam concentrations.	2	3	3
GRAPEFRUIT JUICE Concurrent use of TRIAZOLAM and GRAPEFRUIT JUICE may result in increased bioavailability of triazolam.	1	4	3

Onset: 0=Unspecified 1=Rapid 2=Delayed
Severity: 1=Contraindicated 2=Major 3=Moderate 4=Minor
Evidence: 1=Excellent 2=Good 3=Fair 4=Poor

INTERACTION	ONSET	SEVERITY	EVIDENCE
INDINAVIR Concurrent use of TRIAZOLAM and INDINAVIR may result in an increased risk of serious triazolam adverse effects (excessive or prolonged sedation).	1	1	3
ITRACONAZOLE Concurrent use of TRIAZOLAM and ITRACONAZOLE may result in an increased risk of triazolam toxicity.	1	1	3
JOSAMYCIN Concurrent use of TRIAZOLAM and JOSAMYCIN may result in increased triazolam toxicity (central nervous system depression, poor coordination, lethargy).	2	3	3
KETOCONAZOLE Concurrent use of TRIAZOLAM and KETOCONAZOLE may result in increased triazolam intensity and duration of effect.	1	2	2
MIBEFRADIL Concurrent use of TRIAZOLAM and MIBEFRADIL may result in an increased risk of triazolam toxicity (excessive sedation, confusion).	1	2	3
NEFAZODONE Concurrent use of TRIAZOLAM and NEFAZODONE may result in psychomotor impairment and excessive sedation.	1	3	2
OMEPRAZOLE Concurrent use of TRIAZOLAM and OMEPRAZOLE may result in triazolam toxicity (central nervous system depression, poor coordination, lethargy).	2	3	3
RIFAMPIN Concurrent use of TRIAZOLAM and RIFAMPIN may result in loss of triazolam efficacy.	1	3	3
RITONAVIR Concurrent use of TRIAZOLAM and RITONAVIR may result in an increased risk of extreme sedation and confusion.	2	1	3
ROXITHROMYCIN Concurrent use of TRIAZOLAM and ROXITHROMYCIN may result in increased triazolam toxicity (central nervous system depression, poor coordination, lethargy).	2	3	3
SAQUINAVIR Concurrent use of TRIAZOLAM and SAQUINAVIR may result in an increased risk of triazolam toxicity (excessive sedation, confusion).	1	1	3
THEOPHYLLINE Concurrent use of TRIAZOLAM and THEOPHYLLINE may result in decreased triazolam effectiveness.	1	3	2
TROLEANDOMYCIN Concurrent use of TRIAZOLAM and TROLEANDOMYCIN may result in increased triazolam toxicity (central nervous system depression, poor coordination, lethargy).	2	3	3

Trifluoperazine

INTERACTION	ONSET	SEVERITY	EVIDENCE
BELLADONNA Concurrent use of TRIFLUOPERAZINE and BELLADONNA may result in increased manic, agitated reactions, or enhanced antispasmodic effects resulting in cardiorespiratory failure, especially in cases of belladonna overdose.	1	3	2
BENZTROPINE Concurrent use of TRIFLUOPERAZINE and BENZTROPINE may result in decreased trifluoperazine serum concentrations, decreased trifluoperazine effectiveness, enhanced antispasmodic effects (intestinal blockage, high fever, sedation, dry mouth).	2	3	3
CABERGOLINE Concurrent use of TRIFLUOPERAZINE and CABERGOLINE may result in the decreased therapeutic effect of both drugs.	1	3	3
CISAPRIDE Concurrent use of TRIFLUOPERAZINE and CISAPRIDE may result in cardiotoxicity (irregular heartbeat, cardiac arrest).	1	1	3
DROPERIDOL Concurrent use of TRIFLUOPERAZINE and DROPERIDOL may result in an increased risk of cardiotoxicity (irregular heartbeat, cardiac arrest).	1	2	3
ETHANOL Concurrent use of TRIFLUOPERAZINE and ETHANOL may result in increased central nervous system depression and an increased risk of movement disorders.	1	3	2
FOSPHENYTOIN Concurrent use of TRIFLUOPERAZINE and FOSPHENYTOIN may result in increased or decreased phenytoin levels and possibly reduced trifluoperazine levels.	2	4	3
GREPAFLOXACIN Concurrent use of TRIFLUOPERAZINE and GREPAFLOXACIN may result in an increased risk of cardiotoxicity (irregular heartbeat, cardiac arrest).	2	1	3
HALOFANTRINE Concurrent use of TRIFLUOPERAZINE and HALOFANTRINE may result in cardiotoxicity (irregular heartbeat, cardiac arrest).	2	2	3
IBUTILIDE Concurrent use of TRIFLUOPERAZINE and IBUTILIDE may result in an increased risk of cardiac irregularities.	1	2	3
LEVODOPA Concurrent use of TRIFLUOPERAZINE and LEVODOPA may result in loss of levodopa efficacy.	1	3	2

Onset: 0=Unspecified 1=Rapid 2=Delayed
Severity: 1=Contraindicated 2=Major 3=Moderate 4=Minor
Evidence: 1=Excellent 2=Good 3=Fair 4=Poor

INTERACTION	ONSET	SEVERITY	EVIDENCE
LEVOMETHADYL Concurrent use of TRIFLUOPERAZINE and LEVOMETHADYL may result in an increased risk of cardiotoxicity (irregular heartbeat, cardiac arrest).	2	1	3
LITHIUM Concurrent use of TRIFLUOPERAZINE and LITHIUM may result in weakness, movement disorders, brain disorders, and brain damage.	2	2	1
MEPERIDINE Concurrent use of TRIFLUOPERAZINE and MEPERIDINE may result in an increase in central nervous system and respiratory depression.	1	3	2
ORPHENADRINE Concurrent use of TRIFLUOPERAZINE and ORPHENADRINE may result in decreased trifluoperazine serum concentrations, decreased trifluoperazine effectiveness, enhanced antispasmodic effects (intestinal blockage, high fever, sedation, dry mouth).	2	3	3
PHENYTOIN Concurrent use of TRIFLUOPERAZINE and PHENYTOIN may result in increased or decreased phenytoin levels and possibly reduced trifluoperazine levels.	2	4	3
PORFIMER Concurrent use of TRIFLUOPERAZINE and PORFIMER may result in excessive intracellular damage in photosensitized tissues.	2	3	3
PROCYCLIDINE Concurrent use of TRIFLUOPERAZINE and PROCYCLIDINE may result in decreased trifluoperazine serum concentrations, decreased trifluoperazine effectiveness, enhanced antispasmodic effects (intestinal blockage, high fever, sedation, dry mouth).	2	3	3
SPARFLOXACIN Concurrent use of TRIFLUOPERAZINE and SPARFLOXACIN may result in irregular heartbeat.	2	1	3
TRAMADOL Concurrent use of TRIFLUOPERAZINE and TRAMADOL may result in an increased risk of seizures.	1	2	3
TRIHEXYPHENIDYL Concurrent use of TRIFLUOPERAZINE and TRIHEXYPHENIDYL may result in decreased trifluoperazine serum concentrations, decreased trifluoperazine effectiveness, enhanced antispasmodic effects (intestinal blockage, high fever, sedation, dry mouth).	2	3	3

Trimipramine

INTERACTION	ONSET	SEVERITY	EVIDENCE
ACENOCOUMAROL Concurrent use of TRIMIPRAMINE and ACENOCOUMAROL may result in increased risk of bleeding.	2	3	3

INTERACTION	ONSET	SEVERITY	EVIDENCE
AMPRENAVIR Concurrent use of TRIMIPRAMINE and AMPRENAVIR may result in increased trimipramine serum concentrations and potential toxicity (antispasmodic effects, sedation, confusion, cardiac irregularities).	2	2	3
ANISINDIONE Concurrent use of TRIMIPRAMINE and ANISINDIONE may result in an increased risk of bleeding.	2	3	3
BEPRIDIL Concurrent use of TRIMIPRAMINE and BEPRIDIL may result in cardiac irregularities.	1	1	3
BETHANIDINE Concurrent use of TRIMIPRAMINE and BETHANIDINE may result in decreased bethanidine effectiveness.	1	3	3
CIMETIDINE Concurrent use of TRIMIPRAMINE and CIMETIDINE may result in trimipramine toxicity (dry mouth, blurred vision, urinary retention).	2	3	3
CISAPRIDE Concurrent use of TRIMIPRAMINE and CISAPRIDE may result in cardiotoxicity (irregular heartbeat, cardiac arrest).	1	1	3
CLONIDINE Concurrent use of TRIMIPRAMINE and CLONIDINE may result in decreased clonidine effectiveness.	2	2	3
CLORGYLINE Concurrent use of TRIMIPRAMINE and CLORGYLINE may result in neurotoxicity, seizures, or serotonin syndrome (high blood pressure, high fever, spasms, mental status changes).	2	2	3
DICUMAROL Concurrent use of TRIMIPRAMINE and DICUMAROL may result in an increased risk of bleeding.	2	3	3
DROPERIDOL Concurrent use of TRIMIPRAMINE and DROPERIDOL may result in an increased risk of cardiotoxicity (irregular heartbeat, cardiac arrest).	1	2	3
EPINEPHRINE Concurrent use of TRIMIPRAMINE and EPINEPHRINE may result in high blood pressure, cardiac irregularities, and rapid heartbeat.	1	2	2
ETILEFRINE Concurrent use of TRIMIPRAMINE and ETILEFRINE may result in high blood pressure, cardiac irregularities, and rapid heartbeat.	1	2	2

Onset: 0=Unspecified 1=Rapid 2=Delayed
Severity: 1=Contraindicated 2=Major 3=Moderate 4=Minor
Evidence: 1=Excellent 2=Good 3=Fair 4=Poor

INTERACTION	ONSET	SEVERITY	EVIDENCE
FLUOXETINE Concurrent use of TRIMIPRAMINE and FLUOXETINE may result in trimipramine toxicity (dry mouth, urinary retention, sedation).	2	3	3
GREPAFLOXACIN Concurrent use of TRIMIPRAMINE and GREPAFLOXACIN may result in an increased risk of cardiotoxicity (irregular heartbeat, cardiac arrest).	2	1	3
GUANADREL Concurrent use of TRIMIPRAMINE and GUANADREL may result in decreased guanadrel effectiveness.	2	3	3
HALOFANTRINE Concurrent use of TRIMIPRAMINE and HALOFANTRINE may result in cardiotoxicity (irregular heartbeat, cardiac arrest).	2	2	3
IBUTILIDE Concurrent use of TRIMIPRAMINE and IBUTILIDE may result in an increased risk of cardiac irregularities.	1	2	3
ISOCARBOXAZID Concurrent use of TRIMIPRAMINE and ISOCARBOXAZID may result in neurotoxicity, seizures, or serotonin syndrome (high blood pressure, high fever, spasms, mental status changes).	2	1	3
LEVOMETHADYL Concurrent use of TRIMIPRAMINE and LEVOMETHADYL may result in an increased risk of cardiotoxicity (irregular heartbeat, cardiac arrest).	2	1	3
METHOXAMINE Concurrent use of TRIMIPRAMINE and METHOXAMINE may result in high blood pressure, cardiac irregularities, and rapid heartbeat.	1	2	2
MIDODRINE Concurrent use of TRIMIPRAMINE and MIDODRINE may result in high blood pressure, cardiac irregularities, and rapid heartbeat.	1	2	2
MOCLOBEMIDE Concurrent use of TRIMIPRAMINE and MOCLOBEMIDE may result in neurotoxicity, seizures, or serotonin syndrome (high blood pressure, high fever, spasms, mental status changes).	2	2	3
NOREPINEPHRINE Concurrent use of TRIMIPRAMINE and NOREPINEPHRINE may result in high blood pressure, cardiac irregularities, and rapid heartbeat.	1	2	2
OXILOFRINE Concurrent use of TRIMIPRAMINE and OXILOFRINE may result in high blood pressure, cardiac irregularities, and rapid heartbeat.	1	2	2

INTERACTION	ONSET	SEVERITY	EVIDENCE
PHENELZINE Concurrent use of TRIMIPRAMINE and PHENELZINE may result in neurotoxicity, seizures, or serotonin syndrome (high blood pressure, high fever, spasms, mental status changes).	2	2	3
PHENINDIONE Concurrent use of TRIMIPRAMINE and PHENINDIONE may result in an increased risk of bleeding.	2	3	3
PHENPROCOUMON Concurrent use of TRIMIPRAMINE and PHENPROCOUMON may result in an increased risk of bleeding.	2	3	3
PHENYLEPHRINE Concurrent use of TRIMIPRAMINE and PHENYLEPHRINE may result in high blood pressure, cardiac irregularities, and rapid heartbeat.	1	2	2
PIMOZIDE Concurrent use of TRIMIPRAMINE and PIMOZIDE may result in an increased risk of cardiotoxicity (irregular heartbeat, cardiac arrest).	1	1	3
PROCARBAZINE Concurrent use of TRIMIPRAMINE and PROCARBAZINE may result in neurotoxicity, seizures.	2	2	3
SELEGILINE Concurrent use of TRIMIPRAMINE and SELEGILINE may result in neurotoxicity, seizures, or serotonin syndrome (high blood pressure, high fever, spasms, mental status changes).	2	2	3
SPARFLOXACIN Concurrent use of TRIMIPRAMINE and SPARFLOXACIN may result in irregular heartbeat.	2	1	3
TRANYLCYPROMINE Concurrent use of TRIMIPRAMINE and TRANYLCYPROMINE may result in neurotoxicity, seizures, or serotonin syndrome (high blood pressure, high fever, spasms, mental status changes).	2	2	3
WARFARIN Concurrent use of TRIMIPRAMINE and WARFARIN may result in an increased risk of bleeding.	2	3	3

Valproic Acid

INTERACTION	ONSET	SEVERITY	EVIDENCE
CHOLESTYRAMINE Concurrent use of VALPROIC ACID and CHOLESTYRAMINE may result in decreased serum valproic acid concentrations.	1	3	3

Onset: 0=Unspecified 1=Rapid 2=Delayed
Severity: 1=Contraindicated 2=Major 3=Moderate 4=Minor
Evidence: 1=Excellent 2=Good 3=Fair 4=Poor

INTERACTION	ONSET	SEVERITY	EVIDENCE
CLOMIPRAMINE Concurrent use of VALPROIC ACID and CLOMIPRAMINE may result in increased risk of clomipramine toxicity (agitation, confusion, hallucinations, urinary retention, rapid heartbeat, seizures, coma).	2	3	3
FELBAMATE Concurrent use of VALPROIC ACID and FELBAMATE may result in increased valproic acid levels.	2	3	3
FOSPHENYTOIN Concurrent use of VALPROIC ACID and FOSPHENYTOIN may result in altered valproate levels or altered phenytoin levels.	2	3	3
LAMOTRIGINE Concurrent use of VALPROIC ACID and LAMOTRIGINE may result in lamotrigine toxicity (fatigue, drowsiness, poor coordination) and an increased risk of severe, life-threatening skin peeling.	2	3	3
PHENOBARBITAL Concurrent use of VALPROIC ACID and PHENOBARBITAL may result in phenobarbital toxicity or decreased valproic acid effectiveness.	2	3	1
PHENYTOIN Concurrent use of VALPROIC ACID and PHENYTOIN may result in altered valproate levels or altered phenytoin levels.	2	3	3
PRIMIDONE Concurrent use of VALPROIC ACID and PRIMIDONE may result in severe central nervous system depression.	1	2	3
TOPIRAMATE Concurrent use of VALPROIC ACID and TOPIRAMATE may result in decreased topiramate or valproic acid concentrations.	2	3	3
ZIDOVUDINE Concurrent use of VALPROIC ACID and ZIDOVUDINE may result in increased zidovudine plasma concentrations and potential zidovudine toxicity (weakness, fatigue, nausea, blood abnormalities).	2	3	3

Venlafaxine

INTERACTION	ONSET	SEVERITY	EVIDENCE
ALMOTRIPTAN Concurrent use VENLAFAXINE and ALMOTRIPTAN may result in weakness, exaggerated reflexes, and/or incoordination.	0	3	3
CIMETIDINE Concurrent use of VENLAFAXINE and CIMETIDINE may result in an increased risk of venlafaxine toxicity (nausea, drowsiness, dizziness, ejaculatory disturbances).	2	4	3

INTERACTION	ONSET	SEVERITY	EVIDENCE
CLORGYLINE Concurrent use of VENLAFAXINE and CLORGYLINE may result in central nervous system toxicity or serotonin syndrome (high blood pressure, high fever, spasms, mental status changes).	1	1	2
DEXFENFLURAMINE Concurrent use of VENLAFAXINE and DEXFENFLURAMINE may result in serotonin syndrome (high blood pressure, high fever, spasms, mental status changes).	1	2	3
ETHANOL Concurrent use of VENLAFAXINE and ETHANOL may result in an increased risk of central nervous system effects.	1	4	3
FENFLURAMINE Concurrent use of VENLAFAXINE and FENFLURAMINE may result in serotonin syndrome (high blood pressure, high fever, spasms, mental status changes).	1	2	3
FURAZOLIDONE Concurrent use of VENLAFAXINE and FURAZOLIDONE may result in weakness, exaggerated reflexes, and incoordination.	2	1	3
IPRONIAZID Concurrent use of VENLAFAXINE and IPRONIAZID may result in central nervous system toxicity or serotonin syndrome (high blood pressure, high fever, spasms, mental status changes).	1	1	2
ISOCARBOXAZID Concurrent use of VENLAFAXINE and ISOCARBOXAZID may result in central nervous system toxicity or serotonin syndrome (high blood pressure, high fever, spasms, mental status changes).	1	1	2
MOCLOBEMIDE Concurrent use of VENLAFAXINE and MOCLOBEMIDE may result in central nervous system toxicity or serotonin syndrome (high blood pressure, high fever, spasms, mental status changes).	1	1	2
NIALAMIDE Concurrent use of VENLAFAXINE and NIALAMIDE may result in central nervous system toxicity or serotonin syndrome (high blood pressure, high fever, spasms, mental status changes).	1	1	2
PARGYLINE Concurrent use of VENLAFAXINE and PARGYLINE may result in central nervous system toxicity or serotonin syndrome (high blood pressure, high fever, spasms, mental status changes).	1	1	2

Onset: 0=Unspecified **1**=Rapid **2**=Delayed
Severity: **1**=Contraindicated **2**=Major **3**=Moderate **4**=Minor
Evidence: **1**=Excellent **2**=Good **3**=Fair **4**=Poor

INTERACTION	ONSET	SEVERITY	EVIDENCE
PAROXETINE Concurrent use of VENLAFAXINE and PAROXETINE may result in an increased risk of serotonin syndrome (high blood pressure, high fever, spasms, mental status changes).	1	2	3
PHENELZINE Concurrent use of VENLAFAXINE and PHENELZINE may result in central nervous system toxicity or serotonin syndrome (high blood pressure, high fever, spasms, mental status changes).	1	1	2
PROCARBAZINE Concurrent use of VENLAFAXINE and PROCARBAZINE may result in central nervous system toxicity or serotonin syndrome (high blood pressure, high fever, spasms, mental status changes).	1	1	2
SELEGILINE Concurrent use of VENLAFAXINE and SELEGILINE may result in central nervous system toxicity or serotonin syndrome (high blood pressure, high fever, spasms, mental status changes).	1	1	2
SIBUTRAMINE Concurrent use of VENLAFAXINE and SIBUTRAMINE may result in an increased risk of serotonin syndrome (high blood pressure, hypothermia, spasms, mental status changes).	1	2	3
TOLOXATONE Concurrent use of VENLAFAXINE and TOLOXATONE may result in central nervous system toxicity or serotonin syndrome (high blood pressure, high fever, spasms, mental status changes).	1	1	2
TRAMADOL Concurrent use of VENLAFAXINE and TRAMADOL may result in an increased risk of seizures and serotonin syndrome (high blood pressure, high fever, spasms, mental status changes).	1	2	2
TRANYLCYPROMINE Concurrent use of VENLAFAXINE and TRANYLCYPROMINE may result in central nervous system toxicity or serotonin syndrome (high blood pressure, high fever, spasms, mental status changes).	1	1	2

Zaleplon

INTERACTION	ONSET	SEVERITY	EVIDENCE
ETHANOL Concurrent use of ZALEPLON and ETHANOL may result in impaired psychomotor functions.	1	3	3

Ziprasidone

INTERACTION	ONSET	SEVERITY	EVIDENCE
ACECAINIDE Concurrent use of ZIPRASIDONE and ACECAINIDE may result in an increased risk of cardiotoxicity (irregular heartbeat, cardiac arrest).	2	1	3
AJMALINE Concurrent use of ZIPRASIDONE and AJMALINE may result in an increased risk of cardiotoxicity (irregular heartbeat, cardiac arrest).	2	1	3
AMIODARONE Concurrent use of ZIPRASIDONE and AMIODARONE may result in an increased risk of cardiotoxicity (irregular heartbeat, cardiac arrest).	2	1	3
ARSENIC TRIOXIDE Concurrent use of ZIPRASIDONE and ARSENIC TRIOXIDE may result in an increased risk of cardiotoxicity (irregular heartbeat, cardiac arrest).	2	1	3
AZIMILIDE Concurrent use of ZIPRASIDONE and AZIMILIDE ay result in an increased risk of cardiotoxicity (irregular heartbeat, cardiac arrest).	2	1	3
BRETYLIUM Concurrent use of ZIPRASIDONE and BRETYLIUM may result in an increased risk of cardiotoxicity (irregular heartbeat, cardiac arrest).	2	1	3
CHLORPROMAZINE Concurrent use of ZIPRASIDONE and CHLORPROMAZINE may result in an increased risk of cardiotoxicity (irregular heartbeat, cardiac arrest).	2	1	3
DISOPYRAMIDE Concurrent use of ZIPRASIDONE and DISOPYRAMIDE may result in an increased risk of cardiotoxicity (irregular heartbeat, cardiac arrest).	2	1	3
DOFETILIDE Concurrent use of ZIPRASIDONE and DOFETILIDE may result in an increased risk of cardiotoxicity (irregular heartbeat, cardiac arrest).	2	1	3
DOLASETRON Concurrent use of ZIPRASIDONE and DOLASETRON may result in an increased risk of cardiotoxicity (irregular heartbeat, cardiac arrest).	2	1	3
DROPERIDOL Concurrent use of ZIPRASIDONE and DROPERIDOL may result in an increased risk of cardiotoxicity (irregular heartbeat, cardiac arrest).	2	1	3

Onset: 0=Unspecified 1=Rapid 2=Delayed
Severity: 1=Contraindicated 2=Major 3=Moderate 4=Minor
Evidence: 1=Excellent 2=Good 3=Fair 4=Poor

INTERACTION	ONSET	SEVERITY	EVIDENCE
GATIFLOXACIN Concurrent use of ZIPRASIDONE and GATIFLOXACIN may result in an increased risk of cardiotoxicity (irregular heartbeat, cardiac arrest).	2	1	3
HALOFANTRINE Concurrent use of ZIPRASIDONE and HALOFANTRINE may result in an increased risk of cardiotoxicity (irregular heartbeat, cardiac arrest).	2	1	3
IBUTILIDE Concurrent use of ZIPRASIDONE and IBUTILIDE may result in an increased risk of cardiotoxicity (irregular heartbeat, cardiac arrest).	2	1	3
LEVOMETHADYL Concurrent use of ZIPRASIDONE and LEVOMETHADYL may result in an increased risk of cardiotoxicity (irregular heartbeat, cardiac arrest).	2	1	3
MEFLOQUINE Concurrent use of ZIPRASIDONE and MEFLOQUINE may result in an increased risk of cardiotoxicity (irregular heartbeat, cardiac arrest).	2	1	3
MESORIDAZINE Concurrent use of ZIPRASIDONE and MESORIDAZINE may result in an increased risk of cardiotoxicity (irregular heartbeat, cardiac arrest).	2	1	3
MORICIZINE Concurrent use of ZIPRASIDONE and MORICIZINE may result in an increased risk of cardiotoxicity (irregular heartbeat, cardiac arrest).	2	1	3
MOXIFLOXACIN Concurrent use of ZIPRASIDONE and MOXIFLOXACIN may result in an increased risk of cardiotoxicity (irregular heartbeat, cardiac arrest).	2	1	3
PENTAMIDINE Concurrent use of ZIPRASIDONE and PENTAMIDINE may result in an increased risk of cardiotoxicity (irregular heartbeat, cardiac arrest).	2	1	3
PIMOZIDE Concurrent use of ZIPRASIDONE and PIMOZIDE may result in an increased risk of cardiotoxicity (irregular heartbeat, cardiac arrest).	2	1	3
PIRMENOL Concurrent use of ZIPRASIDONE and PIRMENOL may result in an increased risk of cardiotoxicity (irregular heartbeat, cardiac arrest).	2	1	3
PRAJMALINE Concurrent use of ZIPRASIDONE and PRAJMALINE may result in an increased risk of cardiotoxicity (irregular heartbeat, cardiac arrest).	2	1	3

INTERACTION	ONSET	SEVERITY	EVIDENCE
PROBUCOL Concurrent use of ZIPRASIDONE and PROBUCOL may result in an increased risk of cardiotoxicity (irregular heartbeat, cardiac arrest).	2	1	3
PROCAINAMIDE Concurrent use of ZIPRASIDONE and PROCAINAMIDE may result in an increased risk of cardiotoxicity (irregular heartbeat, cardiac arrest).	2	1	3
QUINIDINE Concurrent use of ZIPRASIDONE and QUINIDINE may result in an increased risk of cardiotoxicity (irregular heartbeat, cardiac arrest).	2	1	3
RECAINAM Concurrent use of ZIPRASIDONE and RECAINAM may result in an increased risk of cardiotoxicity (irregular heartbeat, cardiac arrest).	2	1	3
SEMATILIDE Concurrent use of ZIPRASIDONE and SEMATILIDE may result in an increased risk of cardiotoxicity (irregular heartbeat, cardiac arrest).	2	1	3
SOTALOL Concurrent use of ZIPRASIDONE and SOTALOL may result in an increased risk of cardiotoxicity (irregular heartbeat, cardiac arrest).	2	1	3
SPARFLOXACIN Concurrent use of ZIPRASIDONE and SPARFLOXACIN may result in an increased risk of cardiotoxicity (irregular heartbeat, cardiac arrest).	2	1	3
TACROLIMUS Concurrent use of ZIPRASIDONE and TACROLIMUS may result in an increased risk of cardiotoxicity (irregular heartbeat, cardiac arrest).	2	1	3
TEDISAMIL Concurrent use of ZIPRASIDONE and TEDISAMIL may result in an increased risk of cardiotoxicity (irregular heartbeat, cardiac arrest).	2	1	3
THIORIDAZINE Concurrent use of ZIPRASIDONE and THIORIDAZINE may result in an increased risk of cardiotoxicity (irregular heartbeat, cardiac arrest).	2	1	3

Zolpidem

INTERACTION	ONSET	SEVERITY	EVIDENCE
ETHANOL Concurrent use of ZOLPIDEM and ETHANOL may result in increased sedation.	1	3	3

Onset: 0=Unspecified 1=Rapid 2=Delayed
Severity: 1=Contraindicated 2=Major 3=Moderate 4=Minor
Evidence: 1=Excellent 2=Good 3=Fair 4=Poor

INTERACTION	ONSET	SEVERITY	EVIDENCE
KETOCONAZOLE Concurrent use of ZOLPIDEM and KETOCONAZOLE may result in increased plasma concentrations and effects of zolpidem.	1	3	3
RIFAMPIN Concurrent use of ZOLPIDEM and RIFAMPIN may result in decreased plasma concentration and effects of zolpidem.	1	3	3

Section 3

Common Prescription Drugs

Because patients with psychological disorders are often under simultaneous treatment for other medical problems, this section presents you with brief descriptions of the most commonly prescribed Rx drugs and their customary uses. Based primarily on government-approved product labeling as submitted for publication in *Physicians' Desk Reference*®, the information is organized alphabetically by each medication's leading brand name and cross-referenced by the generic name. To see whether a drug is likely to interact with a patient's psychotropic regimen, check the appropriate listings in Section 2 of this book.

Generic name:

Abacavir

See Ziagen, page 625.

Generic name:

Abacavir, Lamivudine, and Zidovudine

See Trizivir, page 608.

Generic name:

Acarbose

See Precose, page 559.

Brand name:

Accolate

Pronounced: ACK-o-late
Generic name: Zafirlukast

Accolate is prescribed to *prevent* asthma attacks. Unlike some of the inhaled medications used to relieve attacks in progress, it is not a steroid. Instead, it works by blocking the action of certain types of leukotrienes—natural compounds that cause swelling and constriction in the lungs. Taken in tablet form, it is used for long-term treatment.

Brand name:

AccuNeb

See Proventil, page 567.

Brand name:

Accupril

Pronounced: AK-you-prill
Generic name: Quinapril hydrochloride

Accupril is used in the treatment of high blood pressure. It can be taken alone or in combination with a thiazide type of water pill such as HydroDIURIL. Accupril is in a family of drugs known as "ACE inhibitors." It works by preventing a chemical in the blood called angiotensin I from converting into a more potent form that increases salt and water retention in the body. Accupril also enhances blood flow throughout the blood vessels. Along with other drugs, Accupril is also prescribed in the treatment of congestive heart failure.

Brand name:

Accuretic

Pronounced: AK-you-REH-tik
Generic ingredients: Quinapril hydrochloride, Hydrochlorothiazide

Accuretic combines two types of blood pressure medication. The first, quinapril hydrochloride, is an ACE (angiotensin-converting enzyme) inhibitor. It works by preventing a chemical in the blood called angiotensin I from converting into a more potent form (angiotensin II) that increases salt and water retention in the body and causes the blood vessels to constrict—-two actions that tend to increase blood pressure.

To aid in clearing excess water from the body, Accuretic also contains hydrochlorothiazide, a diuretic that promotes production of urine. Diuretics often wash too much potassium out of the body along with the water. However, the ACE inhibitor part of Accuretic tends to keep potassium in the body, thereby canceling this unwanted effect.

Accuretic is not used for the initial treatment of high blood pressure. It is saved for later use, when a single blood pressure medication is not sufficient for the job. In addition, some doctors are using Accuretic along with other drugs to treat congestive heart failure.

Brand name:

Accutane

Pronounced: ACC-u-tane
Generic name: Isotretinoin

Accutane, a chemical cousin of vitamin A, is prescribed for the treatment of severe, disfiguring cystic acne that has not cleared up in response to milder medications such as antibiotics. It works on the oil glands within the skin, shrinking them and diminishing their output. The patient takes Accutane by mouth every day for several months, then stops. The antiacne effect can last even after the course of medication is finished.

Generic name:

Acebutolol

See Sectral, page 579.

Brand name:

Aceon

Pronounced: A-see-on
Generic name: Perindopril erbumine

Aceon is used in the treatment of high blood pressure. It can be taken alone or in combination with thiazide diuretics that help rid the body of excess water. Aceon belongs to a family of drugs called angiotensin converting enzyme (ACE) inhibitors. It works by preventing a chemical in the blood called angiotensin I from converting into a more potent form that increases salt and water retention in the body. Aceon also improves the flow of blood through the circulatory system.

Generic name:

Acetaminophen with Codeine

See Tylenol with Codeine, page 609.

Generic name:

Acetaminophen with Oxycodone

See Percocet, page 550.

Generic name:

Acetazolamide

See Diamox, page 445.

Generic name:

Acetic acid

See Aci-Jel, page 380.

Generic name:

Acetic acid and Hydrocortisone

See VoSoL HC, page 620.

Brand name:

Achromycin V

See Tetracycline, page 596.

Brand name:

Aci-Jel

Pronounced: ASS-ee-jel
Generic ingredient: Acetic acid

In some cases of vaginitis, the level of acidity in the vagina becomes too low. Applying Aci-Jel internally restores the acidity and keeps it within the normal range.

Brand name:

AcipHex

Pronounced: ASS-ih-fex
Generic name: Rabeprazole sodium

AcipHex blocks acid production in the stomach. It is prescribed for the short-term (4 to 8 weeks) treatment of sores and inflammation in the upper digestive canal (esophagus). This condition, known as gastro-esophageal reflux disease (GERD), is caused by the backflow of stomach acid into the esophagus over a prolonged period of time. Because GERD can be chronic, doctors sometimes continue to prescribe AcipHex to prevent a relapse after the initial course of treatment.

AcipHex can also be prescribed for the short-term (up to 4 weeks) treatment of duodenal ulcers (ulcers that form just outside the stomach at the top of the small intestine), and for Zollinger-Ellison syndrome, a disease which causes the stomach to produce too much acid. The drug is classified as a "proton pump inhibitor." It works by blocking a specific enzyme essential to the production of stomach acid. It begins reducing acid within an hour of administration.

Brand name:

Aclovate

Pronounced: AK-low-vait
Generic name: Alclometasone dipropionate

Aclovate, a synthetic steroid medication of the cortisone family, is spread on the skin to relieve certain types of itchy rashes, including psoriasis.

Generic name:

Acrivastine with Pseudoephedrine

See Semprex-D, page 579.

Brand name:

Actigall

Pronounced: AK-ti-gawl
Generic name: Ursodiol
Other brand name: Urso

Actigall is used to help dissolve certain kinds of gallstones. For people who suffer from gallstones but do not want to undergo surgery to remove them, Actigall treatment may be a good alternative. It is also recommended if age, infirmity, or a poor reaction to anesthesia makes someone a poor candidate for surgery.

Actigall is also used to prevent gallstones in people on rapid-weight-loss diets. And under the brand name Urso, its active ingredient is prescribed to treat liver disease caused by hardening and blockage of the bile ducts (primary biliary cirrhosis).

Brand name:

Activella and femhrt

Generic ingredients: Estrogen, Progestin

These medications are designed for use in hormone replacement therapy. Both combine a form of estrogen with a substance that acts like progesterone. Both relieve the symptoms of menopause, and both are prescribed to prevent osteoporosis in postmenopausal women. (Activella is also used for vaginal atrophy.)

Estrogen, when taken by itself, poses an increased risk of uterine cancer. The progestin in these products largely counteracts this effect.

Brand name:

Actonel

Pronounced: AK-ton-ell
Generic name: Risedronate

Although our bones seem solid and stable, they actually undergo constant renewal. Specialized cells called *osteoclasts* draw used calcium out of the bones while other cells called *osteoblasts* replace it. Especially after menopause, this process can get out of balance. Calcium starts to leach out of the bones faster than it can be replaced, leading to the brittle-bone disease called osteoporosis.

Actonel combats this problem by reducing the activity of the osteoclasts and slowing the loss of calcium from the bones. It is prescribed for postmenopausal women, both to prevent osteoporosis and to strengthen the bones once the disease has begun. It is also used in the treatment of Paget's disease, a condition in which patches of bone become softened and enlarged.

Both Actonel and a similar drug called Fosamax are members of the family of drugs called bisphosphonates.

Brand name:

Actos

Pronounced: ACK-toes
Generic name: Pioglitazone hydrochloride

Actos is used to control high blood sugar in type 2 diabetes. This form of the illness usually stems from the body's inability to make good use of insulin, the natural hormone that helps to transfer sugar out of the blood and into the cells, where it's converted to energy. Actos works by improving the body's response to its natural supply of insulin, rather than increasing its insulin output. Actos also reduces the production of unneeded sugar in the liver.

Actos (and the similar drug Avandia) can be used alone or in combination with insulin injections or other oral diabetes medications such as DiaBeta, Micronase, Glucotrol, or Glucophage.

Brand name:
Actron

See Orudis, page 545.

Generic name:
Acyclovir

See Zovirax, page 628.

Brand name:
Adalat

See Procardia, page 564.

Generic name:
Adapalene

See Differin, page 446.

Brand name:
Adipex-P

Pronounced: ADD-i-pecks
Generic name: Phentermine hydrochloride
Other brand name: Ionamin

Adipex-P, an appetite suppressant, is prescribed for short-term use (a few weeks) as part of an overall weight reduction program that also includes dieting, exercise, and counseling. The drug is for use only by excessively overweight individuals who have a condition—-such as diabetes, high blood pressure, or high cholesterol—-that could lead to serious medical problems.

Brand name:
Advair Diskus

Pronounced: AD-vare
Generic ingredients: Fluticasone propionate, Salmeterol

Advair Diskus is an oral inhaler that contains two types of asthma medication. One is fluticasone propionate, a steroid that reduces inflammation in the lungs. The other, salmeterol, is a long-acting bronchodilator that opens up the airways. Together, the two ingredients provide better control of asthma than either does individually.

Brand name:

Advicor

Pronounced: AD-vih-core
Generic ingredients: Lovastatin, Niacin

Advicor is a cholesterol-lowering drug. Excess cholesterol in the bloodstream can lead to hardening of the arteries and heart disease. Advicor lowers total cholesterol and LDL ("bad") cholesterol, while raising the amount of HDL ("good") cholesterol.

Advicor is a combination of two cholesterol-fighting ingredients: extended-release niacin and lovastatin (Mevacor). It is prescribed only when other drugs and a program of diet, exercise, and weight reduction have been unsuccessful in lowering cholesterol levels.

Brand name:

Advil

See Motrin, page 524.

Brand name:

AeroBid

Pronounced: AIR-oh-bid
Generic name: Flunisolide
Other brand names: AeroBid-M, Nasalide

AeroBid is prescribed for people who need long-term treatment to control and prevent the symptoms of asthma. It contains an anti-inflammatory steroid type of medication and may reduce or eliminate the need for other corticosteroids. A nasal-spray form of the drug (Nasalide) is available for relief of hay fever.

Brand name:

Agenerase

Pronounced: ah-JEN-eh-race
Generic name: Amprenavir

Agenerase is one of the many drugs now used to combat human immunodeficiency virus (HIV) infection. HIV undermines the immune system, reducing the body's ability to fight off other infections and eventually leading to the deadly condition known as acquired immune deficiency syndrome (AIDS).

Agenerase slows the progress of HIV by interfering with an important step in the virus's reproductive cycle. The drug is a member of the group of "protease inhibitors" famous for having successfully halted the advance of the virus in many HIV-positive individuals. Agenerase is prescribed only as part of a "drug cocktail" that attacks the virus on several fronts. It is not used alone.

Brand name:

Aggrenox

Pronounced: AG-reh-noks
Generic ingredients: Aspirin, Extended-release dipyridamole

Aggrenox is prescribed to stave off a stroke in people who have had a "mini-stroke" (transient ischemic attack) or a full-scale stroke due to a blood clot blocking an artery in the brain.

Both the ingredients in Aggrenox prevent the formation of clots by interfering with the tendency of blood platelets to clump together. However, the two ingredients together are more effective at preventing strokes than either ingredient taken alone. Aggrenox doesn't eliminate the possibility of a stroke; but it does reduce the odds by almost six percentage points during the first two years of treatment.

Brand name:

Aktob

See Tobrex, page 599.

Brand name:

Alamast

Pronounced: allah-mast
Generic name: Pemirolast
Alamast is taken to prevent the itchy eyes caused by allergies such as

hay fever. It works by inhibiting the release of certain inflammatory agents, such as histamine and leukotrienes, that the body produces in response to an allergen.

Generic name:

Albuterol

See Proventil, page 567.

Generic name:

Alclometasone

See Aclovate, page 381.

Brand name:

Aldactazide

Pronounced: al-DAK-tah-zide
Generic ingredients: Spironolactone, Hydrochlorothiazide

Aldactazide is used in the treatment of high blood pressure and other conditions that require the elimination of excess fluid from the body. These conditions include congestive heart failure, cirrhosis of the liver, and kidney disease. Aldactazide combines two diuretic drugs that help the body produce and eliminate more urine. Spironolactone, one of the ingredients, helps to minimize the potassium loss that can be caused by the hydrochlorothiazide component.

Brand name:

Aldactone

Pronounced: al-DAK-tone
Generic name: Spironolactone

Aldactone flushes excess salt and water from the body and controls high blood pressure. It is used in the diagnosis and treatment of hyperaldosteronism, a condition in which the adrenal gland secretes too much aldosterone (a hormone that regulates the body's salt and potassium levels). It is also used in treating other conditions that require the elimination of excess fluid from the body. These conditions include congestive heart failure, high blood pressure, cirrhosis of the liver, kidney disease, and unusually low potassium levels in the blood. When used for high blood pressure, Aldactone can be taken alone or with other high blood pressure medications.

Brand name:

Aldomet

Pronounced: AL-doe-met
Generic name: Methyldopa

Aldomet is used to treat high blood pressure. It is effective when used alone or with other high blood pressure medications.

Generic name:

Alendronate

See Fosamax, page 473.

Brand name:

Alesse

See Oral Contraceptives, page 542.

Brand name:

Aleve

See Anaprox, page 392.

Brand name:

Allegra

Pronounced: ah-LEG-rah
Generic name: Fexofenadine hydrochloride
Other brand name: Allegra-D

Allegra relieves the itchy, runny nose, sneezing, and itchy, red, watery eyes that come with hay fever. Its effect begins in 1 hour and lasts 12 hours, peaking around the second or third hour. Allegra is one of the new type of antihistamines that rarely cause drowsiness. It is also used to relieve the itching and welts of hives.

In addition, to the antihistamine in Allegra, Allegra-D also contains the nasal decongestant pseudoephedrine.

Generic name:

Allopurinol

See Zyloprim, page 629.

Generic name:

Almotriptan

See Axert, page 401.

Brand name:

Alora

See Estrogen Patches, page 462.

Generic name:

Alprostadil

See Caverject, page 418.

Brand name:

Altace

Pronounced: AL-tayce
Generic name: Ramipril

Altace is used in the treatment of high blood pressure. It is effective when used alone or in combination with other high blood pressure medications, especially thiazide-type water pills (diuretics). Altace works by preventing the conversion of a chemical in the blood called angiotensin I into a more potent substance that increases salt and water retention in the body. It also enhances blood flow in the circulatory system. It is a member of the group of drugs called ACE inhibitors.

Altace is also prescribed to reduce the chances of heart attack, stroke, and heart-related death in people 55 years or older who are in danger of such an event. Typical candidates include those who suffer from coronary artery disease, poor circulation, stroke, or diabetes and have at least one other risk factor, such as high blood pressure, high cholesterol levels, low HDL ("good") cholesterol, or cigarette smoking.

For those who do suffer a heart attack and develop heart failure, Altace can be prescribed to prevent the condition from getting worse.

Brand name:
Alupent

Pronounced: AL-yew-pent
Generic name: Metaproterenol sulfate

Alupent is a bronchodilator prescribed for the prevention and relief of bronchial asthma and bronchial spasms (wheezing) associated with bronchitis and emphysema. Alupent Inhalation Solution is also used to treat acute asthmatic attacks in children 6 years of age and older.

Generic name:
Amantadine

See Symmetrel, page 587.

Brand name:
Amaryl

Pronounced: AM-a-ril
Generic name: Glimepiride

Amaryl is an oral medication used to treat type 2 (non-insulin-dependent) diabetes when diet and exercise alone fail to control abnormally high levels of blood sugar. Like other diabetes drugs classified as sulfonylureas, Amaryl lowers blood sugar by stimulating the pancreas to produce more insulin. Amaryl is often prescribed along with the insulin-boosting drug Glucophage. It may also be used in conjunction with insulin and other diabetes drugs.

Generic name:
Amcinonide

See Cyclocort, page 436.

Brand name:

Amerge

Pronounced: ah-MERJ
Generic name: Naratriptan hydrochloride

Amerge is used for relief of classic migraine headaches. It's helpful whether or not the headache is preceded by an aura (visual disturbances, usually sensations of halos or flickering lights). The drug works only during an actual attack. It will not reduce the number of headaches that develop.

Generic name:

Amiloride with Hydrochlorothiazide

See Moduretic, page 521.

Generic name:

Amlodipine

See Norvasc, page 539.

Generic name:

Amlodipine with Benazepril

See Lotrel, page 505.

Generic name:

Amoxicillin

See Amoxil, page 391.

Generic name:

Amoxicillin, Clarithromycin, and Lansoprazole

See Prevpac, page 562.

Generic name:
Amoxicillin with Clavulanate

See Augmentin, page 398.

Brand name:
Amoxil

Pronounced: a-MOX-il
Generic name: Amoxicillin
Other brand names: Trimox, Wymox

Amoxil, an antibiotic, is used to treat a wide variety of infections, including: gonorrhea, middle ear infections, skin infections, upper and lower respiratory tract infections, and infections of the genital and urinary tract. In combination with other drugs such as Prevacid and Biaxin, it is also used to treat duodenal ulcers caused by *H. pylori* bacteria (sores in the wall of the small intestine near the exit from the stomach).

Generic name:
Ampicillin

Pronounced: AM-pi-sill-in
Brand name: Principen

Ampicillin is a penicillin-like antibiotic prescribed for a wide variety of infections, including gonorrhea and other genital and urinary infections, respiratory infections, and gastrointestinal infections, as well as meningitis (inflamed membranes of the spinal cord or brain).

Generic name:
Amprenavir

See Agenerase, page 385.

Generic name:
Anakinra

See Kineret, page 492.

Brand name:

Anaprox

Pronounced: AN-uh-procks
Generic name: Naproxen sodium
Other brand names: Aleve, Naprelan

Anaprox and Naprelan are nonsteroidal anti-inflammatory drugs used to relieve mild to moderate pain and menstrual cramps. They are also prescribed for relief of the inflammation, swelling, stiffness, and joint pain associated with rheumatoid arthritis and osteoarthritis (the most common form of arthritis), and for ankylosing spondylitis (spinal arthritis), tendinitis, bursitis, acute gout, and other conditions. Anaprox also may be prescribed for juvenile arthritis.

The over-the-counter form of naproxen sodium, Aleve, is used for temporary relief of minor aches and pains, and to reduce fever.

Brand name:

Anaspaz

See Levsin, page 498.

Generic name:

Anastrozole

See Arimidex, page 395.

Generic name:

Androderm

See Testosterone Patches, page 595.

Brand name:

AndroGel

Pronounced: AN-droe-jel
Generic name: Testosterone gel

AndroGel is a hormone replacement product for men suffering from hypogonadism, a low level of the male hormone testosterone. This condition is marked by symptoms such as impotence and decreased interest in sex, lowered mood, fatigue, and decreases in bone density and lean body mass. Testosterone replacement therapy helps correct these problems. AndroGel, applied daily to the skin, provides an especially convenient way of taking the hormone, which was previously administered only by injection or skin patch.

Brand name:

Android

Pronounced: AN-droyd
Generic name: Methyltestosterone
Other brand name: Testred

Android, a synthetic male sex hormone, is given to help develop and/or maintain male sex characteristics in boys and men who, for some reason, are not producing enough of the hormone on their own. A relatively short course of Android is sometimes used to try to trigger changes in boys whose puberty seems delayed. Android may also be given to women who have certain advanced, inoperable forms of breast cancer.

Brand name:

Anexsia

See Vicodin, page 617.

Brand name:

Anolor 300

See Fioricet, page 467.

Brand name:

Ansaid

Pronounced: AN-sed
Generic name: Flurbiprofen

Ansaid, a nonsteroidal anti-inflammatory drug, is used to relieve the inflammation, swelling, stiffness, and joint pain associated with rheumatoid arthritis and osteoarthritis (the most common form of arthritis).

Generic name:

Antipyrine, Benzocaine, and Glycerin

See Auralgan, page 398.

Brand name:

Antivert

Pronounced: AN-tee-vert
Generic name: Meclizine hydrochloride
Other brand name: Bonine

Antivert, an antihistamine, is prescribed for the management of nausea, vomiting, and dizziness associated with motion sickness.

Antivert may also be prescribed for the management of vertigo (a spinning sensation or a feeling that the ground is tilted) due to diseases affecting the vestibular system (the bony labyrinth of the ear, which contains the sensors that control balance).

Brand name:

Anzemet

Pronounced: ANN-zuh-met
Generic name: Dolasetron mesylate

Anzemet is used to prevent the nausea and vomiting that often accompany cancer chemotherapy and usually trouble patients who've received anesthesia during surgery. The drug works by blocking the action of one of the brain's chemical messengers, serotonin, on the nerves that trigger vomiting.

Brand name:

Arava

Pronounced: ah-RAV-ah
Generic name: Leflunomide

Arava is used in the treatment of rheumatoid arthritis. It reduces the pain, stiffness, inflammation, and swelling associated with this disease, and staves off the joint damage that ultimately results.

Brand name:

Arimidex

Pronounced: AR-i-mi-deks
Generic name: Anastrozole

Arimidex is a first-line treatment of breast cancer in postmenopausal women. It slows the growth of advanced cancer within the breast and cancer that has spread to other parts of the body. Arimidex is also used to treat advanced breast cancer in postmenopausal women whose disease has spread to other parts of the body following treatment with tamoxifen (Nolvadex), another anticancer drug.

Arimidex combats the kind of breast cancer that thrives on estrogen. One of the hormones produced by the adrenal gland is converted to a form of estrogen by an enzyme called aromatase. Arimidex suppresses this enzyme and thereby reduces the level of estrogen circulating in the body.

Brand name:

Armour Thyroid

Pronounced: ARE-more THIGH-roid
Generic name: Natural thyroid hormones TC and TD

Armour Thyroid is prescribed when the thyroid gland is unable to produce enough hormone. It is also used to treat or prevent goiter (enlargement of the thyroid gland), and is given in a "suppression test" to diagnose an overactive thyroid.

Brand name:

Artane

Pronounced: AR-tane
Generic name: Trihexyphenidyl hydrochloride

Artane is used, in conjunction with other drugs, for the relief of certain symptoms of Parkinson's disease, a brain disorder that causes muscle tremor, stiffness, and weakness. It is also used to control certain side effects induced by antipsychotic drugs such as Thorazine and Haldol. Artane works by correcting the chemical imbalance that causes Parkinson's disease.

Brand name:
Arthrotec

Pronounced: ARE-throw-teck
Generic ingredients: Diclofenac sodium, Misoprostol

Arthrotec is designed to relieve the symptoms of arthritis in people who are also prone to ulcers. It contains diclofenac, a nonsteroidal anti-inflammatory drug (NSAID) for control of the inflammation, swelling, stiffness, and joint pain associated with rheumatoid arthritis and osteoarthritis. However, since NSAIDs can cause stomach ulcers in susceptible people, Arthrotec also contains misoprostol, a synthetic prostaglandin that serves to reduce the production of stomach acid, thereby protecting the stomach lining and thus preventing ulcers.

Brand name:
Asacol

See Rowasa, page 577.

Generic name:
Aspirin with Extended-release dipyridamole

See Aggrenox, page 385.

Brand name:
Astelin

Pronounced: AST-eh-linn
Generic name: Azelastine hydrochloride

Astelin is an antihistamine nasal spray. It is prescribed for the relief of hay fever symptoms such as itchy, runny nose and sneezing, and can also be used to relieve cases of congested, runny nose and postnasal drip unrelated to allergies.

Brand name:
Atacand

Pronounced: AT-uh-kand
Generic name: Candesartan cilexetil

Atacand controls high blood pressure. It works by blocking the effect of a hormone called angiotensin II. Unopposed, this substance prompts the blood vessels to contract, an action that tends to raise blood pressure. Atacand relaxes and expands the blood vessels, allowing pressure to drop. The drug may be prescribed alone or with other blood pressure medications.

Brand name:
Atacand HCT

Pronounced: AT-uh-kand HCT
Generic name: Candesartan cilexetil, Hydrochlorothiazide

Atacand HCT is a combination medication used in the treatment of high blood pressure. One component, candesartan, belongs to a class of blood pressure medications that work by preventing the hormone angiotensin II from constricting the blood vessels. This allows the blood to flow more freely and helps keep blood pressure down. The other component, hydrochlorothiazide, is a diuretic that increases the output of urine. This removes excess fluid from the body and helps lower blood pressure. Doctors usually prescribe Atacand HCT in place of its individual components. It can also be prescribed along with other blood pressure medications.

Generic name:
Atenolol

See Tenormin, page 593.

Generic name:
Atenolol with Chlorthalidone

See Tenoretic, page 592.

Generic name:
Atorvastatin

See Lipitor, page 500.

Brand name:
Atrovent

Pronounced: AT-row-vent
Generic name: Ipratropium bromide

Atrovent inhalation aerosol and solution are prescribed for long-term treatment of bronchial spasms (wheezing) associated with chronic obstructive pulmonary disease, including chronic bronchitis and emphysema. When inhaled, Atrovent opens the air passages, allowing more oxygen to reach the lungs.

Atrovent nasal spray relieves runny nose. The 0.03% spray is used for year-round runny nose due to allergies and other causes. The 0.06% spray is prescribed for hay fever and for runny nose due to colds. The spray does not relieve nasal congestion or sneezing.

Brand name:
A/T/S

See Erythromycin, Topical, page 460.

Brand name:
Augmentin

Pronounced: awg-MENT-in
Generic ingredients: Amoxicillin, Clavulanate potassium

Augmentin is used in the treatment of lower respiratory, middle ear, sinus, skin, and urinary tract infections that are caused by certain specific bacteria. These bacteria produce a chemical enzyme called beta lactamase that makes some infections particularly difficult to treat.

Augmentin ES-600, a stronger, oral-suspension form of the drug, is prescribed for certain stubborn ear infections that previous treatment has failed to clear up in children two and under, or those attending day care.

Brand name:
Auralgan

Pronounced: Aw-RAL-gan
Generic ingredients: Antipyrine, Benzocaine, Glycerin
Other brand name: Auroto Otic

Auralgan is prescribed to reduce the inflammation and congestion and relieve the pain and discomfort of severe middle ear infections. This drug may be used in combination with an antibiotic for curing the infection.

Auralgan is also used to remove excessive or impacted earwax.

Generic name:
Auranofin

See Ridaura, page 573.

Brand name:
Auroto Otic

See Auralgan, page 398.

Brand name:
Avalide

Pronounced: AV-a-lide
Generic name: Irbesartan, Hydrochlorothiazide

Avalide is a combination medication used to treat high blood pressure. One component, irbesartan, belongs to a class of blood pressure medications that prevents the hormone angiotensin II from constricting the blood vessels, thereby allowing blood to flow more freely and keeping blood pressure down. The other component, hydrochlorothiazide, is a diuretic that increases the output of urine, removing excess fluid from the body and thus lowering blood pressure.

Combinations such as Avalide are usually prescribed only when treatment with a single medication fails to lower blood pressure sufficiently. Avalide can be combined with yet other blood pressure medicines if pressure remains too high.

Brand name:
Avandia

Pronounced: AH-van-DEE-ah
Generic name: Rosiglitazone maleate

Avandia is used to hold down blood sugar levels in people with type 2 diabetes (also known as "non-insulin dependent" or "adult onset" diabetes).

Blood sugar levels are ordinarily controlled by the body's natural supply of insulin, which helps sugar move out of the bloodstream and into the cells. In type 2 diabetes, the buildup of sugar in the blood is often due not to a lack of insulin, but to the body's inability to make proper use of it. Avandia works first by decreasing sugar production, then by helping the body make more efficient use of whatever insulin is available. It does not increase the actual amount of insulin in circulation.

Avandia can be used alone or in conjunction with metformin (Glucophage) or a member of the sulfonylurea class of diabetes drugs (Diabinese, Micronase, Orinase). It takes effect slowly. Patients may not see a reduction in blood sugar levels for the first 2 weeks of therapy, and it may take 2 to 3 months for the medication to deliver maximum results.

Brand name:
Avapro

Pronounced: AVE-ah-pro
Generic name: Irbesartan

Avapro is used to treat high blood pressure. A member of the family of drugs called angiotensin II receptor antagonists, it works by preventing the hormone angiotensin II from narrowing the blood vessels, an action that tends to raise blood pressure. Avapro may be prescribed alone or with other blood pressure medications.

Brand name:
AVC

Pronounced: A VEE CEE
Generic name: Sulfanilamide

AVC is used to treat yeast infections caused by *Candida albicans*, a type of fungus. AVC rapidly relieves vulvovaginitis—the itching, redness, and irritation of the external sex organs (vulva) and the thick, cottage cheese-like discharge that usually accompany yeast infections.

Brand name:
Avelox

Pronounced: AV-eh-locks
Generic name: Moxifloxacin hydrochloride

Avelox, an antibiotic, is prescribed to treat sinus and lung infections. It kills bacteria that can cause sinusitis, pneumonia, and secondary infections in chronic bronchitis. It also fights skin infections caused by staph or strep.

Avelox is a member of the quinolone family of antibiotics. Like all antibiotics, Avelox works only against bacteria. It will not cure an infection caused by a virus.

Brand name:
Avita

See Retin-A and Renova, page 572.

Brand name:
Axert

Pronounced: AKS-ert
Generic name: Almotriptan

Axert is a migraine treatment. It relieves the type of migraine that's accompanied by an aura (a set of symptoms that includes visual disturbances, speech difficulties, tingling, numbness, and weakness), as well as the kind that lacks an aura.

Axert is a member of a family of drugs called selective serotonin receptor agonists. These medications are thought to work by stopping abnormal dilation of blood vessels in the head, fighting inflammation, and reducing pain transmissions along certain nerve pathways near the brain.

Axert relieves migraines already in progress, but it won't prevent them from starting. It has not been tested for other types of headache, such as cluster headache, and should be used only for migraine attacks.

Brand name:

Axid

Pronounced: AK-sid
Generic name: Nizatidine

Axid is prescribed for the treatment of duodenal ulcers and noncancer-ous stomach ulcers. Full-dose therapy for these problems lasts no longer than 8 weeks. However, doctors sometimes prescribe Axid at a reduced dosage after a duodenal ulcer has healed. The drug is also prescribed for the heartburn and the inflammation that result when acid stomach contents flow backward into the esophagus. Axid belongs to a class of drugs known as histamine H-2 blockers.

Generic name:

Azatadine with Pseudoephedrine

See Trinalin, page 607.

Generic name:

Azelaic acid

See Azelex, page 402.

Generic name:

Azelastine

See Astelin, page 396.

Brand name:

Azelex

Pronounced: AY-zuh-lecks
Generic name: Azelaic acid
Other brand name: Finevin

Azelex helps clear up mild to moderate acne. The skin eruptions and inflammation of acne typically begin during puberty, when oily secre-tions undergo an increase.

Generic name:

Azithromycin

See Zithromax, page 626.

Brand name:

Azmacort

Pronounced: AZ-ma-court
Generic name: Triamcinolone acetonide
Other brand names: Nasacort, Nasacort AQ

Azmacort and Nasacort are metered-dose inhalers containing the anti-inflammatory steroid medication, triamcinolone acetonide; Nasacort AQ is a metered-dose pump spray. Azmacort is used as long-term therapy to control bronchial asthma attacks. Nasacort and Nasacort AQ are prescribed to relieve the symptoms of hay fever and other nasal allergies. Nasacort is also used in the treatment of nasal polyps (projecting masses of tissue in the nose).

Brand name:

Azulfidine

Pronounced: A-ZUL-fi-deen
Generic name: Sulfasalazine

Azulfidine, an anti-inflammatory medicine, is prescribed for the treatment of mild to moderate ulcerative colitis (a long-term, progressive bowel disease) and as an added treatment in severe ulcerative colitis (chronic inflammation and ulceration of the lining of large bowel and rectum, the main symptom of which is bloody diarrhea).

Azulfidine EN-tabs are prescribed for people with ulcerative colitis who cannot take the regular Azulfidine tablet because of symptoms of stomach and intestinal irritation such as nausea and vomiting when taking the first few doses of the drug, or for those in whom a reduction in dosage does not lessen the stomach or intestinal side effects. The EN-tabs are also prescribed for adults and children with rheumatoid arthritis who fail to get relief from salicylates (such as aspirin) or other nonsteroidal anti-inflammatory drugs (such as ibuprofen).

Generic name:
Baclofen

See Lioresal, page 499.

Brand name:
Bactrim

Pronounced: BAC-trim
Generic ingredients: Trimethoprim, Sulfamethoxazole
Other brand name: Septra

Bactrim, an antibacterial combination drug, is prescribed for the treatment of certain urinary tract infections, severe middle ear infections in children, long-lasting or frequently recurring bronchitis in adults that has increased in seriousness, inflammation of the intestine due to a severe bacterial infection, and travelers' diarrhea in adults. Bactrim is also prescribed for the treatment of *Pneumocystis carinii* pneumonia, and for prevention of this type of pneumonia in people with weakened immune systems.

Brand name:
Bactroban

Pronounced: BAC-tro-ban
Generic name: Mupirocin

Bactroban is prescribed for the treatment of impetigo, a bacterial infection of the skin. An antibiotic ointment applied to the skin, it kills the staph and strep germs responsible for the problem.

Generic name:
Balsalazide

See Colazal, page 429.

Generic name:
Beclomethasone

Pronounced: BECK-low-METH-ah-sone
Brand names: Beconase AQ Nasal Spray, Beconase Inhalation Aerosol, Qvar Inhalation Aerosol, Vancenase AQ Nasal Spray and Double

Strength Nasal Spray, Vancenase Nasal Inhaler and PocketHaler Nasal Inhaler, Vanceril Inhalation Aerosol and Double Strength Inhalation Aerosol, Vanceril Inhaler

Beclomethasone is a type of steroid used for respiratory problems. Beclovent and Vanceril are prescribed for the prevention of recurring symptoms of bronchial asthma. Beconase and Vancenase are used to relieve the symptoms of hay fever and to prevent regrowth of nasal polyps following surgical removal.

Brand name:

Beconase

See Beclomethasone, page 404.

Brand name:

Bellatal

See Donnatal, page 452.

Generic name:

Benazepril

See Lotensin, page 504.

Generic name:

Benazepril with Hydrochlorothiazide

See Lotensin HCT, page 504.

Brand name:

Bentyl

Pronounced: BEN-til
Generic name: Dicyclomine hydrochloride

Bentyl is prescribed for the treatment of functional bowel/irritable bowel syndrome (abdominal pain, accompanied by diarrhea and constipation associated with stress). It works by quelling the spasms associated with this condition.

Brand name:

BenzaClin

Pronounced: BEN-za-klin
Generic ingredients: Benzoyl peroxide, Clindamycin

BenzaClin is an acne treatment. Both its ingredients—the antibiotic clindamycin and the antibacterial agent benzoyl peroxide—attack the bacteria that help cause acne.

Brand name:

Benzac W

See Desquam-E, page 443.

Brand name:

Benzagel

See Desquam-E, page 443.

Brand name:

Benzamycin

Pronounced: BEN-za-MI-sin
Generic ingredients: Erythromycin, Benzoyl peroxide

A combination of the antibiotic erythromycin and the antibacterial agent benzoyl peroxide, Benzamycin is effective in stopping the bacteria that cause acne and in reducing acne infection.

Brand name:

BenzaShave

See Desquam-E, page 443.

Generic name:

Benzonatate

See Tessalon, page 594.

Generic name:
Benzoyl peroxide
See Desquam-E, page 443.

Generic name:
Benztropine
See Cogentin, page 428.

Generic name:
Bepridil
See Vascor, page 614.

Brand name:
Betagan
Pronounced: BAIT-ah-gan
Generic name: Levobunolol hydrochloride

Betagan eyedrops are given to treat chronic open-angle glaucoma (increased pressure inside the eye). This medication is in a class called beta blockers. It works by lowering pressure within the eyeball.

Generic name:
Betaine
See Cystadane, page 436.

Generic name:
Betamethasone
See Diprolene, page 450.

Generic name:
Betaxolol
See Betoptic, page 408.

Brand name:
Betimol

See Timoptic, page 599.

Brand name:
Betoptic

Pronounced: bet-OP-tick
Generic name: Betaxolol hydrochloride

Betoptic Ophthalmic Solution and Betoptic S Ophthalmic Suspension contain a medication that lowers internal eye pressure. They are used to treat open-angle glaucoma (high pressure of the fluid in the eye).

Brand name:
Bextra

Pronounced: BEK-struh
Generic name: Valdecoxib

Bextra is a member of the relatively new class of painkillers called COX-2 inhibitors. It is prescribed for the relief of osteoarthritis, rheumatoid arthritis, and painful menstruation (dysmenorrhea).

COX-2 inhibitors are part of a larger group of medications called nonsteroidal anti-inflammatory drugs (NSAIDs). All the drugs in this category (including such familiar remedies as aspirin, Motrin, and Naprosyn) relieve pain and inflammation by limiting the effect of a natural enzyme called COX-2. Unlike the older NSAIDs, however, the new COX-2 inhibitors do not interfere with COX-1, a related enzyme that exerts a protective effect on the lining of the stomach. As a result, Bextra and other COX-2 inhibitors are less likely to cause the bleeding and ulcers that sometimes accompany sustained use of the older NSAIDs.

Brand name:
Biaxin

Pronounced: buy-AX-in
Generic name: Clarithromycin
Other brand name: Biaxin XL

Biaxin, an antibiotic chemically related to erythromycin, is used to treat certain bacterial infections of the respiratory tract, including:

Strep throat
Pneumonia
Sinusitis (inflamed sinuses)
Tonsillitis (inflamed tonsils)
Acute middle ear infections
Acute flare-ups of chronic bronchitis (inflamed airways)

Biaxin is also prescribed to treat infections of the skin. Combined with Prilosec or Prevacid and amoxicillin, it is used to cure ulcers near the exit from the stomach (duodenal ulcers) caused by *H. pylori* bacteria. It can also be prescribed to combat *Mycobacterium avium* infections in people with AIDS.

Biaxin is available in tablet and suspension form, and in extended-release tablets (Biaxin XL). The extended-release form is used only for sinus inflammation and flare-ups of bronchitis.

Generic name:

Bicalutamide

See Casodex, page 418.

Generic name:

Bimatoprost

See Lumigan, page 506.

Generic name:

Bismuth subsalicylate, Metronidazole, and Tetracycline

See Helidac Therapy, page 479.

Brand name:

Bleph-10

See Sodium Sulamyd, page 582.

Brand name:

Bonine

See Antivert, page 394.

Brand name:

Brethine

Pronounced: Breath-EEN
Generic name: Terbutaline sulfate

Brethine is a bronchodilator (a medication that opens the bronchial tubes), prescribed for the prevention and relief of the bronchial spasms that constrict the airway in asthma patients. This medication is also used for the relief of bronchial spasm associated with bronchitis and emphysema.

Brand name:

Brevicon

See Oral Contraceptives, page 542.

Generic name:

Bromocriptine

See Parlodel, page 547.

Brand name:

Brontex

See Tussi-Organidin NR, page 609.

Generic name:

Budesonide

See Rhinocort, page 573.

Generic name:

Bumetanide

See Bumex, page 411.

Brand name:

Bumex

Pronounced: BYOO-meks
Generic name: Bumetanide

Bumex is used to lower the amount of excess salt and water in the body by increasing the output of urine. It is prescribed in the treatment of edema, or fluid retention, associated with congestive heart failure and liver or kidney disease. It is also occasionally prescribed, along with other drugs, to treat high blood pressure.

Generic name:

Bupropion for smoking

See Zyban, page 628.

Generic name:

Butalbital, Acetaminophen, and Caffeine

See Fioricet, page 467.

Generic name:

Butalbital, Aspirin, and Caffeine

See Fiorinal, page 467.

Generic name:

Butalbital, Codeine, Aspirin, and Caffeine

See Fiorinal with Codeine, page 467.

Generic name:

Butoconazole

See Mycelex-3, page 525.

Brand name:

Cafergot

Pronounced: KAF-er-got
Generic ingredients: Ergotamine tartrate, Caffeine

Cafergot is prescribed for the relief or prevention of vascular headaches—for example, migraine, migraine variants, or cluster headaches.

Brand name:

Calan

Pronounced: CAL-an
Generic name: Verapamil hydrochloride
Other brand names: Calan SR, Covera-HS, Isoptin, Isoptin SR, Verelan, Verelan PM

Verapamil-based medications can be prescribed for several heart and blood pressure problems. The fast-acting brands (Calan and Isoptin) are taken for angina (chest pain due to clogged cardiac arteries), as well as irregular heartbeat and high blood pressure. The longer-acting brands (Calan SR, Isoptin SR, Verelan, and Verelan PM) are typically used only for high blood pressure. Covera-HS is prescribed for both high blood pressure and angina.

Verapamil is a type of medication called a calcium channel blocker. It eases the heart's workload by slowing down the passage of nerve impulses through it, and hence the contractions of the heart muscle. This improves blood flow through the heart and throughout the body, reduces blood pressure, corrects irregular heartbeat, and helps prevent angina pain.

Some doctors also prescribe verapamil to prevent migraine headache and asthma and to treat manic depression and panic attacks, but the drug is not officially approved for these purposes.

Generic name:

Calcitonin-salmon

See Miacalcin, page 516.

Generic name:

Calcitriol

See Rocaltrol, page 575.

Brand name:

Canasa

See Rowasa, page 577.

Generic name:

Candesartan

See Atacand, page 396.

Generic name:

Candesartan with Hydrochlorothiazide

See Atacand HCT, page 397.

Brand name:

Capoten

Pronounced: KAP-o-ten
Generic name: Captopril

Capoten is used in the treatment of high blood pressure and congestive heart failure. When prescribed for high blood pressure, it is effective used alone or combined with diuretics. If it is prescribed for congestive heart failure, it is used in combination with digitalis and diuretics. Capoten is in a family of drugs known as "ACE (angiotensin converting enzyme) inhibitors." It works by preventing a chemical in the blood called angiotensin I from converting into a more potent form that increases salt and water retention in the body. Capoten also enhances blood flow throughout the blood vessels.

In addition, Capoten is used to improve survival in certain people who have suffered heart attacks and to treat kidney disease in diabetics.

Some doctors also prescribe Capoten for angina pectoris (crushing chest pain), Raynaud's phenomenon (a disorder of the blood vessels that causes the fingers to turn white when exposed to cold), and rheumatoid arthritis.

Brand name:

Capozide

Pronounced: KAP-oh-zide
Generic ingredients: Captopril, Hydrochlorothiazide

Capozide is used in the treatment of high blood pressure. It combines an ACE inhibitor with a thiazide diuretic. Captopril, the ACE inhibitor, works by preventing a chemical in the blood called angiotensin I from converting into a more potent form that increases salt and water retention in the body. Captopril also enhances blood flow throughout the blood vessels. Hydrochlorothiazide, the diuretic, helps the body produce and eliminate more urine, which helps in lowering blood pressure.

Generic name:

Captopril

See Capoten, page 413.

Generic name:

Captopril with Hydrochlorothiazide

See Capozide, page 414.

Brand name:

Carac

See Efudex, page 455.

Brand name:

Carafate

Pronounced: CARE-uh-fate
Generic name: Sucralfate

Carafate Tablets and Suspension are used for the short-term treatment (up to 8 weeks) of an active duodenal ulcer (an open sore in the intestinal wall near the exit from the stomach). Carafate Tablets are also used for longer-term therapy at a reduced dosage after a duodenal ulcer has healed.

Carafate helps ulcers heal by forming a protective coating over them.

Some doctors also prescribe Carafate for ulcers in the mouth and esophagus that develop during cancer therapy, for digestive tract irritation caused by drugs, for long-term treatment of stomach ulcers, and to relieve pain following tonsil removal.

Generic name:

Carbamazepine

See Tegretol, page 591.

Brand name:

Carbatrol

See Tegretol, page 591.

Generic name:

Carbidopa with Levodopa

See Sinemet CR, page 581.

Generic name:

Carbinoxamine or Brompheniramine and Pseudoephedrine

See Rondec, page 576.

Brand name:

Cardene

Pronounced: CAR-deen
Generic name: Nicardipine hydrochloride

Cardene, a type of medication called a calcium channel blocker, is prescribed for the treatment of chronic stable angina (chest pain that results when clogged arteries reduce the heart's oxygen supply, brought on by exertion) and for high blood pressure. When used to treat angina, Cardene is sometimes combined with beta-blocking medications such as Tenormin or Inderal. If it is used to treat high blood pressure, Cardene may be combined with other high blood pressure medications. Calcium channel blockers ease the workload of the heart by slowing down the passage of nerve impulses through the heart and its resulting muscle contractions This improves blood flow through the heart and throughout the body. By expanding the blood vessels, calcium channel blockers also reduce blood pressure.

Cardene SR, a long-acting form of the drug, is prescribed only for high blood pressure.

Some doctors also prescribe Cardene to prevent migraine headache and to treat congestive heart failure. In combination with other drugs, such as Amicar, Cardene is also prescribed to manage neurological problems following certain kinds of stroke.

Brand name:

Cardizem

Pronounced: CAR-di-zem
Generic name: Diltiazem hydrochloride
Other brand names: Cardizem CD, Cardizem SR, Dilacor XR, Tiazac

Cardizem and Cardizem CD (a controlled release form of diltiazem) are used in the treatment of angina pectoris (chest pain that results when clogged arteries reduce the heart's oxygen supply) and chronic stable angina (a type brought on by exertion). Cardizem CD is also used to treat high blood pressure. Another controlled release form, Cardizem SR, is used only in the treatment of high blood pressure. Cardizem, a calcium channel blocker, dilates blood vessels and slows the heart to reduce blood pressure and the pain of angina.

Doctors sometimes prescribe Cardizem for loss of circulation in the fingers and toes (Raynaud's phenomenon), for involuntary movements (tardive dyskinesia), and to prevent heart attack.

Tiazac and Dilacor XR are used in the treatment of high blood pressure and chronic stable angina. They may be taken alone or combined with other blood pressure medications.

Brand name:

Cardura

Pronounced: car-DUHR-uh
Generic name: Doxazosin mesylate

Cardura is used in the treatment of benign prostatic hyperplasia, a condition in which the prostate gland grows larger, pressing on the urethra and threatening to block the flow of urine from the bladder. The drug relieves symptoms such as a weak stream, dribbling, incomplete emptying of the bladder, frequent urination, and burning during urination.

Cardura is also used in the treatment of high blood pressure. It is effective when used alone or in combination with other blood pressure medications, such as diuretics, beta-blocking medications, calcium channel blockers or ACE inhibitors.

Doctors also prescribe Cardura, along with other drugs such as digitalis and diuretics, for treatment of congestive heart failure.

Generic name:
Carisoprodol

See Soma, page 582.

Generic name:
Carteolol

See Cartrol, page 417.

Brand name:
Cartrol

Pronounced: KAR-troll
Generic name: Carteolol hydrochloride

Cartrol, a type of medication known as a beta blocker, is used in the treatment of high blood pressure. It is effective when used alone or when combined with other high blood pressure medications, particularly with a thiazide-type diuretic such as HydroDIURIL. Beta blockers decrease the force and rate of heart contractions, thus lowering blood pressure.

Generic name:
Carvedilol

See Coreg, page 431.

Brand name:

Casodex

Pronounced: KAY-so-dex
Generic name: Bicalutamide

Casodex is used in the treatment of advanced prostate cancer. It belongs to a class of drugs known as antiandrogens. These drugs block the effect of male hormones.

Casodex is prescribed along with a drug, such as Lupron, that mimics the effect of natural luteinizing hormone-releasing hormone (LHRH).

Brand name:

Cataflam

See Voltaren, page 620.

Brand name:

Catapres

Pronounced: KAT-uh-press
Generic name: Clonidine hydrochloride

Catapres is prescribed for high blood pressure. It is effective when used alone or with other high blood pressure medications.

Doctors also prescribe Catapres for alcohol, nicotine, or benzodiazepine (tranquilizer) withdrawal; migraine headaches; smoking cessation programs; Tourette's syndrome (tics and uncontrollable utterances); narcotic/methadone detoxification; premenstrual tension; and diabetic diarrhea.

Brand name:

Caverject

Pronounced: CA-vur-jekt
Generic name: Alprostadil
Other brand names: Edex, Muse

Caverject is used to treat male impotence. Doctors also use the drug to help diagnose the exact nature of a patient's impotence.

Caverject and the similar brand Edex are both taken by injection. A third brand, Muse, is taken as a small suppository inserted in the penis.

Brand name:
Ceclor

Pronounced: SEE-klor
Generic name: Cefaclor

Ceclor, a cephalosporin antibiotic, is used in the treatment of ear, nose, throat, respiratory tract, urinary tract, and skin infections caused by specific bacteria, including staph, strep, and *E. coli*. Uses include treatment of sore or strep throat, pneumonia, and tonsillitis. Ceclor CD, an extended release form of the drug, is also used for flare-ups of chronic bronchitis.

Brand name:
Cedax

Pronounced: SEE-daks
Generic name: Ceftibuten

Cedax cures mild-to-moderate bacterial infections of the throat, ear, and respiratory tract. Among these infections are strep throat, tonsillitis, and acute otitis media (middle ear infection) in children and adults. Cedax is also prescribed for acute flare-ups of chronic bronchitis in adults. Cedax is a cephalosporin antibiotic.

Generic name:
Cefaclor

See Ceclor, page 419.

Generic name:
Cefadroxil

See Duricef, page 453.

Generic name:
Cefdinir

See Omnicef, page 541.

Generic name:

Cefixime

See Suprax, page 586.

Generic name:

Cefprozil

See Cefzil, page 420.

Generic name:

Ceftibuten

See Cedax, page 419.

Brand name:

Ceftin

Pronounced: SEF-tin
Generic name: Cefuroxime axetil

Ceftin, a cephalosporin antibiotic, is prescribed for mild to moderately severe bacterial infections of the throat, lungs, ears, skin, sinuses, and urinary tract, and for gonorrhea. Ceftin tablets are also prescribed in the early stages of Lyme disease.

Generic name:

Ceftriaxone

See Rocephin, page 576.

Generic name:

Cefuroxime

See Ceftin, page 420.

Brand name:

Cefzil

Pronounced: SEFF-zil
Generic name: Cefprozil

Cefzil, a cephalosporin antibiotic, is prescribed for mild to moderately severe bacterial infections of the throat, ear, sinuses, respiratory tract, and skin. Among these infections are strep throat, tonsillitis, bronchitis, and pneumonia.

Brand name:
Celebrex

Pronounced: SELL-eh-breks
Generic name: Celecoxib

Celebrex is prescribed for acute pain, menstrual cramps, and the pain and inflammation of osteoarthritis and rheumatoid arthritis. It is the first of a new class of nonsteroidal anti-inflammatory drugs (NSAIDs) called "COX-2 inhibitors." Like older NSAIDs such as Motrin and Naprosyn, Celebrex is believed to fight pain and inflammation by inhibiting the effect of a natural enzyme called COX-2. Unlike the older medications, however, it does not interfere with a similar substance, called COX-1, which exerts a protective effect on the lining of the stomach. Celebrex is therefore less likely to cause the bleeding and ulcers that sometimes accompany sustained use of the older NSAIDs.

Celebrex has also been found to reduce the number of colorectal polyps (growths in the wall of the lower intestine and rectum) in people who suffer from the condition called familial adenomatous polyposis (FAP), an inherited tendency to develop large numbers of colorectal polyps that eventually become cancerous.

Generic name:
Celecoxib

See Celebrex, page 421.

Brand name:
Cenestin

See Premarin, page 560.

Generic name:
Cephalexin

See Keflex, page 491.

Generic name:
Cephradine

See Velosef, page 615.

Brand name:
Cetacort

See Hydrocortisone Skin Preparations, page 482.

Generic name:
Cetirizine

See Zyrtec, page 630.

Generic name:
Cetirizine with Pseudoephedrine

See Zyrtec-D, page 630.

Generic name:
Chlordiazepoxide with Clidinium

See Librax, page 499.

Generic name:
Chlorhexidine

See Peridex, page 552.

Generic name:
Chlorothiazide

See Diuril, page 451.

Generic name:

Chlorpheniramine with Pseudoephedrine

See Deconamine, page 440.

Generic name:

Chlorpropamide

See Diabinese, page 445.

Generic name:

Chlorthalidone

See Thalitone, page 596.

Generic name:

Chlorzoxazone

See Parafon Forte DSC, page 547.

Generic name:

Cholestyramine

See Questran, page 568.

Generic name:

Choline magnesium trisalicylate

See Trilisate, page 606.

Brand name:

Chronulac Syrup

Pronounced: KRON-yoo-lak
Generic name: Lactulose

Chronulac treats constipation. In people who are chronically constipated, Chronulac increases the number and frequency of bowel movements.

Generic name:

Ciclopirox

See Loprox, page 502.

Generic name:

Cilostazol

See Pletal, page 557.

Generic name:

Cimetidine

See Tagamet, page 588.

Brand name:

Cipro

Pronounced: SIP-roh
Generic name: Ciprofloxacin hydrochloride

Cipro is used to treat infections of the lower respiratory tract, the abdomen, the skin, the bones and joints, and the urinary tract, including cystitis (bladder inflammation) in women. It is also prescribed for severe sinus or bronchial infections, infectious diarrhea, typhoid fever, inhalational anthrax, infections of the prostate gland, and some sexually transmitted diseases such as gonorrhea. Additionally, some doctors prescribe Cipro for certain serious ear infections, tuberculosis, and some of the infections common in people with AIDS.

Because Cipro is effective only for certain types of bacterial infections, before beginning treatment the doctor may perform tests to identify the specific organisms causing the infection.

Cipro is available as a tablet and an oral suspension and as a suspension to be used externally in the ear.

Generic name:

Ciprofloxacin

See Cipro, page 424.

Brand name:

Clarinex

Pronounced: CLAR-in-ecks
Generic name: Desloratadine

Clarinex is an antihistamine used to relieve the symptoms of hay fever (seasonal allergic rhinitis). Like many of the newer members of the antihistamine family, Clarinex causes less drowsiness than do older products such as Benadryl.

Generic name:

Clarithromycin

See Biaxin, page 408.

Brand name:

Claritin

Pronounced: CLAR-i-tin
Generic name: Loratadine

Claritin is an antihistamine that relieves the sneezing, runny nose, stuffiness, itching, and tearing eyes caused by hay fever. It is also prescribed for relief of the swollen, red, itchy patches of skin labeled chronic hives. Like many of the newer members of the antihistamine family, Claritin causes less drowsiness than do older products such as Benadryl.

Brand name:

Claritin-D

Pronounced: CLAR-i-tin dee
Generic ingredients: Loratadine, Pseudoephedrine sulfate

Claritin-D is an antihistamine and decongestant that relieves the sneezing, runny nose, stuffiness, and itchy, tearing eyes caused by hay fever. Two versions are available: Claritin-D 12 Hour for twice-daily dosing and Claritin-D 24 Hour for once-a-day use.

Brand name:
Cleocin T

Pronounced: KLEE-oh-sin tee
Generic name: Clindamycin phosphate

Cleocin T is an antibiotic used to treat acne.

Brand name:
Cleocin Vaginal

Pronounced: KLEE-oh-sin
Generic name: Clindamycin phosphate

Cleocin Vaginal products (cream and ovules) are used to treat bacterial vaginosis, an infection of the vagina. The infection, which is probably sexually transmitted, often produces a gray or yellow discharge with a fishy smell that increases if the external genitals are washed with alkaline soap.

Before prescribing Cleocin, doctors typically test the vaginal discharge in the laboratory and examine it under the microscope to make certain that the patient does not have a yeast infection or another sexually transmitted disease (STD) such as chlamydia, gonorrhea, or herpes simplex.

Brand name:
Climara

See Estrogen Patches, page 462.

Brand name:
Clinac BPO

See Desquam-E, page 443.

Generic name:
Clindamycin

See Cleocin T, page 426.
See Cleocin Vaginal, page 426.

Generic name:
Clindamycin and Benzoyl peroxide

See BenzaClin, page 406.

Brand name:
Clinoril

Pronounced: CLIN-or-il
Generic name: Sulindac

Clinoril, a nonsteroidal anti-inflammatory drug, is used to relieve the inflammation, swelling, stiffness, and joint pain associated with rheumatoid arthritis, osteoarthritis (the most common form of arthritis), and ankylosing spondylitis (stiffness and progressive arthritis of the spine). It is also used to treat bursitis, tendinitis, acute gouty arthritis, and other types of pain.

The safety and effectiveness of this medication in the treatment of people with severe, incapacitating rheumatoid arthritis have not been established.

Generic name:
Clobetasol

See Temovate, page 592.

Brand name:
Clomid

See Clomiphene Citrate, page 427.

Generic name:
Clomiphene Citrate

Pronounced: KLAHM-if-een SIT-rate
Brand names: Clomid, Serophene

Clomiphene is prescribed for the treatment of ovulatory failure in women who wish to become pregnant and whose husbands are fertile and potent.

Generic name:

Clonidine

See Catapres, page 418.

Generic name:

Clopidogrel

See Plavix, page 556.

Generic name:

Clotrimazole

See Gyne-Lotrimin, page 479.

Generic name:

Clotrimazole with Betamethasone

See Lotrisone, page 505.

Brand name:

Cogentin

Pronounced: co-JEN-tin
Generic name: Benztropine mesylate

Cogentin is given to help relieve the symptoms of "parkinsonism": the muscle rigidity, tremors, and difficulties with posture and balance that occur in Parkinson's disease and that sometimes develop as unwanted side effects of antipsychotic drugs such as Haldol and Thorazine.

Cogentin is an "anticholinergic" medication, a drug that controls spasms. It reduces the symptoms of parkinsonism, but it is not a cure.

Brand name:

Co-Gesic

See Vicodin, page 617.

Brand name:

Colazal

Pronounced: KOHL-a-zahl
Generic name: Balsalazide disodium

Colazal is used in the treatment of mild to moderate ulcerative colitis (chronic inflammation and ulceration of the lower intestine). It is an anti-inflammatory medicine specially formulated to release the active ingredient, mesalamine, directly to the lining of the colon. Its ability to provide relief without the severe side effects found with similar drugs is believed to be due to this localized drug delivery mechanism.

Generic name:

Colesevelam

See WelChol, page 621.

Brand name:

Colestid

Pronounced: Koh-LESS-tid
Generic name: Colestipol hydrochloride

Colestid, in conjunction with diet, is used to help lower high levels of cholesterol in the blood. The reduces the chances of developing clogged arteries and heart disease. The drug is available in plain and orange-flavored granules and in tablet form.

Generic name:

Colestipol

See Colestid, page 429.

Generic name:

Colistin, Neomycin, Hydrocortisone, and Thonzonium

See Cortisporin-TC Otic, page 432.

Brand name:
Colyte

Pronounced: KOE-lite
Generic ingredients: Polyethylene glycol, Electrolytes
Other brand name: GoLYTELY

Colyte is used to clean the bowel before an examination of the upper part of the rectum (colonoscopy) or a barium enema X-ray.

Brand name:
CombiPatch

Pronounced: KOM-bee-patch
Generic name: Estradiol and norethindrone acetate

A remedy for the symptoms of menopause, CombiPatch combines the hormones estrogen (estradiol) and progestin (norethindrone acetate) in a slow-release patch that's applied to the skin. The product eases such symptoms of menopause as feelings of warmth in the face, neck, and chest, and the sudden intense episodes of heat and sweating known as "hot flashes." It is also prescribed to relieve external vaginal irritation and internal vaginal dryness.

CombiPatch can also be used as an estrogen supplement by women unable to produce sufficient amounts of estrogen on their own. Problems prompting the need for supplementation include ovarian failure, hypogonadism (impaired hormone production), and surgical removal of the ovaries.

Brand name:
Combivir

Pronounced: KOM-bi-veer
Generic ingredients: Lamivudine, Zidovudine

Combivir is used to fight the human immunodeficiency virus (HIV) that causes AIDS. It is a combination product containing the two AIDS drugs, lamivudine (Epivir) and zidovudine (Retrovir). It is intended for use with additional AIDS drugs.

HIV does its damage by slowly destroying the immune system, eventually leaving the body defenseless against infections. The drugs in Combivir interfere with the virus's ability to reproduce, thus staving off the decline of the immune system and preserving better health.

Brand name:

Comtan

Pronounced: COM-tan
Generic name: Entacapone

Comtan is used for Parkinson's disease. It is prescribed when doses of the combination drug levodopa/carbidopa (Sinemet) begin to wear off too soon. By extending the effect of each dose of Sinemet, it frees the patient from the stiffness and tremors of Parkinson's for a longer period of time.

Comtan works by inhibiting the effect of an enzyme that breaks down the levodopa in Sinemet. It has no effect on Parkinson's disease when used by itself.

Brand name:

Condylox

Pronounced: CON-de-lox
Generic name: Podofilox

Condylox solution and gel are used to treat external genital warts. The gel formulation is also used to treat warts around the anus.

Generic name:

Conjugated estrogens

See Premarin, page 560.

Brand name:

Coreg

Pronounced: KOE-regg
Generic name: Carvedilol

Coreg lowers blood pressure and increases the output of the heart. It is prescribed for people with congestive heart failure to increase survival and reduce the need for hospitalization. It is also used to control high blood pressure.Whe prescribed for heart failure, it can be used alone or with other drugs such as digitalis. For hypertension , it is often prescribed along with a diuretic. Coreg is a member of the beta blocker family of drugs.

Brand name:

Corgard

Pronounced: CORE-guard
Generic name: Nadolol

Corgard is used in the treatment of angina pectoris (chest pain, usually caused by lack of oxygen to the heart due to clogged arteries) and to reduce high blood pressure.

When prescribed for high blood pressure, it is effective when used alone or in combination with other high blood pressure medications. Corgard is a type of drug known as a beta blocker. It decreases the force and rate of heart contractions, reducing the heart's demand for oxygen and lowering blood pressure.

Brand name:

Cormax

See Temovate, page 592.

Brand name:

Cortisporin Ophthalmic Suspension

Pronounced: KORE-ti-SPORE-in
Generic ingredients: Polymyxin B sulfate, Neomycin sulfate,
Hydrocortisone

Cortisporin Ophthalmic Suspension is a combination of the steroid drug, hydrocortisone, and two antibiotics. It is prescribed to relieve inflammatory conditions such as irritation, swelling, redness, and general eye discomfort, and to treat superficial bacterial infections of the eye.

Brand name:

Cortisporin-TC Otic

Pronounced: COURT-i-spore-in
Generic ingredients: Colistin sulfate, Neomycin sulfate, Hydrocortisone
acetate, Thonzonium bromide

Cortisporin-TC is a liquid suspension used to treat external ear infections. They may also be prescribed after ear surgery such as a mastoidectomy.

The ingredients colistin sulfate and neomycin sulfate are antibiotics used to treat the bacterial infection itself, while hydrocortisone acetate is a steroid that helps reduce the inflammation, swelling, itching, and other skin reactions associated with an ear infection; thonzonium bromide facilitates the drug's effects.

Brand name:
Corzide

Pronounced: CORE-zide
Generic ingredients: Nadolol, Bendroflumethiazide

Corzide is a combination drug used in the treatment of high blood pressure. It combines a beta blocker and a thiazide diuretic. Nadolol, the beta blocker, decreases the force and rate of heart contractions, thereby reducing blood pressure. Bendroflumethiazide, the diuretic, helps the body produce and eliminate more urine, which removes excess fluid and thus helps to lower blood pressure.

Brand name:
Coumadin

Pronounced: COO-muh-din
Generic name: Warfarin sodium

Coumadin is an anticoagulant (blood thinner). It is prescribed to:
Prevent and/or treat a blood clot that has formed within a blood vessel or in the lungs.
Prevent and/or treat blood clots associated with certain heart conditions or replacement of a heart valve.
Aid in the prevention of blood clots that may form in blood vessels anywhere in the body after a heart attack.
Reduce the risk of death, another heart attack, or stroke after a heart attack.

Brand name:
Covera-HS

See Calan, page 412.

Brand name:

Cozaar

Pronounced: CO-zahr
Generic name: Losartan potassium

Cozaar is used in the treatment of high blood pressure. It is effective when used alone or with other high blood pressure medications, such as diuretics that help the body get rid of water.

Cozaar is the first of a new class of blood pressure medications called angiotensin II receptor antagonists. Cozaar works, in part, by preventing the hormone angiotensin II from constricting the blood vessels, which tends to raise blood pressure.

Brand name:

Creon

See Pancrease, page 547.

Brand name:

Crixivan

Pronounced: CRIX-i-van
Generic name: Indinavir sulfate

Crixivan is used in the treatment of human immunodeficiency virus (HIV) infection. HIV causes the immune system to break down so that it can no longer fight off other infections. This leads to the fatal disease known as acquired immune deficiency syndrome (AIDS).

HIV thrives by taking over the immune system's vital CD4 cells (white blood cells) and using their inner workings to make additional copies of itself. Crixivan belongs to a class of HIV drugs called protease inhibitors, which work by interfering with an important step in the virus's reproductive cycle. Although Crixivan cannot eliminate HIV already present in the body, it can reduce the amount of virus available to infect other cells.

Crixivan can be taken alone or in combination with other HIV drugs such as Retrovir. Because Crixivan and Retrovir attack the virus in different ways, the combination is likely to be more effective than either drug alone.

Brand name:

Crolom

Pronounced: CROW-lum
Generic name: Cromolyn sodium

Crolom is an eyedrop that relieves the itching, tearing, discharge, and redness caused by seasonal and chronic allergies. The drug works by preventing certain cells in the body from releasing histamine and other substances that can cause an allergic reaction. It may be prescribed alone or with a steroid medication.

Generic name:

Cromolyn, inhaled

See Intal, page 487.

Generic name:

Cromolyn, ocular

See Crolom, page 435.

Brand name:

Cutivate

Pronounced: KYOOT-i-vait
Generic name: Fluticasone propionate

Cutivate cream and ointment are prescribed for relief of inflamed, itchy rashes and other inflammatory skin conditions.

Brand name:

Cyclessa

See Oral Contraceptives, page 542.

Generic name:

Cyclobenzaprine

See Flexeril, page 468.

Brand name:

Cyclocort

Pronounced: SIKE-low-court
Generic name: Amcinonide

Cyclocort is prescribed for the relief of the inflammatory and itchy symptoms of skin disorders that are responsive to corticosteroid treatment.

Generic name:

Cyclophosphamide

See Cytoxan, page 437.

Generic name:

Cyclosporine

See Sandimmune, page 578.

Generic name:

Cyproheptadine

See Periactin, page 551.

Brand name:

Cystadane

Pronounced: SIST-uh-dane
Generic name: Betaine anhydrous

Cystadane is prescribed to reduce dangerously high blood levels of the naturally occurring amino acid homocysteine. Excessive levels of homocysteine can lead to formation of clots within the blood vessels, brittle bones (osteoporosis), other bone abnormalities, and dislocation of the lens of the eye. Homocysteine is also linked with an increased risk of heart disease and heart attack.

When homocysteine levels are so high that the substance appears in the urine, the condition is called homocystinuria. The problem is usually the result of an inherited lack of the enzymes needed to process homocysteine and generally shows up within the first months or years of life.

Early signs of homocystinuria include delays in development, failure to thrive, seizures, and sluggishness.

Brand name:

Cytotec

Pronounced: SITE-oh-tek
Generic name: Misoprostol

Cytotec, a synthetic prostaglandin (hormone-like substance), reduces the production of stomach acid and protects the stomach lining. People who take nonsteroidal anti-inflammatory drugs (NSAIDs) may be given Cytotec tablets to help prevent stomach ulcers.

Aspirin and other NSAIDs such as Motrin, Naprosyn, Feldene, and others, which are widely used to control the pain and inflammation of arthritis, are generally hard on the stomach. If an NSAID is needed for a prolonged period of time and the patient is elderly or has ever had a stomach ulcer, the doctor may prescribe Cytotec for as long as the patient takes the NSAID.

Brand name:

Cytoxan

Pronounced: sigh-TOKS-an
Generic name: Cyclophosphamide

Cytoxan, an anticancer drug, works by interfering with the growth of malignant cells. It may be used alone but is often given with other anti-cancer medications.

Cytoxan is used in the treatment of the following types of cancer:

Breast cancer
Leukemias (cancers affecting the white blood cells)
Malignant lymphomas (Hodgkin's disease or cancer of the lymph nodes)
Multiple myeloma (a malignant condition or cancer of the plasma cells)
Advanced mycosis fungoides (cancer of the skin and lymph nodes)
Neuroblastoma (a malignant tumor of the adrenal gland or sympathetic nervous system)
Ovarian cancer (adenocarcinoma)
Retinoblastoma (a malignant tumor of the retina)

In addition, Cytoxan may sometimes be given to children who have "minimal change" nephrotic syndrome (kidney damage resulting in loss of protein in the urine) and who have not responded well to treatment with steroid medications.

Brand name:

Dantrium

Pronounced: DAN-tree-um
Generic name: Dantrolene sodium

Dantrium is given to relieve muscle spasm caused by conditions such as cerebral palsy, multiple sclerosis, spinal cord injury, or stroke. Dantrium does not cure these conditions, but it may enhance the effect of other treatment, such as physical therapy.

In addition, Dantrium is used to prevent or manage malignant hyperthermia, a life-threatening rapid rise in body temperature that sometimes develops as a reaction to anesthesia. Some doctors also prescribe Dantrium for heat stroke and muscle pain caused by exercise.

Generic name:

Dantrolene

See Dantrium, page 438.

Brand name:

Darvocet-N

Pronounced: DAR-voe-set en
Generic ingredients: Propoxyphene napsylate, Acetaminophen
Other brand names: Darvon-N (propoxyphene napsylate), Darvon (propoxyphene hydrochloride), Darvon Compound-65 (propoxyphene hydrochloride, aspirin, and caffeine)

Darvocet-N and its companion products all contain propoxyphene, a mild narcotic painkiller, and all are prescribed for the relief of mild to moderate pain. In addition, Darvocet-N and Darvon Compound-65 contain extra ingredients capable of reducing fever.

Brand name:

Darvon

See Darvocet-N, page 438.

Brand name:
Darvon Compound-65

See Darvocet-N, page 438.

Brand name:
Darvon-N

See Darvocet-N, page 438.

Brand name:
Daypro

Pronounced: DAY-pro
Generic name: Oxaprozin

Daypro is a nonsteroidal anti-inflammatory drug used to relieve the inflammation, swelling, stiffness, and joint pain associated with rheumatoid arthritis and osteoarthritis (the most common kind of arthritis).

Brand name:
DDAVP

Pronounced: dee-dee-ai-vee-pee
Generic name: Desmopressin acetate
Other brand name: Stimate

DDAVP nasal spray, nose drops, and tablets are given to prevent or control the frequent urination and loss of water associated with diabetes insipidus (a rare condition characterized by very large quantities of diluted urine and excessive thirst). They are also used to treat frequent passage of urine and increased thirst in people with certain brain injuries, and those who have undergone surgery in the pituitary region of the brain. DDAVP nasal spray and nose drops are also prescribed to help stop some types of bedwetting.

Stimate nasal spray is used to stop bleeding in certain types of hemophilia (failure of the blood to clot).

Brand name:
Decadron Tablets

Pronounced: DECK-uh-drohn
Generic name: Dexamethasone

Decadron, a corticosteroid drug, is used to reduce inflammation and relieve symptoms in a variety of disorders, including rheumatoid arthritis and severe cases of asthma. It may be given to people to treat primary or secondary adrenal cortex insufficiency (lack of sufficient adrenal hormone). It is also given to help treat the following disorders:

Severe allergic conditions such as drug-induced allergies
Blood disorders such as various anemias
Certain cancers (along with other drugs)
Skin diseases such as severe psoriasis
Collagen (connective tissue) diseases such as systemic lupus erythematosus
Digestive tract disease such as ulcerative colitis
High serum levels of calcium associated with cancer
Fluid retention due to nephrotic syndrome (a condition in which damage to the kidneys causes the body to lose protein in the urine)
Eye diseases such as allergic conjunctivitis
Lung diseases such as tuberculosis (along with other drugs)

Brand name:

Deconamine

Pronounced: dee-CON-uh-meen
Generic ingredients: Chlorpheniramine maleate, d-Pseudoephedrine hydrochloride

Deconamine is an antihistamine and decongestant used for the temporary relief of persistent runny nose, sneezing, and nasal congestion caused by upper respiratory infections (the common cold), sinus inflammation, or hay fever. It is also used to help clear nasal passages and shrink swollen membranes and to drain the sinuses and relieve sinus pressure.

Brand name:

Deltasone

Pronounced: DELL-tuh-zone
Generic name: Prednisone

Deltasone, a steroid drug, is used to reduce inflammation and alleviate symptoms in a variety of disorders, including rheumatoid arthritis and severe cases of asthma. It may be given to treat primary or secondary adrenal cortex insufficiency (lack of sufficient adrenal hormone in the body). It is used in treating all of the following:

Abnormal adrenal gland development
Allergic conditions (severe)
Blood disorders
Certain cancers (along with other drugs)
Diseases of the connective tissue including systemic lupus erythematosus
Eye diseases of various kinds
Flare-ups of multiple sclerosis
Fluid retention due to "nephrotic syndrome" (a condition in which damage to the kidneys causes protein to be lost in the urine)
Lung diseases, including tuberculosis
Meningitis (inflamed membranes around the brain)
Prevention of organ rejection
Rheumatoid arthritis and related disorders
Severe flare-ups of ulcerative colitis or enteritis (inflammation of the intestines)
Skin diseases
Thyroid gland inflammation
Trichinosis (with complications)

Brand name:

Demerol

Pronounced: DEM-er-awl
Generic name: Meperidine hydrochloride

Demerol, a narcotic analgesic, is prescribed for the relief of moderate to severe pain. Like other painkillers in this category, it can lead to mental and physical dependence if taken too long.

Brand name:

Demulen

See Oral Contraceptives, page 542.

Brand name:

Denavir

Pronounced: DEN-a-veer
Generic name: Penciclovir

Denavir cream is used to treat recurrent cold sores on the lips and face. It works by interfering with the growth of the herpesvirus responsible for the sores.

Brand name:

Depakene

Pronounced: DEP-uh-keen
Generic name: Valproic acid

Depakene, an epilepsy medicine, is used to treat certain types of seizures and convulsions. It may be prescribed alone or with other anticonvulsant medications.

Brand name:

Depo-Provera

Pronounced: DE-po pro-VEH-ra
Generic name: Medroxyprogesterone acetate

Depo-Provera Contraceptive Injection is given in the buttock or upper arm to prevent pregnancy. It is more than 99 percent effective; the chances of becoming pregnant during the first year of use are less than 1 in 100. The injection is given every 3 months (13 weeks) by a doctor. Depo-Provera works by preventing the release of hormones called gonadotropins from the pituitary gland in the brain. Without these hormones, the monthly release of an egg from the ovary cannot occur. If no egg is released, pregnancy is impossible. Depo-Provera also causes changes in the lining of the uterus that make pregnancy less likely even if an egg is released.

In higher doses, Depo-Provera is also used in the treatment of certain cancers including cancer of the endometrium (lining of the uterus) and kidney cancer.

Generic name:

Desloratadine

See Clarinex, page 425.

Generic name:

Desmopressin

See DDAVP, page 439.

Brand name:

Desogen

See Oral Contraceptives, page 542.

Generic name:

Desonide

See Tridesilon, page 605.

Brand name:

DesOwen

See Tridesilon, page 605.

Generic name:

Desoximetasone

See Topicort, page 602.

Brand name:

Desquam-E

Pronounced: DES-kwam ee
Generic name: Benzoyl peroxide
Other brand names: Benzac W, Benzagel, BenzaShave, Clinac BPO, Triaz

Desquam-E gel is used to treat acne. It can be used alone or with other treatments, including antibiotics and products that contain retinoic acid, sulfur, or salicylic acid.

Brand name:

Detrol

Pronounced: DEE-troll
Generic name: Tolterodine tartrate
Other brand name: Detrol LA

Detrol combats symptoms of overactive bladder, including frequent urination, urgency (increased need to urinate), and urge incontinence
(inability to control urination). The drug works by blocking the nerve
impulses that prompt the bladder to contract.

Generic name:

Dexamethasone

See Decadron Tablets, page 439.

Generic name:

Dexamethasone with Neomycin

See Neodecadron Ophthalmic Ointment and Solution, page 530.

Generic name:

Dexchlorpheniramine

See Polaramine, page 557.

Brand name:

DiaBeta

See Micronase, page 518.

Brand name:

Diabinese

Pronounced: dye-AB-in-eez
Generic name: Chlorpropamide

Diabinese is an oral antidiabetic medication used to treat type 2 (non-insulin-dependent) diabetes. Diabetes (a buildup of sugar in the blood) occurs when the body fails to produce enough insulin or is unable to use it properly. Insulin expedites the transfer of sugar into the cells, where it's converted to energy.

There are two forms of diabetes: type 1 (insulin-dependent) and type 2 (non-insulin-dependent). Type 1 usually requires insulin injection for life, while type 2 diabetes can usually be treated by dietary changes and oral antidiabetic medications such as Diabinese. Diabinese is thought to control diabetes by stimulating the pancreas to secrete more insulin. Occasionally, type 2 diabetics must take insulin injections on a temporary basis, especially during stressful periods or times of illness.

Brand name:

Diamox

Pronounced: DYE-uh-mocks
Generic name: Acetazolamide

Diamox controls fluid secretion. It is used in the treatment of glaucoma (excessive pressure in the eyes), epilepsy (for both brief and unlocalized seizures), and fluid retention due to congestive heart failure or drugs. It is also used to prevent or relieve the symptoms of acute mountain sickness in climbers attempting a rapid climb and those who feel sick even though they are making a gradual climb.

Generic name:

Diclofenac

See Voltaren, page 620.

Generic name:

Diclofenac with Misoprostol

See Arthrotec, page 396.

Generic name:

Dicyclomine

See Bentyl, page 405.

Generic name:

Didanosine

See Videx, page 617.

Brand name:

Didronel

Pronounced: DIE-droe-nel
Generic name: Etidronate disodium

Didronel tablets are prescribed for the treatment of Paget's bone disease, which causes pain, bone fractures, and problems in the circulatory and nervous systems. Didronel can decrease pain, increase the ability to move, and slow the progression of the disease.

Didronel is also prescribed following hip replacement and spinal cord injury to prevent abnormal bone formation and inflammation.

Generic name:

Diethylpropion

See Tenuate, page 593.

Generic name:

Diethylstilbestrol (DES)

Pronounced: dye-ETH-il-stil-BESS-trole

Diethylstilbestrol (DES), a synthetic estrogen (female hormone), is often given to ease symptoms of some inoperable kinds of breast cancer and prostate cancer.

Brand name:

Differin

Pronounced: DIFF-er-in
Generic name: Adapalene

Differin is prescribed for the treatment of acne. Its exact mode of action is unknown, but it appear to modulate the cellular differentiation, hardening, and inflammatory processes that contribute to acne.

Generic name:

Diflorasone

See Psorcon, page 568.

Brand name:

Diflucan

Pronounced: Dye-FLEW-can
Generic name: Fluconazole

Diflucan is used to treat fungal infections called candidiasis (also known as thrush or yeast infections). These include vaginal infections, throat infections, and fungal infections elsewhere in the body, such as infections of the urinary tract, peritonitis (inflammation of the lining of the abdomen), and pneumonia. Diflucan is also prescribed to guard against candidiasis in some people receiving bone marrow transplants, and is used to treat meningitis (brain or spinal cord inflammation) caused by another type of fungus.

In addition, Diflucan is now being prescribed for fungal infections in kidney and liver transplant patients, and fungal infections in patients with AIDS.

Generic name:

Diflunisal

See Dolobid, page 451.

Generic name:

Digoxin

See Lanoxin, page 494.

Generic name:

Dihydrocodeine, Aspirin, and Caffeine

See Synalgos-DC, page 587.

Generic name:
Dihydroergotamine

See Migranal, page 519.

Brand name:
Dilacor XR

See Cardizem, page 416.

Brand name:
Dilantin

Pronounced: dye-LAN-tin
Generic name: Phenytoin sodium

Dilantin is an antiepileptic drug, prescribed to control grand mal seizures (a type of seizure in which the individual experiences a sudden loss of consciousness immediately followed by generalized convulsions) and temporal lobe seizures (a type of seizure caused by disease in the cortex of the temporal [side] lobe of the brain affecting smell, taste, sight, hearing, memory, and movement).

Dilantin may also be used to prevent and treat seizures occurring during and after neurosurgery (surgery of the brain and spinal cord).

Brand name:
Dilaudid

Pronounced: Dye-LAW-did
Generic name: Hydromorphone hydrochloride

Dilaudid, a narcotic analgesic, is prescribed for the relief of moderate to severe pain such as that due to:

Biliary colic (pain caused by an obstruction in the gallbladder or bile duct)
Burns
Cancer
Heart attack
Injury (soft tissue and bone)
Renal colic (sharp lower back and groin pain usually caused by the passage of a stone through the ureter)
Surgery

Generic name:

Diltiazem

See Cardizem, page 416.

Brand name:

Diovan

Pronounced: DYE-oh-van
Generic name: Valsartan
Other brand name: Diovan HCT

Diovan is one of a new class of blood pressure medications called angiotensin II receptor antagonists. Diovan works by preventing the hormone angiotensin II from narrowing the blood vessels, which tends to raise blood pressure. Diovan may be prescribed alone or with other blood pressure medications, such as diuretics that help the body get rid of excess water. Diovan HCT is just such a combination. It contains Diovan plus the common diuretic hydrochlorothiazide.

Brand name:

Dipentum

Pronounced: dye-PENT-um
Generic name: Olsalazine sodium

Dipentum is an anti-inflammatory drug used to maintain long-term freedom from symptoms of ulcerative colitis (chronic inflammation and ulceration of the large intestine and rectum). It is prescribed for people who cannot take sulfasalazine (Azulfidine).

Generic name:

Diphenoxylate with Atropine

See Lomotil, page 501.

Generic name:

Dipivefrin

See Propine, page 565.

Brand name:

Diprolene

Pronounced: dye-PROH-leen
Generic name: Betamethasone dipropionate
Other brand name: Diprosone

Diprolene, a synthetic cortisone-like steroid available in cream, gel, lotion, or ointment form, is used to treat certain itchy rashes and other inflammatory skin conditions. Its sister product Diprosone is available only as a cream.

Brand name:

Diprosone

See Diprolene, page 450.

Generic name:

Dipyridamole

See Persantine, page 552.

Generic name:

Dirithromycin

See Dynabac, page 453.

Brand name:

Disalcid

Pronounced: dye-SAL-sid
Generic name: Salsalate

Disalcid, a nonsteroidal anti-inflammatory drug, is used to relieve the symptoms of rheumatoid arthritis, osteoarthritis (the most common form of arthritis), and other rheumatic disorders (conditions that involve pain and inflammation in joints and the tissues around them).

Generic name:

Disopyramide

See Norpace, page 538.

Brand name:

Ditropan

Pronounced: DYE-tro-pan
Generic name: Oxybutynin chloride
Other brand name: Ditropan XL

Ditropan relaxes the bladder muscle and reduces spasms. It is used to treat the urgency, frequency, leakage, incontinence, and painful or difficult urination caused by neurogenic bladder (altered bladder function due to a nervous system abnormality).

Brand name:

Diuril

Pronounced: DYE-your-il
Generic name: Chlorothiazide

Diuril is used in the treatment of high blood pressure and other conditions that require the elimination of excess fluid from the body. These conditions include congestive heart failure, cirrhosis of the liver, corticosteroid and estrogen therapy, and kidney disease. When used for high blood pressure, Diuril can be used alone or with other high blood pressure medications. Diuril contains a form of thiazide, a diuretic that prompts the body to eliminate more fluid, which helps lower blood pressure.

Generic name:

Dolasetron

See Anzemet, page 394.

Brand name:

Dolobid

Pronounced: DOLL-oh-bid
Generic name: Diflunisal

Dolobid, a nonsteroidal anti-inflammatory drug, is used to treat mild to moderate pain and to relieve the inflammation, swelling, stiffness, and joint pain associated with rheumatoid arthritis and osteoarthritis (the most common form of arthritis).

Brand name:

Donnatal

Pronounced: DON-nuh-tal
Generic ingredients: Phenobarbital, Hyoscyamine sulfate, Atropine sulfate, Scopolamine hydrobromide
Other brand name: Bellatal

Donnatal is a mild antispasmodic medication; it has been used with other drugs for relief of cramps and pain associated with various stomach, intestinal, and bowel disorders, including irritable bowel syndrome, acute colitis, and duodenal ulcer.

One of its ingredients, phenobarbital, is a mild sedative.

Generic name:

Dornase alfa

See Pulmozyme, page 568.

Brand name:

Doryx

Pronounced: DORE-icks
Generic name: Doxycycline hyclate
Other brand names: Vibramycin, Vibra-Tabs

Doxycycline is a broad-spectrum tetracycline antibiotic used against a wide variety of bacterial infections, including Rocky Mountain spotted fever and other fevers caused by ticks, fleas, and lice; urinary tract infections; trachoma (chronic infections of the eye); and some gonococcal infections in adults. It is an approved treatment for inhalational anthrax. It is also used with other medications to treat severe acne and amoebic dysentery (diarrhea caused by severe parasitic infection of the intestines).

Doxycycline may also be taken for the prevention of malaria on foreign trips of less than 4 months' duration. Occasionally doctors prescribe doxycycline to treat early Lyme disease and to prevent "traveler's diarrhea." These are not yet officially approved uses for this drug.

Generic name:

Dorzolamide

See Trusopt, page 608.

Generic name:

Doxazosin

See Cardura, page 416.

Generic name:

Doxycycline

See Doryx, page 452.

Brand name:

Duricef

Pronounced: DUHR-i-sef
Generic name: Cefadroxil monohydrate

Duricef, a cephalosporin antibiotic, is used in the treatment of nose, throat, urinary tract, and skin infections that are caused by specific bacteria, including staph, strep, and *E. coli.*

Brand name:

Dyazide

Pronounced: DYE-uh-zide
Generic ingredients: Hydrochlorothiazide, Triamterene
Other brand names: Maxzide, Maxzide-25 MG

Dyazide is a combination of diuretic drugs used in the treatment of high blood pressure and other conditions that require the elimination of excess fluid from the body. When used for high blood pressure, Dyazide can be taken alone or with other high blood pressure medications. Diuretics help the body produce and eliminate more urine, which helps lower blood pressure. Triamterene, one of the ingredients of Dyazide, helps to minimize the potassium loss that can be caused by the other component, hydrochlorothiazide. Maxzide and Maxzide-25 MG contain the same combination of ingredients.

Brand name:

Dynabac

Pronounced: DYE-na-bak
Generic name: Dirithromycin

Dynabac cures certain mild-to-moderate skin infections and respiratory infections such as strep throat, tonsillitis, pneumonia, and flare-ups of chronic bronchitis. Dynabac is part of the same family of drugs as the commonly prescribed antibiotic erythromycin.

Brand name:
Dynacin

See Minocin, page 519.

Brand name:
DynaCirc

Pronounced: DYE-na-serk
Generic name: Isradipine
Other brand name: DynaCirc CR

DynaCirc, a type of medication called a calcium channel blocker, is prescribed for the treatment of high blood pressure. It is effective when used alone or with a thiazide-type diuretic to flush excess water from the body. Calcium channel blockers ease the workload of the heart by slowing down the passage of nerve impulses through the heart muscle, thereby slowing the beat. This improves blood flow through the heart and throughout the body and reduces blood pressure. A controlled-release version of this drug (DynaCirc CR) maintains lower blood pressure for 24 hours.

Generic name:
Echothiophate

See Phospholine Iodide, page 554.

Brand name:
EC-Naprosyn

See Naprosyn, page 528.

Generic name:
Econazole

See Spectazole Cream, page 583.

Brand name:
Edex

See Caverject, page 418.

Brand name:
E.E.S.

See Erythromycin, Oral, page 459.

Generic name:
Efavirenz

See Sustiva, page 586.

Brand name:
Efudex

Pronounced: EFF-you-decks
Generic name: Fluorouracil
Other brand name: Carac

Efudex and Carac are prescribed for the treatment of actinic or solar keratoses (small red horny growths or flesh-colored wartlike growths caused by overexposure to ultraviolet radiation or the sun). Such growths may develop into skin cancer. When conventional methods are impractical—as when the affected sites are hard to get at—the 5 percent strength of Efudex is useful in the treatment of superficial basal cell carcinomas, or slow-growing malignant tumors of the face usually found at the edge of the nostrils, eyelids, or lips. Efudex is available in cream and solution forms. Carac comes in cream form only.

Brand name:
Eldepryl

Pronounced: ELL-dep-rill
Generic name: Selegiline hydrochloride

Eldepryl is prescribed along with Sinemet (levodopa/carbidopa) for people with Parkinson's disease. It is used when Sinemet no longer seems to be working well. Eldepryl has no effect when taken by itself; it works only in combination with levodopa or Sinemet.

Parkinson's disease, which causes muscle rigidity and difficulty with walking and talking, involves the progressive degeneration of a particular type of nerve cell. Early on, levodopa or Sinemet alone may alleviate the symptoms of the disease. In time, however, these medications begin to lose their effect; their action seems to switch on and off at random, and the individual may begin to experience side effects such as involuntary movements and "freezing" in mid-motion.

Eldepryl may be prescribed at this stage of the disease to help restore the effectiveness of Sinemet. When a patient begins to take Eldepryl, the dosage of Sinemet may need to be reduced.

Brand name:
Elidel

Pronounced: ELL-ih-dell
Generic name: Pimecrolimus

Elidel is a non-steroidal cream that relieves mild to moderate symptoms of eczema, a skin condition marked by itchy red patches that often crust, scale, and ooze. Elidel is approved for use in adults and children over 2 years old; it can be used for short-term treatment or on-and-off treatment over longer periods of time. Elidel is considered an effective alternative for people who cannot tolerate or do not respond to conventional eczema therapies.

Brand name:
Elocon

Pronounced: ELL-oh-con
Generic name: Mometasone furoate

Elocon is a cortisone-like steroid available in cream, ointment, and lotion form. It is used to treat certain itchy rashes and other inflammatory skin conditions.

Brand name:
E-Mycin

See Erythromycin, Oral, page 459.

Generic name:
Enalapril

See Vasotec, page 615.

Generic name:

Enalapril with Felodipine

See Lexxel, page 498.

Generic name:

Enalapril with Hydrochlorothiazide

See Vaseretic, page 614.

Brand name:

Enbrel

Pronounced: EN-brell
Generic name: Etanercept

Enbrel is used to treat the symptoms of moderate to severe rheumatoid arthritis when other drugs have proved inadequate. It is the first in a new class of drugs designed to block the action of tumor necrosis factor (TNF), a naturally occurring protein responsible for much of the joint inflammation that plagues the victims of rheumatoid arthritis.

In clinical trials, Enbrel provided the majority of patients with significant relief. In addition, it can be taken along with other drugs commonly used to treat rheumatoid arthritis, including methotrexate (Rheumatrex), steroids such as hydrocortisone and prednisone, nonsteroidal anti-inflammatory drugs such as Motrin and Naprosyn, aspirin, and other pain-killers. It is also prescribed for patients with psoriatic arthritis.

Brand name:

Enduron

Pronounced: EN-duh-ron
Generic name: Methyclothiazide

Enduron is used in the treatment of high blood pressure and other conditions that require the elimination of excess fluid from the body. These conditions include congestive heart failure, cirrhosis of the liver, side effects of steroid and estrogen therapy, and kidney disease. When used for high blood pressure, Enduron can be used alone or with other high blood pressure medications. Enduron contains a form of thiazide, a diuretic that prompts the body to produce and eliminate more urine, which helps lower blood pressure.

Generic name:

Entacapone

See Comtan, page 431.

Brand name:

Epitol

See Tegretol, page 591.

Brand name:

Epivir

Pronounced: EPP-ih-veer
Generic name: Lamivudine

Epivir is one of the drugs used to fight infection with the human immu-nodeficiency virus (HIV), the deadly cause of AIDS. Doctors turn to Epivir as the infection gets worse. The drug is taken along with Retrovir, another HIV medication.

HIV does its damage by slowly destroying the immune system, even-tually leaving the body defenseless against infections. Like other drugs for HIV, Epivir interferes with the virus's ability to reproduce. This staves off the collapse of the immune system.

Generic name:

Eprosartan

See Teveten, page 596.

Generic name:

Ergoloid mesylates

See Hydergine, page 481.

Generic name:

Ergotamine with Caffeine

See Cafergot, page 412.

Brand name:

Erycette

See Erythromycin, Topical, page 460.

Brand name:

Eryc

See Erythromycin, Oral, page 459.

Brand name:

Ery-Tab

See Erythromycin, Oral, page 459.

Brand name:

Erythrocin

See Erythromycin, Oral, page 459.

Generic name:

Erythromycin, Oral

Pronounced: er-ITH-row MY-sin
Brand names: E.E.S., E-Mycin, ERYC, Ery-Tab, Erythrocin, PCE

Erythromycin is an antibiotic used to treat many kinds of infections, including:

Acute pelvic inflammatory disease
Gonorrhea
Intestinal parasitic infections
Legionnaires' disease
Listeriosis
Pinkeye
Rectal infections
Reproductive tract infections
Skin infections
Syphilis
Upper and lower respiratory tract infections
Urinary tract infections
Whooping cough

Erythromycin is also prescribed to prevent rheumatic fever in people who are allergic to penicillin and sulfa drugs. It is prescribed before colorectal surgery to prevent infection.

Generic name:
Erythromycin, Topical

Pronounced: err-rith-ro-MY-sin
Brand names: A/T/S, Erycette, T-Stat

Topical erythromycin (applied directly to the skin) is used for the treatment of acne.

Generic name:
Erythromycin with Benzoyl peroxide

See Benzamycin, page 406.

Generic name:
Erythromycin ethylsuccinate with Sulfisoxazole

See Pediazole, page 549.

Brand name:
Eryzole

See Pediazole, page 549.

Brand name:
Esclim

See Estrogen Patches, page 462.

Brand name:
Esgic

See Fioricet, page 467.

Brand name:
Esidrix

See HydroDIURIL, page 482.

Generic name:
Esomeprazole

See Nexium, page 531.

Brand name:
Estraderm

See Estrogen Patches, page 462.

Generic name:
Estradiol

See Estrogen Patches, page 462.

Generic name:
Estradiol and Norethindrone acetate

See CombiPatch, page 430.

Generic name:
Estradiol Vaginal Ring

See Estring, page 461.

Brand name:
Estring

Pronounced: ESST-ring
Generic name: Estradiol vaginal ring

Estring is an estrogen replacement system for relief of the vaginal problems that often occur after menopause, including vaginal dryness, burning, and itching, and difficult or painful intercourse. Estring is also

prescribed for postmenopausal urinary problems such as difficulty urinating or urinary urgency.

Brand name:

Estrogen Patches

Generic name: Estradiol
Other brand names: Alora, Climara, Esclim, Estraderm, Vivelle, Vivelle-Dot

All of these products are used to reduce symptoms of menopause,
including feelings of warmth in the face, neck, and chest; the sudden
intense episodes of heat and sweating known as "hot flashes"; dry, itchy
external genitals; and vaginal irritation. They are also prescribed for
other conditions that cause low levels of estrogen, and some doctors prescribe them for teenagers who fail to mature at the usual rate.

Along with diet, calcium supplements, and exercise, Estraderm,
Climara, and Vivelle are prescribed to prevent osteoporosis, a condition
in which the bones become brittle and easily broken. Climara may also
be used to treat certain types of abnormal bleeding from the uterus.

Generic name:

Estrogen with Progestin

See Activella and femhrt, page 381.

Generic name:

Estropipate

See Ogen, page 541.

Generic name:

Etanercept

See Enbrel, page 457.

Generic name:

Ethinyl estradiol and Norelgestromin

See Ortho Evra, page 544.

Brand name:
Ethmozine

Pronounced: ETH-moe-zeen
Generic name: Moricizine hydrochloride

Ethmozine is prescribed for the treatment of certain life-threatening heartbeat irregularities.

Generic name:
Etidronate

See Didronel, page 446.

Generic name:
Etodolac

See Lodine, page 500.

Brand name:
Eulexin

Pronounced: you-LEKS-in
Generic name: Flutamide

Eulexin is used along with drugs such as Lupron to treat prostate cancer. Eulexin belongs to a class of drugs known as antiandrogens. It blocks the effect of the male hormone testosterone. Giving Eulexin with Lupron, which reduces the body's testosterone levels, is one way of treating prostate cancer. For some forms of prostate cancer, radiation therapy is administered along with the drugs.

Brand name:
Evista

Pronounced: Eve-IST-ah
Generic name: Raloxifene hydrochloride

Evista is prescribed to treat and prevent osteoporosis, the brittle-bone disease that strikes some women after menopause. A variety of factors promote osteoporosis. The more factors that apply to an individual, the greater her chances of developing the disease. These factors include:

Caucasian or Asian descent
Slender build
Early menopause
Smoking
Drinking
A diet low in calcium
An inactive lifestyle
Osteoporosis in the family

Generic name:
Famciclovir

See Famvir, page 464.

Generic name:
Famotidine

See Pepcid, page 550.

Brand name:
Famvir

Pronounced: FAM-veer
Generic name: Famciclovir

Famvir tablets are used to treat herpes zoster, commonly referred to as "shingles," in adults. Shingles is a painful rash with raised, red pimples on the trunk of the body, usually the back. Because it is caused by the same virus that causes chickenpox, only people who have had chickenpox can get shingles. When prescribed for shingles, Famvir works best in people age 50 or over.

Famvir is also prescribed to treat attacks of genital herpes and to prevent future flare-ups. For people with HIV infections, it is used as a treatment for both genital and oral herpes.

Brand name:
Fareston

Pronounced: FAIR-es-tahn
Generic name: Toremifene citrate

Fareston is used to treat advanced breast cancer in women who have passed menopause. Some forms of breast cancer are stimulated by estrogen. Fareston slows the progression of such cancers by blocking the sites where estrogen normally acts on the tumor.

Generic name:

Felbamate

See Felbatol, page 465.

Brand name:

Felbatol

Pronounced: FELL-ba-tohl
Generic name: Felbamate

Felbatol, a relatively new epilepsy medication, is used alone or with other drugs to treat partial seizures with or without generalization (seizures in which consciousness may be retained or lost). It is also used with other medications to treat seizures associated with Lennox-Gastaut syndrome (a childhood condition characterized by brief loss of awareness and muscle tone).

Felbatol is prescribed only when other medications have failed to control severe cases of epilepsy.

Brand name:

Feldene

Pronounced: FELL-deen
Generic name: Piroxicam

Feldene, a nonsteroidal anti-inflammatory drug, is used to relieve the inflammation, swelling, stiffness, and joint pain associated with rheumatoid arthritis and osteoarthritis (the most common form of arthritis). It is prescribed both for sudden flare-ups and for long-term treatment.

Generic name:

Felodipine

See Plendil, page 556.

Brand name:
femhrt

See Activella and femhrt, page 381.

Generic name:
Fenofibrate

See Tricor, page 605.

Generic name:
Fenoprofen

See Nalfon, page 527.

Brand name:
Fertinex

Pronounced: FUR-tin-ecks
Generic name: Urofollitropin

Fertinex contains the female hormone called follicle-stimulating hormone (FSH). It is used to promote development of eggs in the ovaries of women who have difficulty producing eggs on their own. Fertinex therapy is usually followed by an injection of another hormone, human chorionic gonadotropin (Profasi), which triggers release of the egg. Fertinex is also given to produce many eggs in women going through in vitro fertilization.

Before prescribing Fertinex, the doctor will do a careful workup to make certain that the patient's infertility is not the result of a problem outside the ovaries, and that there's no other reason, such as pregnancy, to avoid the use of Fertinex.

Generic name:
Fexofenadine

See Allegra, page 387.

Generic name:
Finasteride for baldness

See Propecia, page 565.

Generic name:

Finasteride for prostate problems

See Proscar, page 566.

Brand name:

Finevin

See Azelex, page 402.

Brand name:

Fioricet

Pronounced: fee-OAR-i-set
Generic ingredients: Butalbital, Acetaminophen, Caffeine
Other brand names: Anolor 300, Esgic, Esgic-Plus

Fioricet, a strong, non-narcotic pain reliever and relaxant, is prescribed for the relief of tension headache symptoms caused by muscle contractions in the head, neck, and shoulder area. It combines a sedative barbiturate (butalbital), a non-aspirin pain reliever (acetaminophen), and caffeine.

Brand name:

Fiorinal

Pronounced: fee-OR-i-nahl
Generic ingredients: Butalbital, Aspirin, Caffeine

Fiorinal, a strong, non-narcotic pain reliever and muscle relaxant, is prescribed for the relief of tension headache symptoms caused by stress or muscle contraction in the head, neck, and shoulder area. It combines a non-narcotic, sedative barbiturate (butalbital) with a pain reliever (aspirin) and a stimulant (caffeine).

Brand name:

Fiorinal with Codeine

Pronounced: fee-OR-i-nahl with KO-deen
Generic ingredients: Butalbital, Codeine phosphate, Aspirin, Caffeine

Fiorinal with Codeine, a strong narcotic pain reliever and muscle relaxant, is prescribed for the relief of tension headache caused by stress and muscle contraction in the head, neck, and shoulder area. It combines a sedative-barbiturate (butalbital), a narcotic pain reliever and cough suppressant (codeine), a non-narcotic pain and fever reliever (aspirin), and a stimulant (caffeine).

Brand name:

Flagyl

Pronounced: FLAJ-ill
Generic name: Metronidazole

Flagyl is an antibacterial drug prescribed for certain vaginal and urinary tract infections in men and women; amebic dysentery and liver abscess; and infections of the abdomen, skin, bones and joints, brain, lungs, and heart caused by certain bacteria.

Generic name:

Flavoxate

See Urispas, page 612.

Generic name:

Flecainide

See Tambocor, page 589.

Brand name:

Flexeril

Pronounced: FLEX-eh-rill
Generic name: Cyclobenzaprine hydrochloride

Flexeril is a muscle relaxant prescribed to relieve muscle spasms resulting from injuries such as sprains, strains, or pulls. Combined with rest and physical therapy, Flexeril provides relief of muscular stiffness and pain.

Brand name:

Flomax

Pronounced: FLOW-maks
Generic name: Tamsulosin hydrochloride

Flomax is used to treat the symptoms of an enlarged prostate—a condition technically known as benign prostatic hyperplasia or BPH. The walnut-sized prostate gland surrounds the urethra (the duct that drains the bladder). If the gland becomes enlarged, it can squeeze the urethra, interfering with the flow of urine. This can cause difficulty in starting urination, a weak flow of urine, and the need to urinate urgently or more frequently. Flomax doesn't shrink the prostate. Instead, it relaxes the muscle around it, freeing the flow of urine and decreasing urinary symptoms.

Brand name:

Flonase

See Fluticasone, page 470.

Brand name:

Flovent

See Fluticasone, page 470.

Brand name:

Floxin

Pronounced: FLOCKS-in
Generic name: Ofloxacin

Floxin is an antibiotic. Floxin tablets have been used effectively to treat lower respiratory tract infections, including chronic bronchitis and pneumonia, sexually transmitted diseases (except syphilis), pelvic inflammatory disease, and infections of the urinary tract, prostate gland, and skin. Floxin Otic solution is used to treat ear infections.

Generic name:

Fluconazole

See Diflucan, page 447.

Generic name:

Flunisolide

See AeroBid, page 384.

Generic name:

Fluocinonide

See Lidex, page 499.

Generic name:

Fluorometholone

See FML, page 471.

Generic name:

Fluorouracil

See Efudex, page 455.

Generic name:

Fluoxymesterone

See Halotestin, page 479.

Generic name:

Flurbiprofen

See Ansaid, page 393.

Generic name:

Flutamide

See Eulexin, page 463.

Generic name:

Fluticasone

Pronounced: flue-TICK-uh-zone
Brand names: Flonase, Flovent, Flovent Diskus, Flovent Rotadisk

Flonase nasal spray is a remedy for the stuffy, runny, itchy nose that plagues many allergy-sufferers. It can be used either for seasonal attacks of hay fever or for year-round allergic conditions. Flonase is a steroid medication. It works by relieving inflammation within the nasal passages.

The Flovent, Flovent Rotadisk, and Flovent Diskus oral inhalers are used to prevent flare-ups of asthma. (They will not, however, relieve an acute attack.) They sometimes serve as a replacement for the steroid tablets that many people take to control asthma.

Generic name:
Fluticasone and Salmeterol

See Advair Diskus, page 383.

Generic name:
Fluticasone for skin conditions

See Cutivate, page 435.

Generic name:
Fluvastatin

See Lescol, page 495.

Brand name:
FML

Generic name: Fluorometholone

FML is a steroid (cortisone-like) eye ointment that is used to treat inflammation of the eyelid and the eye itself.

Brand name:
Follistim

Pronounced: FAHL-i-stim
Generic name: Follitropin beta for injection

Follistim contains "follicle stimulating hormone" (FSH). This is the natural hormone that prompts a new egg to ripen inside a follicle (egg sac) within the ovaries each month. Follistim injections are given to stimulate production of eggs for use in Assisted Reproductive Technology (ART), a procedure in which the egg is removed from the body and fertilized in the laboratory. Follistim is also used to promote ovulation and pregnancy in infertile patients if the problem is not due to primary ovarian failure (lack of viable eggs).

A second hormone—human chorionic gonadotropin (HCG)—is needed to bring an egg to full maturity. Follistim treatments therefore end with an injection of HCG.

Generic name:
Follitropin beta for Injection

See Follistim, page 471.

Brand name:
Foradil

Pronounced: FOUR-a-dil
Generic name: Formoterol

Foradil is an asthma medication. It relaxes the muscles in the walls of the airways, allowing them to expand. When taken on a twice-daily basis, it helps to control asthma and can be used to prevent tightening of the airways (bronchospasm) in patients who need regular treatment with short-acting inhalers, including those with nighttime asthma.

Taken on an as-needed basis, Foradil can also be used to prevent exercise-induced bronchospasm (also called "exercise-induced asthma") in adults and children 12 years of age and older.

Generic name:
Formoterol

See Foradil, page 472.

Brand name:
Fortovase

Pronounced: FORT-o-vace
Generic name: Saquinavir

Fortovase is used in the treatment of advanced human immunodeficiency virus (HIV) infection. HIV causes the immune system to break down so that it can no longer fight off other infections. This leads to the fatal disease known as acquired immune deficiency syndrome (AIDS).

Fortovase belongs to a class of HIV drugs called protease inhibitors, which work by interfering with an important step in the virus's reproductive cycle. Fortovase is used in combination with other HIV drugs called nucleoside analogues (Retrovir or Hivid, for example). The combination produces an increase in the immune system's vital CD4 cells (white blood cells) and reduces the amount of virus in the bloodstream.

Brand name:

Fosamax

Pronounced: FAH-suh-max
Generic name: Alendronate sodium

Fosamax is prescribed for the prevention and treatment of osteoporosis, the brittle bone disease, in postmenopausal women. It is also used to increase bone mass in men with osteoporosis, and is prescribed for both men and women who have developed a form of osteoporosis sometimes caused by steroid medications such as prednisone. This drug can also be used to relieve Paget's disease of bone, a painful condition that weakens and deforms the bones.

Generic name:

Fosfomycin

See Monurol, page 523.

Generic name:

Fosinopril

See Monopril, page 522.

Generic name:

Fosinopril with Hydrochlorothiazide

See Monopril-HCT, page 523.

Brand name:

Fulvicin P/G

See Gris-PEG, page 478.

Generic name:

Furosemide

See Lasix, page 494.

Generic name:

Gabapentin

See Neurontin, page 530.

Brand name:

Gantrisin

Pronounced: GAN-tris-in
Generic name: Sulfisoxazole acetyl

Gantrisin is a children's medication prescribed for the treatment of severe, repeated, or long-lasting urinary tract infections. These include pyelonephritis (bacterial kidney inflammation), pyelitis (inflammation of the part of the kidney that drains urine into the ureter), and cystitis (inflammation of the bladder).

This drug is also used to treat bacterial meningitis, and is prescribed as a preventive measure for children who have been exposed to meningitis.

Some middle ear infections are treated with Gantrisin in combination with penicillin or erythromycin.

Toxoplasmosis (parasitic disease transmitted by infected cats, their feces or litter boxes, and by undercooked meat) can be treated with Gantrisin in combination with pyrimethamine (Daraprim).

Malaria that does not respond to the drug chloroquine (Aralen) can be treated with Gantrisin in combination with other drug treatment.

Gantrisin is also used in the treatment of bacterial infections such as trachoma and inclusion conjunctivitis (eye infections), nocardiosis (bacterial disease affecting the lungs, skin, and brain), and chancroid (venereal disease causing enlargement and ulceration of lymph nodes in the groin).

Brand name:

Garamycin Ophthalmic

Pronounced: gar-uh-MY-sin
Generic name: Gentamicin sulfate

Garamycin Ophthalmic, an antibiotic, is applied to the eye for treatment of infections such as conjunctivitis (pinkeye) and other eye infections.

Generic name:

Gatifloxacin

See Tequin, page 593.

Generic name:

Gemfibrozil

See Lopid, page 501.

Generic name:

Gentamicin

See Garamycin Ophthalmic, page 475.

Generic name:

Glimepiride

See Amaryl, page 389.

Generic name:

Glipizide

See Glucotrol, page 476.

Brand name:

Glucophage

Pronounced: GLEW-co-fahj
Generic name: Metformin hydrochloride

Glucophage is an oral antidiabetic medication used to treat type 2 (non-insulin-dependent) diabetes. Diabetes develops when the body proves unable to burn sugar and the unused sugar builds up in the bloodstream. Glucophage lowers the amount of sugar in the blood by decreasing sugar production and absorption and helping the body respond better to its own insulin, which promotes the burning of sugar. It does not, however, increase the body's production of insulin.

Glucophage is sometimes prescribed along with insulin or certain other oral antidiabetic drugs such as Micronase or Glucotrol. It is also used alone.

Standard Glucophage tablets are taken two or three times daily. An extended-release form (Glucophage XR) is available for once-daily dosing.

Brand name:
Glucotrol

Pronounced: GLUE-kuh-troll
Generic name: Glipizide

Glucotrol is an oral antidiabetic medication used to treat type 2 (non-insulin-dependent) diabetes. In diabetics either the body does not make enough insulin or the insulin that is produced no longer works properly.

There are actually two forms of diabetes: type 1 (insulin-dependent) and type 2 (non-insulin-dependent). Type 1 usually requires insulin injections for life, while type 2 diabetes can usually be treated by dietary changes and/or oral antidiabetic medications such as Glucotrol. Glucotrol is thought to control diabetes by stimulating the pancreas to secrete more insulin. Occasionally, type 2 diabetics must take insulin injections on a temporary basis, especially during stressful periods or times of illness.

Brand name:
Glucovance

Pronounced: GLUE-coe-vance
Generic ingredients: Glyburide, Metformin

Glucovance is used in the treatment of type 2 (noninsulin dependent) diabetes. Diabetes develops when the body's ability to burn sugar declines and the unused sugar builds up in the bloodstream. Ordinarily, sugar is moved out of the blood and into the body's cells by the hormone insulin. A buildup occurs when the body either fails to make enough insulin or doesn't respond to it properly.

Glucovance is a combination of 2 drugs—glyburide (DiaBeta, Micronase) and metformin (Glucophage)—that attack high blood sugar levels in several ways. The glyburide component stimulates the pancreas to produce more insulin and helps the body use it properly. The metformin component also encourages proper insulin utilization, and in addition works to decrease sugar production and absorption. Glucovance is prescribed when diet and exercise prove insufficient to keep sugar levels under control.

Generic name:
Glyburide

See Micronase, page 518.

Generic name:
Glyburide with Metformin

See Glucovance, page 476.

Brand name:
Glynase

See Micronase, page 518.

Brand name:
GoLYTELY

See Colyte, page 430.

Generic name:
Goserelin

See Zoladex, page 627.

Generic name:
Granisetron

See Kytril, page 492.

Brand name:

Grisactin

See Gris-PEG, page 478.

Generic name:

Griseofulvin

See Gris-PEG, page 478.

Brand name:

Gris-PEG

Pronounced: GRISS-peg
Generic name: Griseofulvin
Other brand names: Grisactin, Fulvicin P/G

Gris-PEG is prescribed for the treatment of the following ringworm infections:

Athlete's foot
Barber's itch (inflammation of the facial hair follicles)
Ringworm of the body
Ringworm of the groin and thigh
Ringworm of the nails
Ringworm of the scalp

Because Gris-PEG is effective for only certain types of fungal infections, before treatment the doctor may perform tests to identify the source of infection.

Generic name:

Guaifenesin with Codeine

See Tussi-Organidin NR, page 609.

Generic name:

Guanfacine

See Tenex, page 592.

Brand name:

Gyne-Lotrimin

Pronounced: GUY-nuh-LOW-trim-in
Generic name: Clotrimazole
Other brand names: Lotrimin, Mycelex, Mycelex-7

Clotrimazole, the active ingredient in these medications, is used to treat fungal infections. In preparations for the skin, it is effective against ringworm, athlete's foot, and jock itch. In vaginal creams and tablets, it is used against vaginal yeast infections. In lozenge form, it is prescribed to treat oral yeast infections and to prevent them in people with weak immune systems.

Brand name:

Habitrol

See Nicotine Patches, page 532.

Brand name:

Halotestin

Pronounced: HA-lo-TES-tin
Generic name: Fluoxymesterone

Halotestin is a male hormone used to ease the symptoms of advanced, recurrent breast cancer in women who are between 1 and 5 years past menopause or who have a type of breast tumor that is promoted by female hormones. Halotestin is also prescribed for men who have too little of the male hormone testosterone.

Brand name:

Helidac Therapy

Pronounced: HEL-i-dak
Generic ingredients: Bismuth subsalicylate, Metronidazole, Tetracycline hydrochloride

Helidac is a drug combination that cures the infection responsible for most stomach ulcers. Although ulcers used to be blamed on stress and spicy food, doctors now know that a germ called *Helicobacter pylori* is the actual culprit in a majority of cases.

Brand name:
Hivid

Pronounced: HIV-id
Generic name: Zalcitabine

Hivid is one of the drugs used against the human immunodeficiency virus (HIV)—the deadly cause of AIDS. HIV does its damage by slowly undermining the immune system, finally leaving the body without any defense against infection. Hivid staves off collapse of the immune system by interfering with the virus's ability to reproduce.

Hivid is often combined with a protease inhibitor (such as Crixivan, Invirase, or Norvir) as part of the "cocktail" of drugs that has proven so effective in halting or even reversing the progress of HIV. Hivid can also be combined with the HIV drug Retrovir, provided the patient has not already been taking Retrovir for more than 3 months. For people with advanced cases of HIV, Hivid is sometimes prescribed by itself when other drugs don't work or can't be tolerated.

Brand name:
Humalog

See Insulin, page 486.

Generic name:
Human chorionic gonadotropin

See Profasi, page 564.

Brand name:
Humegon

See Pergonal, page 551.

Brand name:
Humulin

See Insulin, page 486.

Brand name:

Hydergine

Pronounced: HY-der-jeen
Generic name: Ergoloid mesylates

Hydergine helps relieve symptoms of declining mental capacity seen in some people over age 60. The symptoms include reduced understanding and motivation, and a decline in self-care and interpersonal skills.

Brand name:

Hydrocet

See Vicodin, page 617.

Generic name:

Hydrochlorothiazide

See HydroDIURIL, page 482.

Generic name:

Hydrochlorothiazide with Triamterene

See Dyazide, page 453.

Generic name:

Hydrocodone with Acetaminophen

See Vicodin, page 617.

Generic name:

Hydrocodone with Chlorpheniramine polistirex

See Tussionex, page 608.

Generic name:

Hydrocodone with Ibuprofen

See Vicoprofen, page 617.

Generic name:

Hydrocortisone Skin Preparations

Pronounced: hi-droh-COURT-i-zone
Brand names: Cetacort, Hytone, Nutracort

Hydrocortisone creams and lotions contain a steroid medication that relieves a variety of itchy rashes and inflammatory skin conditions.

Brand name:

HydroDIURIL

Pronounced: High-dro-DYE-your-il
Generic name: Hydrochlorothiazide
Other brand name: Esidrix

HydroDIURIL is used in the treatment of high blood pressure and other conditions that require the elimination of excess fluid (water) from the body. These conditions include congestive heart failure, cirrhosis of the liver, corticosteroid and estrogen therapy, and kidney disorders. When used for high blood pressure, HydroDIURIL can be used alone or with other high blood pressure medications. HydroDIURIL contains a form of thiazide, a diuretic that prompts the body to produce and eliminate more urine, which helps lower blood pressure.

Generic name:

Hydromorphone

See Dilaudid, page 448.

Generic name:

Hydroxychloroquine

See Plaquenil, page 556.

Generic name:

Hyoscyamine

See Levsin, page 498.

Brand name:

Hytone

See Hydrocortisone Skin Preparations, page 482.

Brand name:

Hytrin

Pronounced: HIGH-trin
Generic name: Terazosin hydrochloride

Hytrin is prescribed to reduce high blood pressure. It may be used alone or in combination with other blood pressure lowering drugs, such as HydroDIURIL (a diuretic) or Inderal, a beta blocker.

Hytrin is also prescribed to relieve the symptoms of benign prostatic hyperplasia or BPH. BPH is an enlargement of the prostate gland that surrounds the urinary canal. It leads to the following symptoms:

a weak or interrupted stream when urinating
a feeling that the bladder cannot be completely emptied
a delay when starting to urinate
a need to urinate often, especially at night
a feeling that urgency when urination is needed

Hytrin relaxes the tightness of a certain type of muscle in the prostate and at the opening of the bladder. This can reduce the severity of the symptoms.

Brand name:

Hyzaar

Pronounced: HIGH-zahr
Generic ingredients: Losartan potassium, Hydrochlorothiazide

Hyzaar is a combination medication used in the treatment of high blood pressure. One component, losartan, belongs to a new class of blood pressure medications that work by preventing the hormone angiotensin II from constricting the blood vessels, thus allowing blood to flow more freely and keeping the blood pressure down. The other component, hydrochlorothiazide, is a diuretic that increases the output of urine, removing excess fluid from the body and thus lowering blood pressure.

Generic name:
Ibuprofen

See Motrin, page 524.

Brand name:
Iletin

See Insulin, page 486.

Brand name:
Imdur

Pronounced: IM-duhr
Generic name: Isosorbide mononitrate
Other brand names: Ismo, Monoket

Imdur is prescribed to prevent angina pectoris (crushing chest pain that results when partially clogged arteries restrict the flow of needed oxygen-rich blood to the heart muscle). This medication does not relieve angina attacks already underway.

Brand name:
Imitrex

Pronounced: IM-i-trex
Generic name: Sumatriptan succinate

Imitrex is prescribed for the treatment of a migraine attack with or without the presence of an aura (visual disturbances, usually sensations of halos or flickering lights, which precede an attack). The injectable form is also used to relieve cluster headache attacks. (Cluster headaches come on in waves, then disappear for long periods of time. They are limited to one side of the head, and occur mainly in men.)

Imitrex cuts headaches short. It will not reduce the number of attacks.

Brand name:
Imodium

Pronounced: i-MOH-dee-um
Generic name: Loperamide hydrochloride

Imodium is prescribed for the control and relief of symptoms of diarrhea not known to be caused by a specific germ, and for diarrhea associated with long-term inflammatory bowel disease. This drug is also prescribed for reducing the volume of discharge from an ileostomy (a surgical opening of the small intestine onto the abdominal wall for purposes of elimination).

Some doctors also prescribe Imodium, along with antibiotics such as Septra or Bactrim, to treat traveler's diarrhea.

Generic name:
Indapamide

See Lozol, page 506.

Brand name:
Inderal

Pronounced: IN-der-al
Generic name: Propranolol hydrochloride
Other brand name: Inderal LA

Inderal, a type of medication known as a beta blocker, is used in the treatment of high blood pressure, angina pectoris (chest pain, usually caused by lack of oxygen to the heart due to clogged arteries), changes in heart rhythm, prevention of migraine headache, hereditary tremors, hypertrophic subaortic stenosis (a condition related to exertional angina), and tumors of the adrenal gland. It is also used to reduce the risk of death from recurring heart attack.

When used for the treatment of high blood pressure, it is effective alone or combined with other high blood pressure medications, particularly thiazide-type diuretics. Beta blockers decrease the force and rate of heart contractions, reducing the heart's demand for oxygen and lowering blood pressure.

Brand name:
Inderide

Pronounced: IN-deh-ride
Generic ingredients: Propranolol hydrochloride, Hydrochlorothiazide
Other brand name: Inderide LA

Inderide is used in the treatment of high blood pressure. It combines a beta blocker (propranolol) with a thiazide diuretic (hydrochlorothiazide).

Beta blockers decrease the force and rate of heart contractions, thus lowering blood pressure. Diuretics help the body produce and eliminate more urine, which also helps lower blood pressure.

Generic name:

Indinavir

See Crixivan, page 434.

Brand name:

Indocin

Pronounced: IN-doh-sin
Generic name: Indomethacin

Indocin, a nonsteroidal anti-inflammatory drug, is used to relieve the inflammation, swelling, stiffness and joint pain associated with moderate or severe rheumatoid arthritis and osteoarthritis (the most common form of arthritis), and ankylosing spondylitis (arthritis of the spine). It is also used to treat bursitis, tendinitis (acute painful shoulder), acute gouty arthritis, and other kinds of pain.

Generic name:

Indomethacin

See Indocin, page 486.

Generic name:

Insulin

Pronounced: IN-suh-lin
Brand names: Humalog, Humulin, Iletin, Novolin, Velosulin

Insulin is prescribed for diabetes mellitus when diet modifications and oral medications fail to correct the condition. Insulin is a hormone produced by the pancreas, a large gland that lies near the stomach. This hormone is necessary for the body's correct use of food, especially sugar. Insulin apparently works by helping sugar penetrate the cell wall, where it is then utilized by the cell. In people with diabetes, the body either does not make enough insulin, or the insulin that is produced cannot be used properly.

There are actually two forms of diabetes: type 1 (insulin-dependent) and type 2 (non-insulin-dependent). Type 1 usually requires insulin injections for life, while type 2 diabetes can usually be treated by dietary changes and/or oral antidiabetic medications such as Diabinese, Glucotrol, and Glucophage. Occasionally, type 2 diabetics must take insulin injections on a temporary basis, especially during stressful periods or times of illness.

The various available types of insulin differ in several ways: in the source (animal, human, or genetically engineered), in the time requirements for the insulin to take effect, and in the length of time the insulin remains working.

Regular insulin is manufactured from beef and pork pancreas, begins working within 30 to 60 minutes, and lasts for 6 to 8 hours. Variations of insulin have been developed to satisfy the needs of individual patients. For example, zinc suspension insulin is an intermediate-acting insulin that starts working within 1 to 1-1/2 hours and lasts approximately 24 hours. Insulin combined with zinc and protamine is a longer-acting insulin that takes effect within 4 to 6 hours and lasts up to 36 hours. The time and course of action may vary considerably in different individuals or at different times in the same individual. The genetically engineered insulin lispro injection works faster and for a shorter length of time than human regular insulin and should be used along with a longer-acting insulin. It is available only by prescription.

Animal-based insulin is a very safe product. However, some components may cause an allergic reaction. Therefore, genetically engineered human insulin has been developed to lessen the chance of an allergic reaction. It is structurally identical to the insulin produced by the human pancreas. However, some human insulin may be produced in a semi-synthetic process that begins with animal-based ingredients, and may cause an allergic reaction.

Brand name:

Intal

Pronounced: IN-tahl
Generic name: Cromolyn sodium
Other brand name: Nasalcrom

Intal contains the antiasthmatic/antiallergic medication cromolyn sodium.

Different forms of the drug are used to manage bronchial asthma, to prevent asthma attacks, and to prevent and treat seasonal and chronic allergies.

The drug works by preventing certain cells in the body from releasing substances that can cause allergic reactions or prompt too much bronchial activity. It also helps prevent bronchial constriction caused by exercise, aspirin, cold air, and certain environmental pollutants such as sulfur dioxide.

Brand name:

Ionamin

See Adipex-P, page 383.

Generic name:

Ipratropium

See Atrovent, page 398.

Generic name:

Irbesartan

See Avapro, page 400.

Generic name:

Irbesartan with Hydrochlorothiazide

See Avalide, page 399.

Brand name:

Ismo

See Imdur, page 484.

Generic name:

Isometheptene, Dichloralphenazone, and Acetaminophen

See Midrin, page 519.

Brand name:

Isoptin

See Calan, page 412.

Brand name:

Isopto Carpine

See Pilocar, page 554.

Brand name:

Isordil

Pronounced: ICE-or-dill
Generic name: Isosorbide dinitrate
Other brand name: Sorbitrate

Isordil is prescribed to relieve or prevent angina pectoris (suffocating chest pain). Angina pectoris occurs when the arteries and veins become constricted and sufficient oxygen does not reach the heart. Isordil dilates the blood vessels by relaxing the muscles in their walls. Oxygen flow improves as the vessels relax, and chest pain subsides.

In swallowed capsules or tablets, Isordil helps to increase the amount of exercise patients can do before chest pain begins.

In chewable or sublingual (held under the tongue) tablets, Isordil can help relieve chest pain that has already started or prevent pain expected from a strenuous activity such as walking up a hill or climbing stairs.

Generic name:

Isosorbide dinitrate

See Isordil, page 489.

Generic name:

Isosorbide mononitrate

See Imdur, page 484.

Generic name:

Isotretinoin

See Accutane, page 378.

Generic name:

Isradipine

See DynaCirc, page 454.

Generic name:

Itraconazole

See Sporanox, page 583.

Brand name:

Kadian

See MS Contin, page 524.

Brand name:

Kaletra

Pronounced: cuh-LEE-tra
Generic ingredients: Lopinavir, Ritonavir

Kaletra combats the human immunodeficiency virus (HIV). HIV is the deadly virus that undermines the infection-fighting capacity of the body's immune system, eventually leading to AIDS.

Kaletra is a combination of two drugs, lopinavir and ritonavir (Norvir), both of which fall into the drug category known as protease inhibitors. When taken along with other HIV drugs, Kaletra lowers the amount of the virus circulating in the bloodstream. However, it does not completely eradicate the virus, and the patient may continue to develop the rare infections that attack when the immune system weakens. It's also important to remember that Kaletra does not eliminate the danger of transmitting the virus to others.

Brand name:

Kaon-CL

See Micro-K, page 517.

Brand name:

K-Dur

See Micro-K, page 517.

Brand name:

Keflex

Pronounced: KEF-lecks
Generic name: Cephalexin hydrochloride
Other brand name: Keftab

Keflex and Keftab are cephalosporin antibiotics. They are prescribed for bacterial infections of the respiratory tract, the middle ear, the bones, the skin, and the reproductive and urinary systems. Because the drugs are effective for only certain types of bacterial infections, before beginning treatment the doctor may perform tests to identify the organisms causing the infection.

Keflex is available in capsules and an oral suspension form for use in children. Keftab, available only in tablet form, is prescribed exclusively for adults.

Brand name:

Keftab

See Keflex, page 491.

Brand name:

Keppra

Pronounced: kep-rah
Generic name: Levetiracetam

Keppra helps reduce the frequency of partial epileptic seizures, a form of epilepsy in which neural disturbances are limited to a specific region of the brain and the victim remains conscious throughout the attack. The drug is used along with other epilepsy medications, never by itself.

Generic name:

Ketoconazole

See Nizoral, page 536.

Generic name:

Ketoprofen

See Orudis, page 545.

Generic name:

Ketorolac

See *Toradol*, page 602.

Generic name:

Ketotifen

See *Zaditor*, page 623.

Brand name:

Kineret

Pronounced: KIN-eh-ret
Generic name: Anakinra

Kineret is used to relieve the symptoms of rheumatoid arthritis. It is usually prescribed after other antirheumatic drugs have failed to make an improvement. Kineret can be prescribed alone or in combination with other drugs for rheumatoid arthritis.

Kineret works by blocking the effects of interleukin-1, an inflammatory compound released by the immune system. While fighting inflammation, Kineret may also affect the immune system's ability to fight infection.

Brand name:

Klor-Con

See *Micro-K*, page 517.

Brand name:

K-Tab

See *Micro-K*, page 517.

Brand name:

Kytril

Pronounced: KIE-tril
Generic name: Granisetron hydrochloride

Kytril is prescribed to prevent the nausea and vomiting associated with radiation therapy and chemotherapy for cancer.

Generic name:
Labetalol

See Normodyne, page 538.

Generic name:
Lactulose

See Chronulac Syrup, page 423.

Brand name:
Lamictal

Pronounced: LAM-ic-tal
Generic name: Lamotrigine

Lamictal is prescribed to control partial epileptic seizures, a form of epilepsy in which neural disturbances are limited to a specific region of the brain and the victim remains conscious throughout the attack. This drug is used in combination with other antiepileptic medications or as a replacement for a medication such as Tegretol, Dilantin, phenobarbital, or Mysoline.

Brand name:
Lamisil

Pronounced: LAM-ih-sill
Generic name: Terbinafine hydrochloride

Lamisil fights fungal infections. In tablet form, it's used for fungus of the toenail or fingernail. The cream and the solution are used for other fungal infections such as athlete's foot, jock itch, and ringworm. The solution is also used to treat tinea versicolor, a fungal infection that produces brown, tan, or white spots on the trunk of the body.

Generic name:
Lamivudine

See Epivir, page 458.

Generic name:

Lamivudine and Zidovudine

See Combivir, page 430.

Generic name:

Lamotrigine

See Lamictal, page 493.

Brand name:

Lanoxin

Pronounced: la-NOCKS-in
Generic name: Digoxin

Lanoxin is used in the treatment of congestive heart failure, certain types of irregular heartbeat, and other heart problems. It improves the strength and efficiency of the heart, which leads to better circulation of blood and reduction of the uncomfortable swelling that is common in people with congestive heart failure. Lanoxin is usually prescribed along with a water pill (to help relieve swelling) and a drug called an ACE inhibitor (to further improve circulation). It belongs to a class of drugs known as digitalis glycosides.

Generic name:

Lansoprazole

See Prevacid, page 561.

Brand name:

Lasix

Pronounced: LAY-six
Generic name: Furosemide

Lasix is a diuretic (water pill) used in the treatment of high blood pressure and other conditions that require the elimination of excess fluid from the body. These conditions include congestive heart failure, cirrhosis of the liver, and kidney disease. When used to treat high blood pressure, Lasix is effective alone or in combination with other high blood pressure medications. Diuretics help the body produce and eliminate more urine, which helps lower blood pressure. Lasix is classified as a "loop diuretic" because of its point of action in the kidneys.

Lasix is also used with other drugs in people with fluid accumulation in the lungs.

Generic name:

Latanoprost

See Xalatan, page 621.

Generic name:

Leflunomide

See Arava, page 394.

Brand name:

Lescol

Pronounced: LESS-cahl
Generic name: Fluvastatin sodium

Lescol reduces "bad" LDL cholesterol—and increases "good" HDL cholesterol—in the blood, and can lower the risk of developing clogged arteries and heart disease. It is also prescribed to slow the accumulation of plaque in the arteries of people who already have coronary heart disease, and can also be prescribed when a patient is released from the hospital after a heart attack. Doctors prescribe the drug only when patients have been unable to reduce their blood cholesterol level sufficiently with a low-fat, low-cholesterol diet alone.

Generic name:

Leuprolide acetate

See Lupron Depot, page 507.

Generic name:

Levalbuterol

See Xopenex, page 622.

Brand name:
Levaquin

Pronounced: LEAV-ah-kwin
Generic name: Levofloxacin

Levaquin cures a variety of bacterial infections, including several types of sinus infection and pneumonia. It is also prescribed for flare-ups of chronic bronchitis, acute kidney infections, certain urinary infections, and skin infections. Levaquin is a member of the quinolone family of antibiotics.

Brand name:
Levbid

See Levsin, page 498.

Generic name:
Levetiracetam

See Keppra, page 491.

Brand name:
Levlen

See Oral Contraceptives, page 542.

Brand name:
Levlite

See Oral Contraceptives, page 542.

Generic name:
Levobunolol

See Betagan, page 407.

Generic name:

Levodopa

Pronounced: lee-voh-DOE-puh

Levodopa (L-dopa) relieves the symptoms of parkinsonism (a nerve disorder characterized by tremors, drooling, stooped posture, a shuffling walk, and muscle weakness). Levodopa is also used in elderly people whose parkinsonism is related to hardening of the arteries in the brain.

Some doctors also prescribe levodopa for male sexual dysfunction, shingles, restless leg syndrome, and periodic leg movements.

Generic name:

Levofloxacin

See Levaquin, page 496.

Generic name:

Levonorgestrel and Ethinyl Estradiol

See Preven, page 562.

Generic name:

Levonorgestrel implants

See Norplant, page 539.

Brand name:

Levothroid

See Synthroid, page 588.

Generic name:

Levothyroxine

See Synthroid, page 588.

Brand name:

Levoxyl

See Synthroid, page 588.

Brand name:

Levsin

Pronounced: LEV-sin
Generic name: Hyoscyamine sulfate
Other brand names: Anaspaz, Levbid, Levsinex, NuLev

Levsin is an antispasmodic medication given to help treat various stomach, intestinal, and urinary tract disorders that involve cramps, colic, or other painful muscle contractions. Because Levsin has a drying effect, it may also be used to dry a runny nose or to dry excess secretions before anesthesia is administered.

Together with morphine or other narcotics, Levsin is prescribed for the pain of gallstones or kidney stones. For inflammation of the pancreas, Levsin may be used to help control excess secretions and reduce pain. Levsin may also be taken in Parkinson's disease to help reduce muscle rigidity and tremors and to help control drooling and excess sweating. The drug is sometimes prescribed during treatment for peptic ulcer.

Doctors also give Levsin as part of the preparation for certain diagnostic x-rays (for example, of the stomach, intestines, or kidneys).

Levsin comes in several forms, including regular tablets, tablets to be dissolved under the tongue, tablets that dissolve on the tongue (NuLev), sustained-release capsules (Levsinex Timecaps), and sustained-release tablets (Levbid), as well as liquid, drops, and an injectable solution.

Brand name:

Levsinex

See Levsin, page 498.

Brand name:

Lexxel

Pronounced: LECKS-ell
Generic ingredients: Enalapril maleate, Felodipine

Lexxel is used to treat high blood pressure. It combines two blood pressure drugs: an ACE inhibitor and a calcium channel blocker. The ACE inhibitor (enalapril) lowers blood pressure by preventing a chemical in the blood called angiotensin I from converting to a more potent form that narrows the blood vessels and increases salt and water retention. The calcium channel blocker (felodipine) also works to keep the blood vessels open, and eases the heart's workload by reducing the force and rate of the heartbeat.

Lexxel can be prescribed alone or in combination with other blood pressure medicines, especially water pills (diuretics) such as HydroDIURIL or Esidrix.

Brand name:
Librax

Pronounced: LIB-racks
Generic ingredients: Chlordiazepoxide hydrochloride, Clidinium bromide

Librax is used, in combination with other therapy, for the treatment of peptic ulcer, irritable bowel syndrome (spastic colon), and acute enterocolitis (inflammation of the colon and small intestine). Librax is a combination of a benzodiazepine (chlordiazepoxide) and an antispasmodic medication (clidinium).

Brand name:
Lidex

Pronounced: LYE-decks
Generic name: Fluocinonide

Lidex is a steroid medication that relieves the itching and inflammation of a wide variety of skin problems, including redness and swelling.

Generic name:
Linezolid

See Zyvox, page 630.

Brand name:
Lioresal

Pronounced: lye-OAR-eh-sal
Generic name: Baclofen

Lioresal is a muscle relaxant that helps relieve the symptoms and pain of muscle spasms caused by multiple sclerosis (MS), particularly in muscles that control joints. It also relieves pain due to rhythmic expansion and contraction of muscles (clonus) and pain due to muscular stiffness. Lioresal may also be of some help to people with spinal cord injuries and diseases.

Brand name:

Lipitor

Pronounced: LIP-ih-tor
Generic name: Atorvastatin calcium

Lipitor is a cholesterol-lowering drug. Doctors may prescribe it along with a special diet if blood cholesterol or triglyceride levels are high enough to pose a risk of heart disease, and the patient has been unable to lower the readings by diet alone.

The drug works by helping to clear harmful low density lipoprotein (LDL) cholesterol out of the blood and by limiting the body's ability to form new LDL cholesterol.

Generic name:

Lisinopril

See Zestril, page 625.

Generic name:

Lisinopril with Hydrochlorothiazide

See Zestoretic, page 624.

Brand name:

Lodine

Pronounced: LOW-deen
Generic name: Etodolac

Lodine, a nonsteroidal anti-inflammatory drug, is available in regular and extended-release forms (Lodine XL). Both forms are used to relieve the inflammation, swelling, stiffness, and joint pain of osteoarthritis (the most common form of arthritis) and rheumatoid arthritis. Regular Lodine is also used to relieve pain in other situations.

Brand name:
Loestrin

See Oral Contraceptives, page 542.

Generic name:
Lomefloxacin

See Maxaquin, page 509.

Brand name:
Lomotil

Pronounced: loe-MOE-till
Generic ingredients: Diphenoxylate hydrochloride, Atropine sulfate

Lomotil is used, along with other drugs, in the treatment of diarrhea. It should not be used for antibiotic-induced diarrhea (pseudomembranous colitis) or diarrhea caused by enterotoxin-producing bacteria.

Brand name:
Lo/Ovral

See Oral Contraceptives, page 542.

Generic name:
Loperamide

See Imodium, page 484.

Brand name:
Lopid

Pronounced: LOH-pid
Generic name: Gemfibrozil

Lopid is prescribed, along with a special diet, for treatment of people with very high levels of serum triglycerides (a fatty substance in the blood) who are at risk of developing pancreatitis (inflammation of the pancreas) and who do not respond adequately to a strict diet.

This drug can also be used to reduce the risk of coronary heart disease in people who have failed to respond to weight loss, diet, exercise, and other triglyceride- or cholesterol-lowering drugs.

Generic name:

Lopinavir and Ritonavir

See Kaletra, page 490.

Brand name:

Lopressor

Pronounced: low-PRESS-or
Generic name: Metoprolol tartrate
Other brand name: Toprol-XL

Lopressor, a type of medication known as a beta blocker, is used in the treatment of high blood pressure, angina pectoris (chest pain, usually caused by lack of oxygen to the heart due to clogged arteries), and heart attack. When prescribed for high blood pressure, it is effective when used alone or in combination with other high blood pressure medications. Beta blockers decrease the force and rate of heart contractions, thereby reducing the demand for oxygen and lowering blood pressure.

Occasionally doctors prescribe Lopressor for the treatment of aggressive behavior, prevention of migraine headache, and relief of temporary anxiety.

An extended-release form of this drug, called Toprol-XL, is prescribed for high blood pressure, angina, and heart failure.

Brand name:

Loprox

Pronounced: LOW-prox
Generic name: Ciclopirox

Loprox cream and lotion are prescribed for the treatment of the following fungal skin infections:

Athlete's foot
Fungal infection of the groin (jock itch)
Fungal infection of non-hairy parts of the skin
Candidiasis (yeastlike fungal infection of the skin)
Tinea versicolor—infection of the skin that is characterized by brown or
    tan patches on the trunk.

Loprox gel is used for athlete's foot, fungal infections of the non-hairy parts of the skin, and certain scalp inflammations (seborrheic dermatitis of the scalp).

Brand name:
Lorabid

Pronounced: LOR-a-bid
Generic name: Loracarbef

Lorabid is a carbacephem antibiotic. It is used to treat mild-to-moderate bacterial infections of the lungs, ears, throat, sinuses, skin, urinary tract, and kidneys.

Generic name:
Loracarbef

See Lorabid, page 503.

Generic name:
Loratadine

See Claritin, page 425.

Generic name:
Loratadine with Pseudoephedrine

See Claritin-D, page 425.

Brand name:
Lorcet

See Vicodin, page 617.

Brand name:
Lortab

See Vicodin, page 617.

Generic name:

Losartan

See Cozaar, page 434.

Generic name:

Losartan with Hydrochlorothiazide

See Hyzaar, page 483.

Brand name:

Lotensin

Pronounced: Lo-TEN-sin
Generic name: Benazepril hydrochloride

Lotensin is used in the treatment of high blood pressure. It is effective when used alone or in combination with thiazide diuretics. Lotensin is in a family of drugs called ACE (angiotensin-converting enzyme) inhibitors. It works by preventing a chemical in the blood called angiotensin I from converting into a more potent form that increases salt and water retention in the body. Lotensin also enhances blood flow throughout the circulatory system.

Brand name:

Lotensin HCT

Pronounced: lo-TEN-sin
Generic ingredients: Benazepril hydrochloride, Hydrochlorothiazide

Lotensin HCT combines two types of blood pressure medication. The first, benazepril hydrochloride, is an ACE (angiotensin-converting enzyme) inhibitor. It works by preventing a chemical in the blood called angiotensin I from converting into a more potent form (angiotensin II) that increases salt and water retention in the body and causes the blood vessels to constrict——two actions that tend to increase blood pressure.

To aid in clearing excess water from the body, Lotensin HCT also contains hydrochlorothiazide, a diuretic that promotes production of urine. Diuretics often wash too much potassium out of the body along with the water. However, the ACE inhibitor part of Lotensin HCT tends to keep potassium in the body, thereby canceling this unwanted effect.

Lotensin HCT is not used for the initial treatment of high blood pressure. It is saved for later use, when a single blood pressure medication is not sufficient for the job. In addition, some doctors are using Lotensin HCT along with other drugs to treat congestive heart failure.

Brand name:

Lotrel

Pronounced: LOW-trel
Generic names: Amlodipine, Benazepril Hydrochloride

Lotrel is used in the treatment of high blood pressure. It is a combination medicine that is used when treatment with a single drug has not been successful or has caused side effects.

One component, amlodipine, is a calcium channel blocker. It eases the workload of the heart by slowing down the passage of nerve impulses and hence the contractions of the heart muscle. This improves blood flow through the heart and throughout the body and reduces blood pressure. The other component, benazepril, is an angiotensin-converting enzyme (ACE) inhibitor. It works by preventing the transformation of a hormone called angiotensin I into a more potent substance that increases salt and water retention in the body.

Brand name:

Lotrimin

See Gyne-Lotrimin, page 479.

Brand name:

Lotrisone

Pronounced: LOE-trih-sone
Generic ingredients: Clotrimazole, Betamethasone dipropionate

Lotrisone cream and lotion contain a combination of a steroid (betamethasone) and an antifungal drug (clotrimazole). Lotrisone is used to treat skin infections caused by fungus, such as athlete's foot, jock itch, and ringworm of the body.

Betamethasone treats symptoms (such as itching, redness, swelling, and inflammation) that result from fungus infections, while clotrimazole treats the cause of the infection by inhibiting the growth of certain yeast and fungus organisms. If the infection is not inflamed, the doctor may prescribe a different medication.

Generic name:

Lovastatin

See Mevacor, page 515.

Generic name:

Lovastatin and Extended-release Niacin

See Advicor, page 384.

Brand name:

Low-Ogestrel

See Oral Contraceptives, page 542.

Brand name:

Lozol

Pronounced: LOW-zoll
Generic name: Indapamide

Lozol is used in the treatment of high blood pressure, either alone or in combination with other high blood pressure medications. Lozol is also used to relieve salt and fluid retention. During pregnancy, doctors may prescribe Lozol to relieve fluid retention caused by a specific condition or when fluid retention causes extreme discomfort that is not relieved by rest.

Brand name:

Lumigan

Pronounced: LOO-mi-gan
Generic name: Bimatoprost

Lumigan is an eye drop that combats high pressure inside the eyeball. It is prescribed for a condition called open-angle glaucoma (a gradual increase of pressure in the eye). It is typically used after other remedies have caused problems or fail to work. It lowers pressure by promoting drainage of the fluid (aqueous humor) that fills the eye.

Brand name:

Lupron Depot

Pronounced: LU-pron DEE-poe
Generic name: Leuprolide acetate

Lupron is a synthetic version of the naturally occurring gonadotropin releasing hormone (GnRH). Lupron suppresses shedding of the endometrium (lining of the uterus) during menstruation and is used to treat endometriosis, a condition in which cells from the endometrium grow outside of the uterus. Endometriosis causes painful growths to form around the outside of the uterus, fallopian tubes, and ovaries.

Two forms of Lupron—Lupron Depot 3.75 and Lupron Depot 11.5—are prescribed to relieve the pain of endometriosis and shrink the growths. (The hormonal medication norethindrone acetate is often added to the regimen.) Three other forms of Lupron—Lupron Depot 7.5, Lupron Depot 22.5, and Lupron Depot 30—are prescribed to relieve the symptoms of advanced prostate cancer.

The first two forms of Lupron are also used before surgery, along with iron, to treat anemia caused by fibroids (tumors) in the uterus when iron alone is not effective. Some doctors also prescribe Lupron for infertility and for early puberty.

Brand name:

Luride

Pronounced: LUHR-ide
Generic name: Sodium fluoride

Luride is prescribed to strengthen children's teeth against decay during the period when the teeth are still developing.

Studies have shown that children who live where the drinking water contains a certain level of fluoride have fewer cavities than others. Fluoride helps prevent cavities in three ways: by increasing the teeth's resistance to dissolving on contact with acid, by strengthening teeth, and by slowing down the growth of mouth bacteria.

Luride may be given to children who live where the water fluoride level is 0.6 parts per million or less.

Brand name:

Macrobid

See Macrodantin, page 508.

Brand name:
Macrodantin

Pronounced: Mack-row-DAN-tin
Generic name: Nitrofurantoin
Other brand name: Macrobid

Nitrofurantoin, an antibacterial drug, is prescribed for the treatment of urinary tract infections caused by certain strains of bacteria.

Brand name:
Materna

See Stuartnatal Plus, page 584.

Brand name:
Mavik

Pronounced: MA-vick
Generic name: Trandolapril

Mavik controls high blood pressure. It is effective when used alone or combined with other high blood pressure medications such as diuretics that help rid the body of excess water. Mavik is also used to treat heart failure or dysfunction following a heart attack.

Mavik is in a family of drugs known as ACE (angiotensin converting enzyme) inhibitors. It works by preventing a chemical in the blood called angiotensin I from converting into a more potent form that increases salt and water retention in the body. ACE inhibitors also expand the blood vessels, further reducing blood pressure.

Brand name:
Maxalt

Pronounced: MAX-alt
Generic name: Rizatriptan benzoate
Other brand name: Maxalt-MLT

Maxalt is prescribed for the treatment of a migraine attack with or without the presence of an aura (visual disturbances, usually sensations of halos or flickering lights, which precede an attack). It cuts headaches short, but won't prevent attacks.

Brand name:
Maxaquin

Pronounced: MAX-ah-kwin
Generic name: Lomefloxacin hydrochloride

Maxaquin is a quinolone antibiotic used to treat lower respiratory infections, including chronic bronchitis, and urinary tract infections, including cystitis (inflammation of the inner lining of the bladder). Maxaquin is also given before bladder surgery and prostate biopsy to prevent the infections that sometimes follow these operations.

Brand name:
Maxidone

See Vicodin, page 617.

Brand name:
Maxzide

See Dyazide, page 453.

Generic name:
Meclizine

See Antivert, page 394.

Generic name:
Meclofenamate

Pronounced: meh-cloh-FEN-uh-mate

Meclofenamate, a nonsteroidal anti-inflammatory drug, is used for the relief of mild to moderate pain. It is also used in the treatment of menstrual pain and heavy menstrual blood loss (when the cause is unknown) and to relieve the inflammation, swelling, stiffness, and joint pain associated with rheumatoid arthritis and osteoarthritis (the most common form of arthritis).

Brand name:

Medrol

Pronounced: MED-rohl
Generic name: Methylprednisolone

Medrol, a corticosteroid drug, is used to reduce inflammation and improve symptoms in a variety of disorders, including rheumatoid arthritis, acute gouty arthritis, and severe cases of asthma. Medrol may be prescribed to treat primary or secondary adrenal cortex insufficiency (inability of the adrenal gland to produce sufficient hormone). It is also given to help treat the following disorders:

Severe allergic conditions (including drug-induced allergic states)
Blood disorders (leukemia and various anemias)
Certain cancers (along with other drugs)
Skin diseases (including severe psoriasis)
Connective tissue diseases such as systemic lupus erythematosus
Digestive tract diseases such as ulcerative colitis
High serum levels of calcium associated with cancer
Fluid retention due to nephrotic syndrome (a condition in which damage to the kidney causes loss of protein in urine)
Various eye diseases
Lung diseases such as tuberculosis
Worsening of multiple sclerosis

Generic name:

Medroxyprogesterone

See Provera, page 567.

Generic name:

Medroxyprogesterone acetate for contraception

See Depo-Provera, page 442.

Generic name:

Mefenamic acid

See Ponstel, page 558.

Brand name:
Megace

Pronounced: MEG-ace
Generic name: Megestrol acetate

Megace is a synthetic drug that has the same effect as the female hormone progesterone. In tablet form it is used to treat cancer of the breast and uterus. Megace is usually prescribed when a tumor cannot be removed by surgery or has recurred after surgery, or when other drugs or radiation therapy are ineffective. Megace Oral Suspension is used to treat lack or loss of appetite, malnutrition and wasting away, and unexplained, significant weight loss in people with AIDS.

Generic name:
Megestrol acetate

See Megace, page 511.

Generic name:
Meloxicam

See Mobic, page 520.

Generic name:
Menotropins

See Pergonal, page 551.

Generic name:
Meperidine

See Demerol, page 441.

Brand name:
Meridia

Pronounced: mer-ID-dee-uh
Generic name: Sibutramine hydrochloride

Meridia helps the seriously overweight shed pounds and keep them off. It is especially recommended for those who in addition to being overweight have other health problems such as high blood pressure, diabetes, or high cholesterol. It is used in conjunction with a low-calorie diet.

Meridia works by boosting levels of certain chemical messengers in the nervous system, including serotonin, dopamine, and norepinephrine.

Generic name:

Mesalamine

See Rowasa, page 577.

Generic name:

Metaproterenol

See Alupent, page 389.

Generic name:

Metformin

See Glucophage, page 475.

Generic name:

Methazolamide

See Neptazane, page 530.

Generic name:

Methenamine

See Urised, page 611.

Brand name:

Methergine

Pronounced: METH-er-jin
Generic name: Methylergonovine maleate

Methergine, a blood-vessel constrictor, is given to prevent or control excessive bleeding following childbirth. It works by causing the uterine muscles to contract, thereby reducing the mother's blood loss.

Methergine comes in tablet and injectable forms.

Generic name:

Methocarbamol

See Robaxin, page 575.

Generic name:

Methotrexate

Pronounced: meth-oh-TREX-ate
Brand name: Rheumatrex

Methotrexate is an anticancer drug used in the treatment of lymphoma (cancer of the lymph nodes) and certain forms of leukemia. It is also given to treat some forms of cancers of the uterus, breast, lung, head, neck, and ovary. Methotrexate is also given to treat rheumatoid arthritis when other treatments have proved ineffective, and is sometimes used to treat very severe and disabling psoriasis (a skin disease characterized by thickened patches of red, inflamed skin often covered by silver scales).

Generic name:

Methyclothiazide

See Enduron, page 457.

Generic name:

Methyldopa

See Aldomet, page 387.

Generic name:

Methylergonovine

See Methergine, page 512.

Generic name:

Methylprednisolone

See Medrol, page 510.

Generic name:

Methyltestosterone

See Android, page 393.

Generic name:

Methysergide

See Sansert, page 578.

Generic name:

Metoclopramide

See Reglan, page 570.

Generic name:

Metolazone

See Zaroxolyn, page 624.

Generic name:

Metoprolol

See Lopressor, page 502.

Brand name:

MetroCream

See MetroGel, page 514.

Brand name:

MetroGel

Pronounced: MET-roh-jell
Generic name: Metronidazole
Other brand names: MetroCream, MetroLotion

MetroGel is a preparation of the drug metronidazole used for the treatment of a skin condition called rosacea (red eruptions, usually on the face). The cream and lotion forms of metronidazole are used for the same problem. All are for external (topical) use only.

Brand name:

Metrogel-Vaginal

Pronounced: MET-roh-jell VA-jin-al
Generic name: Metronidazole

Metrogel-Vaginal is used to treat bacterial vaginosis, a bacteria-caused inflammation of the vagina accompanied by pain and a vaginal discharge.

Brand name:

MetroLotion

See MetroGel, page 514.

Generic name:

Metronidazole

See Flagyl, page 468.

Generic name:

Metronidazole cream, gel, and lotion

See MetroGel, page 514.

Generic name:

Metronidazole vaginal gel

See Metrogel-Vaginal, page 515.

Brand name:

Mevacor

Pronounced: MEV-uh-core
Generic name: Lovastatin

Mevacor is used, along with diet, to lower cholesterol levels in people with primary hypercholesterolemia (too much cholesterol in the bloodstream). High cholesterol levels foster the buildup of artery-clogging plaque, which can be especially dangerous when it collects in the vessels serving the muscles of the heart. Mevacor is prescribed to prevent this problem—called coronary heart disease—or to slow its advance if the arteries are already clogging up.

Generic name:

Mexiletine

See Mexitil, page 516.

Brand name:

Mexitil

Pronounced: MEX-ih-till
Generic name: Mexiletine hydrochloride

Mexitil is used to treat severe irregular heartbeat (arrhythmia). Irregular heart rhythms are generally divided into two main types: heartbeats that are faster than normal (tachycardia) and heartbeats that are slower than normal (bradycardia). Arrhythmias are often caused by drugs or disease but can occur in otherwise healthy people with no history of heart disease or other illness.

Brand name:

Miacalcin

Pronounced: my-ah-CAL-sin
Generic name: Calcitonin-salmon

Miacalcin is a synthetic form of calcitonin, a naturally occurring hormone produced by the thyroid gland. Miacalcin reduces the rate of calcium loss from bones. Since less calcium passes from the bones to the blood, Miacalcin also helps control blood calcium levels.

Miacalcin Nasal Spray is used to treat postmenopausal osteoporosis (bone loss occurring after menopause) in women who cannot or will not take estrogen.

Brand name:
Micardis

Pronounced: MY-car-diss
Generic name: Telmisartan

Micardis controls high blood pressure. It works by blocking the effects of a hormone called angiotensin II. Unopposed, this substance tends to constrict the blood vessels while promoting retention of salt and water—actions that tend to raise blood pressure. Micardis prevents these effects and thus keeps blood pressure lower. It can be prescribed alone or with other high blood pressure medications, such as diuretics that help rid the body of excess water.

Brand name:
Micardis HCT

Pronounced: my-CAR-diss
Generic name: Telmisartan, Hydrochlorothiazide

Micardis HCT is a combination medication used in the treatment of high blood pressure. One component, telmisartan, belongs to a class of blood pressure medications that work by preventing the hormone angiotensin II from constricting the blood vessels. This allows the blood to flow more freely and helps keep blood pressure down. The other component of Micardis HCT, hydrochlorothiazide, is a diuretic that increases the output of urine. This removes excess fluid from the body and helps lower blood pressure. Doctors usually prescribe Micardis HCT in place of its individual components. It can also be prescribed along with other blood pressure medications.

Generic name:
Miconazole

See Monistat, page 522.

Brand name:
Micro-K

Pronounced: MY-kroe kay
Generic name: Potassium chloride
Other brand names: Klor-Con, K-Dur, K-Tab, Kaon-CL, Slow-K

Micro-K is used to treat or prevent low potassium levels in people who may face potassium loss caused by digitalis (Lanoxin), non-potassium-sparing diuretics (such as Diuril and Dyazide), and certain diseases.

Potassium plays an essential role in the proper functioning of a wide range of systems in the body, including the kidneys, muscles, and nerves. As a result, a potassium deficiency may have a wide range of effects, including dry mouth, thirst, reduced urination, weakness, fatigue, drowsiness, low blood pressure, restlessness, muscle cramps, abnormal heart rate, nausea, and vomiting.

Micro-K and its sister products are slow-release potassium formulations.

Brand name:

Micronase

Pronounced: MIKE-roh-naze
Generic name: Glyburide
Other brand names: DiaBeta, Glynase

Micronase is an oral antidiabetic medication used to treat type 2 diabetes, the kind that occurs when the body either does not make enough insulin or fails to use insulin properly. Insulin transfers sugar from the bloodstream to the body's cells, where it is then used for energy.

There are two forms of diabetes: type 1 and type 2. Type 1 diabetes results from a complete shutdown of normal insulin production and usually requires insulin injections for life, while type 2 diabetes can usually be treated by dietary changes, exercise, and/or oral antidiabetic medications such as Micronase. This medication controls diabetes by stimulating the pancreas to produce more insulin and by helping insulin to work better. Type 2 diabetics may need insulin injections, sometimes only temporarily during stressful periods such as illness, or on a long-term basis if an oral antidiabetic medication fails to control blood sugar.

Micronase can be used alone or along with a drug called metformin (Glucophage) if diet plus either drug alone fails to control sugar levels.

Brand name:

Micronor

See Oral Contraceptives, page 542.

Brand name:
Midrin

Pronounced: MID-rin
Generic ingredients: Isometheptene mucate, Dichloralphenazone,
Acetaminophen

Midrin is prescribed for the treatment of tension headaches. It is also used to treat vascular headaches such as migraine.

Brand name:
Migranal

Pronounced: MY-grah-nal
Generic name: Dihydroergotamine mesylate

Migranal Nasal Spray is used for relief of migraine headache attacks, whether or not preceded by an aura (visual disturbances, usually including sensations of halos or flickering lights).

This nasally administered remedy contains the same active ingredient as D.H.E. 45, an injectable form of the drug. It constricts the blood vessels, and may defeat migraine through this action.

Brand name:
Minipress

Pronounced: MIN-ee-press
Generic name: Prazosin hydrochloride

Minipress is used to treat high blood pressure. It is effective used alone or with other high blood pressure medications such as diuretics or beta-blocking medications (drugs that ease heart contractions) such as Tenormin.

Minipress is also prescribed for the treatment of benign prostatic hyperplasia (BPH), an abnormal enlargement of the prostate gland.

Brand name:
Minocin

Pronounced: MIN-o-sin
Generic name: Minocycline hydrochloride
Other brand name: Dynacin

Minocin is a form of the antibiotic tetracycline. It is given to help treat many different kinds of infection, including:

Acne
Amebic dysentery
Anthrax (when penicillin cannot be given)
Cholera
Gonorrhea (when penicillin cannot be given)
Plague
Respiratory infections such as pneumonia
Rocky Mountain spotted fever
Syphilis (when penicillin cannot be given)
Urinary tract infections caused by certain microbes

Generic name:

Minocycline

See Minocin, page 519.

Brand name:

Mirapex

Pronounced: MERE-a-pecks
Generic name: Pramipexole dihydrochloride

Although it is not a cure, Mirapex eases the symptoms of Parkinson's disease—a progressive disorder marked by muscle rigidity, weakness, shaking, tremor, and eventually difficulty with walking and talking. Parkinson's disease results from a shortage of the chemical messenger dopamine in certain areas of the brain. Mirapex is believed to work by boosting the action of whatever dopamine is available. The drug can be used with other Parkinson's medications such as Eldepryl and Sinemet.

Generic name:

Misoprostol

See Cytotec, page 437.

Brand name:

Mobic

Pronounced: MOH-bik
Generic name: Meloxicam

Mobic is a nonsteroidal anti-inflammatory drug (NSAID) in prescription form. It is used to relieve the pain and stiffness of osteoarthritis.

Generic name:

Modafinil

See Provigil, page 567.

Brand name:

Modicon

See Oral Contraceptives, page 542.

Brand name:

Moduretic

Pronounced: mod-your-ET-ik
Generic ingredients: Amiloride, Hydrochlorothiazide

Moduretic is a diuretic combination used in the treatment of high blood pressure and congestive heart failure, conditions which require the elimination of excess fluid (water) from the body. When used for high blood pressure, Moduretic can be used alone or with other high blood pressure medications. Diuretics help the body produce and eliminate more urine, which helps lower blood pressure. Amiloride, one of the ingredients, helps minimize the potassium loss that can be caused by the other component, hydrochlorothiazide.

Generic name:

Moexipril

See Univasc, page 611.

Generic name:

Moexipril with Hydrochlorothiazide

See Uniretic, page 610.

Generic name:

Mometasone furoate

See Elocon, page 456.

Generic name:

Mometasone furoate monohydrate

See Nasonex, page 529.

Brand name:

Monistat

Pronounced: MON-ih-stat
Generic name: Miconazole nitrate

Monistat is available in several formulations, including Monistat 3 vaginal suppositories, Monistat 7 vaginal cream and suppositories, and Monistat-Derm skin cream. Monistat's active ingredient, Miconazole, fights fungal infections.

Monistat 3 and Monistat 7 are used for vaginal yeast infections. Monistat-Derm is used for skin infections such as athlete's foot, ringworm, jock itch, yeast infection on the skin (cutaneous candidiasis), and tinea versicolor (a common skin condition that produces patches of white, tan, or brown finely flaking skin over the neck and trunk).

Brand name:

Monoket

See Imdur, page 484.

Brand name:

Monopril

Pronounced: MON-oh-prill
Generic name: Fosinopril sodium

Monopril is a high blood pressure medication known as an ACE inhibitor. It is effective when used alone or in combination with other medications for the treatment of high blood pressure. Monopril is also prescribed for heart failure.

Monopril works by preventing the conversion of a chemical in the blood called angiotensin I into a more potent substance that increases salt and water retention in the body and causes blood vessels to constrict—two actions that tend to increase blood pressure. Monopril also enhances blood flow in the circulatory system.

Brand name:

Monopril-HCT

Pronounced: MON-oh-prill
Generic ingredients: Fosinopril sodium, Hydrochlorothiazide

Monopril-HCT is used to treat high blood pressure. It usually is prescribed after other blood pressure medications have failed to do the job. Monopril-HCT combines two types of blood pressure medicine. The first, fosinopril sodium, is an ACE (angiotensin-converting enzyme) inhibitor. It works by preventing a chemical in the blood called angiotensin I from converting into a more potent form (angiotensin II) that increases salt and water retention in the body and causes blood vessels to constrict—two actions that tend to increase blood pressure. To aid in clearing water from the body, Monopril-HCT also contains hydrochlorothiazide, a diuretic that promotes the production of urine.

Generic name:

Montelukast

See Singulair, page 581.

Brand name:

Monurol

Pronounced: MON-your-all
Generic name: Fosfomycin tromethamine

Monurol is an antibiotic used to treat bladder infections (cystitis) in women. Produced in dry granule form, Monurol is taken as a single dose mixed with water.

Generic name:

Moricizine

See Ethmozine, page 463.

Generic name:

Morphine

See MS Contin, page 524.

Brand name:

Motrin

Generic name: Ibuprofen
Other brand name: Advil

Motrin is a nonsteroidal anti-inflammatory drug available in both prescription and nonprescription forms. Prescription Motrin is used in adults for relief of the symptoms of rheumatoid arthritis and osteoarthritis, treatment of menstrual pain, and relief of mild to moderate pain. In children aged 6 months and older it can be given to reduce fever and relieve mild to moderate pain. It is also used to relieve the symptoms of juvenile arthritis.

Motrin IB tablets, caplets, and gelcaps; Children's Motrin Suspension; and Advil tablets and caplets are available without a prescription. Check the packages for uses, dosage, and other information on these products.

Generic name:

Moxifloxacin

See Avelox, page 401.

Brand name:

MS Contin

Pronounced: em-ess KON-tin
Generic name: Morphine sulfate
Other brand name: Kadian

MS Contin, a controlled-release tablet containing morphine, is used to relieve moderate to severe pain. While regular morphine is usually given every 4 hours, MS Contin is typically taken every 12 hours—only twice a day. The Kadian brand may be taken once or twice a day. The drugs are intended for people who need a morphine painkiller for more than just a few days.

Generic name:

Mupirocin

See Bactroban, page 404.

Brand name:

Muse

See Caverject, page 418.

Brand name:

Mycelex

See Gyne-Lotrimin, page 479.

Brand name:

Mycelex-3

Pronounced: MI-seh-lecks
Generic name: Butoconazole nitrate

Mycelex-3 Vaginal Cream is an antifungal medication that cures yeast-like infections of the vulva and vagina.

Brand name:

Mycolog-II

Pronounced: MY-koe-log too
Generic ingredients: Nystatin, Triamcinolone acetonide
Other brand names: Myco-Triacet II, Mytrex

Mycolog-II Cream and Ointment are prescribed for the treatment of candidiasis (a yeast-like fungal infection) of the skin. The combination of an antifungal (nystatin) and a steroid (triamcinolone acetonide) provides greater benefit than nystatin alone during the first few days of treatment. Nystatin kills the fungus or prevents its growth; triamcinolone helps relieve the redness, swelling, itching, and other discomfort that can accompany a skin infection.

Brand name:
Myco-Triacet II

See Mycolog-II, page 525.

Brand name:
Mykrox

See Zaroxolyn, page 624.

Brand name:
Mysoline

Pronounced: MY-soh-leen
Generic name: Primidone

Mysoline is used to treat epileptic and other seizures. It can be used alone or with other anticonvulsant drugs. It is chemically similar to barbiturates.

Brand name:
Mytrex

See Mycolog-II, page 525.

Generic name:
Nabumetone

See Relafen, page 571.

Generic name:
Nadolol

See Corgard, page 432.

Generic name:
Nadolol with Bendroflumethiazide

See Corzide, page 433.

Generic name:
Nafarelin

See Synarel, page 587.

Brand name:
Nalfon

Pronounced: NAL-fahn
Generic name: Fenoprofen calcium

Nalfon, a nonsteroidal anti-inflammatory drug, is used to relieve the inflammation, swelling, stiffness, and joint pain associated with rheumatoid arthritis and osteoarthritis (the most common form of arthritis). It is also used to relieve mild to moderate pain.

Generic name:
Naltrexone

See ReVia, page 573.

Generic name:
Naphazoline with Pheniramine

See Naphcon-A, page 527.

Brand name:
Naphcon-A

Pronounced: NAFF-kon ay
Generic ingredients: Naphazoline hydrochloride, Pheniramine maleate
Other brand name: Opcon-A

Naphcon-A, an eyedrop containing both a decongestant and an antihistamine, is used to relieve itchy, red eyes caused by ragweed, pollen, and animal hair.

Brand name:
Naprelan

See Anaprox, page 392.

Brand name:
Naprosyn

Pronounced: NA-proh-sinn
Generic name: Naproxen
Other brand name: EC-Naprosyn

Naprosyn, a nonsteroidal anti-inflammatory drug, is used to relieve the inflammation, swelling, stiffness, and joint pain associated with rheumatoid arthritis, osteoarthritis (the most common form of arthritis), juvenile arthritis, ankylosing spondylitis (spinal arthritis), tendinitis, bursitis, and acute gout; it is also used to relieve menstrual cramps and other types of mild to moderate pain.

Generic name:
Naproxen

See Naprosyn, page 528.

Generic name:
Naproxen sodium

See Anaprox, page 392.

Generic name:
Naratriptan

See Amerge, page 390.

Brand name:
Nasacort

See Azmacort, page 403.

Brand name:

Nasalcrom

See Intal, page 487.

Brand name:

Nasalide

See AeroBid, page 384.

Brand name:

Nasonex

Pronounced: NAZE-oh-necks
Generic name: Mometasone furoate monohydrate

Nasonex nasal spray prevents and relieves the runny, stuffy nose that accompanies hay fever and year-round allergies. It contains a steroid medication that fights inflammation.

Brand name:

Natalins

See Stuartnatal Plus, page 584.

Generic name:

Nateglinide

See Starlix, page 584.

Brand name:

Necon

See Oral Contraceptives, page 542.

Generic name:

Nedocromil

See Tilade, page 598.

Generic name:
Nelfinavir

See Viracept, page 618.

Brand name:
Neodecadron Ophthalmic Ointment and Solution

Pronounced: Nee-oh-DECK-uh-drohn
Generic ingredients: Dexamethasone sodium phosphate, Neomycin sulfate

Neodecadron is a steroid and antibiotic combination that is used to treat inflammatory eye conditions in which there is also a bacterial infection or the possibility of a bacterial infection. Dexamethasone (the steroid) decreases inflammation. Neomycin, the antibiotic, kills some of the more common bacteria.

Brand name:
Neoral

See Sandimmune, page 578.

Brand name:
Neptazane

Pronounced: NEP-tuh-zayne
Generic name: Methazolamide

Neptazane, anhydrase is used to treat the eye condition called chronic open-angle glaucoma. This type of glaucoma is caused by a gradual block-age of the outflow of fluid in the front compartment of the eye over a period of years, causing a slow rise in pressure. It rarely occurs before the age of 40. Neptazane is also used for the type called acute angle-closure glaucoma when pressure within the eye must be lowered before surgery.

Brand name:
Neurontin

Pronounced: NUHR-on-tin
Generic name: Gabapentin

Neurontin, an epilepsy medication, is used with other medications to treat partial seizures (the type in which the victim remains conscious). It may be prescribed whether or not the seizures eventually become general and result in loss of consciousness.

Generic name:

Nevirapine

See Viramune, page 619.

Brand name:

Nexium

Pronounced: NECKS-ee-um
Generic name: Esomeprazole magnesium

Nexium relieves heartburn and other symptoms caused by the backflow of stomach acid into the canal to the stomach (the esophagus)—a condition known as gastroesophageal reflux disease. It is also prescribed to heal the damage (erosive esophagitis) that reflux disease can cause.

Prescribed in combination with the antibiotics Biaxin and Amoxil, Nexium is also used to treat the infection that causes most duodenal ulcers (ulcers occurring just beyond the exit from the stomach).

Like its sister drug Prilosec, Nexium works by reducing the production of stomach acid.

Generic name:

Niacin

See Niaspan, page 531.

Brand name:

Niaspan

Pronounced: NYE-uh-span
Generic name: Niacin

Although the niacin in Niaspan is one of the B-complex vitamins, this drug isn't taken to prevent deficiencies. In large doses, niacin also lowers cholesterol, and Niaspan extended-release tablets are designed specifically for this purpose.

Excessive levels of cholesterol in the blood can lead to clogged arteries and increased risk of heart attack. Niaspan is prescribed, along with a low-fat, low cholesterol diet, to reduce blood cholesterol levels, combat clogged arteries, and lower the chance of repeated heart attacks. It is used only when diet alone fails to do the job, and is often taken along with another type of cholesterol-lowering drug known as a bile acid sequestrant (Colestid, Questran, WelChol). It can also be combined with any of the cholesterol-lowering "statin" drugs (Lescol, Lipitor, Mevacor, Pravachol, Zocor).

Niaspan is also used to reduce very high levels of the blood fats known as triglycerides, a condition that can cause painful inflammation of the pancreas.

Generic name:
Nicardipine

See Cardene, page 415.

Brand name:
NicoDerm CQ

See Nicotine Patches, page 532.

Generic name:
Nicotine Inhalation System

See Nicotrol Inhaler, page 533.

Generic name:
Nicotine nasal spray

See Nicotrol NS, page 534.

Category:
Nicotine Patches

Brand names: Habitrol, NicoDerm CQ, Nicotrol

Nicotine patches, which are available under several brand names, are designed to help people quit smoking by reducing the craving for tobacco. Each adhesive patch contains a specific amount of nicotine embedded in a pad or gel.

Nicotine, the habit-forming ingredient in tobacco, is a stimulant and a mood lifter. When people give up smoking, lack of nicotine makes them crave cigarettes and may also cause anger, anxiety, concentration problems, irritability, frustration, or restlessness.

When a nicotine patch is worn, a specific amount of nicotine steadily travels out of the patch, through the skin, and into the bloodstream, keeping a constant low level of nicotine in the body. Although the resulting level of nicotine is less than smoking would deliver, it may be enough to prevent craving for cigarettes or development of other withdrawal symptoms.

Habitrol patches are round and come in three strengths: 21, 14, or 7 milligrams of nicotine per patch. Habitrol patches are worn 24 hours a day.

NicoDerm CQ patches are rectangular and come in three strengths: 21, 14, or 7 milligrams of nicotine per patch. NicoDerm CQ patches are worn 24 hours a day.

Nicotrol patches are rectangular and deliver 15 milligrams of nicotine per patch. Nicotrol patches are applied in the morning, worn all day, and removed at bedtime. They are not worn during sleep. Nicotrol is available over-the-counter.

Brand name:
Nicotrol

See Nicotine Patches, page 532.

Brand name:
Nicotrol Inhaler

Pronounced: NICK-o-trole
Generic name: Nicotine inhalation system

A quit-smoking aid, the Nicotrol Inhaler provides a substitute source of nicotine when people first give up cigarettes. A sudden decline in nicotine levels can cause such withdrawal symptoms as nervousness, restlessness, irritability, anxiety, depression, dizziness, drowsiness, concentration problems, sleep disturbances, increased appetite, weight gain, headache, constipation, fatigue, muscle aches, and a craving for tobacco. Nicotrol Inhaler prevents these symptoms and, through a familiar hand-to-mouth ritual, acts as a replacement for cigarettes. (Most of the nicotine in the product is, however, deposited in the mouth instead of the lungs.)

Brand name:

Nicotrol NS

Pronounced: NIK-oh-troll
Generic name: Nicotine nasal spray

Nicotrol NS is used to relieve withdrawal symptoms in people who are attempting to give up smoking. A sudden decline in nicotine levels can cause such withdrawal symptoms as nervousness, restlessness, irritability, anxiety, depression, dizziness, drowsiness, concentration problems, sleep disturbances, increased appetite, weight gain, headache, constipation, fatigue, muscle aches, and a craving for tobacco. Used as part of a comprehensive smoking cessation program, Nicotrol Inhaler prevents these symptoms.

Generic name:

Nifedipine

See Procardia, page 564.

Brand name:

Nilandron

Pronounced: nigh-LAND-ron
Generic name: Nilutamide

Nilandron is used for advanced prostate cancer—cancer that has begun to spread beyond the prostate gland. An "antiandrogen" drug, it blocks the effects of the male hormone testosterone, which is known to encourage prostate cancer. The drug is part of a treatment program that begins with removal of the testes, a major—but not the only—source of testosterone.

Generic name:

Nilutamide

See Nilandron, page 534.

Generic name:

Nimodipine

See Nimotop, page 535.

Brand name:

Nimotop

Pronounced: NIM-oh-top
Generic name: Nimodipine

Nimotop is used to prevent and treat problems caused by a burst blood vessel in the head (subarachnoid hemorrhage).

It is also occasionally prescribed for certain types of migraine headaches, stroke, and age-related memory problems such as Alzheimer's disease.

Nimotop belongs to a class of drugs known as calcium channel blockers which are frequently prescribed for high blood pressure and the crushing chest pain of angina.

Generic name:

Nisoldipine

See Sular, page 585.

Brand name:

Nitro-Bid

See Nitroglycerin, page 535.

Brand name:

Nitro-Dur

See Nitroglycerin, page 535.

Generic name:

Nitrofurantoin

See Macrodantin, page 508.

Generic name:

Nitroglycerin

Pronounced: NIGHT-row-GLISS-err-in
Brand names: Nitro-Bid, Nitro-Dur, Nitrolingual Spray, Nitrostat Tablets, Transderm-Nitro

Nitroglycerin is prescribed to prevent and treat angina pectoris (suffocating chest pain). This condition occurs when the coronary arteries become constricted and are not able to carry sufficient oxygen to the heart muscle. Nitroglycerin is thought to improve oxygen flow by relaxing muslcles in the walls of arteries and veins, thus allowing them to dilate.

Nitroglycerin is used in different forms. As a patch or ointment, nitroglycerin may be applied to the skin. The patch and the ointment are for *prevention* of chest pain.

Swallowing nitroglycerin in capsule or tablet form also helps to *prevent* chest pain from occurring.

In the form of sublingual (held under the tongue) or buccal (held in the cheek) tablets, or in oral spray (sprayed on or under the tongue), nitroglycerin helps relieve chest pain that has *already begun*. The spray can also prevent anginal pain. The type of nitroglycerin prescribed depends on the patient's condition.

Brand name:

Nitrolingual Spray

See Nitroglycerin, page 535.

Brand name:

Nitrostat Tablets

See Nitroglycerin, page 535.

Generic name:

Nizatidine

See Axid, page 402.

Brand name:

Nizoral

Pronounced: NYE-zore-al
Generic name: Ketoconazole

Nizoral, a broad-spectrum antifungal drug available in tablet form, may be given to treat several fungal infections within the body, including oral thrush and candidiasis.

It may also be given to treat severe, hard-to-treat fungal skin infections that have not cleared up after treatment with creams, ointments, or the oral drug griseofulvin (Fulvicin, Grisactin).

Brand name:

Nolvadex

Pronounced: NOLL-vah-decks
Generic name: Tamoxifen citrate

Nolvadex, an anticancer drug, is given to treat breast cancer. It also has proved effective when cancer has spread to other parts of the body. Nolvadex is most effective in stopping the kind of breast cancer that thrives on estrogen.

Nolvadex is also prescribed to reduce the risk of invasive breast cancer following surgery and radiation therapy for ductal carcinoma in situ (a localized cancer that can be totally removed surgically). The drug can also be used to reduce the odds of breast cancer in women at high risk of developing the disease. It does not completely eliminate the risk, but in a five-year study of over 1,500 high-risk women, it slashed the number of cases by 44 percent.

Brand name:

Norco

See Vicodin, page 617.

Brand name:

Nordette

See Oral Contraceptives, page 542.

Generic name:

Norfloxacin

See Noroxin, page 538.

Brand name:

Norgesic

Pronounced: nor-JEE-zic
Generic ingredients: Orphenadrine citrate, Aspirin, Caffeine
Other brand name: Norgesic Forte

Norgesic is prescribed, along with rest, physical therapy, and other measures, for the relief of mild to moderate pain caused by severe muscle disorders.

Brand name:

Norinyl

See Oral Contraceptives, page 542.

Brand name:

Normodyne

Pronounced: NORM-oh-dine
Generic name: Labetalol hydrochloride
Other brand name: Trandate

Normodyne is used in the treatment of high blood pressure. It is effective when used alone or in combination with other high blood pressure medications, especially thiazide diuretics such as HydroDIURIL and "loop" diuretics such as Lasix.

Brand name:

Noroxin

Pronounced: Nor-OX-in
Generic name: Norfloxacin

Noroxin is an antibacterial medication used to treat infections of the urinary tract, including cystitis (inflammation of the inner lining of the bladder caused by a bacterial infection), prostatitis (inflammation of the prostate gland), and certain sexually transmitted diseases, such as gonorrhea.

Brand name:

Norpace

Pronounced: NOR-pace
Generic name: Disopyramide phosphate
Other brand name: Norpace CR

Norpace is used to treat severe irregular heartbeat. It relaxes an overactive heart and improves the efficiency of the heart's pumping action.

Brand name:
Norplant

Pronounced: NOR-plant
Generic name: Levonorgestrel implants

Norplant is a birth control method consisting of 6 thin, flexible plastic capsules implanted just beneath the skin in a woman's upper, inner arm. The implants are inserted by a physician. Each set prevents pregnancy for 5 years, but can be removed by the doctor at any time. The Norplant capsules contain progestin, a synthetic version of the naturally occurring female hormone progesterone, which they release slowly and continuously into the bloodstream. This constant release of progestin prevents the ovaries from releasing eggs for fertilization. Norplant also works by thickening the mucus in the vagina near the opening of the uterus. The thick mucus makes it difficult for sperm to enter the uterus during sexual intercourse.

Norplant is more than 99 percent effective in preventing pregnancy. Overall, fewer than one woman in 100 becomes pregnant during the first year of Norplant use.

Brand name:
Norvasc

Pronounced: NOR-vask
Generic name: Amlodipine besylate

Norvasc is prescribed for angina, a condition characterized by episodes of crushing chest pain that usually results from a lack of oxygen in the heart muscle due to clogged arteries. Norvasc is also prescribed for high blood pressure. It is a type of medication called a calcium channel blocker. These drugs dilate blood vessels and slow the heart to reduce blood pressure and the pain of angina.

Brand name:
Norvir

Pronounced: NOR-veer
Generic name: Ritonavir

Norvir is prescribed to slow the progress of HIV (human immunodeficiency virus) infection. HIV causes the immune system to break down so that it can no longer respond effectively to infection, leading to the fatal disease known as acquired immune deficiency syndrome

(AIDS). Without treatment, HIV takes over certain human cells, especially white blood cells, and uses the inner workings of the infected cell to make additional copies of itself. Norvir belongs to a class of HIV drugs called protease inhibitors, which work by interfering with an important step in this reproduction process. Although Norvir cannot get rid of HIV already present in the body, it can reduce the amount of virus available to infect other cells.

Norvir is used in combination with other HIV drugs called nucleoside analogues (Retrovir, Hivid, and others). These two types of drugs act against HIV in different ways, thus improving the odds of success.

Brand name:
Novolin

See Insulin, page 486.

Brand name:
NuLev

See Levsin, page 498.

Brand name:
Nutracort

See Hydrocortisone Skin Preparations, page 482.

Generic name:
Nystatin with Triamcinolone

See Mycolog-II, page 525.

Generic name:
Ofloxacin

See Floxin, page 469.

Brand name:

Ogen

Pronounced: OH-jen
Generic name: Estropipate
Other brand name: Ortho-Est

Ogen and Ortho-Est are estrogen replacement drugs. The tablets are used to reduce symptoms of menopause, including feelings of warmth in face, neck, and chest, and the sudden intense episodes of heat and sweating known as "hot flashes." They also may be prescribed for teenagers who fail to mature at the usual rate.

In addition, either the tablets or Ogen vaginal cream can be used for other conditions caused by lack of estrogen, such as dry, itchy external genitals and vaginal irritation.

Along with diet, calcium supplements, and exercise, Ogen and Ortho-Est tablets are also prescribed to prevent osteoporosis, a condition in which the bones become brittle and easily broken.

Some doctors also prescribe these drugs to treat breast cancer and cancer of the prostate.

Brand name:

Ogestrel

See Oral Contraceptives, page 542.

Generic name:

Olsalazine

See Dipentum, page 449.

Generic name:

Omeprazole

See Prilosec, page 562.

Brand name:

Omnicef

Pronounced: OM-knee-seff
Generic name: Cefdinir
Omnicef is a member of the family of antibiotics known as cephalosporins.

It is used to treat mild to moderate infections, including:

Acute flare-ups of chronic bronchitis
Middle ear infections (otitis media)
Throat and tonsil infections (pharyngitis/tonsillitis)
Pneumonia
Sinus infections
Skin infections

Generic name:
Ondansetron

See Zofran, page 626.

Brand name:
Opcon-A

See Naphcon-A, page 527.

Category:
Oral Contraceptives

Brand names: Alesse, Brevicon, Cyclessa, Demulen, Desogen, Levlen, Levlite, Loestrin, Lo/Ovral, Low-Ogestrel, Micronor, Modicon, Necon, Nordette, Norinyl, Ogestrel, Ortho-Cept, Ortho-Cyclen, Ortho-Novum, Ortho Tri-Cyclen, Ovcon, Ovral, Tri-Norinyl, Triphasil, Trivora, Yasmin, Zovia

Oral contraceptives (also known as "The Pill") are highly effective means of preventing pregnancy. Oral contraceptives consist of synthetic forms of two hormones produced naturally in the body: either progestin alone or estrogen and progestin. Estrogen and progestin regulate a woman's menstrual cycle, and the fluctuating levels of these hormones play an essential role in fertility.

To reduce side effects, oral contraceptives are available in a wide range of estrogen and progestin concentrations. Progestin-only products (such as Micronor) are usually prescribed for women who should avoid estrogens; however, they may not be as effective as estrogen/progestin contraceptives.

One variety of the Pill—the Ortho Tri-Cyclen 28-day Dialpak—is also used in the treatment of moderate acne in women aged 15 and older. It is taken just as it would be for contraception.

Brand name:
Orap

Pronounced: OH-rap
Generic name: Pimozide

Orap is prescribed for people with severe cases of the neurological disorder known as Tourette's syndrome if they have not been helped sufficiently by Haldol (haloperidol), the first-choice medication. Orap helps suppress the physical and verbal symptoms—twitches, jerks, and bizarre outbursts—that are associated with Tourette's syndrome.

Brand name:
Orinase

Pronounced: OR-in-aze
Generic name: Tolbutamide

Orinase is an oral antidiabetic medication used to treat type 2 (non-insulin-dependent) diabetes. Diabetes occurs when the body does not make enough insulin, or when the insulin that is produced no longer works properly. Insulin works by helping sugar get inside the body's cells, where it is then used for energy.

There are two forms of diabetes: type 1 (insulin-dependent) and type 2 (non-insulin-dependent). Type 1 diabetes usually requires taking insulin injections for life, while type 2 diabetes can usually be treated by dietary changes, exercise, and/or oral antidiabetic medications such as Orinase. Orinase controls diabetes by stimulating the pancreas to secrete more insulin and by helping insulin work better.

Occasionally, type 2 diabetics must take insulin injections temporarily during stressful periods or times of illness. When diet, exercise, and an oral antidiabetic medication fail to reduce symptoms and/or blood sugar levels, a person with type 2 diabetes may require long-term insulin injections.

Generic name:
Orlistat

See Xenical, page 621.

Generic name:
Orphenadrine, Aspirin, and Caffeine

See Norgesic, page 537.

Brand name:

Ortho-Cept

See Oral Contraceptives, page 542.

Brand name:

Ortho-Cyclen

See Oral Contraceptives, page 542.

Brand name:

Ortho-Est

See Ogen, page 541.

Brand name:

Ortho Evra

Pronounced: OR-thoe EV-rah
Generic ingredients: Ethinyl estradiol, Norelgestromin

Ortho Evra is a contraceptive skin patch. It contains estrogen and progestin, the same hormones found in many birth control pills. Fertility depends on regular fluctuations in the levels of these hormones. Contraceptives such as Ortho Evra reduce fertility by eliminating the fluctuations. Once applied to the skin, the Ortho Evra patch releases a steady supply of estrogen and progestin through the skin and into the bloodstream.

Brand name:

Ortho-Novum

See Oral Contraceptives, page 542.

Brand name:

Ortho Tri-Cyclen

See Oral Contraceptives, page 542.

Brand name:

Orudis

Pronounced: Oh-ROO-dis
Generic name: Ketoprofen
Other brand names: Actron, Orudis KT, Oruvail

Orudis, a nonsteroidal anti-inflammatory drug, is used to relieve the inflammation, swelling, stiffness, and joint pain associated with rheumatoid arthritis and osteoarthritis (the most common form of arthritis). It is also used to relieve mild to moderate pain, as well as menstrual pain.

Oruvail, an extended-release form of the drug, is used to treat the signs and symptoms of rheumatoid arthritis and osteoarthritis over the long term, not severe attacks that come on suddenly.

Actron and Orudis KT are over-the-counter forms of the drug. They are used to relieve minor aches and pains associated with the common cold, headache, toothache, muscle aches, backache, minor arthritis, and menstrual cramps. They are also used to reduce fever.

Brand name:

Oruvail

See Orudis, page 545.

Generic name:

Oseltamivir

See Tamiflu, page 589.

Brand name:

Ovcon

See Oral Contraceptives, page 542.

Brand name:

Ovral

See Oral Contraceptives, page 542.

Generic name:

Oxaprozin

See Daypro, page 439.

Generic name:

Oxcarbazepine

See Trileptal, page 605.

Generic name:

Oxiconazole

See Oxistat, page 546.

Brand name:

Oxistat

Pronounced: OX-ee-stat
Generic name: Oxiconazole nitrate

Oxistat is used to treat fungal skin diseases, including athlete's foot (tinea pedis), jock itch (tinea cruris), ringworm (tinea corporis), and tinea versicolor, which appears as patches on the skin. It is available as a cream or lotion.

Generic name:

Oxybutynin

See Ditropan, page 451.

Generic name:

Oxycodone and Aspirin

See Percodan, page 551.

Generic name:

Paclitaxel

See Taxol, page 590.

Brand name:

Pancrease

Pronounced: PAN-kree-ace
Generic name: Pancrelipase
Other brand names: Creon, Pancrease MT, Viokase, Ultrase

Pancrease is used to treat pancreatic enzyme deficiency. It is often prescribed for people with cystic fibrosis, chronic inflammation of the pancreas, or blockages of the pancreas or common bile duct caused by cancer. It is also taken by people who have had their pancreas removed or who have had gastrointestinal bypass surgery. Pancrease helps with the digestion of proteins, starches, and fats.

Generic name:

Pancrelipase

See Pancrease, page 547.

Generic name:

Pantoprazole

See Protonix, page 566.

Brand name:

Parafon Forte DSC

Pronounced: PAIR-a-fahn FOR-tay
Generic name: Chlorzoxazone

Parafon Forte DSC is prescribed, along with rest and physical therapy, for the relief of discomfort associated with severe, painful muscle spasms.

Brand name:

Parlodel

Pronounced: PAR-luh-del
Generic name: Bromocriptine mesylate

Parlodel inhibits the secretion of the hormone prolactin from the pituitary gland. It also mimics the action of dopamine, a shortage of which leads to Parkinson's disease. It is used to treat a variety of medical conditions, including:

Infertility in some women

Menstrual problems such as the abnormal stoppage or absence of flow, with or without excessive production of milk

Growth hormone overproduction leading to acromegaly, a condition characterized by an abnormally large skull, jaw, hands, and feet

Parkinson's disease

Pituitary gland tumors

Some doctors also prescribe Parlodel to treat cocaine addiction, the eye condition known as glaucoma, erection problems in certain men, restless leg syndrome, and a dangerous reaction to major tranquilizers called neuroleptic malignant syndrome.

Brand name:

PCE

See Erythromycin, Oral, page 459.

Brand name:

Pediapred

Pronounced: PEE-dee-uh-pred
Generic name: Prednisolone sodium phosphate

Pediapred, a steroid drug, is used to reduce inflammation and improve symptoms in a variety of disorders, including rheumatoid arthritis, acute gouty arthritis, and severe cases of asthma. It may be given to people to treat primary or secondary adrenal cortex insufficiency (lack of or insufficient adrenal cortical hormone in the body). It is also given to help treat the following disorders:

Blood disorders such as leukemia and various anemias

Certain cancers (along with other drugs)

Connective tissue diseases such as systemic lupus erythematosus

Digestive tract diseases such as ulcerative colitis

Eye diseases of various kinds

Fluid retention due to nephrotic syndrome (a condition in which damage to the kidneys causes a loss of protein in the urine)

High blood levels of calcium associated with cancer

Lung diseases such as tuberculosis

Severe allergic conditions such as drug-induced allergic reactions

Severe skin eruptions

Studies have shown that high doses of Pediapred are effective in controlling severe symptoms of multiple sclerosis, although they do not affect the ultimate outcome or natural history of the disease.

Brand name:
Pediazole

Pronounced: PEE-dee-uh-zole
Generic ingredients: Erythromycin ethylsuccinate, Sulfisoxazole acetyl
Other brand name: Eryzole

Pediazole is a combination of two antibacterial agents, the macrolide antibiotic erythromycin and the sulfa drug sulfisoxazole. It is prescribed for the treatment of severe middle ear infections in children.

Generic name:
Pemirolast

See Alamast, page 385.

Generic name:
Penciclovir

See Denavir, page 442.

Brand name:
Penicillin VK

See Penicillin V Potassium, page 549.

Generic name:
Penicillin V Potassium

Brand names: Penicillin VK, Veetids
Penicillin V potassium is used to treat infections, including dental infection, infections in the heart, middle ear infections, rheumatic fever, scarlet fever, skin infections, and upper and lower respiratory tract infections.

Penicillin V works against only certain types of bacteria—it is ineffective against fungi, viruses, and parasites.

Brand name:

Pentasa

See Rowasa, page 577.

Generic name:

Pentoxifylline

See Trental, page 604.

Brand name:

Pepcid

Pronounced: PEP-sid
Generic name: Famotidine
Other brand names: Pepcid AC, Pepcid RPD

Pepcid is prescribed for the short-term treatment of active duodenal ulcer (in the upper intestine) for 4 to 8 weeks and for active, benign gastric ulcer (in the stomach) for 6 to 8 weeks. It is prescribed for maintenance therapy, at reduced dosage, after a duodenal ulcer has healed. It is also used for short-term treatment of GERD, a condition in which the acid contents of the stomach flow back into the food canal (esophagus), and for the resulting inflammation of the esophagus. And it is prescribed for certain diseases that cause the stomach to produce excessive quantities of acid, such as Zollinger-Ellison syndrome. Pepcid belongs to a class of drugs known as histamine H-2 blockers.

An over-the-counter formulation, Pepcid AC, is used to relieve and prevent heartburn, acid indigestion, and sour stomach. Pepcid RPD is a preparation that dissolves rapidly in the mouth.

Brand name:

Percocet

Pronounced: PERK-o-set
Generic ingredients: Acetaminophen, Oxycodone hydrochloride
Other brand names: Roxicet, Tylox

Percocet, a narcotic analgesic, is used to treat moderate to moderately severe pain. It contains two drugs—acetaminophen and oxycodone. Acetaminophen is used to reduce both pain and fever. Oxycodone, a narcotic analgesic, is used for its calming effect and for pain.

Brand name:

Percodan

Pronounced: PERK-o-dan
Generic ingredients: Oxycodone, Aspirin

Percodan combines two pain-killing drugs: the narcotic analgesic oxycodone, and the common pain reliever aspirin. It is prescribed for moderate to moderately severe pain.

Generic name:

Pergolide

See Permax, page 552.

Brand name:

Pergonal

Pronounced: PER-go-nal
Generic name: Menotropins
Other brand name: Humegon

Pergonal is a synthetic version of two female hormones, luteinizing hormone (LH) and follicle-stimulating hormone (FSH). It is used to stimulate the follicles in the ovaries to cause ovulation, or release of an egg, in women who are having difficulty getting pregnant. It is usually followed by 1 injection of human chorionic gonadotropin (Profasi). In addition, Pergonal is given to produce many eggs in women undergoing *in vitro* fertilization.

Pergonal is also used to stimulate the production of sperm in men with some forms of male infertility.

Brand name:

Periactin

Pronounced: pair-ee-AK-tin
Generic name: Cyproheptadine hydrochloride

Periactin is an antihistamine given to help relieve cold- and allergy-related symptoms such as hay fever, nasal inflammation, stuffy nose, red and inflamed eyes, hives, and swelling. Periactin may also be given after epinephrine to help treat anaphylaxis, a life-threatening allergic reaction.

Some doctors prescribe Periactin to treat cluster headache and to stimulate appetite in underweight people.

Brand name:

Peridex

Pronounced: PAIR-i-decks
Generic name: Chlorhexidine gluconate

Peridex is an oral rinse used to treat gingivitis, a condition in which the gums become red and swollen. Peridex is also used to control gum bleeding caused by gingivitis. It is not effective for the more serious form of gum disease known as periodontitis

Generic name:

Perindopril

See Aceon, page 379.

Brand name:

Permax

Pronounced: PER-maks
Generic name: Pergolide mesylate

Permax is given, along with another drug, to help relieve the symptoms of Parkinson's disease.

In Parkinson's disease, the brain cells receive too little of a natural chemical messenger called dopamine. This results in tremor, rigid muscles, difficulty with walking and talking, and other distressing symptoms.

People with Parkinson's disease are given medication to increase the amount of dopamine reaching their brain; the medication may be levodopa, or, more commonly, a levodopa-carbidopa combination, such as Sinemet.

The role of Permax is to increase the effectiveness of Sinemet so that people need less of it.

Brand name:

Persantine

Pronounced: per-SAN-teen
Generic name: Dipyridamole

Persantine helps reduce the formation of blood clots in people who have had heart valve surgery. It is used in combination with blood thinners such as Coumadin.

Some doctors also prescribe Persantine in combination with other drugs, such as aspirin, to reduce the damage from a heart attack and prevent a recurrence, to treat angina, and to prevent complications during heart bypass surgery.

Brand name:
Phenaphen with Codeine

See Tylenol with Codeine, page 609.

Generic name:
Phenazopyridine

See Pyridium, page 568.

Brand name:
Phenergan with Codeine

Pronounced: FEN-er-gan
Generic ingredients: Promethazine hydrochloride, Codeine phosphate

Phenergan with Codeine is used to relieve coughs and other symptoms of allergies and the common cold. Promethazine, an antihistamine, helps reduce itching and swelling and dries up secretions from the nose, eyes, and throat. It also has sedative effects and helps control nausea and vomiting. Codeine, a narcotic analgesic, helps relieve pain and stops coughing.

Generic name:
Phenobarbital, Hyoscyamine, Atropine, and Scopolamine

See Donnatal, page 452.

Generic name:
Phentermine

See Adipex-P, page 383.

Generic name:
Phenytoin

See Dilantin, page 448.

Brand name:
Phospholine Iodide

Pronounced: FOS-foh-lin I-o-dide
Generic name: Echothiophate iodide

Phospholine Iodide is used to treat chronic open-angle glaucoma, a partial loss of vision or blindness resulting from a gradual increase in pressure of fluid in the eye. Because the vision loss occurs slowly, people often do not experience any symptoms and do not realize that their vision has declined. By the time the loss is noticed, it may be irreversible. Phospholine Iodide helps by reducing fluid pressure in the eye.

Phospholine Iodide is also used to treat secondary glaucoma (such as glaucoma following surgery to remove cataracts), for subacute or chronic angle-closure glaucoma after iridectomy (surgical removal of a portion of the iris) or when someone cannot have surgery or refuses it. The drug is also prescribed for children with accommodative esotropia ("cross-eye").

Brand name:
Pilocar

Pronounced: PYE-low-car
Generic name: Pilocarpine hydrochloride
Other brand names: Isopto Carpine, Pilopine HS Gel

Pilocar causes constriction of the pupils (miosis) and reduces pressure within the eye. It is used to treat the increased pressure of open-angle glaucoma and to lower eye pressure before surgery for the more severe condition called acute angle-closure glaucoma. It can be used alone or in combination with other medications. Glaucoma, one of the leading causes of blindness in the United States, is characterized by increased pressure in the eye that can damage the optic nerve and cause loss of vision. It results from insufficient drainage of the eyeball through a field called the "angle."

Generic name:
Pilocarpine

See Pilocar, page 554.

Brand name:

Pilopine HS Gel

See Pilocar, page 554.

Generic name:

Pimecrolimus

See Elidel, page 456.

Generic name:

Pimozide

See Orap, page 543.

Generic name:

Pindolol

Pronounced: PIN-doh-loll

Pindolol, a type of medication known as a beta blocker, is used in the treatment of high blood pressure. It is effective alone or combined with other high blood pressure medications, particularly with a thiazide-type diuretic (a "water pill" that increases urine output to remove excess fluid from the body). Beta blockers decrease the force and rate of heart contractions.

Generic name:

Pioglitazone

See Actos, page 382.

Generic name:

Piroxicam

See Feldene, page 465.

Brand name:

Plaquenil

Pronounced: PLAK-en-ill
Generic name: Hydroxychloroquine sulfate

Plaquenil is prescribed for the prevention and treatment of certain forms of malaria. Plaquenil is also used to treat the symptoms of rheumatoid arthritis such as swelling, inflammation, stiffness, and joint pain. It is also prescribed for lupus erythematosus, a chronic inflammation of the connective tissue.

Brand name:

Plavix

Pronounced: PLA-vicks
Generic name: Clopidogrel bisulfate

Plavix keeps blood platelets slippery and discourages formation of clots, thereby improving blood flow to the heart, brain, and body. The drug is prescribed to reduce the risk of heart attack, stroke, and serious circulation problems in people with hardening of the arteries or unstable angina (dangerous chest pain), and in people who've already suffered a heart attack or stroke.

Brand name:

Plendil

Pronounced: PLEN-dill
Generic name: Felodipine

Plendil is prescribed for the treatment of high blood pressure. It is effective alone or in combination with other high blood pressure medications. A type of medication called a calcium channel blocker, Plendil eases the workload of the heart by slowing down the passage of nerve impulses through the heart, thereby reducing the rate its beats. This improves blood flow through the heart and throughout the body, reduces blood pressure, and helps prevent angina pain (chest pain, often accompanied by a feeling of choking, usually caused by lack of oxygen in the heart due to clogged arteries).

Brand name:
Pletal

Pronounced: PLAT-tal
Generic name: Cilostazol

Pletal helps relieve the painful leg cramps caused by "intermittent claudication," a condition that results when arteries clogged with fatty plaque are unable to deliver an adequate blood supply to the muscles of the legs. Pletal helps the blood get through by dilating the blood vessels and preventing blood cells from clumping together.

Generic name:
Podofilox

See Condylox, page 431.

Brand name:
Polaramine

Pronounced: poll-AR-ah-meen
Generic name: Dexchlorpheniramine maleate

Polaramine is an antihistamine that relieves allergy symptoms, including: nasal stuffiness and inflammation and eye irritation caused by hay fever and other allergies; itching, swelling, and redness from hives and other rashes; allergic reactions to blood transfusions; and, with other medications, anaphylactic shock (severe allergic reaction).

Antihistamines work by decreasing the effects of histamine, a chemical the body releases in response to certain irritants. Histamine narrows air passages in the lungs and contributes to inflammation. Antihistamines reduce itching and swelling and dry up secretions from the nose, eyes, and throat.

Generic name:
Polyethylene glycol with Electrolytes

See Colyte, page 430.

Generic name:
Polymyxin B, Neomycin, and Hydrocortisone

See Cortisporin Ophthalmic Suspension, page 432.

Brand name:
Ponstel

Pronounced: PON-stel
Generic name: Mefenamic acid

Ponstel, a nonsteroidal anti-inflammatory drug, is used for the relief of moderate pain (when treatment will not last for more than 7 days) and for the treatment of menstrual pain.

Generic name:
Potassium chloride

See Micro-K, page 517.

Generic name:
Pramipexole

See Mirapex, page 520.

Brand name:
Prandin

Pronounced: PRAN-din
Generic name: Repaglinide

Prandin is used to reduce blood sugar levels in people with type 2 diabetes (the kind that does not require insulin shots). It works by promoting the production of insulin, the hormone responsible for transporting sugar out of the bloodstream and into the cells, where it supplies energy. Prandin is prescribed when diet and exercise alone fail to correct the problem. A combination of Prandin and a second diabetes drug called Glucophage can be prescribed if either drug alone proves insufficient.

Brand name:

Pravachol

Pronounced: PRAV-a-coll
Generic name: Pravastatin sodium

Pravachol is a cholesterol-lowering drug. Doctor prescribe it along with a cholesterol-lowering diet when blood cholesterol levels are dangerously high and the patient has not been able to lower it by diet alone.

High cholesterol can lead to heart problems. By lowering cholesterol, Pravachol improves a patient's chances of avoiding a heart attack, heart surgery, and death from heart disease. In people who already have hardening of the arteries, it slows progression of the disease and cuts the risk of acute attacks.

The drug works by helping to clear harmful low-density lipoprotein (LDL) cholesterol out of the blood and by limiting the body's ability to form new LDL cholesterol.

Generic name:

Pravastatin

See Pravachol, page 559.

Generic name:

Prazosin

See Minipress, page 519.

Brand name:

Precose

Pronounced: PREE-cohs
Generic name: Acarbose

Precose is an oral medication used to treat type 2 (noninsulin-dependent) diabetes when high blood sugar levels cannot be controlled by diet alone. Precose works by slowing the body's digestion of carbohydrates so that blood sugar levels won't surge upward after a meal. Precose may be taken alone or in combination with certain other diabetes medications such as Diabinese, Micronase, Glucophage, and Insulin.

Brand name:
Pred Forte

Pronounced: PRED FORT
Generic name: Prednisolone acetate

Pred Forte contains a steroid medication that eases redness, irritation, and swelling due to inflammation of the eye.

Generic name:
Prednisolone acetate

See Pred Forte, page 560.

Generic name:
Prednisolone sodium phosphate

See Pediapred, page 548.

Generic name:
Prednisone

See Deltasone, page 440.

Brand name:
Premarin

Pronounced: PREM-uh-rin
Generic name: Conjugated estrogens
Other brand names: Cenestin, Premphase, Prempro,

Premarin is an estrogen replacement drug. The tablets are used to reduce symptoms of menopause, including feelings of warmth in the face, neck, and chest, and the sudden intense episodes of heat and sweating known as "hot flashes." Cenestin tablets, containing a synthetic form of conjugated estrogens, may also be prescribed for these symptoms.

In addition to the symptoms of menopause, Premarin tablets are prescribed for teenagers who fail to mature at the usual rate, and to relieve the symptoms of certain types of cancer, including some forms of breast and prostate cancer.

In addition, either the tablets or Premarin vaginal cream can be used for other conditions caused by lack of estrogen, such as dry, itchy external genitals and vaginal irritation.

Along with diet, calcium supplements, and exercise, Premarin tablets are also prescribed to prevent osteoporosis, a condition in which the bones become brittle and easily broken.

The addition of progesterone to estrogen-replacement therapy has been shown to reduce the risk of uterine cancer. Prempro combines estrogen and progesterone in a single tablet taken once daily. Premphase is a 28-day supply of tablets. The first 14 contain only estrogen. The second 14 supply both estrogen and progesterone. Both Prempro and Premphase are prescribed to reduce the symptoms of menopause, including vaginal problems, and to prevent osteoporosis.

Brand name:

Premphase

See Premarin, page 560.

Brand name:

Prempro

See Premarin, page 560.

Brand name:

Prevacid

Pronounced: PREH-va-sid
Generic name: Lansoprazole

Prevacid blocks the production of stomach acid. It is prescribed for the short-term treatment (up to 4 weeks) of duodenal ulcers, (ulcers in the intestinal wall near the exit from the stomach). It is also used for up to 8 weeks in the treatment of stomach ulcers, gastroesophageal reflux disease (backflow of acid into the canal to the stomach), and a condition called erosive esophagitis (severe inflammation of the canal). Once a duodenal ulcer or case of esophagitis has cleared up, the doctor may continue prescribing Prevacid to prevent a relapse. Prevacid is also prescribed to reduce the risk of stomach ulcers in people who develop this problem while taking nonsteroidal anti-inflammatory drugs such as Advil, Motrin, and Naprosyn. The drug is also used for long-term treatment of certain diseases marked by excessive acid production, such as Zollinger-Ellison syndrome.

Prevacid is also prescribed as part of a combination treatment to eliminate the *H. pylori* infection that causes most cases of duodenal ulcer.

Brand name:

Preven

Pronounced: PREH-vin
Generic name: Levonorgestrel and Ethinyl Estradiol

The Preven Emergency Contraception Kit provides "morning after" birth control following a contraceptive failure (for instance, a broken condom) or unprotected intercourse.

The hormone pills in the Preven kit can prevent a pregnancy, but will not end one that's already begun. They work primarily by inhibiting ovulation (release of an egg) and possibly by blocking fertilization and implantation of the egg in the lining of the uterus.

Brand name:

Prevpac

Pronounced: PREV-pack
Generic name: Amoxicillin, Clarithromycin, and Lansoprazole

Prevpac is a prepackaged combination of drugs designed to cure duodenal ulcers (ulcers in the intestinal wall near the exit from the stomach) caused by *H. pylori* bacteria, the most common source of ulcers. With two antibiotics and an acid-blocking agent, Prevpac will eradicate the *H. pylori* infection and improve the odds of remaining ulcer-free. This type of therapy is usually reserved for people with an active ulcer and those who've had one for at least a year.

Brand name:

Prilosec

Pronounced: PRY-low-sek
Generic name: Omeprazole

Prilosec is prescribed for the short-term treatment (4 to 8 weeks) of stomach ulcer, duodenal ulcer (near the exit from the stomach), and erosive esophagitis (inflammation of the esophagus), and for the treatment of heartburn and other symptoms of gastroesophageal reflux disease (backflow of acid stomach contents into the canal leading to the stomach). It is also used to maintain healing of erosive esophagitis and for the long-term treatment of conditions in which too much stomach acid is secreted, including Zollinger-Ellison syndrome, multiple endocrine adenomas (benign tumors), and systemic mastocytosis (cancerous cells).

Combined with the antibiotic clarithromycin (Biaxin) (and sometimes with the antibiotic amoxicillin as well), Prilosec is also used to cure patients whose ulcers are caused by infection with the germ *H. pylori*, the most common source of duodenal ulcers.

Generic name:

Primidone

See Mysoline, page 526.

Brand name:

Principen

See Ampicillin, page 391.

Brand name:

Prinivil

See Zestril, page 625.

Brand name:

Prinzide

See Zestoretic, page 624.

Generic name:

Procainamide

See Procanbid, page 563.

Brand name:

Procanbid

Pronounced: PROH-can
Generic name: Procainamide hydrochloride
Other brand names: Pronestyl, Pronestyl-SR

Procanbid is used to treat severe irregular heartbeats (arrhythmias). Arrhythmias are generally divided into two main types: heartbeats that are faster than normal (tachycardia), and heartbeats that are slower than normal (bradycardia). Irregular heartbeats are often caused by drugs or disease but can occur in otherwise healthy people with no history of heart disease or other illness.

Brand name:

Procardia

Pronounced: pro-CAR-dee-uh
Generic name: Nifedipine
Other brand names: Procardia XL, Adalat, Adalat CC

Procardia and Procardia XL are used to treat angina (chest pain caused by lack of oxygen to the heart due to clogged arteries or spasm of the arteries). Procardia XL is also used to treat high blood pressure. Procardia and Procardia XL are calcium channel blockers. They ease the workload of the heart by relaxing the muscles in the walls of the arteries, allowing them to dilate. This improves blood flow through the heart and throughout the body, reduces blood pressure, and helps prevent angina. Procardia XL is taken once a day and provides a steady rate of medication over a 24-hour period.

Brand name:

Profasi

Pronounced: PRO-fah-see
Generic name: Human chorionic gonadotropin

Profasi is an infertility treatment that brings on ovulation, or release of an egg from the ovary, in women who do not ovulate on their own. It is used after therapy with another drug, Pergonal or Humegon (menotropins).

Profasi is also given to boys to treat undescended or underdeveloped testicles. It is used in men to stimulate the production of testosterone.

Some doctors also use human chorionic gonadotropin in men with erection problems or lack of sexual desire, and in the therapy of male "menopause."

Generic name:

Promethazine with Codeine

See Phenergan with Codeine, page 553.

Brand name:

Pronestyl

See Procanbid, page 563.

Generic name:

Propafenone

See Rythmol, page 577.

Brand name:

Propecia

Pronounced: pro-PEE-she-ah
Generic name: Finasteride

Propecia is a remedy for baldness in men with mild to moderate hair loss on the top of the head and the front of the mid-scalp area. It increases hair growth, improves hair regrowth, and slows down hair loss. It works only on scalp hair and does not affect hair on other parts of the body.

Improvement can be seen as early as 3 months after starting therapy with Propecia, but for many men it takes longer. The improvement lasts only as long as therapy continues; when it stops, new hair growth ceases and hair loss resumes.

Propecia is a low-dose form of Proscar, a drug prescribed for prostate enlargement.

Brand name:

Propine

Pronounced: PROH-peen
Generic name: Dipivefrin hydrochloride

Propine is used to treat chronic open-angle glaucoma, the most common form of the disease. In glaucoma, the fluid inside the eyeball is under abnormally high pressure, a condition which can cause vision problems or even blindness.

Propine belongs to a class of medication called "prodrugs," drugs that generally are not active by themselves, but are converted in the body to an active form. This makes for better absorption, stability, and comfort and reduces side effects.

Generic name:

Propoxyphene

See Darvocet-N, page 438.

Generic name:

Propranolol

See Inderal, page 485.

Generic name:

Propranolol with Hydrochlorothiazide

See Inderide, page 485.

Brand name:

Proscar

Pronounced: PRAHS-car
Generic name: Finasteride

Proscar is prescribed to help shrink an enlarged prostate.

The prostate, a chestnut-shaped gland present in males, produces a liquid that forms part of the semen. This gland completely surrounds the upper part of the urethra, the tube through which urine flows out of the bladder. Many men over age 50 suffer from a benign (noncancerous) enlargement of the prostate. The enlarged gland squeezes the urethra, obstructing the normal flow of urine. Resulting problems may include difficulty in starting urination, weak flow of urine, and the need to urinate urgently or frequently. Sometimes surgical removal of the prostate is necessary.

By shrinking the enlarged prostate, Proscar may alleviate the various associated urinary problems, making surgery unnecessary.

Some doctors are also prescribing Proscar for baldness and as a preventive measure against prostate cancer.

Brand name:

Protonix

Pronounced: PRO-ton-iks
Generic name: Pantoprazole sodium

Protonix blocks the production of stomach acid. It is prescribed to heal a condition called erosive esophagitis (a severe inflammation of the passage to the stomach) brought on by a persistent backflow of stomach acid (gastroesophageal reflux disease). Later, it may be prescribed to maintain healing and prevent a relapse.

Protonix is a member of the "proton pump inhibitor" class of acid blockers, which includes AcipHex, Nexium, Prilosec, and Prevacid.

Brand name:
Proventil

Pronounced: Proh-VEN-till
Generic name: Albuterol sulfate
Other brand names: AccuNeb, Proventil HFA, Ventolin HFA, Volmax Extended-Release Tablets

Drugs containing albuterol are prescribed for the prevention and relief of bronchial spasms that narrow the airway. This especially applies to the treatment of asthma. Some brands of this medication are also used for the prevention of bronchial spasm due to exercise.

Brand name:
Provera

Pronounced: pro-VAIR-uh
Generic name: Medroxyprogesterone acetate

Provera is derived from the female hormone progesterone. It is prescribed for problems such as failure to menstruate or abnormal menstruation. Provera is also prescribed to prevent abnormal growth of the uterine lining in women taking estrogen replacement therapy.

Other forms of medroxyprogesterone, such as Depo-Provera, are used as a contraceptive injection and are prescribed in the treatment of endometrial cancer.

Some doctors also prescribe Provera to treat endometriosis, menopausal symptoms, premenstrual tension, sexual aggressive behavior in men, and sleep apnea (temporary failure to breath while sleeping).

Brand name:
Provigil

Pronounced: PRO-vi-jil
Generic name: Modafinil

Provigil is a stimulant drug used to prevent the excessive daytime sleepiness suffered by people with narcolepsy.

Brand name:

Psorcon

Pronounced: SORE-kon
Generic name: Diflorasone diacetate

Psorcon is prescribed for the relief of the inflammation and itching of skin disorders that respond to the application of steroids (hormones produced by the body that have potent anti-inflammatory effects).

Psorcon is available in ointment and cream forms, and in emollient ointment and cream.

Brand name:

Pulmozyme

Pronounced: PULL-muh-zime
Generic name: Dornase alfa

Pulmozyme inhalation solution reduces the number of respiratory infections that require injectable antibiotics in people with cystic fibrosis. It is also used to make breathing easier by thinning the mucus in the lungs.

Brand name:

Pyridium

Pronounced: pie-RI-di-um
Generic name: Phenazopyridine hydrochloride

Pyridium is a urinary tract analgesic that helps relieve the pain, burning, urgency, frequency, and irritation caused by infection, trauma, catheters, or various surgical procedures in the lower urinary tract. Pyridium is indicated for short-term use and can only relieve symptoms; it is not a treatment for the underlying cause of the symptoms.

Brand name:

Questran

Pronounced: KWEST-ran
Generic name: Cholestyramine
Other brand name: Questran Light

Questran is used to lower cholesterol levels in the blood of people with primary hypercholesterolemia (too much LDL cholesterol).

Hypercholesterolemia is a genetic condition characterized by a lack of the LDL receptors that remove cholesterol from the bloodstream.

This drug can be used to lower cholesterol levels in people who also have hypertriglyceridemia, a condition in which an excess of fat is stored in the body.

This drug may also be prescribed to relieve itching associated with gallbladder obstruction.

It is available in two forms: Questran and Questran Light.

Brand name:

Quibron-T/SR

See Theo-Dur, page 597.

Generic name:

Quinapril

See Accupril, page 377.

Generic name:

Quinapril with Hydrochlorothiazide

See Accuretic, page 378.

Brand name:

Quinidex Extentabs

Pronounced: KWIN-i-deks Eks-TEN-tabs
Generic name: Quinidine sulfate

Quinidex Extentabs are used to correct certain types of irregular heart rhythms and to slow an abnormally fast heartbeat.

Generic name:

Quinidine sulfate

See Quinidex Extentabs, page 569.

Brand name:

Qvar Inhalation Aerosol

See Beclomethasone, page 404.

Generic name:

Rabeprazole

See AcipHex, page 380.

Generic name:

Raloxifene

See Evista, page 463

Generic name:

Ramipril

See Altace, page 388.

Generic name:

Ranitidine

See Zantac, page 623.

Brand name:

Reglan

Pronounced: REG-lan
Generic name: Metoclopramide hydrochloride

Reglan increases the contractions of the stomach and small intestine, helping the passage of food. It is given to treat the symptoms of diabetic gastroparesis, a condition in which the stomach does not contract. These symptoms include vomiting, nausea, heartburn, feeling of indigestion, persistent fullness after meals, and appetite loss. Reglan is also used, for short periods, to treat heartburn in people with gastroesophageal reflux disease (backflow of stomach contents into the esophagus). In addition, it is given to prevent nausea and vomiting caused by cancer chemotherapy and surgery.

Brand name:
Relafen

Pronounced: REL-ah-fen
Generic name: Nabumetone

Relafen, a nonsteroidal anti-inflammatory drug, is used to relieve the inflammation, swelling, stiffness, and joint pain associated with rheumatoid arthritis and osteoarthritis (the most common form of arthritis).

Brand name:
Relenza

Pronounced: rell-EN-zuh
Generic name: Zanamivir

Relenza is an antiviral drug that hastens recovery from the flu. Victims who begin taking Relenza within the first 2 days of their illness typically start to feel improvement a day earlier than would otherwise. The drug is believed to work by interfering with the spread of virus particles inside the respiratory tract.

Brand name:
Renova

See Retin-A and Renova, page 572.

Generic name:
Repaglinide

See Prandin, page 558.

Brand name:
Requip

Pronounced: REE-kwip
Generic name: Ropinirole hydrochloride

Requip helps relieve the signs and symptoms of Parkinson's disease. Caused by a deficit of dopamine (one of the brain's chief chemical messengers), this disorder is marked by progressive muscle stiffness, tremor, and fatigue. Requip works by stimulating dopamine receptors in the brain, thus promoting better, easier movement.

Requip can be taken with or without levodopa (usually prescribed as Sinemet), another drug used to treat the symptoms of Parkinson's disease.

Brand names:
Retin-A and Renova

Pronounced: Ret-in-A, Re-NO-va
Generic name: Tretinoin
Other brand name: Avita

Retin-A, Avita, and Renova contain the skin medication tretinoin. Retin-A and Avita are used in the treatment of acne. Renova is prescribed to reduce fine wrinkles, discoloration, and roughness on facial skin (as part of a comprehensive program of skin care and sun avoidance).

Retin-A is available in liquid, cream, or gel form, and in a stronger gel called Retin-A Micro. Avita comes only as a gel. Renova is available in cream form only.

Brand name:
Retrovir

Pronounced: reh-troh-VEER
Generic name: Zidovudine

Retrovir is prescribed for adults infected with human immunodeficiency virus (HIV). HIV causes the immune system to break down so that it can no longer respond effectively to infection, leading to the fatal disease known as acquired immune deficiency syndrome (AIDS). Retrovir slows down the progress of HIV. Combining Retrovir with other drugs such as Epivir and Crixivan can further slow the progression.

Retrovir is also prescribed for HIV-infected children over 3 months of age who have symptoms of HIV or who have no symptoms but, through testing, have shown evidence of impaired immunity.

Retrovir taken during pregnancy often prevents transmission of HIV from mother to child. Signs and symptoms of HIV disease are significant weight loss, fever, diarrhea, infections, and problems with the nervous system.

Brand name:

ReVia

Pronounced: reh-VEE-uh
Generic name: Naltrexone hydrochloride

ReVia is prescribed to treat alcohol dependence and narcotic addiction. ReVia is not a cure. Patients must be ready to make a change and be willing to undertake a comprehensive treatment program that includes professional counseling, support groups, and close medical supervision.

Brand name:

Rheumatrex

See Methotrexate, page 513.

Brand name:

Rhinocort

Pronounced: RYE-no-kort
Generic name: Budesonide

Rhinocort is an anti-inflammatory steroid medication. It is prescribed for relief of the symptoms of hay fever and other nasal inflammations. It is taken as a nasal spray.

Brand name:

Ridaura

Pronounced: ri-DOOR-ah
Generic name: Auranofin

Ridaura, a gold preparation, is given to help treat rheumatoid arthritis. Ridaura is taken by mouth, unlike other gold compounds, which are given by injection. It is recommended only for people who have not been helped sufficiently by nonsteroidal anti-inflammatory drugs (Anaprox, Dolobid, Indocin, Motrin, and others). Ridaura should be part of a comprehensive arthritis treatment program that includes non-drug forms of therapy.

The patients most likely to benefit from Ridaura are those with active joint inflammation, especially in the early stages.

Brand name:
Rifadin

Pronounced: RIFF-ah-din
Generic name: Rifampin
Other brand name: Rimactane

Rifadin is used to treat all forms of tuberculosis. Rifadin is used in combination with two other antituberculosis drugs at the start of therapy: isoniazid and pyrazinamide. Later, streptomycin or ethambutol may be added. Rifadin is also used to eliminate a meningitis-causing bacteria in people who are carriers of the disease but have no symptoms of the illness. Rifadin is not effective as a treatment for active meningitis.

Occasionally doctors prescribe rifampin to treat leprosy or Legionnaires' disease.

Generic name:
Rifampin

See Rifadin, page 574.

Generic name:
Rifampin, Isoniazid, and Pyrazinamide

See Rifater, page 574.

Brand name:
Rifater

Pronounced: RIF-a-tur
Generic ingredients: Rifampin, Isoniazid, Pyrazinamide

Rifater is a combination antibiotic used to treat the initial phase of tuberculosis. After a 2-month period, the doctor may prescribe another combination of antituberculosis drugs (Rifamate), which can be continued for longer periods.

Brand name:
Rimactane

See Rifadin, page 574.

Generic name:
Risedronate
See Actonel, page 382.

Generic name:
Ritonavir
See Norvir, page 539.

Generic name:
Rizatriptan
See Maxalt, page 508.

Brand name:
Robaxin
Pronounced: Ro-BAKS-in
Generic name: Methocarbamol

Robaxin is prescribed, along with rest, physical therapy, and other measures, for the relief of pain due to severe muscular injuries, sprains, and strains.

Brand name:
Rocaltrol
Pronounced: Ro-CAL-trol
Generic name: Calcitriol

Rocaltrol is a synthetic form of vitamin D used to treat people on dialysis who have hypocalcemia (abnormally low blood calcium levels) and resulting bone damage. Rocaltrol is also prescribed to treat low blood calcium levels in people who have hypoparathyroidism (decreased functioning of the parathyroid glands). When functioning correctly, these glands help control the level of calcium in the blood.

Rocaltrol is also prescribed for *hyper*parathyroidism (*increased* functioning of the parathyroid glands) and resulting bone disorders in people with kidney disease who are not yet on dialysis.

Brand name:
Rocephin

Pronounced: row-SEF-in
Generic name: Ceftriaxone sodium

Rocephin is a member of the cephalosporin family of antibiotics. It is used to treat infections of the skin, blood, bones, joints, ears, respiratory tract, abdomen, and urinary tract. It is also prescribed for gonorrhea, pelvic inflammatory disease, and meningitis (brain infection), and to protect against infection after surgery.

Generic name:
Rofecoxib

See Vioxx, page 618.

Brand name:
Rondec

Pronounced: RON-dek
Generic ingredients: Carbinoxamine maleate or Brompheniramine maleate, Pseudoephedrine hydrochloride

Rondec is an antihistamine/decongestant that relieves nasal inflammation and runny nose and the symptoms of hay fever and other allergies. Carbinoxamine and brompheniramine, the antihistamines, fight the effects of histamine, a chemical released by the body in response to certain irritants. Histamine narrows air passages in the lungs and contributes to inflammation. Antihistamines reduce itching and swelling and dry up secretions from the nose, eyes, and throat. Pseudoephedrine, the decongestant, reduces nasal congestion and makes breathing easier.

Generic name:
Ropinirole

See Requip, page 571.

Generic name:
Rosiglitazone

See Avandia, page 399

Brand name:

Rowasa

Pronounced: ROH-ace-ah
Generic name: Mesalamine
Other brand names: Asacol, Canasa, Pentasa

Rowasa Suspension Enema, Pentasa, and Asacol are used to treat mild to moderate ulcerative colitis (inflammation of the large intestine and rectum). Rowasa Suspension Enema is also prescribed for inflammation of the lower colon, and inflammation of the rectum.

Rowasa Suppositories and Canasa Suppositories are used to treat inflammation of the rectum.

Brand name:

Roxicet

See Percocet, page 550.

Brand name:

Rynatan

See Trinalin, page 607.

Brand name:

Rythmol

Pronounced: RITH-mol
Generic name: Propafenone

Rythmol is used to help correct certain life-threatening heartbeat irregularities (ventricular arrhythmias) by reducing the excitability of the heart muscle.

Generic name:

Salmeterol

See Serevent, page 580.

Generic name:

Salsalate

See Disalcid, page 450.

Brand name:

Sandimmune

Pronounced: SAN-dim-ewn
Generic name: Cyclosporine
Other brand name: Neoral

Sandimmune suppresses the body's immune system. It is given after transplant surgery to help prevent rejection of organs (kidney, heart, or liver). It is also used to avoid long-term rejection in people previously treated with other immunosuppressant drugs, such as Imuran.

Neoral is a newer formulation of Sandimmune's active ingredient, cyclosporine. In addition to prevention of organ rejection, it is prescribed for certain severe cases of rheumatoid arthritis and psoriasis.

Some doctors also prescribe Sandimmune to treat alopecia areata (localized areas of hair loss), aplastic anemia (shortage of red and white blood cells and platelets), Crohn's disease (chronic inflammation of the digestive tract), and nephropathy (kidney disease). Sandimmune is sometimes used in the treatment of severe skin disorders, including psoriasis and dermatomyositis (inflammation of the skin and muscles causing weakness and rash). The drug is also used in procedures involving bone marrow, the pancreas, and the lungs.

Sandimmune is always given with prednisone or a similar steroid. It is available in capsules and liquid, or as an injection.

Brand name:

Sansert

Pronounced: SAN-surt
Generic name: Methysergide maleate

Sansert tablets are prescribed to prevent or reduce the intensity and frequency of severe "vascular" headaches (the kind caused by constriction and dilation of arteries within the head). Doctors usually prescribe Sansert only if a patient has one or more severe headaches per week, or the headaches are extremely severe and uncontrollable.

Sansert is preventive medication. Sansert is not a painkiller and cannot diminish a headache that has already developed. It should not be used for acute migraine attacks.

Generic name:
Saquinavir

See Fortovase, page 472.

Brand name:
Sectral

Pronounced: SEK-tral
Generic name: Acebutolol hydrochloride

Sectral, a type of medication known as a beta blocker, is used in the treatment of high blood pressure and abnormal heart rhythms. When used to treat high blood pressure, it is effective used alone or in combination with other high blood pressure medications, particularly with a thiazide-type diuretic. Beta blockers decrease the force and rate of heart contractions, thus reducing pressure within the circulatory system.

Generic name:
Selegiline

See Eldepryl, page 455.

Brand name:
Semprex-D

Pronounced: SEM-precks-D
Generic ingredients: Acrivastine, Pseudoephedrine hydrochloride

Semprex-D is an antihistamine and decongestant drug that relieves sneezing, running nose, itching, watery eyes, and stuffy nose caused by seasonal allergies such as hay fever.

Brand name:
Septra

See Bactrim, page 404.

Brand name:

Serevent

Pronounced: SER-ah-vent
Generic name: Salmeterol xinafoate
Other brand name: Serevent Diskus

Serevent relaxes the muscles in the walls of the bronchial tubes, allowing the passageways to expand and carry more air. Taken regularly (twice a day), the drug is used in the treatment of asthma and chronic obstructive pulmonary disease (COPD), including emphysema and chronic bronchitis. A relatively long-acting medication, it is recommended only for the type of asthma patient who needs shorter-acting bronchodilators such as Alupent and Ventolin on a frequent, regular basis.

Serevent is available in an aerosol inhaler and as Serevent Diskus inhalation powder. Both forms of Serevent can be used with or without inhaled or oral steroid therapy.

Brand name:

Serophene

See Clomiphene Citrate, page 427.

Generic name:

Sibutramine

See Meridia, page 511.

Generic name:

Sildenafil

See Viagra, page 616.

Brand name:

Silvadene Cream 1%

Pronounced: SIL-vuh-deen
Generic name: Silver sulfadiazine

Silvadene Cream 1% is applied directly to the skin. The cream is used along with other medications to prevent and treat wound infections in people with second- and third-degree burns. It is effective against a variety of bacteria as well as yeast.

Generic name:

Silver sulfadiazine

See Silvadene Cream 1%, page 580.

Generic name:

Simvastatin

See Zocor, page 626.

Brand name:

Sinemet CR

Pronounced: SIN-uh-met see-are
Generic ingredients: Carbidopa, Levodopa

Sinemet CR is a controlled-release tablet that may be given to help relieve the muscle stiffness, tremor, and weakness caused by Parkinson's disease. It may also be given to relieve Parkinson-like symptoms caused by encephalitis (brain fever), carbon monoxide poisoning, or manganese poisoning.

Sinemet CR contains two drugs, carbidopa and levodopa. The drug that actually produces the anti-Parkinson's effect is levodopa. Carbidopa prevents vitamin B-6 from destroying levodopa, thus allowing levodopa to work more efficiently.

Parkinson's drugs such as Sinemet CR relieve the symptoms of the disease, but are not a permanent cure.

Brand name:

Singulair

Pronounced: sing-you-LAIR
Generic name: Montelukast sodium

Singulair is used for long-term prevention of asthma. It reduces the swelling and inflammation that tend to close up the airways, and relaxes the walls of the bronchial tubes, expanding the airways and permitting more air to pass through.

Brand name:

Slo-bid

See Theo-Dur, page 597

Brand name:

Slow-K

See Micro-K, page 517.

Generic name:

Sodium fluoride

See Luride, page 507.

Brand name:

Sodium Sulamyd

Pronounced: SOH-dee-um SOO-lah-mid
Generic name: Sulfacetamide sodium
Other brand name: Bleph-10

Sodium Sulamyd is used in the treatment of eye inflammations, corneal ulcer, and other eye infections. It may be used along with an oral sulfa drug to treat a serious eye infection called trachoma.

Brand name:

Soma

Pronounced: SOE-muh
Generic name: Carisoprodol

Soma is used, along with rest, physical therapy, and other measures, for the relief of acute, painful muscle strains and spasms.

Brand name:

Sorbitrate

See Isordil, page 489.

Brand name:

Spectazole Cream

Pronounced: SPEK-tah-zole
Generic name: Econazole nitrate

Spectazole cream is prescribed for fungal skin diseases commonly called ringworm (tinea). It is used to treat athlete's foot (tinea pedis), "jock itch" (tinea cruris), a fungus infection of the entire body (tinea corporis), and a skin infection that causes yellow- or brown-colored skin eruptions (tinea versicolor). It is also prescribed for yeast infections of the skin caused by candida fungus (cutaneous candidiasis).

Generic name:

Spironolactone

See Aldactone, page 386.

Generic name:

Spironolactone with Hydrochlorothiazide

See Aldactazide, page 386.

Brand name:

Sporanox

Pronounced: SPORE-ah-nocks
Generic name: Itraconazole

Sporanox capsules are used to treat four types of serious fungal infection: blastomycosis, histoplasmosis, aspergillosis, and onychomycosis. Blastomycosis can affect the lungs, bones, and skin. Histoplasmosis can affect the lungs, heart, and blood. Aspergillosis can affect the lungs, kidneys, and other organs. Onychomycosis affects the nails. Sporanox is also used against fungal infections in people with weak immune systems, such as AIDS patients.

Sporanox oral solution is used to treat candidiasis (fungal infection) of the mouth, throat, and gullet (esophagus), and for other fungal infections in people with weakened immunity and fever.

Brand name:

Starlix

Pronounced: STAR-licks
Generic name: Nateglinide

Starlix combats high blood sugar levels in people with type 2 diabetes (the kind that does not require insulin shots). Insulin speeds the transfer of sugar from the bloodstream to the body's cells, where it's burned to produce energy. In diabetes, the body either fails to make enough insulin, or proves unable to properly use what's available. Starlix attacks the problem from the production angle, stimulating the pancreas to secrete more insulin.

Starlix can be used alone or combined with another diabetes drug, called Glucophage, that tackles the other part of the problem, working to improve the body's response to whatever insulin it makes. Starlix is prescribed only when diet and exercise—or Glucophage alone—have failed to control blood sugar levels.

Generic name:

Stavudine

See Zerit, page 624.

Brand name:

Stimate

See DDAVP, page 439.

Brand name:

Stuartnatal Plus

Pronounced: STU-art NAY-tal plus
Generic ingredients: Prenatal vitamins and minerals
Other brand names: Materna, Natalins

Stuartnatal Plus contains vitamins and minerals, including iron, calcium, zinc, and folic acid. The tablets are given during pregnancy and after childbirth to ensure an adequate supply of these critical nutrients. They may also be prescribed to improve a woman's nutritional status before she becomes pregnant.

Generic name:

Sucralfate

See Carafate, page 414.

Brand name:

Sular

Pronounced: SOO-lar
Generic name: Nisoldipine

Sular controls high blood pressure. A long-acting tablet, Sular may be used alone or in combination with other blood pressure medications.

Sular is a type of medication called a calcium channel blocker. It inhibits the flow of calcium through the smooth muscles of the heart, delaying the passage of nerve impulses, slowing down the heart, and expanding the blood vessels. This eases the heart's workload and reduces blood pressure.

Generic name:

Sulfabenzamide, Sulfacetamide, and Sulfathiazole

See Triple Sulfa, page 607.

Generic name:

Sulfacetamide

See Sodium Sulamyd, page 582.

Generic name:

Sulfanilamide

See AVC, page 400.

Generic name:

Sulfasalazine

See Azulfidine, page 403.

Generic name:

Sulfisoxazole

See Gantrisin, page 474.

Generic name:

Sulindac

See Clinoril, page 427.

Generic name:

Sumatriptan

See Imitrex, page 484.

Brand name:

Sumycin

See Tetracycline, page 596.

Brand name:

Suprax

Pronounced: SUE-praks
Generic name: Cefixime

Suprax, a cephalosporin antibiotic, is prescribed for bacterial infections of the chest, ears, urinary tract, and throat, and for uncomplicated gonorrhea.

Brand name:

Sustiva

Pronounced: suss-TEE-vah
Generic name: Efavirenz

Sustiva is one of the growing number of drugs used to fight HIV infection. HIV, the human immunodeficiency virus, weakens the immune system until it can no longer fight off infections, leading to the fatal disease known as AIDS (acquired immune deficiency syndrome).

Like other drugs for HIV, Sustiva works by impairing the virus's ability to multiply. However, when taken alone it may prompt the virus to become resistant. Sustiva is therefore always taken with at least one other HIV medication, such as Retrovir or Crixivan. Even when used properly, it may remain effective for only a limited time.

Brand name:

Symmetrel

Pronounced: SIM-eh-trell
Generic name: Amantadine hydrochloride

Symmetrel is used to treat or prevent flu caused by the Influenza A virus; to treat Parkinson's disease; and to relieve tremors, jerks, or writhing caused by treatment with other drugs.

Hospital workers—and others in close contact with someone who has or is likely to get flu caused by the Influenza A virus—should have a flu shot each year. If a flu shot is impossible or contraindicated, preventive treatment with Symmetrel may be advisable. A flu shot can still be taken after starting treatment with Symmetrel. Once the body has manufactured enough antibodies to the Influenza A virus, Symmetrel will no longer be needed.

Brand name:

Synalgos-DC

Pronounced: SIN-al-gose dee-cee
Generic ingredients: Dihydrocodeine bitartrate, Aspirin, Caffeine

Synalgos-DC is a narcotic analgesic prescribed for the relief of moderate to moderately severe pain.

Brand name:

Synarel

Pronounced: SIN-er-el
Generic name: Nafarelin acetate

Synarel is used to relieve the symptoms of endometriosis, including menstrual cramps or low back pain during menstruation, painful intercourse, painful bowel movements, and abnormal and heavy menstrual bleeding. Endometriosis is a condition in which fragments of the tissue that lines the uterus are found in the other parts of the pelvic cavity.

Synarel is also used to treat unusually early puberty in children of both sexes. Some doctors prescribe Synarel as a contraceptive for both men and women.

Brand name:

Synthroid

Pronounced: SIN-throid
Generic name: Levothyroxine
Other brand names: Levothroid, Levoxyl, Unithroid

Synthroid, a synthetic thyroid hormone available in tablet or injectable form, may be given in any of the following cases:

If the thyroid gland is not making enough hormone;

If the thyroid is enlarged (a goiter) or there is a risk for developing a goiter;

If the patient needs a "suppression test" to determine whether the thyroid gland is making too much hormone;

If the patient has certain cancers of the thyroid;

If thyroid production is low due to surgery, radiation, certain drugs, or disease of the pituitary gland or the hypothalamus in the brain.

Brand name:

Tagamet

Pronounced: TAG-ah-met
Generic name: Cimetidine
Other brand name: Tagamet HB

Tagamet is prescribed for the treatment of certain kinds of stomach and intestinal ulcers and related conditions. These include: active duodenal (upper intestinal) ulcers; active benign stomach ulcers; erosive gastro-esophageal reflux disease (backflow of acid stomach contents); prevention of upper abdominal bleeding in those who are critically ill; and excess-acid conditions such as Zollinger-Ellison syndrome (a form of peptic ulcer with too much acid). It is also used to prevent a relapse after the healing of active ulcers. Tagamet is a histamine blocker.

Some doctors also use Tagamet to treat acne and to prevent stress-induced ulcers. It may also be used to treat chronic hives, herpesvirus infections (including shingles), abnormal hair growth in women, and overactivity of the parathyroid gland.

An over-the-counter version of the drug, Tagamet HB, is used to relieve heartburn, acid indigestion, and sour stomach.

Brand name:
Tambocor

Pronounced: TAM-ba-kore
Generic name: Flecainide acetate

Tambocor is prescribed to treat certain heart rhythm disturbances, including paroxysmal atrial fibrillation (a sudden attack or worsening of irregular heartbeat in which the upper chamber of the heart beats irregularly and very rapidly) and paroxysmal supraventricular tachycardia (a sudden attack or worsening of an abnormally fast but regular heart rate that occurs in intermittent episodes).

Brand name:
Tamiflu

Pronounced: TAM-ih-floo
Generic name: Oseltamivir phosphate

Tamiflu speeds recovery from the flu. When started during the first 2 days of the illness, it hastens improvement by at least a day. It also can prevent the flu if treatment is started within 2 days after exposure to a flu victim. Tamiflu is one of a new class of antiviral drugs called neuraminidase inhibitors.

As the flu virus takes hold in the body, it forms new copies of itself and spreads from cell to cell. Neuraminidase inhibitors fight the virus by preventing the release of new copies from infected cells. The other drug in this class, Relenza, is taken by inhalation. Tamiflu is taken in liquid or capsule form.

Generic name:
Tamoxifen

See Nolvadex, page 537.

Generic name:
Tamsulosin

See Flomax, page 469.

Brand name:

Tarka

Pronounced: TAR-kah
Generic ingredients: Trandolapril, Verapamil hydrochloride

Tarka is used to treat high blood pressure. It combines two blood pressure drugs: an ACE inhibitor and a calcium channel blocker. The ACE inhibitor (trandolapril) lowers blood pressure by preventing a chemical in the blood called angiotensin I from converting to a more potent form that narrows the blood vessels and increases salt and water retention. The calcium channel blocker (verapamil hydrochloride) also works to keep the blood vessels open, and eases the heart's workload by reducing the force and rate of the heartbeat.

Brand name:

Tasmar

Pronounced: TAZ-mahr
Generic name: Tolcapone

Tasmar helps to relieve the muscle stiffness, tremor, and weakness caused by Parkinson's disease. When taken with Sinemet (levodopa/carbidopa), it sustains the blood levels of dopamine needed for normal muscle function. Because Tasmar has been known to cause liver failure, it is prescribed only when other Parkinson's drugs fail to control the symptoms.

Like all Parkinson's medications, Tasmar can provide long-term relief of symptoms, but won't cure the underlying disease. If symptoms do not improve after 3 weeks of Tasmar therapy, the doctor will discontinue the drug.

Brand name:

Taxol

Pronounced: TACKS-all
Generic name: Paclitaxel

Taxol is used to treat cancer of the ovary and breast cancer that does not respond to other drugs. An extract of the bark of the Pacific yew tree, it works by interfering with the growth of cancer cells.

Some doctors also prescribe Taxol to treat certain kinds of lung cancer.

Generic name:

Tazarotene

See Tazorac, page 591.

Brand name:

Tazorac

Pronounced: TAZZ-o-rack
Generic name: Tazarotene

Tazorac gel comes in two strengths, 0.05% and 0.1%. Both strengths are used to treat the type of psoriasis that causes large plaques on the skin. The 0.1% strength is also used to treat mild to moderate facial acne. The drug is chemically related to vitamin A.

Brand name:

Tegretol

Pronounced: TEG-re-tawl
Generic name: Carbamazepine
Other brand names: Carbatrol, Epitol, Tegretol-XR

Tegretol is used in the treatment of seizure disorders, including certain types of epilepsy. It is also prescribed for trigeminal neuralgia (severe pain in the jaws) and pain in the tongue and throat.

Without official approval, Tegretol is also used to treat alcohol withdrawal, cocaine addiction, and emotional disorders such as depression and abnormally aggressive behavior. The drug is also used to treat migraine headache and "restless legs."

Generic name:

Telmisartan

See Micardis, page 517.

Generic name:

Telmisartan with Hydrochlorothiazide

See Micardis HCT, page 517.

Brand name:

Temovate

Pronounced: TIM-oh-vate
Generic name: Clobetasol propionate
Other brand name: Cormax

Temovate and Cormax relieve the itching and inflammation of moderate to severe skin conditions. The scalp application is used for short-term treatment of scalp conditions; the cream, ointment, emollient cream, and gel are used for short-term treatment of skin conditions on the body. The products contain a steroid medication for external use only.

Brand name:

Tenex

Pronounced: TEN-ex
Generic name: Guanfacine hydrochloride

Tenex is given to help control high blood pressure. This medication reduces nerve impulses to the heart and arteries; this slows the heartbeat, relaxes the blood vessels, and thus reduces blood pressure. Tenex may be given alone or in combination with other high blood pressure medications, especially thiazide diuretics, such as Diuril, Esidrix, or Naturetin.

Generic name:

Tenofovir disoproxil

See Viread, page 619.

Brand name:

Tenoretic

Pronounced: Ten-or-ET-ic
Generic ingredients: Atenolol, Chlorthalidone

Tenoretic is used in the treatment of high blood pressure. It combines a beta-blocker drug and a diuretic. Tenoretic can be used alone or in combination with other high blood pressure medications. Atenolol, the beta blocker, decreases the force and rate of heart contractions. Chlorthalidone, the diuretic, helps the body produce and eliminate more urine, which clears excess fluid from the body and tends to lower blood pressure.

Brand name:

Tenormin

Pronounced: Ten-OR-min
Generic name: Atenolol

Tenormin, a type of medication known as a beta blocker, is used in the treatment of high blood pressure, angina pectoris (chest pain, usually caused by lack of oxygen in the heart muscle due to clogged arteries), and heart attack. When used for high blood pressure it is effective alone or combined with other high blood pressure medications, particularly with a thiazide-type water pill (diuretic). Beta blockers decrease the force and rate of heart contractions.

Without official approval, Tenormin is also used for treatment of alcohol withdrawal, prevention of migraine headache, and bouts of anxiety.

Brand name:

Tenuate

Pronounced: TEN-you-ate
Generic name: Diethylpropion hydrochloride

Tenuate, an appetite suppressant, is prescribed for short-term use (a few weeks) as part of an overall diet plan for weight reduction. It is available in two forms: immediate-release tablets (Tenuate) and controlled-release tablets (Tenuate Dospan). Tenuate should be used with a behavior modification program.

Brand name:

Tequin

Pronounced: TEK-win
Generic name: Gatifloxacin

Tequin is a member of the "quinolone" family of antibiotics. It is used to treat acute sinus infections, pneumonia, complications of chronic bronchitis, kidney and urinary tract infections, and gonorrhea.

Brand name:

Terazol

Pronounced: TER-uh-zawl
Generic name: Terconazole

Terazol is an antifungal medication. It is prescribed to treat candidiasis (a yeast-like fungal infection) of the vulva and vagina.

Generic name:

Terazosin

See Hytrin, page 483.

Generic name:

Terbinafine

See Lamisil, page 493.

Generic name:

Terbutaline

See Brethine, page 410.

Generic name:

Terconazole

See Terazol, page 593.

Brand name:

Tessalon

Pronounced: TESS-ah-lon
Generic name: Benzonatate

Tessalon is taken for relief of a cough. It works by deadening certain receptors in the respiratory tract, thereby dampening the cough reflex.

Generic name:

Testoderm

See Testosterone Patches, page 595.

Brand name:

Testopel

Pronounced: TEST-o-pell
Generic name: Testosterone pellets

Testopel pellets contain testosterone, the sex hormone responsible for growth and maintenance of male physical characteristics. Testosterone is a member of the androgen family of steroids that cause the growth spurt that happens during adolescence. Testopel is used to treat low testosterone levels brought on by age, tumors, injury, radiation, or a condition present from birth. It also is used to stimulate puberty in boys who have a family history of delayed puberty.

In addition, testosterone is sometimes used to treat certain types of breast cancer.

Generic name:

Testosterone gel

See AndroGel, page 392.

Category:

Testosterone Patches

Brand names: Androderm, Testoderm

These patches are prescribed for men with low levels of the male hormone, testosterone. Lack of testosterone can lead to declining interest in sex, as well as impotence, fatigue, depression, and loss of masculine characteristics.

Generic name:

Testosterone pellets

See Testopel, page 595.

Brand name:

Testred

See Android, page 393.

Generic name:

Tetracycline

Pronounced: TET-ra-SY-clin
Brand names: Achromycin V, Sumycin

Tetracycline, a "broad-spectrum" antibiotic, is used to treat bacterial infections such as Rocky Mountain spotted fever, typhus fever, and tick fevers; upper respiratory infections; pneumonia; gonorrhea; amoebic infections; and urinary tract infections. It is also used to help treat severe acne and to treat trachoma (a chronic eye infection) and conjunctivitis (pinkeye). Tetracycline is often a viable alternative for people who are allergic to penicillin.

Brand name:

Teveten

Pronounced: TEH-veh-ten
Generic name: Eprosartan mesylate

Teveten is used to treat high blood pressure. It is a member of the family of drugs called angiotensin II receptor blockers. The hormone angiotensin II makes the blood vessels constrict, causing blood pressure to rise. Teveten works by blocking the receptors that respond to this hormone. The drug may be prescribed alone or in combination with other medications that help lower blood pressure, such as water pills (diuretics) or calcium channel blockers.

Brand name:

Thalitone

Pronounced: THAL-i-tone
Generic name: Chlorthalidone

Thalitone is a diuretic (water pill) used to treat high blood pressure and fluid retention associated with congestive heart failure, cirrhosis of the liver (a disease of the liver caused by damage to its cells), corticosteroid and estrogen therapy, and kidney disease. When used for high blood pressure, Thalitone may be used alone or in combination with other high blood pressure medications. Diuretics rid the body of excess fluid by stiulating the production of urine. This tends to lower blood pressure.

Brand name:
Theo-24

See Theo-Dur, page 597.

Brand name:
Theochron

See Theo-Dur, page 597.

Brand name:
Theo-Dur

Pronounced: THEE-a-door
Generic name: Theophylline
Other brand names: Quibron-T/SR, Slo-bid, T-Phyl, Theo-24,
Theochron, Uni-Dur, Uniphyl

Theo-Dur, an oral bronchodilator medication, is given to treat symptoms
of asthma, chronic bronchitis, and emphysema. The active ingredient of
Theo-Dur, theophylline, is a chemical cousin of caffeine. It opens the
airways by relaxing the smooth muscle that circles the tubes and blood
vessels in the lungs.

Generic name:
Theophylline

See Theo-Dur, page 597.

Generic name:
Thyroid Hormones

See Armour Thyroid, page 395.

Brand name:
Tiazac

See Cardizem, page 416.

Brand name:

Ticlid

Pronounced: TIE-klid
Generic name: Ticlopidine hydrochloride

Ticlid makes the blood less likely to clot. It is prescribed to reduce the risk of stroke in people who have already suffered a stroke or had warning signs of stroke, and who either cannot take aspirin or fail to benefit from aspirin therapy.

Ticlid is also given, along with aspirin, to reduce the chances of a clot forming after a stent (a metal mesh tube) has been inserted in a coronary artery (a procedure used to keep the artery open and relieve the chest pain of angina).

Generic name:

Ticlopidine

See Ticlid, page 598.

Brand name:

Tigan

Pronounced: TIE-gan
Generic name: Trimethobenzamide hydrochloride

Tigan is prescribed to control nausea and vomiting.

Brand name:

Tilade

Pronounced: TILE-aid
Generic name: Nedocromil sodium

Tilade is an anti-inflammatory medication prescribed for use on a regular basis to control symptoms of mild to moderate asthma.

Generic name:

Timolol

See Timoptic, page 599.

Brand name:
Timoptic

Pronounced: Tim-OP-tic
Generic name: Timolol
Other brand names: Betimol, Timoptic-XE

Timoptic is an eyedrop that effectively reduces internal pressure in the eye. Timoptic is used in the treatment of open-angle glaucoma (potentially damaging chronic high pressure in the eye).

Generic name:
Tioconazole

See Vagistat-1, page 612.

Brand name:
Tobradex

Pronounced: TOE-bra-dex
Generic ingredients: Tobramycin, Dexamethasone

Tobradex combines a steroid drug, dexamethasone, and an antibiotic, tobramycin. It is prescribed to control inflammation and infection in the eye.

Generic name:
Tobramycin

See Tobrex, page 599.

Generic name:
Tobramycin and Dexamethasone

See Tobradex, page 599.

Brand name:
Tobrex

Pronounced: TOE-breks
Generic name: Tobramycin
Other brand name: Aktob

Tobrex is an antibiotic applied to the eye to treat bacterial infections.

Generic name:

Tocainide

See Tonocard, page 601.

Generic name:

Tolazamide

See Tolinase, page 600.

Generic name:

Tolbutamide

See Orinase, page 543.

Generic name:

Tolcapone

See Tasmar, page 590.

Brand name:

Tolectin

Pronounced: toe-LEK-tin
Generic name: Tolmetin sodium

Tolectin is a nonsteroidal anti-inflammatory drug used to relieve the inflammation, swelling, stiffness, and joint pain associated with rheumatoid arthritis and osteoarthritis (the most common form of arthritis). It is used for both acute episodes and long-term treatment. It is also used to treat juvenile rheumatoid arthritis.

Brand name:

Tolinase

Pronounced: TAHL-in-ace
Generic name: Tolazamide

Tolinase is an oral antidiabetic drug available in tablet form. It lowers the high blood sugar levels found in diabetics by stimulating the pancreas to release insulin, the hormone that helps transport sugar into the cells, where it is burned to produce energy. Tolinase may be given as a supplement to diet therapy to help control type 2 (non-insulin-dependent) diabetes.

There are two type of diabetes: type 1 (insulin-dependent) and type 2 (non-insulin-dependent). Type 1 diabetes usually requires insulin injection for life; type 2 can usually be controlled by dietary changes, exercise, and oral diabetes medications. Occasionally—during stressful periods or times of illness, or if oral medications fail to work—a type 2 diabetic may need insulin injections.

Generic name:
Tolmetin

See Tolectin, page 600.

Generic name:
Tolterodine

See Detrol, page 444.

Brand name:
Tonocard

Pronounced: TAH-nuh-card
Generic name: Tocainide hydrochloride

Tonocard is used to treat severe irregular heartbeat (arrhythmias). Arrhythmias are generally divided into two main types: heartbeats that are faster than normal (tachycardia), or heartbeats that are slower than normal (bradycardia). Irregular heartbeats are often caused by drugs or disease but can occur in otherwise healthy people with no history of heart disease or other illness. Tonocard works differently from other antiarrhythmic drugs, such as quinidine (Quinidex), procainamide (Procan SR), and disopyramide (Norpace). It is similar to lidocaine (Xylocaine) and is effective in treating severe ventricular arrhythmias (irregular heartbeats that occur in the main chambers of the heart).

Brand name:
Topamax

Pronounced: TOW-pah-macks
Generic name: Topiramate

Topamax is an antiepileptic drug, prescribed to control both the mild attacks known as partial seizures and the severe tonic-clonic convulsions known as grand mal seizures. It is typically added to the treatment regimen when other drugs fail to fully control a patient's attacks.

Brand name:

Topicort

Pronounced: TOP-i-court
Generic name: Desoximetasone

Topicort is a synthetic steroid medication in cream, gel, or ointment form that relieves the inflammation and itching caused by a variety of skin conditions.

Generic name:

Topiramate

See Topamax, page 601.

Brand name:

Toprol-XL

See Lopressor, page 502.

Brand name:

Toradol

Pronounced: TOH-rah-dol
Generic name: Ketorolac tromethamine

Toradol, a nonsteroidal anti-inflammatory drug, is used to relieve moderately severe, acute pain. It is prescribed for a limited amount of time (no more than 5 days), not for long-term therapy.

Generic name:

Toremifene

See Fareston, page 464.

Brand name:

T-Phyl

See Theo-Dur, page 597.

Generic name:

Tramadol

See Ultram, page 610.

Generic name:

Tramadol and Acetaminophen

See Ultracet, page 609.

Brand name:

Trandate

See Normodyne, page 538.

Generic name:

Trandolapril

See Mavik, page 508.

Generic name:

Trandolapril with Verapamil

See Tarka, page 590.

Brand name:

Transderm-Nitro

See Nitroglycerin, page 535.

Brand name:

Travatan

Pronounced: TRAV-a-tan
Generic name: Travoprost

Travatan is an eyedrop that reduces excessive pressure in the eye (often a result of the condition called open-angle glaucoma). Travatan works by promoting drainage of the fluid that fills the eye. It is usually prescribed when other remedies cannot be used or the other drugs have not been effective.

Generic name:

Travoprost

See Travatan, page 603.

Brand name:

Trental

Pronounced: TREN-tall
Generic name: Pentoxifylline

Trental is a medication that reduces the viscosity or "stickiness" of the blood, allowing it to flow more freely. It helps relieve the painful leg cramps caused by "intermittent claudication," a condition that results when hardening of the arteries reduces the leg muscles' blood supply.

Some doctors also prescribe Trental for dementia, strokes, circulatory and nerve problems caused by diabetes, and Raynaud's syndrome (a disorder of the blood vessels in which exposure to cold causes the fingers and toes to turn white). The drug is also used to treat impotence and to increase sperm motility in infertile men.

Generic name:

Tretinoin

See Retin-A and Renova, page 572.

Generic name:

Triamcinolone

See Azmacort, page 403.

Brand name:

Triaz

See Desquam-E, page 443.

Brand name:

Tricor

Pronounced: TRY-core
Generic name: Fenofibrate

Tricor combats high levels of cholesterol and triglycerides. It works by promoting the dissolution and elimination of fat particles in the blood.

Tricor is usually added to a treatment regimen only when other measures have failed to produce adequate results. Often, diet and exercise are enough to bring blood fats under control. Likewise, it's sometimes sufficient to simply treat an underlying problem such as diabetes, underactive thyroid, kidney disease, liver dysfunction, or alcoholism. And in some cases, just discontinuing a medication is enough to do the job. For instance, certain water pills and "beta-blocker" heart medications are capable of causing a massive increase in triglyceride levels. Estrogen replacement therapy is another potential culprit.

Whatever the other treatment measures may be, it's important to remember that Tricor is intended to supplement them, rather than replace them outright. To get the full benefit of the medication, patients need to stick to the diet, exercise program, and other treatments the doctor prescribes. All these efforts to keep cholesterol and triglyceride levels normal are important because together they may lower the risk of heart disease.

Brand name:

Tridesilon

Pronounced: tri-DESS-ill-on
Generic name: Desonide
Other brand name: DesOwen

Tridesilon is a steroid preparation that relieves the itching and inflammation of a variety of skin problems. It is applied directly to the skin.

Generic name:

Trihexyphenidyl

See Artane, page 395.

Brand name:

Trileptal

Pronounced: tri-LEP-tal
Generic name: Oxcarbazepine

Trileptal helps reduce the frequency of partial epileptic seizures, a form of epilepsy in which neural disturbances are limited to a specific region of the brain and the victim remains conscious throughout the attack. Trileptal may be prescribed by itself to treat the problem in adults. It can also be used in combination with other seizure medications in adults and in children as young as four years old.

Brand name:

Trilisate

Pronounced: TRILL-ih-sate
Generic name: Choline magnesium trisalicylate

Trilisate, a nonsteroidal, anti-inflammatory medication, is prescribed for the relief of the signs and symptoms of rheumatoid arthritis (chronic joint inflammation disease), osteoarthritis (degenerative joint disease), and other forms of arthritis. This drug is used in the long-term management of these diseases and especially for flare-ups of severe rheumatoid arthritis.

Trilisate may also be prescribed for the treatment of acute painful shoulder, for mild to moderate pain in general, and for fever.

In children, this medication is prescribed for severe conditions—such as juvenile rheumatoid arthritis—that require relief of pain and inflammation.

Generic name:

Trimethobenzamide

See Tigan, page 598.

Generic name:

Trimethoprim with Sulfamethoxazole

See Bactrim, page 404.

Brand name:

Trimox

See Amoxil, page 391.

Brand name:
Trinalin

Pronounced: TRIN-uh-lin
Generic ingredients: Azatadine maleate, Pseudoephedrine sulfate
Other brand name: Rynatan

Trinalin and Rynatan are long-acting antihistamine/decongestants that relieve nasal stuffiness and middle ear congestion caused by hay fever and ongoing nasal inflammation. They can be used alone or with antibiotics and analgesics such as aspirin or acetaminophen. Azatadine, the antihistamine in these products, reduces itching and swelling and dries up secretions from the nose, eyes, and throat. Pseudoephedrine, the decongestant, reduces nasal congestion and makes breathing easier.

Brand name:
Tri-Norinyl

See Oral Contraceptives, page 542.

Brand name:
Triphasil

See Oral Contraceptives, page 542.

Brand name:
Triple Sulfa

Pronounced: SUL-fuh
Generic ingredients: Sulfathiazole, Sulfacetamide, Sulfabenzamide

Triple Sulfa vaginal cream is used to treat bacterial vaginitis (bacteria-caused inflammation of the vagina with a gray or yellow discharge like a thin flour paste and a fishy odor). Because it is effective only against one type of bacteria, the doctor may run tests before prescribing this medication.

Brand name:
Trivora

See Oral Contraceptives, page 542.

Brand name:

Trizivir

Pronounced: TRY-zuh-vir
Generic ingredients: Abacavir, Lamivudine, Zidovudine

Trizivir combines three drugs used to fight HIV, the deadly virus that undermines the immune system, leaving the body ever more vulnerable to infection, and eventually leading to AIDS. The components of Trizivir are all members of the category of HIV drugs known as nucleoside analogs:

Abacavir (also called Ziagen)
Lamivudine (also called Epivir or 3TC)
Zidovudine (also called Retrovir, AZT, or ZDV)

Trizivir may be prescribed alone or in combination with other HIV drugs. It reduces the amount of HIV in the bloodstream, but does not completely cure the disease. Patients may still develop the rare infections and other complications that accompany HIV. Remember, too, that Trizivir does not reduce the risk of transmitting the virus to others.

Brand name:

Trusopt

Pronounced: TRU-sopt
Generic name: Dorzolamide hydrochloride

Trusopt eye drops are prescribed for the treatment of the excessive pressure in the eyeball known as open-angle glaucoma.

Brand name:

T-Stat

See Erythromycin, Topical, page 460.

Brand name:

Tussionex

Pronounced: TUSS-ee-uh-nex
Generic ingredients: Hydrocodone polistirex, Chlorpheniramine polistirex

Tussionex Extended-Release Suspension is a cough-suppressant/antihistamine combination used to relieve coughs and the upper respiratory symptoms of colds and allergies. Hydrocodone, a mild narcotic similar to codeine, is believed to work directly on the cough center. Chlorpheniramine, an antihistamine, reduces itching and swelling and dries up secretions from the eyes, nose, and throat.

Brand name:
Tussi-Organidin NR

Pronounced: TUSS-ee or-GAN-i-din
Generic ingredients: Guaifenesin, Codeine phosphate
Other brand name: Brontex

Tussi-Organidin NR is used to relieve coughs and chest congestion in adults and children. It contains guaifenesin, which helps thin and loosen mucus in the lungs, making it easier to cough up. It also contains a cough suppressant, the narcotic codeine.

Brand name:
Tylenol with Codeine

Pronounced: TIE-len-awl with CO-deen
Generic ingredients: Acetaminophen, Codeine phosphate
Other brand name: Phenaphen with Codeine

Tylenol with Codeine, a narcotic analgesic, is used to treat mild to moderately severe pain. It contains two drugs—acetaminophen and codeine. Acetaminophen, an antipyretic (fever-reducing) analgesic, is used to reduce pain and fever. Codeine, a narcotic analgesic, relieves moderate to severe pain.

People who are allergic to aspirin can take Tylenol with Codeine.

Brand name:
Tylox

See Percocet, page 550.

Brand name:
Ultracet

Pronounced: UL-tra-set
Generic ingredients: Tramadol hydrochloride, Acetaminophen

Ultracet is used to treat moderate to severe pain for a period of five days or less. It contains two pain-relieving agents. Tramadol, known techni-cally as an opioid analgesic, is a narcotic pain reliever. Acetaminophen is the active ingredient in the over-the-counter pain remedy Tylenol.

Brand name:

Ultram

Pronounced: UL-tram
Generic name: Tramadol hydrochloride

Ultram, known technically as an opioid analgesic, is a narcotic painkiller. It is prescribed to relieve moderate to moderately severe pain.

Brand name:

Ultrase

See Pancrease, page 547.

Brand name:

Uni-Dur

See Theo-Dur, page 597.

Brand name:

Uniphyl

See Theo-Dur, page 597.

Brand name:

Uniretic

Pronounced: you-nih-RET-ick
Generic ingredients: Moexipril hydrochloride, Hydrochlorothiazide

Uniretic combines two types of blood pressure medication. The first, moexipril hydrochloride, is an ACE (angiotensin-converting enzyme) inhibitor. It works by preventing a chemical in the blood called angiotensin I from converting into a more potent form (angiotensin II) that increases salt and water retention in the body and causes the blood vessels to constrict—two actions that tend to increase blood pressure.

To aid in clearing excess water from the body, Uniretic also contains hydrochlorothiazide, a diuretic that promotes production of urine. Diuretics often wash too much potassium out of the body along with the water. However, the ACE inhibitor part of Uniretic tends to keep potassium in the body, thereby canceling this unwanted effect.

Uniretic is not used for the initial treatment of high blood pressure. It is saved for later use, when a single blood pressure medication is not sufficient for the job.

Brand name:
Unithroid

See Synthroid, page 588.

Brand name:
Univasc

Pronounced: YOO-ni-vask
Generic name: Moexipril hydrochloride

Univasc is used in the treatment of high blood pressure. It is effective when used alone or with thiazide diuretics that help rid the body of excess water. Univasc belongs to a family of drugs called angiotensin-converting enzyme (ACE) inhibitors. It works by preventing the transformation of a hormone in the blood called angiotensin I into a more potent substance that increases salt and water retention in the body and causes the blood vessels to constrict—two actions that tend to increase blood pressure.

Brand name:
Urised

Pronounced: YOUR-i-said
Generic ingredients: Methenamine, Methylene blue, Phenyl salicylate, Benzoic acid, Atropine sulfate, Hyoscyamine

Urised relieves lower urinary tract discomfort caused by inflammation or diagnostic procedures. It is used to treat urinary tract infections including cystitis (inflammation of the bladder and ureters), urethritis (inflammation of the urethra), and trigonitis (inflammation of the mucous membrane of the bladder). Methenamine, the major component of this drug, acts as a mild antiseptic by changing into formaldehyde in the urinary tract when it comes in contact with acidic urine.

Brand name:

Urispas

Pronounced: YOUR-eh-spaz
Generic name: Flavoxate hydrochloride

Urispas prevents spasms in the urinary tract and relieves the painful or difficult urination, urinary urgency, excessive nighttime urination, pubic area pain, frequency of urination, and inability to hold urine caused by urinary tract infections. Urispas is taken in combination with antibiotics to treat the infection.

Generic name:

Urofollitropin

See Fertinex, page 466.

Generic name:

Ursodiol

See Actigall, page 381.

Brand name:

Urso

See Actigall, page 381.

Brand name:

Vagistat-1

Pronounced: VAG-i-stat
Generic name: Tioconazole

Vagistat-1 ointment is used to treat repeated bouts of vaginal yeast infection (candidiasis of the vagina). Symptoms include irritation and discharge. Women experiencing these symptoms for the first time should see their doctor to make certain the problem is yeast. If they've had them before, they can use this over-the-counter medication without another trip to the doctor.

Generic name:
Valacyclovir

See *Valtrex, page 614.*

Brand name:
Valcyte

Pronounced: VAL-site
Generic name: Valganciclovir

Valcyte tablets are used in the treatment of an eye disease called cytomegalovirus (CMV) retinitis, one of the many infections that take hold when the immune system is undermined by AIDS. Valcyte is very similar to the CMV medication Cytovene (ganciclovir).

Generic name:
Valdecoxib

See *Bextra, page 408.*

Generic name:
Valganciclovir

See *Valcyte, page 613.*

Generic name:
Valproic acid

See *Depakene, page 442.*

Generic name:
Valsartan

See *Diovan, page 449.*

Brand name:

Valtrex

Pronounced: VAL-trex
Generic name: Valacyclovir hydrochloride

Valtrex is used to treat herpes zoster, (the painful rash known as shingles). It is also prescribed to relieve the sores caused by genital herpes.

Brand name:

Vancenase

See Beclomethasone, page 404.

Brand name:

Vanceril

See Beclomethasone, page 404.

Brand name:

Vascor

Pronounced: VAS-core
Generic name: Bepridil hydrochloride

Vascor, a type of medication called a calcium channel blocker, is prescribed for the treatment of chronic stable angina (severe chest pain, often accompanied by a feeling of choking, brought on by exertion). Vascor is effective used alone or in combination with beta-blocking drugs and/or nitrates. Calcium channel blockers slow down the passage of nerve impulses through the heart and blood vessels. This slows the heartbeat and dilates the blood vessels to reduce blood pressure—actions that ease the workload on the heart and help prevent angina pain.

Brand name:

Vaseretic

Pronounced: Vaz-err-ET-ik
Generic ingredients: Enalapril maleate, Hydrochlorothiazide

Vaseretic is used in the treatment of high blood pressure. It combines an ACE inhibitor with a thiazide diuretic. Enalapril, the ACE inhibitor, works by preventing a chemical in the blood called angiotensin I from converting into a more potent form that increases salt and water retention in the body and constricts the blood vessels—actions that tend to increase blood pressure. Hydrochlorothiazide, a diuretic, rids the body of excess fluid by promoting the production of urine, which also helps in lowering blood pressure.

Brand name:

Vasotec

Pronounced: VAZ-oh-tek
Generic name: Enalapril maleate

Vasotec is a high blood pressure medication known as an ACE inhibitor. It works by preventing a chemical in the blood called angiotensin I from converting into a more potent form that increases salt and water retention in the body and constricts the blood vessels—actions that tend to increase blood pressure. It is effective when used alone or in combination with other medications, especially thiazide-type diuretics. It is also used in the treatment of congestive heart failure, usually in combination with diuretics and digitalis, and is prescribed as a preventive measure in certain conditions that could lead to heart failure.

Brand name:

Veetids

See Penicillin V Potassium, page 549.

Brand name:

Velosef

Pronounced: VELL-oh-seff
Generic name: Cephradine

Velosef, a broad-spectrum cephalosporin antibiotic available in capsule or liquid form, is similar to penicillin. Velosef is given to treat certain infections of the upper or lower respiratory tract, including pharyngitis (strep throat) and pneumonia, as well as middle ear, skin, or urinary tract infections.

Brand name:

Velosulin BR

See Insulin, page 486.

Brand name:

Ventolin HFA

See Proventil, page 567.

Generic name:

Verapamil

See Calan, page 412.

Brand name:

Verelan

See Calan, page 412.

Brand name:

Viagra

Pronounced: vye-AG-ruh
Generic name: Sildenafil citrate

Viagra is the first oral drug for male impotence. It works by dilating blood vessels in the penis, allowing the inflow of blood needed for an erection.

Brand name:

Vibramycin

See Doryx, page 452.

Brand name:

Vibra-Tabs

See Doryx, page 452.

Brand name:
Vicodin

Pronounced: VY-koe-din
Generic ingredients: Hydrocodone bitartrate, Acetaminophen
Other brand names: Anexsia, Co-Gesic, Hydrocet, Lorcet, Lortab,
Maxidone, Norco, Zydone

Vicodin combines a narcotic analgesic (painkiller) and cough reliever with a non-narcotic analgesic for the relief of moderate to moderately severe pain.

Brand name:
Vicoprofen

Pronounced: VY-koe-pro-fen
Generic ingredients: Hydrocodone bitartrate, Ibuprofen

Vicoprofen is a chemical cousin of the well-known painkiller Vicodin. Both products contain the prescription pain medication hydrocodone. However, while Vicodin also includes acetaminophen (the active ingredient in Tylenol), Vicoprofen replaces it with ibuprofen (the active ingredient in Advil).

Vicoprofen relieves acute pain. It is generally prescribed for less than 10 days, and cannot be used in the long-term treatment of osteoarthritis or rheumatoid arthritis.

Brand name:
Videx

Pronounced: VIE-decks
Generic name: Didanosine

Videx is one of the drugs used to fight the human immunodeficiency virus (HIV)—the deadly cause of AIDS. Over a period of years, HIV slowly destroys the immune system, leaving the body defenseless against infection. Videx disrupts reproduction of HIV, thereby staving off the immune system's collapse.

Signs and symptoms of advanced HIV infection include diarrhea, fever, headache, infections, problems with the nervous system, rash, sore throat, and significant weight loss.

Brand name:

Viokase

See Pancrease, page 547.

Brand name:

Vioxx

Pronounced: VYE-ox
Generic name: Rofecoxib

Vioxx is a new kind of painkiller used in the treatment of osteoarthritis, painful menstruation (dysmenorrhea), and other types of acute pain. It is a member of the family of nonsteroidal anti-inflammatory drugs (NSAIDs) called "COX-2 inhibitors." Other drugs in this family include Celebrex and Bextra.

Like older NSAIDs such as aspirin, Motrin, and Naprosyn, these newer drugs are believed to fight pain and inflammation by inhibiting the effect of a natural enzyme called COX-2. Unlike the older medications, however, the newer drugs do not interfere with a similar substance, called COX-1, which exerts a protective effect on the lining of the stomach. The COX-2 inhibitors are therefore less likely to cause the bleeding and ulcers that sometimes accompany sustained use of the older NSAIDs.

Although COX-2 inhibitors offer many of the same benefits as aspirin, they do not share its blood-thinning effects. People taking low-dose aspirin to reduce the risk of a heart attack will need to continue taking it in addition to Vioxx.

Brand name:

Viracept

Pronounced: VYE-ruh-sept
Generic name: Nelfinavir mesylate

Viracept is one of the drugs prescribed to fight HIV, the human immunodeficiency virus that causes AIDS (acquired immune deficiency syndrome). Once inside the body, HIV spreads through certain key cells in the immune system, weakening the body's ability to fight off other infections. Viracept works by interfering with an important step in the virus's reproductive cycle. This slows the spread of the virus and prolongs the strength of the immune system.

Viracept belongs to the new class of drugs that has successfully reversed the course of HIV infection in many people. Called protease inhibitors, these drugs work better when used in combination with other HIV medications called nucleoside analogues (Retrovir, Hivid, and others) that act against the virus in other ways.

Brand name:

Viramune

Pronounced: VIE-ruh-mewn
Generic name: Nevirapine

Viramune is prescribed for advanced cases of HIV. HIV—the human immunodeficiency virus that causes AIDS—undermines the immune system over a period of years, eventually leaving the body defenseless against infection. Viramune is generally prescribed only after the immune system has declined and infections have begun to appear. It is always taken with at least one other HIV medication such as Retrovir or Videx. If taken alone, it can cause the virus to become resistant. Even if used properly, it may be effective for only a limited time.

Like other drugs for HIV, Viramune works by impairing the virus's ability to multiply.

Brand name:

Viread

Pronounced: VEER-ee-ad
Generic name: Tenofovir disoproxil fumarate

Viread is one of the drugs prescribed to fight HIV, the human immuno-deficiency virus that causes AIDS (acquired immune deficiency syndrome). HIV attacks the immune system, slowly destroying the body's ability to fight off infection. Viread staves off the attack by interfering with HIV reverse transcriptase, an enzyme the virus needs to reproduce.

Viread lowers the amount of HIV in the blood and may help increase the number of T cells, important agents of the immune system that kill microscopic foreign invaders. It is used in combination with other anti-HIV drugs when these drugs are not effective by themselves.

Generic name:

Vitamins, Prenatal

See Stuartnatal Plus, page 584.

Brand name:

Vivelle

See Estrogen Patches, page 462.

Brand name:

Volmax

See Proventil, page 567.

Brand name:

Voltaren

Pronounced: vol-TAR-en
Generic name: Diclofenac sodium
Other brand name: Cataflam (Diclofenac potassium)

Voltaren and Cataflam are nonsteroidal anti-inflammatory drugs used to relieve the inflammation, swelling, stiffness, and joint pain associated with rheumatoid arthritis, osteoarthritis (the most common form of arthritis), and ankylosing spondylitis (arthritis and stiffness of the spine). Voltaren-XR, the extended-release form of Voltaren, is used only for long-term treatment. Cataflam is also prescribed for immediate relief of pain and menstrual discomfort.

Brand name:

VoSoL HC

Pronounced: VOE-sol
Generic ingredients: Acetic acid and hydrocortisone

VoSoL HC is prescribed for infection and inflammation of the external ear canal.

Generic name:

Warfarin

See Coumadin, page 433.

Brand name:
WelChol

Pronounced: WELL-call
Generic name: Colesevelam

WelChol is used to lower blood cholesterol levels when diet and exercise prove insufficient. It works by binding with cholesterol-based bile acids to take them out of circulation. This prompts the liver to produce a replacement supply of bile acids, drawing the extra cholesterol it needs out of the bloodstream.

WelChol is sometimes prescribed along with one of the popular "statin" drugs that fight cholesterol in a different way. Among these drugs are Lescol, Lipitor, Mevacor, Pravachol, and Zocor.

Brand name:
Wymox

See Amoxil, page 391.

Brand name:
Xalatan

Pronounced: ZAL-a-tan
Generic name: Latanoprost

Xalatan is used to relieve high pressure within the eye (a hallmark of the condition known as open-angle glaucoma). Xalatan usually is prescribed when other medications have failed to do the job or have caused other problems.

Brand name:
Xenical

Pronounced: ZEN-eh-kal
Generic name: Orlistat

Xenical blocks absorption of dietary fat into the bloodstream, thereby reducing the number of calories obtained from a meal. At the usual dosage level, it cuts fat absorption by almost one-third. Combined with a low-calorie diet, it is used to promote weight loss and discourage the return of unwanted pounds.

The drug is prescribed for the frankly obese and for merely over-weight people who have other health problems such as high blood pressure, diabetes, or high cholesterol levels. Weight status is determined by the body mass index (BMI), a comparison of height to weight.

Brand name:
Xopenex

Pronounced: ZOH-pen-ecks
Generic name: Levalbuterol hydrochloride

Xopenex is a "bronchodilator." It works by relaxing the muscles in the walls of the lungs' many tiny airways (bronchioles), allowing them to expand so patients can get more air. It is prescribed for asthma.

Brand name:
Yasmin

See Oral Contraceptives, page 542.

Brand name:
Yocon

Pronounced: YOE-kon
Generic name: Yohimbine hydrochloride
Other brand name: Yohimex

Yocon is used in the treatment of male impotence. The drug is thought to work by stimulating the release of norepinephrine, one of the body's natural chemical regulators. This results in increased blood flow to the penis.

Generic name:
Yohimbine

See Yocon, page 622.

Brand name:
Yohimex

See Yocon, page 622.

Brand name:

Zaditor

Pronounced: ZA-di-tor
Generic name: Ketotifen fumarate

Zaditor combats the release of chemicals that trigger allergic reactions. Available in eyedrop form, it works within minutes to relieve the itchy eyes brought on by allergies.

Generic name:

Zafirlukast

See Accolate, page 377.

Generic name:

Zalcitabine

See Hivid, page 480.

Generic name:

Zanamivir

See Relenza, page 571.

Brand name:

Zantac

Pronounced: ZAN-tac
Generic name: Ranitidine hydrochloride

Zantac is prescribed for the short-term treatment (4 to 8 weeks) of active duodenal ulcer (near the exit from the stomach) and active benign gastric ulcer (in the stomach itself), and as maintenance therapy for gastric or duodenal ulcer, at a reduced dosage, after the ulcer has healed. It is also used for the treatment of conditions in which the stomach produces too much acid, such as Zollinger-Ellison syndrome and systemic mastocytosis, for gastroesophageal reflux disease (backflow of acid stomach contents into the entry to the stomach) and for healing—and maintaining healing of—erosive esophagitis (severe inflammation of the esophagus).

Some doctors prescribe Zantac to prevent damage to the stomach and duodenum from long-term use of nonsteroidal anti-inflammatory drugs such as Indocin and Motrin, and to treat bleeding of the stomach and intestine. Zantac is also sometimes prescribed for stress-induced ulcers.

Brand name:

Zaroxolyn

Pronounced: Zar-OX-uh-lin
Generic name: Metolazone
Other brand name: Mykrox

Zaroxolyn is a diuretic used in the treatment of high blood pressure and other conditions that require the elimination of excess fluid from the body. These conditions include congestive heart failure and kidney disease. When used for high blood pressure, Zaroxolyn can be used alone or with other high blood pressure medications. Diuretics prompt the body to produce and eliminate more urine, which helps lower blood pressure.

Brand name:

Zerit

Pronounced: ZAIR-it
Generic name: Stavudine

Zerit is one of the drugs used to fight the human immunodeficiency virus (HIV)—the deadly cause of AIDS. It is usually prescribed for people who have already been taking the HIV drug Retrovir for an extended period. HIV attacks the immune system, slowly destroying the body's ability to fight off infection. Zerit helps stave off the attack by disrupting the virus's ability to reproduce.

Signs and symptoms of HIV infection include diarrhea, fever, headache, infections, problems with the nervous system, rash, sore throat, and significant weight loss.

Brand name:

Zestoretic

Pronounced: zest-or-ET-ik
Generic ingredients: Lisinopril, Hydrochlorothiazide
Other brand name: Prinzide

Zestoretic is used in the treatment of high blood pressure. It combines an ACE inhibitor drug with a diuretic. Lisinopril, the ACE inhibitor, works by limiting production of a substance that promotes salt and water retention in the body. Hydrochlorothiazide, a diuretic, prompts the body to produce and eliminate more urine, which helps in lowering blood pressure. Combination products such as Zestoretic are usually not prescribed until therapy is already under way.

Brand name:
Zestril

Pronounced: ZEST-rill
Generic name: Lisinopril
Other brand name: Prinivil

Lisinopril is used in the treatment of high blood pressure. It is effective when used alone or when combined with other high blood pressure medications. It may also be used with other medications in the treatment of heart failure, and may be given within 24 hours of a heart attack to improve chances of survival.

Lisinopril is a type of drug called an ACE inhibitor. It works by reducing production of a substance that increases salt and water retention in the body.

Brand name:
Ziagen

Pronounced: ZYE-a-jen
Generic name: Abacavir sulfate

Ziagen helps to halt the inroads of the human immunodeficiency virus (HIV). Without treatment, HIV gradually undermines the body's immune system, encouraging other infections to take hold until the body succumbs to full-blown acquired immune deficiency syndrome (AIDS).

Like other anti-HIV drugs, Ziagen holds back the advance of the virus by disrupting its reproductive cycle. This medication is used only as part of a "drug cocktail" that attacks the virus on several fronts. It is not prescribed alone.

Generic name:
Zidovudine

See Retrovir, page 572.

Generic name:
Zileuton

See Zyflo, page 629.

Brand name:
Zithromax

Pronounced: ZITH-roh-macks
Generic name: Azithromycin

Zithromax is an antibiotic related to erythromycin. For adults, it is prescribed to treat certain mild to moderate skin infections; upper and lower respiratory tract infections, including pharyngitis (strep throat), tonsillitis, and pneumonia; sexually transmitted infections of the cervix or urinary tract; and genital ulcer disease in men. In children, Zithromax is used to treat middle ear infection, pneumonia, tonsillitis, and strep throat.

Brand name:
Zocor

Pronounced: ZOH-core
Generic name: Simvastatin

Zocor is a cholesterol-lowering drug. Doctors prescribe Zocor in addition to a cholesterol-lowering diet when blood cholesterol levels are too high and a patient has been unable to lower it by diet alone.

In people with high cholesterol and heart disease, Zocor reduces the risk of heart attack, stroke and "mini-stroke" (transient ischemic attack) and can stave off the need for bypass surgery or angioplasty to clear clogged arteries.

Brand name:
Zofran

Pronounced: ZOH-fran
Generic name: Ondansetron hydrochloride
Other brand name: Zofran ODT

Zofran is used for the prevention of nausea and vomiting caused by radiation therapy and chemotherapy for cancer. In some cases, it is also used to prevent these problems following surgery.

Brand name:
Zoladex

Pronounced: ZO-luh-dex
Generic name: Goserelin acetate

Zoladex relieves the symptoms of advanced prostate cancer in men and advanced breast cancer in premenopausal women. In combination with other forms of therapy, it is also prescribed during treatment of early prostate cancer.

In addition, it can be used in the treatment of endometriosis, a condition in which tissue from the lining of the uterus invades the abdomen. If a woman is scheduled for surgical removal of the lining, the drug may be used to thin the lining prior to the operation.

Zoladex works by reducing levels of testosterone in men and estrogen in women. These hormones can encourage the growth of certain cancers.

Generic name:
Zolmitriptan

See Zomig, page 627.

Brand name:
Zomig

Pronounced: ZOE-mig
Generic name: Zolmitriptan

Zomig relieves migraine headaches. It's effective whether or not the headache is preceded by an aura (visual disturbances such as halos and flickering lights). For most people Zomig provides relief within 2 hours, but it will not abort an attack or reduce the number of headaches experienced.

Migraines are thought to be caused by expansion and inflammation of blood vessels in the head. Zomig ends a migraine attack by constricting these blood vessels and reducing inflammation.

Brand name:
Zonegran

Pronounced: ZAH-nah-gran
Generic name: Zonisamide

Zonegran helps reduce the frequency of partial epileptic seizures, a form of epilepsy in which neural disturbances are limited to a specific region of the brain and the victim remains conscious throughout the attack. The drug is used in combination with other antiseizure medications, not by itself.

Generic name:

Zonisamide

See Zonegran, page 627.

Brand name:

Zovia

See Oral Contraceptives, page 542.

Brand name:

Zovirax

Pronounced: zoh-VIGH-racks
Generic name: Acyclovir

Zovirax liquid, capsules, and tablets, are used in the treatment of certain infections with herpesviruses. These include genital herpes, shingles, and chickenpox. This drug may not be appropriate for everyone, and its use should be thoroughly discussed with the doctor.

In ointment form, Zovirax is used to treat initial episodes of genital herpes and certain herpes simplex infections of the skin and mucous membranes.

Some doctors use Zovirax, along with other drugs, in the treatment of AIDS, and for unusual herpes infections such as those following kidney and bone marrow transplants.

Brand name:

Zyban

Pronounced: ZIGH-ban
Generic name: Bupropion hydrochloride

Zyban is a nicotine-free quit-smoking aid. Instead, Zyban has the same active ingredient as the antidepressant medication Wellbutrin. It works by boosting the levels of several chemical messengers in the brain. With more of these chemicals at work, patients experience a reduction in nicotine withdrawal symptoms and a weakening of the urge to smoke. More than a third of the people who take Zyban while participating in a support program are able to quit smoking for at least 1 month. Zyban can also prove helpful when people with conditions such as chronic bronchitis and emphysema decide it's time to quit.

Brand name:

Zydone

See Vicodin, page 617.

Brand name:

Zyflo

Pronounced: ZIGH-flow
Generic name: Zileuton

Zyflo tablets prevent and relieve the symptoms of chronic asthma. The drug works by relaxing the muscles in the walls of the airways, allowing them to open wider, and by reducing inflammation, swelling, and mucus secretion in the lungs.

Brand name:

Zyloprim

Pronounced: ZYE-loe-prim
Generic name: Allopurinol

Zyloprim is used in the treatment of many symptoms of gout, including acute attacks, tophi (collection of uric acid crystals in the tissues, especially around joints), joint destruction, and uric acid stones. Gout is a form of arthritis characterized by increased blood levels of uric acid. Zyloprim works by reducing uric acid production in the body, thus preventing crystals from forming.

Zyloprim is also used to manage increased uric acid levels in the blood of people with certain cancers, such as leukemia. It is also prescribed to manage some types of kidney stones.

Brand name:

Zyrtec

Pronounced: ZEER-tek
Generic name: Cetirizine hydrochloride

Zyrtec is an antihistamine. It is prescribed to treat the sneezing; itchy; runny nose; and itchy, red, watery eyes caused by seasonal allergies such as hay fever. Zyrtec also relieves the symptoms of year-round allergies due to dust, mold, and animal dander. This medication is also used in the treatment of chronic itchy skin and hives.

Brand name:

Zyrtec-D

Pronounced: ZEER-tek
Generic ingredients: Cetirizine hydrochloride, Pseudoephedrine hydrochloride

Zyrtec-D contains the same antihistamine found in regular Zyrtec, plus the decongestant pseudoephedrine. The drug is prescribed to relieve the symptoms of hay fever and similar allergies, whether seasonal or year-round.

Brand name:

Zyvox

Pronounced: ZIGH-vox
Generic name: Linezolid

Zyvox is a member of a new class of antibiotics called oxazolidinones. It is used to treat certain types of pneumonia, some forms of skin infection, and infections involving certain strains of a germ called Enterococcus faecium.

Mental and Emotional Side Effects

It's an unfortunate fact that psychological symptoms are sometimes the result of medications prescribed for an entirely unrelated purpose. These unwanted side effects can confound diagnosis and complicate therapy, leading to additional—perhaps unnecessary—medication. Part 1 of this section lists alphabetically some 175 mental and emotional symptoms and the drugs that can cause them. (For example, you will see here a list of all the drugs that can trigger or exacerbate depression.) Part 2 lists alphabetically the potential psychological side effects of each drug (for example, all the symptoms that can be caused by the antibiotic Cipro).

The information in this section is extracted from the Side Effects Index of *Physicians' Desk Reference*®, a compilation of all adverse events reported in official product labeling as published in *PDR*. The reported incidence of the side effect for each drug is shown in parentheses following the entry. Side effects known to occur in 3 percent of patients or more are marked with a ▲ symbol. Entries are limited to reactions that may be expected to occur at recommended dosage levels in the general patient population. Effects of overdose are not included.

Part 1.
Side Effects by Symptom

Aggression

Advair Diskus
Ambien Tablets (Rare)
Amerge Tablets (Rare)
Aricept Tablets (Frequent)
Celexa (Infrequent)
Celontin Capsules
Claritin-D 12 Hour (Less frequent)
Claritin-D 24 Hour (Fewer than 2%)
Crinone 4% Gel (Less than 5%)
Crinone 8% Gel (Less than 5%)
Depacon Injection
Depakene
Depakote ER Tablets
Depakote Sprinkle Capsules
Depakote Tablets
Evoxac Capsules
▲ Exelon (3%)
Felbatol (Frequent)
Flexeril Tablets
Flovent Diskus
Flovent Inhalation Aerosol
Flovent Rotadisk
Floxin
Foscavir Injection (Between 1% and 5%)
Genotropin Lyophilized Powder
Halcion Tablets
Imitrex Injection
Imitrex Tablets (Rare)
Intron A for Injection (Less than 5%)
Klonopin Tablets (Infrequent)
Levaquin (Less than 5%)
Neurontin
Priftin Tablets (Less than 1%)
Prilosec (Less than 1%)
Pulmicort Respules (Less than 1%)
Pulmicort Turbuhaler Powder (Rare)
Requip Tablets (Infrequent)
Rhinocort Nasal Inhaler (Rare)
Risperdal (1% to 3%)
Symmetrel
Topamax (2.7% to 4%)
Trileptal
Ventolin Inhalation Aerosol (1%)
Versed Syrup (Less than 1%)
Xanax Tablets (Rare)
Zarontin
Zoloft (Infrequent)

Zosyn (1.0% or less)

Agitation

AcipHex Tablets (Rare)
Actiq (Less than 1%)
Advair Diskus
Aggrenox Capsules (Less than 1%)
Akineton
Allegra-D (1.9%)
Aloprim for Injection (Less than 1%)
Ambien Tablets (Infrequent)
AmBisome for Injection (Less common)
Amerge Tablets (Rare)
Amoxil (Rare)
Amphotec (1% to 5%)
Anzemet (Infrequent)
Aricept Tablets
Artane
Ativan Injection (Infrequent)
Ativan Tablets (Less frequent)
Augmentin (Rare)
Betaseron
Bicillin L-A
Bontril
Brevibloc Injection (About 2%)
Buprenex Injectable (Rare)
Carbatrol Capsules
Cardura Tablets (0.5% to 1%)
Catapres Tablets (About 3 in 100 patients)
Catapres-TTS (0.5% or less)
Cedax Oral Suspension (0.1% to 1%)
▲ Celexa (3%)
▲ CellCept (3% to 10%)
▲ Cerebyx Injection (3.3% to 9.5%)
Cipro
Cipro I.V.
Claritin (At least one patient)
Claritin-D 12 Hour (Less frequent)
Claritin-D 24 Hour (Fewer than 2%)
Clorpres Tablets (About 3%)
▲ Clozaril Tablets (4%)
▲ Cognex Capsules (7%)
Combipres Tablets (About 3%)
Compazine
Comtan Tablets (1%)
Comvax
▲ Copaxone (4%)
Crixivan Capsules (Less than 2%)

Cuprimine Capsules
Demerol
Depacon Injection (1% or more)
Depakene (1% or more)
Depakote ER Tablets
(Greater than 1%)
Depakote Sprinkle Capsules
Depakote Tablets (1% to 5%)
Dexedrine
Dilaudid Oral Liquid (Less frequent)
Dilaudid Tablets - 8 mg
(Less frequent)
Dilaudid-HP (Less frequent)
Diprivan (Less than 1%)
Dolophine Tablets
Donnatal (In elderly patients)
▲ Duraclon Injection (3%)
Duragesic Transdermal System (1% or
greater)
Ecotrin Enteric Coated Aspirin
▲ Effexor Tablets (2% to 4.5%)
▲ Effexor XR Capsules (3%)
Eldepryl Capsules
Elspar for Injection (No incidence
data in labeling)
Engerix-B Vaccine (Less than 1%)
Evoxac Capsules (Less than 1%)
Exelon (2% or more)
Famotidine Injection (Infrequent)
Felbatol (Frequent)
Ferrlecit Injection (Greater than 1%)
Flexeril Tablets (Less than 1%)
▲ Flolan for Injection (11%)
Flovent Diskus
Flovent Inhalation Aerosol
Flovent Rotadisk
Floxin
Fludara for Injection
Flumadine (0.3% to 1%)
Fortovase Capsules (Less than 2%)
Foscavir Injection
(Between 1% and 5%)
Gabitril Tablets (1%)
Geodon Capsules (Frequent)
Halcion Tablets
Haldol
Haldol Decanoate
Hivid Tablets (Less than 1%)
Imitrex Injection (Infrequent)
Imitrex Nasal Spray (Infrequent)
Imitrex Tablets (Up to 2%)
▲ Indapamide Tablets (Greater than or
equal to 5%)
▲ Infergen (4% to 6%)

Intron A for Injection (Less than 5%)
Invirase Capsules (Less than 2%)
Ismo Tablets (Fewer than 1%)
Kadian Capsules (Less than 3%)
Kaletra (Less than 2%)
Keflex
Klonopin Tablets
Kytril Injection (Less than 2%)
Lamictal (Infrequent)
Leukeran Tablets (Rare)
Levaquin (0.5% to less than 1.0%)
Levbid
Levsin/Levsinex
Lexxel Tablets
Lodosyn Tablets
Loxitane Capsules
Lufyllin
Lufyllin-GG
Lupron Depot 7.5 mg (Less than 5%)
Lupron Depot—3 Month 11.25 mg
Luvox Tablets (2%)
Maxalt (Infrequent)
Mepergan Injection
Meridia Capsules (Greater than or
equal to 1%)
Merrem I.V. (0.1% to 1.0%)
Miacalcin Nasal Spray (Less than 1%)
Mirapex Tablets (1.1%)
MS Contin Tablets (Less frequent)
MSIR (Less frequent)
Narcan Injection (Infrequent)
Nardil Tablets (Uncommon)
Naropin Injection (Less than 1%)
Navane
Nembutal (Less than 1%)
Neurontin (Infrequent)
Norflex
Norpramin Tablets
Norvasc Tablets (Less than or equal to
0.1%)
Norvir (Less than 2%)
Nubain Injection
Oramorph SR Tablets (Less frequent)
Orthoclone OKT3
OxyContin Tablets (Less than 1%)
Parnate Tablets
Paxil (1.1% to 5%)
Pepcid (Infrequent)
Permax Tablets (Infrequent)
Phrenilin (Infrequent)
Prevacid (Less than 1%)
Prevpac (Less than 1%)
▲ Prograf (3% to 15%)
Proleukin for Injection

ProSom Tablets (Infrequent)
Prozac (Frequent)
Recombivax HB
Reglan
Relafen Tablets (1%)
Remeron (Frequent)
Reminyl (Greater than or equal to 2%)
ReoPro Vials (0.7%)
Requip Tablets (Infrequent)
Rescriptor Tablets (Less than 2%)
Rilutek Tablets (Frequent)
▲ Risperdal (22% to 26%)
Rituxan (1% to 5%)
Roferon-A Injection
▲ Romazicon Injection (3% to 9%)
Roxanol
Roxanol 100
Roxanol-T
Roxicodone Tablets (Less than 3%)
Salagen Tablets (Rare)
Sarafem Pulvules (Frequent)
Sedapap Tablets (Infrequent)
Serentil
Serzone Tablets
▲ Simulect for Injection (3% to 10%)
Sinemet CR Tablets
Sinemet Tablets
Soma Compound (Very rare to
    infrequent)
Soma Compound w/Codeine
    (Infrequent or rare)
Soma Tablets
Sonata Capsules (Infrequent)
Stadol NS Nasal Spray (Less than 1%)
Stelazine
Stimate Nasal Spray
Suprane Liquid for Inhalation (Less
    than 1%)
Surmontil Capsules
Sustiva Capsules (Less than 2%)
Symmetrel (1% to 5%)
Tagamet
Tasmar Tablets (1%)
Tegretol
Tenex Tablets (Less frequent)
Tequin (Less than 0.1%)
Thalomid Capsules
Thioridazine Hydrochloride Tablets
Thiothixene Capsules
Thorazine
Tonocard Tablets (Less than 1%)
▲ Topamax (4% to 4.4%)
Trasylol Injection (1% to 2%)
Trental Tablets

Trileptal (1% to 2%)
▲ Trisenox Injection (5%)
Trovan (Less than 1%)
Twinrix Vaccine (Less than 1%)
▲ Ultram Tablets (1% to 14%)
Valcyte Tablets (Less than 5%)
Valtrex Caplets
Ventolin Inhalation Aerosol (1%)
Versed Injection (Less than 1%)
Versed Syrup (2%)
▲ Vesanoid Capsules (9%)
Vicoprofen Tablets (Less than 1%)
Vistide Injection
Vivactil Tablets
▲ Wellbutrin SR (0.3% to 9%)
▲ Wellbutrin Tablets (31.9%)
Xanax Tablets (Rare; 2.9%)
Zanaflex Tablets (Infrequent)
Zantac Injection
Zantac Tablets, Granules, & Syrup
    (Rare)
Zithromax Capsules & Tablets (1% or
    less)
Zithromax for Oral Suspension (1% or
    less)
▲ Zofran Injection (2% to 6%)
▲ Zofran Tablets & Oral Solution (6%)
▲ Zoloft (6%)
▲ Zometa for Intravenous Infusion
    (12.8%)
Zomig (Infrequent)
▲ Zonegran Capsules (9%)
▲ Zosyn (2.1% to 7.1%)
Zovirax Capsules, Tablets, &
    Suspension
Zovirax for Injection (Approximately
    1%)
Zyban (Frequent)
▲ Zyprexa (23%)
Zyrtec (Less than 2%)
Zyrtec-D (Less than 2%)

Agoraphobia
Luvox Tablets (Infrequent)

Alcohol abuse
Effexor Tablets (Rare)
Effexor XR Capsules (Rare)
Paxil (Infrequent)
Zyprexa (Infrequent)

Anger
Meridia Capsules
Valium Injectable

Antisocial reaction
Zyprexa (Infrequent)

Anxiety
▲ Acel-Imune (9% to (18%)
Aceon Tablets (0.3% to 1%)
AcipHex Tablets
▲ Actonel Tablets (4.3%)
Adalat CC Tablets (Less than 1.0%)
Aerobid (1% to 3%)
Allegra-D (1.4%)
Alphagan Ophthalmic Solution (Less than 3%)
Altace Capsules (Less than 1%)
Ambien Tablets (1%)
▲ AmBisome for Injection (7.4%) to 13.7%)
Amerge Tablets (Infrequent)
Amoxil (Rare)
Androderm (Less than 1%)
AndroGel (Fewer than 1%)
▲ Android Capsules (Among most common)
▲ Angiomax for Injection (6%)
Anzemet (Infrequently)
Arava Tablets (1% to 3%)
▲ Aredia for Injection (14.3%)
▲ Arimidex Tablets (2% to 5%)
▲ Aromasin Tablets (10%)
Arthrotec Tablets (Rare)
Asacol Tablets (2% or greater)
Astelin Nasal Spray (Infrequent)
Astramorph/PF Injection
Atacand HCT Tablets (0.5% or greater)
Atacand Tablets (0.5% or greater)
Augmentin (Rare)
Avalide Tablets (1% or greater)
Avapro Tablets (Less than 1%)
Avelox Tablets (0.05% to 1%)
Avonex
Axert Tablets (Infrequent)
Axid Pulvules (1.6%)
▲ Betapace Tablets (2% to 4%)
▲ Betaseron (15%)
Betaxon Ophthalmic Suspension (Less than 2%)
Bextra Tablets (0.1% to 1.9%)
Biaxin
Bicillin C-R
Bicillin L-A
Brethine Ampuls (Less than 0.5%)
Brethine Tablets (1%)
Brevibloc Injection (Less than 1%)
Brevital
Cardura Tablets (1.1%)

Carnitor Injection (1% to 2%)
▲ Casodex Tablets (2% to 5%)
Cataflam Tablets (Less than 1%)
Catapres Tablets
Catapres-TTS (0.5% or less)
Ceclor CD (0.1% to 1%)
Celebrex Capsules (0.1% to 1.9%)
▲ Celexa (4%)
▲ CellCept (3% to 28.4%)
Chirocaine Injection (1%)
Cipro
Cipro I.V. (1% or less)
Claritin (At least one patient)
Claritin-D 12 Hour (Less frequent)
Claritin-D 24 Hour (Fewer than 2%)
Clomid Tablets
Clorpres Tablets
Clozaril Tablets (1%)
▲ Cognex Capsules (3%)
Colazal Capsules
Combipres Tablets
Comtan Tablets (2%)
▲ Copaxone (23%)
Corlopam Injection (1% to 2%)
Cosopt Ophthalmic Solution
Cozaar Tablets (Less than 1%)
Crixivan Capsules (Less than 2%)
Cuprimine Capsules
Cytotec Tablets (Infrequent)
Cytovene (At least 3 subjects)
D.H.E. 45 Injection (Occasional)
DaunoXome Injection (Less than or equal to 5%)
Delatestryl Injection
Demser Capsules
Depacon Injection (1% to 5%)
Depakene (1% to 5%)
Depakote ER Tablets (1% to 5%)
Depakote Sprinkle Capsules (1% to 5%)
Depakote Tablets (1% to 5%)
Detrol LA Capsules (1%)
Digitek Tablets
Dilaudid Injection
Dilaudid Powder
Dilaudid Rectal Suppositories
Dilaudid Tablets
Diovan Capsules
Diovan HCT Tablets (Greater than 0.2%)
▲ Diphtheria & Tetanus Toxoids (22.6%)
Diprivan (Less than 1%)
▲ Dostinex Tablets (1% to less than 10%)
Doxil Injection (Less than 1% to 5%)

▲ Duraclon Injection (38%)
▲ Duragesic Transdermal System
  (3% to 10%)
  Duramorph Injection
  Dynabac Tablets (0.1% to 1%)
▲ Effexor Tablets (2% to 11.2%)
  Effexor XR Capsules
  Eldepryl Capsules (1 of 49 patients)
  Emcyt Capsules (1%)
  EpiPen Auto-Injector
  EpiPen Jr. Auto-Injector
▲ Epogen for Injection (2% to 7%)
  Ergamisol Tablets (1%)
▲ Esclim Transdermal System
  (Up to 8.3%)
  Estratest
  Estring Vaginal Ring (1% to 3%)
  Etrafon
  Eulexin Capsules (1%)
  Evoxac Capsules (1.3%)
▲ Exelon (5%)
  Famotidine Injection (Infrequent)
▲ Felbatol (5.2% to 5.3%)
  Feldene Capsules (Occasional)
  Femara Tablets (Less frequent)
  Flexeril Tablets (Less than 1%)
▲ Flolan for Injection (7% to 21%)
  Floxin (Less than 1%)
  Fortovase Capsules (2.2%)
▲ Foscavir Injection (5% or greater)
  Gabitril Tablets (1% or more)
  Gamimune N
  Gammar-P I.V.
  Gastrocrom Oral Concentrate (Less
  common)
  Gengraf Capsules (1% to less than
  3%)
  Geodon Capsules
  Glucotrol XL (Less than 3%)
  Gonal-F for Injection
  Haldol
  Haldol Decanoate
  Hivid Tablets (Less than 1%)
  Hycodan
  Hycomine Compound Tablets
  Hycotuss Expectorant Syrup
  Hytrin Capsules (At least 1%)
  Hyzaar
  Imdur Tablets (Less than or equal to
  5%)
  Imitrex Injection (1.1%)
  Imitrex Nasal Spray (Infrequent)
  Imitrex Tablets
▲ Indapamide Tablets (Greater than or
  equal to 5%)

  Indocin Capsules/Suspension/
  Suppositories (Less than 1%)
▲ Infanrix Vaccine (3.3% to 9.2%)
▲ Infergen (10% to 19%)
  Infumorph
▲ Intron A for Injection (Up to 5%)
  Invirase Capsules (Less than 2%)
  IPOL Vaccine
  Ismo Tablets (Fewer than 1%)
▲ Kadian Capsules (Less than 3% to
  6%)
  Kaletra (Less than 2%)
  Keppra Tablets (2%)
  Klonopin Tablets (Infrequent)
  Kytril Injection (Less than 2%)
  Kytril Tablets (2%)
▲ Lamictal (3.8%)
  Lanoxin/Lanoxicaps
  Lariam Tablets
  Lescol Capsules
  Lescol XL Tablets
▲ Leukine (11%)
  Levaquin (0.1% to less than 1.0%)
  Levbid
  Levoxyl Tablets
  Levsin
  Lexxel Tablets
  Lodine XL Extended-Release Tablets
  (Less than 1%)
  Lodosyn Tablets
  Lortab
  Lotensin Tablets (Less than 1%)
  Lotrel Capsules
  Lupron Depot 3.75 mg
  (Less than 5%)
  Lupron Depot—3 Month 11.25 mg
  (Less than 5%)
  Lupron Depot—3 Month 22.5 mg
  (Less than 5%)
  Lupron Injection (Less than 5%)
  Luvox Tablets (1% to 5%)
  Marinol Capsules (Greater than 1%)
  Mavik Tablets (0.3% to 1.0%)
  Maxair (Less than 1%)
  Maxalt (Infrequent)
  Maxidone Tablets
  Maxzide
▲ Mepron Suspension (7%)
▲ Meridia Capsules (4.5%)
  Merrem I.V. (0.1% to 1.0%)
  Mevacor Tablets (0.5% to 1.0%)
  Miacalcin Nasal Spray (Less than 1%)
  Micardis HCT Tablets
  Micardis Tablets (More than 0.3%)

Migranal Nasal Spray (Rare)
Mirapex Tablets (1% or more)
Mobic Tablets (Less than 2%)
Mykrox Tablets (Less than 2%)
Myobloc Injectable Solution (2% or greater)
Naprelan Tablets (Less than 1%)
Nardil Tablets (Less frequent)
Naropin Injection (1% to 5%)
Nascobal Gel
▲ Natrecor for Injection (3%)
Nembutal (Less than 1%)
Neoral (1% to less than 3%)
Nesacaine
Neurontin (Frequent)
▲ Nicotrol Nasal Spray (Over 5%)
▲ Nipent for Injection (3% to 10%)
Norco
Noroxin Tablets (Less frequent)
Norplant System
Norpramin Tablets
Norvasc Tablets (More than 0.1% to 1%)
Norvir (Less than 2%)
▲ Novantrone for Injection (5%)
OptiPranolol (A small number of patients)
OxyContin Tablets (Between 1% and 5%)
Parnate Tablets
▲ Paxil (5% to 5.9%)
Pediazole Suspension
▲ PEG-Intron Powder for Injection (28%)
Pepcid (Infrequent)
▲ Permax Tablets (6.4%)
Phenergan VC Syrup
Phenergan VC with Codeine Syrup
▲ Photofrin for Injection (7%)
Plavix Tablets (1% to 2.5%)
Plendil (0.5% to 1.5%)
Pletal Tablets (Less than 2%)
Polocaine
Polocaine-MPF
Pravachol Tablets
Prevacid (Less than 1%)
Prevpac (Less than 1%)
Prilosec (Less than 1%)
ProAmatine Tablets (Less frequent)
Procardia XL Tablets (1% or less)
▲ Procrit for Injection (2% to 11%)
▲ Prograf (3% to 15%)
▲ Proleukin for Injection (12%)
Prometrium Capsules (Less than 5%)
ProSom Tablets (Frequent)

Protonix (Greater than or equal to 1%)
Proventil HFA Inhalation Aerosol (Less than 3%)
▲ Provigil Tablets (4%)
▲ Prozac (2% to 28%)
Pulmicort Respules (Less than 1%)
Pulmicort Turbuhaler Powder (Rare)
▲ Rapamune (3% to 20%)
Reglan
Relafen Tablets (Less than 1%)
Remeron (Frequent)
Remicade for IV Injection (Less than 2%)
Reminyl (Greater than or equal to 2%)
ReoPro Vials (1.7%)
Requip Tablets (1% or more)
Retrovir Capsules, Tablets & Syrup
Retrovir IV Infusion
Rhinocort Nasal Inhaler (Rare)
Rifater Tablets
▲ Risperdal (12% to 20%)
▲ Roferon-A Injection (5% to 6%)
▲ Romazicon Injection (3% to 9%)
Roxicodone Tablets (Less than 3%)
Rynatan Tablets
Rythmol Tablets (1.5% to 2.0%)
Salagen Tablets (Less than 1%)
Sandimmune (Rare)
Sandostatin Injection (Less than 1%)
▲ Sandostatin LAR Depot (5% to 15%)
▲ Sarafem Pulvules (13%)
Sectral Capsules (Up to 2%)
Sensorcaine Injection
Sensorcaine with Epinephrine Injection
Sensorcaine-MPF Injection
Sensorcaine-MPF with Epinephrine Injection
Serophene Tablets
▲ Serostim for Injection (1% to 10%)
Serzone Tablets
▲ Simulect for Injection (3% to 10%)
Sinemet CR Tablets
Sinemet Tablets
Skelid Tablets (Greater than or equal to 1%)
Sonata Capsules (Less than 1% to 3%)
Soriatane Capsules (Less than 1%)
▲ Sporanox Capsules (3%)
Stadol NS Nasal Spray (1% or greater)
Sular Tablets (Less than or equal to 1%)
Surmontil Capsules

Sustiva Capsules (Less than 2%)
Symmetrel (1% to 5%)
Synercid I.V. (Less than 1%)
Synvisc
Tagamet
Tambocor Tablets (1% to 3%)
Tarka Tablets (0.3% or more)
Tasmar Tablets (1% or more)
▲ Temodar Capsules (7%)
Tenex Tablets (Less frequent)
Tequin (Less than 0.1%)
Testoderm Transdermal Systems
Testopel Pellets
Testred Capsules
Teveten Tablets (Less than 1%)
Thalomid Capsules
Thyrel TRH for Injection (Less
  frequent)
Tikosyn Capsules (Greater than 2%)
Timolol GFS
Timoptic (Less frequent)
Tonocard Tablets (1.1% to 1.5%)
▲ Topamax (2.2% to 9.3%)
Trasylol Injection (1% to 2%)
Travatan Ophthalmic Solution (1% to
  5%)
Trental Tablets (Less than 1%)
Tricor Tablets (Less than 1%)
▲ Trileptal (5% to 7%)
Tripedia Vaccine
▲ Trisenox Injection (30%)
Trovan (Less than 1%)
Tussionex
Ultracet Tablets (At least 1%)
▲ Ultram Tablets (1% to 14%)
Uniretic Tablets (Less than 1%)
Unithroid Tablets
Univasc Tablets (Less than 1%)
Vantin (Less than 1%)
Vascor Tablets (0.5% to 2.0%)
Versed Injection (Less than 1%)
▲ Vesanoid Capsules (17%)
Viadur Implant (Less than 2%)
Viagra Tablets
Vicodin
Vicodin Tuss Expectorant
▲ Vicoprofen Tablets (3% to 9%)
Vioxx (Greater than 0.1% to 1.9%)
Viracept
Vistide Injection
Vivactil Tablets
Voltaren (Less than 1%)
▲ Wellbutrin SR (5% to 6%)
▲ Wellbutrin Tablets (3.1%)

▲ Xanax Tablets (16.6%)
▲ Xenical Capsules (2.8% to 4.4%)
Xopenex Inhalation Solution (2.7%)
Xylocaine Injection
Xylocaine with Epinephrine Injection
Zanaflex Tablets (Frequent)
Zebeta Tablets
▲ Zenapax for Injection (2% to 5%)
Ziac Tablets
Zocor Tablets
▲ Zofran Injection (2% to 6%)
▲ Zofran Tablets & Oral Solution (6%)
Zoladex (1% to 5%)
Zoladex 3-month
▲ Zoloft (4%)
▲ Zometa for Intravenous Infusion (9%
  to 14%)
Zomig (Infrequent)
▲ Zonegran Capsules (3%)
Zosyn (1.2% to 3.2%)
▲ Zyban (8%)
Zydone Tablets
▲ Zyprexa (9%)
Zyrtec (Less than 2%)
Zyrtec-D (Less than 2%)

Anxiety, paradoxical

Halcion Tablets
Valium Injectable
Valium Tablets
Vivactil Tablets

Apathy

Ambien Tablets (Rare)
Bactrim
Betaseron
Bicillin C-R
Campath Ampules
Celexa (Infrequent)
Claritin-D 12 Hour (Less frequent)
Claritin-D 24 Hour (Fewer than 2%)
Cognex Capsules (Infrequent)
D.H.E. 45 Injection
Digitek Tablets
Effexor Tablets (Infrequent)
Effexor XR Capsules (Infrequent)
Eldepryl Capsules
Evoxac Capsules
Exelon (Infrequent)
Felbatol
Gabitril Tablets (Infrequent)
Imitrex Injection
Imitrex Nasal Spray (Rare)
Imitrex Tablets (Rare)
Intron A for Injection (Less than 5%)

Kadian Capsules (Less than 3%)
Klonopin Tablets (Infrequent)
Lamictal (Infrequent)
Lanoxin/Lanoxicaps
Luvox Tablets (Frequent)
Mirapex Tablets (1% or more)
Neurontin (Infrequent)
Nexium (Less than 1%)
Nicotrol Nasal Spray (Under 5%)
Norvasc Tablets (Less than or equal to 0.1%)
Permax Tablets (Infrequent)
Prevacid (Less than 1%)
Prevpac (Less than 1%)
Prilosec (Less than 1%)
ProSom Tablets (Infrequent)
Prozac (Infrequent)
Remeron (Frequent)
Reminyl (Infrequent)
Requip Tablets (Infrequent)
Rilutek Tablets (Infrequent)
Risperdal (Infrequent)
Roferon-A Injection (Infrequent)
Sarafem Pulvules (Infrequent)
Septra
Seroquel Tablets (Infrequent)
Serzone Tablets (Infrequent)
Sonata Capsules (Frequent)
Sustiva Capsules (Less than 2%)
Tambocor Tablets (Less than 1%)
Tasmar Tablets (Infrequent)
Topamax (1.8% to 4.5%)
Trileptal
Zoloft (Infrequent)
Zomig (Rare)
Zyprexa

Argumentativeness
Versed Injection (Less than 1%)

Auditory disturbances
Aralen Tablets
Navelbine Injection
▲ Wellbutrin Tablets (5.3%)

Awareness, altered
Diprivan (Less than 1%)
Halcion Tablets
▲ Tonocard Tablets (1.5% to 11.0%)
Wellbutrin SR (Rare)

Awareness, heightened
Demser Capsules
Imitrex Tablets (Rare)
▲ Marinol Capsules (8% to 24%)

Behavior, hypochondriacal
Celontin Capsules

Behavior, inappropriate
Artane
Ativan Injection (Occasional)
Diprivan (Less than 1%)
Halcion Tablets
ProSom Tablets
Ritalin
Serentil
Symmetrel
Tessalon Capsules (Isolated instances)
Xanax Tablets (Rare)
Zovirax for Injection

Behavior, schizophrenic
Zonegran Capsules (2%)

Behavior, violent
Prozac
Sarafem Pulvules
Tenex Tablets
Zovirax Capsules, Tablets, & Suspension

Behavioral changes
Akineton
Ambien Tablets
Amoxil (Rare)
Augmentin (Rare)
Biaxin
Catapres Tablets
Catapres-TTS (0.5% or less)
Clorpres Tablets
Combipres Tablets
Corgard Tablets (6 of 1000 patients)
Cosopt Ophthalmic Solution
Cytotec Tablets (Infrequent)
Duraclon Injection (Rare)
Eldepryl Capsules
Fortovase Capsules (Less than 2%)
Gastrocrom Oral Concentrate (Less common)
JE-VAX Vaccine (One case)
▲ Klonopin Tablets (5% to 25%)
Monopril Tablets (0.4% to 1.0%)
Nadolol Tablets (6 of 1000 patients)
Neurontin
▲ Orap Tablets (27.7%)
Prevpac
Priftin Tablets
Rifadin
Rifater Tablets
▲ Roferon-A Injection (3%)
Thioridazine Hydrochloride Tablets

Timolol GFS
Timoptic (Less frequent)
Uniphyl Tablets
Valtrex Caplets
Vascor Tablets (0.5% to 2.0%)
Ventolin Inhalation Aerosol (1%)
Versed Syrup (Less than 1%)
Zyprexa

Behavioral deterioration

Depacon Injection
Depakene
Depakote ER Tablets
Depakote Sprinkle Capsules
Depakote Tablets

Bulimia

Paxil (Rare)

Catatonia

Blocadren Tablets
Celexa (Rare)
Compazine
Corgard Tablets
Corzide
Cosopt Ophthalmic Solution
Depacon Injection (1% or more)
Depakene (1% or more)
Depakote ER Tablets (Greater than 1%)
Depakote Sprinkle Capsules
Depakote Tablets (1% to 5%)
Effexor Tablets
Effexor XR Capsules
Etrafon
Haldol
Haldol Decanoate
Inderal Injectable
Inderide
Nadolol Tablets
Normodyne Tablets
Phenergan Injection
Phenergan Suppositories
Phenergan Tablets
Risperdal (Infrequent)
Sectral Capsules
Seroquel Tablets (Infrequent)
Stelazine
Tenoretic Tablets
Tenormin
Thorazine (Rare)
Timolide Tablets
Timolol GFS
Timoptic
Toprol-XL Tablets

Trilafon
Zebeta Tablets
Ziac Tablets

Central nervous system depression

Anaprox (Less than 1%)
Ativan Injection
Cerebyx Injection (Infrequent)
Depacon Injection
Depakene
Depakote ER Tablets
Depakote Tablets
Duranest Injections
EC-Naprosyn (Less than 1%)
ELA-Max Cream
EMLA (Unlikely)
▲ Klonopin Tablets (Most frequent)
Lamictal (Infrequent)
Luvox Tablets (Infrequent)
Naprosyn (Less than 1%)
Nembutal (Less than 1%)
Neurontin
Phenergan VC with Codeine Syrup
Phenergan with Codeine Syrup
Prozac (Infrequent)
Rilutek Tablets (Rare)
Rynatan Tablets
Sarafem Pulvules (Infrequent)
▲ Vesanoid Capsules (3%)
▲ Xanax Tablets (13.8% to 13.9%)
▲ Xylocaine Injection (Among most common)
▲ Xylocaine with Epinephrine Injection (Among most common)

Central nervous system depression, neonatal

Halcion Tablets
Streptomycin Sulfate Injection
Versed Injection

Central nervous system reactions

Attenuvax
Azulfidine
Chibroxin Ophthalmic Solution
Clozaril Tablets
Compazine
Digitek Tablets
Hexalen Capsules
Intron A for Injection (Less than 5%)
Lanoxin/Lanoxicaps
Lariam Tablets
▲ Leukine (11%)

Levbid
Levsin
▲ Nipent for Injection (1% to 11%)
Noroxin Tablets
▲ Novantrone for Injection (30% to 34%)
Orap Tablets
Orthoclone OKT3
Orudis Capsules (Less than 1%)
Oruvail Capsules (Less than 1%)
▲ Paraplatin for Injection (5%)
Roferon-A Injection (Less than 5%)
Serentil
Silvadene Cream 1%
Stelazine

Central nervous system stimulation

Adipex-P
Avelox Tablets
Axert Tablets (Infrequent)
Cafcit
Chibroxin Ophthalmic Solution
Cipro
Cipro I.V.
Claritin-D 12 Hour
Claritin-D 24 Hour
Combivent Inhalation Aerosol
Duranest Injections
Effexor Tablets (Infrequent)
Effexor XR Capsules (Infrequent)
ELA-Max Cream
EMLA (Unlikely)
Floxin
Kytril Injection (Less than 2%)
Lamictal (Rare)
Levaquin
Levo-Dromoran
Lidoderm Patch
Lindane
Lufyllin-GG
Luvox Tablets (2%)
Meridia Capsules (1.5%)
Noroxin Tablets
Paxil (Frequent)
Proventil HFA Inhalation Aerosol
Proventil Inhalation Aerosol
Proventil Repetabs Tablets
Prozac (Infrequent)
Sarafem Pulvules (Infrequent)
Serzone Tablets
Tequin
Trovan
▲ Ultram Tablets (7% to 14%)

Ventolin HFA Inhalation Aerosol
Ventolin Inhalation Aerosol (No incidence data in labeling)
Volmax Extended-Release Tablets
Wellbutrin SR (1% to 2%)
▲ Xylocaine Injection (Among most common)
▲ Xylocaine with Epinephrine Injection (Among most common)
Zyban (Infrequent)
Zyprexa (Infrequent)
Zyrtec-D

Central nervous system stimulation, paradoxical

Halcion Tablets
Librium Capsules
Numorphan

Cognitive dysfunction

Ambien Tablets (Infrequent)
Amerge Tablets (Infrequent)
Anaprox (Less than 1%)
EC-Naprosyn (Rare)
Floxin (Less than 1%)
▲ Naprelan Tablets (3% to 9%)
Naprosyn (Less than 1%)
Orthoclone OKT3
Rescriptor Tablets (Less than 2%)
Risperdal
Ultracet Tablets
Ultram Tablets (Less than 1%)
▲ Xanax Tablets (28.8%)

Coma

AcipHex Tablets
Aggrenox Capsules (Less than 1%)
Aloprim for Injection (Less than 1%)
AmBisome for Injection (Less common)
Arthrotec Tablets (Rare)
Ativan Injection (Less than 1%)
Betaseron
Bicillin C-R
Bicillin L-A
Buprenex Injectable (Infrequent)
Campath Ampules
Cataflam Tablets (Rare)
Cerebyx Injection (Infrequent)
Cognex Capsules (Rare)
Compazine
Copaxone (Infrequent)
DDAVP Injection (Rare)
DDAVP Nasal Spray (Rare)
DDAVP Rhinal Tube (Rare)

Depacon Injection (Rare)
Depakene (Rare)
Depakote ER Tablets (Rare)
Depakote Sprinkle Capsules (Rare)
Depakote Tablets (Rare)
Desmopressin Acetate Injection (Rare)
Ecotrin Enteric Coated Aspirin
Elspar for Injection (No incidence
  data in labeling)
Ergamisol Tablets
Eskalith
Evoxac Capsules (Less than 1%)
Felbatol
Feldene Capsules (Rare)
Fludara for Injection
Foscavir Injection (Less than 1%)
Gabitril Tablets (Infrequent)
Gliadel Wafer (1%)
Ifex for Injection (Occasional)
Indocin Capsules/Suspension/
  Suppositories (Less than 1%)
Indocin I.V. (Less than 1%)
Intron A for Injection (Less than 5%)
Klonopin Tablets
Levaquin (Less than 0.3%)
Levbid
Levo-Dromoran
Levsin
Lithium
Lithobid Slow-Release Tablets
Lodine XL Extended-Release Tablets
Luvox Tablets (Rare)
LYMErix Vaccine (Greater than 1%)
Matulane Capsules
Motrin (Rare; less than 1%)
Nardil Tablets (Less frequent)
Naropin Injection (Less than 1%)
Oncaspar
Orthoclone OKT3
Permax Tablets (Infrequent)
Pfizerpen for Injection
PhosLo
Podocon-25 Liquid
Ponstel Capsules (Rare)
Prograf
Proleukin for Injection (1%)
Prozac (Rare)
ReoPro Vials (0.4%)
Requip Tablets (Infrequent)
Rilutek Tablets (Infrequent)
Risperdal (Rare)
Roferon-A Injection (Rare to
  infrequent)
Rythmol Tablets (Less than 1%)

Sarafem Pulvules (Rare)
Stimate Nasal Spray
Streptomycin Sulfate Injection
  (Occasional)
Symmetrel
Tonocard Tablets (Less than 1%)
▲ Trisenox Injection (5%)
Valtrex Caplets
▲ Vesanoid Capsules (3%)
Voltaren (Rare)
Wellbutrin SR
Wellbutrin Tablets
Zoloft (Rare)
Zovirax Capsules, Tablets, &
  Suspension
Zovirax for Injection (Approximately
  1%)
Zyban
Zyprexa (Infrequent)

Combativeness

Diprivan (Less than 1%)
Orthoclone OKT3
Versed Injection
Zosyn (1.0% or less)

Confusion

AcipHex Tablets (Rare)
Actimmune (Rare)
▲ Actiq (1% to 6%)
Adalat CC Tablets (Less than 1.0%)
Aggrenox Capsules (1.1%)
Agrylin Capsules (1% to 5%)
Aldoclor Tablets
Aldomet Tablets
Aldoril Tablets
Alferon N Injection (One patient to
  3%)
Ambien Tablets (Frequent)
▲ AmBisome for Injection (8.6% to
  12.9%)
Amerge Tablets (Rare)
Amicar
Amoxil (Rare)
▲ Amphotec (5% or more)
Ancobon Capsules
Androderm (Less than 1%)
Angiomax for Injection (Rare)
Anzemet (Infrequently)
Apligraf (1.8%)
Aricept Tablets
Arimidex Tablets (2% to 5%)
▲ Arixtra Injection (3.1%)
▲ Aromasin Tablets (2% to 5%)
Artane

Arthrotec Tablets (Rare)
Asacol Tablets
Astelin Nasal Spray
Ativan Injection (1.3%)
Augmentin (Rare)
Avalide Tablets
Avelox Tablets (0.05% to 1%)
Avonex
Axid Pulvules (Rare)
Azactam for Injection (Less than 1%)
Benadryl Parenteral
Betagan
▲ Betaseron (4%)
Bextra Tablets (0.1% to 1.9%)
Biaxin
Bicillin C-R
Bicillin L-A
Brevibloc Injection (About 2%)
Campath Ampules
Captopril Tablets
Carbatrol Capsules
Cardene I.V. (Rare)
Cardura Tablets (Less than 0.5%)
▲ Casodex Tablets (2% to 5%)
Ceclor (Rare)
Ceclor CD
Cefzil (Less than 1%)
Celexa (Frequent)
▲ CellCept (13.5%)
Celontin Capsules
Cerebyx Injection (Infrequent)
Chibroxin Ophthalmic Solution
Chirocaine Injection (Less than 1%)
Cipro
Cipro I.V. (1% or less)
Claritin (At least one patient)
Claritin-D 12 Hour (Less frequent)
Claritin-D 24 Hour (Fewer than 2%)
▲ Clozaril Tablets (3%)
Cogentin Tablets
▲ Cognex Capsules (7%)
Copaxone (2%)
Cosopt Ophthalmic Solution
Covera-HS Tablets (Less than 2%)
Cozaar Tablets (Less than 1%)
Cytotec Tablets
Cytovene (At least 3 subjects)
D.H.E. 45 Injection
Dantrium Capsules (Less frequent)
Daranide Tablets
DaunoXome Injection (Less than or equal to 5%)
Demser Capsules
Depacon Injection (1% to 5%)

Depakene (1% to 5%)
Depakote ER Tablets (1% to 5%)
Depakote Sprinkle Capsules (1% to 5%)
Depakote Tablets (1% to 5%)
▲ DepoCyt Injection (4% to 14%)
Diamox (Occasional)
Didronel Tablets
Digitek Tablets
▲ Dilantin (Among most common)
Diovan HCT Tablets
Diprivan (Less than 1%)
Ditropan XL (2% to 5%)
Diuril
Dolobid Tablets (Less than 1 in 100)
Dostinex Tablets
Doxil Injection (Less than 1%)
▲ Duraclon Injection (13.2% to 38%)
▲ Duragesic Transdermal System (10% or more)
Duranest Injections
Dyazide Capsules
Ecotrin Enteric Coated Aspirin
Edecrin
Effexor Tablets (2%)
Effexor XR Capsules (Frequent)
ELA-Max Cream
▲ Eldepryl Capsules (3 of 49 patients)
Elspar for Injection (No incidence data in labeling)
EMLA (Unlikely)
Enalaprilat Injection
Ergamisol Tablets (Less frequent)
Ery-Tab Tablets (Isolated reports)
Erythrocin Stearate (Isolated reports)
Erythromycin (Isolated reports)
Eskalith
Etrafon
Eulexin Capsules (1%)
Evoxac Capsules (Less than 1%)
▲ Exelon (8%)
Famotidine Injection (Infrequent)
Famvir Tablets (Infrequent)
Felbatol
Feldene Capsules (Occasional)
▲ Flolan for Injection (6%)
Floxin (Less than 1%)
Fludara for Injection
Flumadine (Less than 0.3%)
Fortovase Capsules (Less than 2%)
▲ Foscavir Injection (5% or greater)
▲ Gabitril Tablets (5%)
Gengraf Capsules (1% to less than 3%)

Geodon Capsules (Frequent)
▲ Gliadel Wafer (10%)
Glucotrol XL (Less than 1%)
Grifulvin V (Occasional)
Gris-PEG Tablets (Occasional)
Halcion Tablets (0.5% to 0.9%)
Haldol
Haldol Decanoate
Herceptin I.V. (At least one of 958 patients)
Hivid Tablets (Less than 1%)
HydroDIURIL Tablets
Hyzaar
▲ Ifex for Injection (Among most common)
Imdur Tablets (Less than or equal to 5%)
Imitrex Injection (Infrequent)
Imitrex Nasal Spray (Infrequent)
Imitrex Tablets (Infrequent)
Indocin Capsules/Suspension/Suppositories (Less than 1%)
▲ Infergen (4%)
Innohep Injection (Greater than or equal to 1%)
▲ Intron A for Injection (Up to 12%)
Invirase Capsules (Less than 2%)
Ismo Tablets (Fewer than 1%)
Isoptin SR Tablets (1% or less)
Kadian Capsules (Less than 3%)
Kaletra (Less than 2%)
Keflex
Keppra Tablets (1% or more)
Klonopin Tablets (1%)
K-Phos
Lamictal (1.8%)
Lanoxin/Lanoxicaps
Lariam Tablets
Leukeran Tablets (Rare)
Levaquin (Less than 0.3%)
Levbid
Levo-Dromoran
▲ Levorphanol Tartrate Tablets (3% to 9%)
Levsin
Lexxel Tablets
Librium Capsules (Some patients)
Librium for Injection
Lidoderm Patch
Limbitrol (Less common)
Lithium
Lithobid Slow-Release Tablets
Lodine (Less than 1%)

Lodine XL Extended-Release Tablets (Less than 1%)
Lodosyn Tablets
Lopid Tablets
Lovenox Injection (2.2%)
Loxitane Capsules
Lupron Depot 3.75 mg
Lupron Depot—4 Month 30 mg (Less than 5%)
Luvox Tablets
Macrobid Capsules (Rare)
Macrodantin Capsules (Rare)
Marinol Capsules (Greater than 1%)
Matulane Capsules
Maxair (Less than 1%)
Maxalt (Infrequent)
Megace Oral Suspension (1% to 3%)
Meridia Capsules
Merrem I.V. (0.1% to 1.0%)
Mexitil Capsules (1.9% to 2.6%)
Midamor Tablets (Less than or equal to 1%)
Migranal Nasal Spray (Infrequent)
Mintezol
▲ Mirapex Tablets (4% to 10%)
Mobic Tablets (Less than 2%)
Moduretic Tablets (Less than or equal to 1%)
Monopril HCT
Monopril Tablets (0.2% to 1.0%)
Motofen Tablets (1 in 200 to 1 in 600)
Motrin (Less than 1%)
Myambutol Tablets
Mycobutin Capsules (More than one patient)
Myobloc Injectable Solution (2% or greater)
Naprelan Tablets (Less than 1%)
Naropin Injection (Less than 1%)
Natrecor for Injection (At least 1%)
Nebcin
Nembutal (Less than 1%)
Neoral (1% to less than 3%)
Neptazane Tablets (Occasional)
Neurontin
Nexium (Less than 1%)
▲ Nicotrol Nasal Spray (3%)
Norflex (Infrequent)
Noroxin Tablets
Norpramin Tablets
Norvir (Less than 2%)
Nubain Injection (1% or less)
NuLev
Numorphan

Oncaspar (Less than 1%)
Oramorph SR Tablets
Orthoclone OKT3
Orudis Capsules (Less than 1%)
Oruvail Capsules (Less than 1%)
OxyContin Tablets (Between 1% and 5%)
Parnate Tablets
Paxil (1%)
Pepcid (Infrequent)
Periactin Tablets (No incidence data in labeling)
▲ Permax Tablets (11.1%)
Phenergan Suppositories
Phenergan Syrup (Rare)
Phenergan VC Syrup (Rare)
Phenergan VC with Codeine Syrup (Rare)
Phenergan with Codeine Syrup (Rare)
Phenergan with Dextromethorphan Syrup (Rare)
PhosLo
▲ Photofrin for Injection (8%)
Phrenilin
Ponstel Capsules (Occasional)
Prevacid (Less than 1%)
Prevpac (Less than 1% to 3%)
Prilosec (Less than 1%)
Primaxin (Less than 0.2%)
Prinivil Tablets (0.3% to 1.0%)
Prinzide Tablets
ProAmatine Tablets (Less frequent)
▲ Prograf (3% to 15%)
▲ Proleukin for Injection (34%)
Prometrium Capsules (Less than 5%)
ProSom Tablets (2%)
Protonix (Less than 1%)
Provigil Tablets (1%)
Prozac (Frequent)
Quinaglute Dura-Tabs Tablets
Quinidex Extentabs
▲ Rapamune (3% to 20%)
Reglan (Less frequent)
Relafen Tablets (Less than 1%)
Remeron (2%)
Remicade for IV Injection (Less than 2%)
Reminyl (Greater than or equal to 2%)
ReoPro Vials (0.6%)
▲ Requip Tablets (5%)
Rescriptor Tablets (Less than 2%)
Retrovir Capsules, Tablets & Syrup
Retrovir IV Infusion
Rifadin

Rifamate Capsules
Rifater Tablets
Rilutek Tablets (Infrequent)
Risperdal (Infrequent)
Robaxin Injectable
Robaxin Tablets
Robinul Injectable
Robinul Tablets
▲ Roferon-A Injection (Less than 4% to 8%)
Romazicon Injection (Less than 1%)
Roxanol
Roxanol 100
Roxanol-T
Roxicodone Intensol
Roxicodone Oral Solution
Roxicodone Tablets (Less than 3%)
Rynatan Tablets
Rythmol Tablets (Less than 1%)
Salagen Tablets (Less than 1%)
Sandimmune (2% or less)
▲ Sandostatin LAR Depot (5% to 15%)
Sarafem Pulvules (Frequent)
Sedapap Tablets (Infrequent)
Sensorcaine Injection
Sensorcaine-MPF Injection
Sensorcaine-MPF with Epinephrine Injection
Serentil
Seroquel Tablets (Infrequent)
▲ Serzone Tablets (7% to 8%)
▲ Sinemet CR Tablets (3.7%)
Sinemet Tablets
Sinequan (Infrequent)
Soma Compound (Very rare)
Soma Compound w/Codeine (Very rare)
Soma Tablets
Sonata Capsules (Infrequent)
▲ Stadol NS Nasal Spray (3-9%)
Sterile FUDR (Remote possibility)
Sular Tablets (Less than or equal to 1%)
Surmontil Capsules
Sustiva Capsules (Less than 2%)
Symmetrel (0.1% to 5%)
Synercid I.V. (Less than 1%)
Tagamet (Occasional)
Talacen Caplets
Talwin Nx Tablets
Tambocor Tablets (Less than 1%)
Tamiflu
Tarka Tablets
▲ Tasmar Tablets (10% to 11%)

Taxotere for Injection Concentrate
Tegretol
▲ Temodar Capsules (5%)
Tenex Tablets (3% or less)
Tequin (Less than 0.1%)
Tessalon Capsules
Thalomid Capsules
Timolide Tablets (Less than 1%)
Timolol GFS
Timoptic (Less frequent)
▲ Tonocard Tablets (2.1% to 11.2%)
▲ Topamax (8.9% to 15%)
Toprol-XL Tablets
Transderm Scop (Infrequent)
Tranxene (Less common)
▲ Trasylol Injection (4%)
Trental Tablets (Less than 1%)
Tricor Tablets (Less than 1%)
Trileptal (1% to 2%)
Trilisate Liquid (Rare)
Trilisate Tablets (Rare)
▲ Trisenox Injection (5%)
Trovan (Less than 1%)
Ultracet Tablets (At least 1%)
Ultram Tablets (1% to 5%)
Uroqid-Acid No. 2 Tablets
Valcyte Tablets (Less than 5%)
Valium Injectable
Valium Tablets (Infrequent)
Valtrex Caplets
Vantin (Less than 1%)
Vaseretic Tablets
Vasotec I.V. Injection
Vasotec Tablets (0.5% to 1%)
Verelan Capsules (1% or less)
Verelan PM Capsules (2% or less)
Versed Injection (Less than 1%)
Versed Syrup (Less than 1%)
▲ Vesanoid Capsules (14%)
Vicoprofen Tablets (Less than 3%)
Vioxx
Vistide Injection
Vivactil Tablets
Wellbutrin SR
▲ Wellbutrin Tablets (8.4%)
▲ Xanax Tablets (9.9% to 10.4%)
Xeloda Tablets (Less than 5%)
▲ Xylocaine Injection (Among most
   common)
▲ Xylocaine with Epinephrine Injection
   (Among most common)
Zantac Injection (Rare)
Zantac Tablets, Granules, & Syrup
   (Rare)
Zestoretic Tablets

Zestril Tablets (0.3% to 1.0%)
Zoloft (Infrequent)
▲ Zometa for Intravenous Infusion
   (12.8%)
▲ Zonegran Capsules (6%)
Zosyn (1.0% or less)
Zovirax Capsules, Tablets, &
   Suspension
Zovirax for Injection (Approximately
   1%)
Zyban (Infrequent)
Zyprexa
Zyrtec (Less than 2%)
Zyrtec-D (Less than 2%)

Confusion, nocturnal

Etrafon
Thioridazine Hydrochloride Tablets
   (Extremely rare)
Trilafon

Consciousness, disorders of

Amerge Tablets (Rare)
▲ Betapace Tablets (2% to 4%)
Comtan Tablets
Hexalen Capsules
Intron A for Injection (Less than 5%)
Neoral
Permax Tablets
Reglan
Sandimmune
Symmetrel (Uncommon)
Tasmar Tablets (Four cases)
Valtrex Caplets
Zovirax Capsules, Tablets, &
   Suspension

Delirium

AcipHex Tablets
Amicar
Ativan Injection (1.3%)
Betaseron
Brevital
Catapres Tablets
Catapres-TTS (0.5% or less)
▲ CellCept (3% to 10%)
Cerebyx Injection
Cipro
Cipro I.V.
Clorpres Tablets
Clozaril Tablets
Cognex Capsules (Infrequent)
Combipres Tablets
Digitek Tablets
Diprivan (Less than 1%)

Duraclon Injection (Rare)
Effexor Tablets
Effexor XR Capsules
Evoxac Capsules
Exelon (Infrequent)
Famvir Tablets (Infrequent)
Geodon Capsules (Frequent)
Lamictal (Rare)
Lanoxin/Lanoxicaps
Levaquin (Less than 0.3%)
Luvox Tablets (Infrequent)
Merrem I.V. (0.1% to 1.0%)
Nardil Tablets (Less frequent)
Orthoclone OKT3 (Less than 1%)
Paxil (Rare)
PhosLo
Prograf
Quinaglute Dura-Tabs Tablets
Quinidex Extentabs
Remeron (Infrequent)
Remicade for IV Injection
 (Less than 2%)
Reminyl (Infrequent)
Requip Tablets (Infrequent)
Rilutek Tablets (Infrequent)
Risperdal (Rare)
Romazicon Injection (Less than 1%)
Seroquel Tablets (Rare)
Symmetrel
Tasmar Tablets (Rare)
Topamax (Infrequent)
Trileptal
Vistide Injection
Wellbutrin SR
Wellbutrin Tablets
Zovirax Capsules, Tablets, &
 Suspension
Zovirax for Injection
Zyban
Zyprexa (Infrequent)

Delusions

Ambien Tablets (Rare)
Aricept Tablets (Frequent)
Artane (Rare)
Betaseron
Celexa (Rare)
Clozaril Tablets (Less than 1%)
Effexor Tablets (Rare)
Effexor XR Capsules (Rare)
Eldepryl Capsules
Etrafon
Evoxac Capsules
Exelon (2% or more)

Felbatol
Flexeril Tablets (Rare)
Gabitril Tablets (Infrequent)
Halcion Tablets
Lamictal (Rare)
Limbitrol
Lodosyn Tablets
▲ Lupron Depot 3.75 mg (Among most
 frequent)
Lupron Depot—3 Month 11.25 mg
 (Less than 5%)
Lupron Depot—3 Month 22.5 mg
 (Less than 5%)
Luvox Tablets (Infrequent)
Mirapex Tablets (1%)
Norpramin Tablets
Nubain Injection (1% or less)
Paxil (Rare)
Permax Tablets (Infrequent)
Prozac (Rare)
Remeron (Infrequent)
Requip Tablets (Infrequent)
Rilutek Tablets (Infrequent)
Salagen Tablets (Rare)
Sarafem Pulvules (Rare)
Seroquel Tablets (Infrequent)
Sinemet CR Tablets
Sinemet Tablets
Sonata Capsules (Rare)
Stadol NS Nasal Spray (Less than 1%)
Surmontil Capsules
Sustiva Capsules
Symmetrel
Tasmar Tablets (Infrequent)
Topamax (Infrequent)
Trileptal
Vivactil Tablets
Wellbutrin SR
Wellbutrin Tablets (1.2%)
Zoloft (Infrequent)
Zyban

Dementia

Ambien Tablets (Rare)
Betaseron
Depacon Injection (Several reports)
Depakene (Several reports)
Depakote ER Tablets (Several reports)
Depakote Sprinkle Capsules (Several
 reports)
Depakote Tablets (Several reports)
Effexor Tablets (Rare)
Effexor XR Capsules (Rare)
Evoxac Capsules

Exelon (Infrequent)
Foscavir Injection (Between 1% and 5%)
Hivid Tablets (Less than 1%)
Lodosyn Tablets
Lupron Depot—4 Month 30 mg (Less than 5%)
Remeron (Rare)
Requip Tablets (Infrequent)
Rilutek Tablets (Rare)
Sinemet CR Tablets
Sinemet Tablets
▲ Vesanoid Capsules (3%)
Vistide Injection
Zanaflex Tablets (Rare)

Depersonalization
Ambien Tablets (Rare)
Anzemet (Infrequently)
Astelin Nasal Spray (Infrequent)
Avelox Tablets (0.05% to 1%)
Avonex
Betaseron
Biaxin
Buprenex Injectable (Infrequent)
Cardura Tablets (Less than 0.5%)
Celexa (Infrequent)
Cerebyx Injection (Infrequent)
Cipro (Less than 1%)
Cipro I.V. (1% or less)
Copaxone (Infrequent)
Duragesic Transdermal System (Less than 1%)
Effexor Tablets (1%)
Effexor XR Capsules (Frequent)
Evoxac Capsules (Less than 1%)
Exelon (Infrequent)
Gabitril Tablets (Frequent)
Halcion Tablets
Helixate Concentrate
Hivid Tablets (Less than 1%)
Indocin Capsules/Suspension/Suppositories (Less than 1%)
Klonopin Tablets (Infrequent)
Kogenate FS
Lamictal (Infrequent)
Luvox Tablets (Infrequent)
Marinol Capsules (Greater than 1%)
Maxalt (Rare)
Neurontin (Infrequent)
Norvasc Tablets (More than 0.1% to 1%)
Nubain Injection (1% or less)

OxyContin Tablets (Less than 1%)
Paxil (Infrequent)
Prevacid (Less than 1%)
Prevpac
Prozac (Infrequent)
Remeron (Infrequent)
Requip Tablets (Infrequent)
Rilutek Tablets (Infrequent)
Romazicon Injection (1% to 3%)
Sarafem Pulvules (Infrequent)
Seroquel Tablets (Infrequent)
Serzone Tablets (Infrequent)
Sonata Capsules (Less than 1% to 2%)
Tambocor Tablets (Less than 1%)
Tequin (Less than 0.1%)
Topamax (1.6% to 1.8%)
Trovan (Less than 1%)
Ultracet Tablets (Less than 1%)
Wellbutrin SR (Infrequent)
Wellbutrin Tablets (Infrequent)
Xanax Tablets
Zanaflex Tablets (Infrequent)
Zoloft (Infrequent)
Zyban (Infrequent)
Zyprexa (Infrequent)
Zyrtec (Less than 2%)

Depression
8-MOP Capsules
Accupril Tablets (0.5% to 1.0%)
Accuretic Tablets (Greater than 0.5%)
Accutane Capsules
Aceon Tablets (2.0%)
AcipHex Tablets
▲ Actimmune (3%)
Activella Tablets
▲ Actonel Tablets (6.8%)
Adalat CC Tablets (Less than 1.0%)
Adderall XR Capsules (0.7%)
Advair Diskus
Aerobid (1% to 3%)
▲ Agenerase (9% to 16%)
Agrylin Capsules (1% to 5%)
Aldoclor Tablets
Aldomet Tablets
Aldoril Tablets
Alesse-21 Tablets
Alesse-28 Tablets
Alferon N Injection (One patient to 3%)
Alora Transdermal System
Alphagan Ophthalmic Solution (Less than 3%)

Altace Capsules (Less than 1%)
Ambien Tablets (2%)
AmBisome for Injection (Less common)
Amerge Tablets (Infrequent)
Amphotec (1% to 5%)
▲ Androderm (3%)
AndroGel (Up to 1%)
▲ Android Capsules (Among most common)
Arava Tablets (1% to 3%)
▲ Aricept Tablets (3%)
▲ Arimidex Tablets (2.4% to 5.3%)
▲ Aromasin Tablets (13%)
Arthrotec Tablets (Rare)
Asacol Tablets
Astelin Nasal Spray (Infrequent)
Atacand HCT Tablets (0.5% or greater)
Atacand Tablets (0.5% or greater)
Ativan Injection (1.3%)
Ativan Tablets (Less frequent)
Avalide Tablets
Avapro Tablets (Less than 1%)
Avelox Tablets
Avonex
Axert Tablets (Rare)
Aygestin Tablets
Azmacort Inhalation Aerosol
Azulfidine (Rare)
Bactrim
Beconase AQ Nasal Spray
Beconase Inhalation Aerosol
Betagan
Betapace Tablets (1% to 4%)
Betaseron
Betimol Ophthalmic Solution
Betoptic S Ophthalmic Suspension (Rare)
Bextra Tablets (0.1% to 1.9%)
Blocadren Tablets
Brevibloc Injection (Less than 1%)
Brevicon 28-Day Tablets
▲ Campath Ampules (1% to 7%)
Captopril Tablets
Carbatrol Capsules
Cardizem
Cardura Tablets (1%)
▲ Carnitor Injection (5% to 6%)
Carteolol
▲ Casodex Tablets (4%)
Cataflam Tablets (Less than 1%)
Catapres Tablets (About 1 in 100 patients)

Catapres-TTS (0.5% or less)
Celebrex Capsules (0.1% to 1.9%)
Celestone Soluspan Injectable Suspension
Celexa (Frequent)
▲ CellCept (3% to 15.6%)
Celontin Capsules
▲ Cenestin Tablets (28%)
Cerebyx Injection (Infrequent)
Chibroxin Ophthalmic Solution
Cipro (Less than 1%)
Cipro I.V. (1% or less)
Claritin (At least one patient)
Claritin-D 12 Hour (Less frequent)
Claritin-D 24 Hour (Fewer than 2%)
Climara Transdermal System
Clinoril Tablets (Less than 1%)
Clomid Tablets (Fewer than 1%)
Clorpres Tablets (About 1%)
Clozaril Tablets (1%)
Cogentin
▲ Cognex Capsules (4%)
Colazal Capsules
▲ CombiPatch (8% to 9%)
Combipres Tablets (About 1%)
Concerta
Copaxone (At least 2%)
Coreg Tablets (Greater than 2%)
Corgard Tablets
Cortone
Corzide
Cosopt Ophthalmic Solution (Less than 1%)
Cozaar Tablets (Less than 1%)
▲ Crinone 4% Gel (19%)
▲ Crinone 8% Gel (11% to 15%)
Crixivan Capsules (Less than 2%)
Cyclessa Tablets
Cylert
Cytovene (At least 3 subjects)
Dantrium Capsules (Less frequent)
Daranide Tablets
▲ DaunoXome Injection (3% to 7%)
DDAVP Nasal Spray
DDAVP Rhinal Tube
Decadron
Delatestryl Injection
Demser Capsules
▲ Depacon Injection (4% to 5%)
▲ Depakene (5%)
Depakote ER Tablets (Greater than 1%)
▲ Depakote Sprinkle Capsules (4% to 5%)
Depakote Tablets (1% to 5%)

Depo-Provera Contraceptive Injection
(1% to 5%)
Desmopressin Acetate Rhinal Tube
Desogen Tablets
Didronel Tablets
Digitek Tablets
Dilaudid Oral Liquid (Less frequent)
Dilaudid Tablets - 8 mg (Less
frequent)
Dilaudid-HP (Less frequent)
Diovan HCT Tablets (Greater than
0.2%)
Dipentum Capsules (1.5%)
Diprivan (Less than 1%)
Dolobid Tablets (Less than 1 in 100)
▲ Dostinex Tablets (3%)
Doxil Injection (Less than 1% to 5%)
Duraclon Injection (1%)
▲ Duragesic Transdermal System (3% to
10%)
Duranest Injections
Dynabac Tablets (0.1% to 1%)
DynaCirc (0.5% to 1%)
Effexor Tablets (1%)
▲ Effexor XR Capsules (3%)
Eldepryl Capsules
Eligard (Less than 2%)
Elmiron Capsules
Elspar for Injection (No incidence
data in labeling)
Enalaprilat Injection
Enbrel for Injection (Infrequent)
Ergamisol Tablets (1% to 2%)
Esclim Transdermal System
Estinyl Tablets
Estrace
Estratest
Estring Vaginal Ring (At least 1
report)
Estrostep 21 Tablets
Estrostep Fe Tablets
Eulexin Capsules (1%)
▲ Evista Tablets (6.4%)
Evoxac Capsules (1% to 3%)
▲ Exelon (6%)
Famotidine Injection (Infrequent)
Fareston Tablets
▲ Felbatol (5.3%)
Feldene Capsules (Occasional)
Femara Tablets (Less frequent)
▲ femhrt Tablets (5.8%)
Flexeril Tablets (Less than 1%)
▲ Flolan for Injection (13% to 37%)
Florinef Acetate Tablets

Flovent Diskus
Flovent Inhalation Aerosol
Flovent Rotadisk
Floxin (Less than 1%)
Fludara for Injection (Up to 1%)
Flumadine (0.3% to 1%)
Focalin Tablets
Fortovase Capsules (2.7%)
▲ Foscavir Injection (5% or greater)
▲ Gabitril Tablets (3%)
Gastrocrom Oral Concentrate
(Less common)
Gengraf Capsules (Rare)
▲ Gliadel Wafer (3%)
Glucotrol XL (Less than 3%)
Halcion Tablets (0.5% to 0.9%)
Haldol
Haldol Decanoate
▲ Herceptin I.V. (6%)
Hivid Tablets (0.4%)
Hydrocortone
Hytrin Capsules (0.3%)
Hyzaar
Imdur Tablets (Less than or equal to
5%)
Imitrex Injection (Rare)
Imitrex Nasal Spray (Infrequent)
Imitrex Tablets (Infrequent)
Indapamide Tablets (Less than 5%)
Inderal
Inderide
Indocin
Capsules/Suspension/Suppositories
(Greater than 1%)
▲ Infergen (18% to 26%)
▲ Intron A for Injection (2% to 40%)
Invirase Capsules (Less than 2%)
Iopidine 0.5% Ophthalmic Solution
(Less than 3%)
Kadian Capsules (Less than 3%)
Kaletra (Less than 2%)
▲ Keppra Tablets (4%)
▲ Klonopin Tablets (4% to 7%)
▲ Lamictal (4.2%)
Lanoxin/Lanoxicaps
Lariam Tablets
Lescol Capsules
Lescol XL Tablets
Levaquin (Less than 0.3%)
Levlen
Levlite
Levo-Dromoran
Levora Tablets
Lexxel Tablets

Lidoderm Patch
Lipitor Tablets (Less than 2%)
Lo/Ovral
Lodine (1% to 3%)
Lodine XL Extended-Release Tablets (1% to 3%)
Loestrin
Lopid Tablets
Low-Ogestrel-28 Tablets
Lunelle Monthly Injection
▲ Lupron Depot 3.75 mg (10.8%)
▲ Lupron Depot—3 Month 11.25 mg (10.8% to 22%)
Lupron Depot—3 Month 22.5 mg (Less than 5%)
Lupron Depot—4 Month 30 mg (Less than 5%)
Lupron Injection (Less than 5%)
Luvox Tablets (2%)
LYMErix Vaccine (1.02%)
Macrobid Capsules (Rare)
Macrodantin Capsules (Rare)
Marinol Capsules (Less than 1%)
Matulane Capsules
Maxair (Less than 1%)
Maxalt (Infrequent)
Maxzide
Megace Oral Suspension (1% to 3%)
Menest Tablets
▲ Meridia Capsules (4.3%)
Merrem I.V. (0.1% to 1.0%)
Metadate
Methylin
MetroGel-Vaginal Gel (Less than 1%)
Mevacor Tablets (0.5% to 1.0%)
Mexitil Capsules (2.4%)
Miacalcin Nasal Spray (1% to 3%)
Micardis HCT Tablets
Micardis Tablets (More than 0.3%)
Microgestin Fe
Midamor Tablets (Less than or equal to 1%)
Migranal Nasal Spray (Rare)
Minipress Capsules (1% to 4%)
Minizide Capsules (Rare)
Mintezol
Mirapex Tablets (1% or more)
▲ Mirena Intrauterine System (5% or more)
Mithracin
Moban (Less frequent)
Mobic Tablets (Less than 2%)
Modicon
Moduretic Tablets (Less than or equal

to 1%)
Monopril HCT (Less than 2%)
Monopril Tablets (0.4% to 1.0%)
Motofen Tablets
Motrin (Less than 1%)
MS Contin Tablets (Less frequent)
MSIR (Less frequent)
Mykrox Tablets (Less than 2%)
▲ Mylotarg for Injection (8% to 13%)
Nadolol Tablets
Naprelan Tablets (Less than 1%)
Naropin Injection
Nasacort Nasal Inhaler
Necon
Neoral (Rare)
Nesacaine
Neurontin (1.8%)
Nicotrol Nasal Spray (Under 5%)
▲ Nilandron Tablets (8.6%)
Nimotop Capsules (Up to 1.4%)
▲ Nipent for Injection (3% to 10%)
Nizoral Tablets (Rare)
Nolvadex Tablets (Infrequent)
Nordette-28 Tablets
Norinyl
Normodyne Tablets
Noroxin Tablets (Less frequent)
Norvasc Tablets (More than 0.1% to 1%)
Norvir (Less than 2%)
Novarel for Injection
Nubain Injection (1% or less)
Numorphan
Ogen Tablets
Ogestrel Tablets
OptiPranolol (A small number of patients)
Oramorph SR Tablets (Less frequent)
▲ Orap Tablets (2 of 20 patients)
Ortho Dienestrol Cream
Ortho Tri-Cyclen
Ortho-Cept
Ortho-Cyclen
Ortho-Est Tablets
Ortho-Novum
▲ Ortho-Prefest Tablets (5%)
Orudis Capsules (Greater than 1%)
Oruvail Capsules (Greater than 1%)
Ovcon
Ovral
Ovrette Tablets
Oxandrin Tablets
Oxsoralen-Ultra Capsules
OxyContin Tablets (Less than 1%)

Paxil (Frequent)
Pediazole Suspension
▲ PEG-Intron Powder for Injection (29%)
Pentasa Capsules (Less than 1%)
Pepcid (Infrequent)
▲ Permax Tablets (3.2%)
Phrenilin
▲ Plavix Tablets (3.6%)
Plendil (0.5% to 1.5%)
Polocaine
Polocaine-MPF
Ponstel Capsules (Occasional)
Pravachol Tablets
Prednisone
Pregnyl for Injection
Prelone Syrup
Premarin
Premphase Tablets
▲ Prempro Tablets (6% to 11%)
Prevacid (Less than 1%)
Prevpac (Less than 1%)
Prilosec (Less than 1%)
Prinivil Tablets (Greater than 1%)
Prinzide Tablets (0.3% to 1%)
Procanbid Extended-Release Tablets (Occasional)
Procardia Capsules (Less than 0.5%)
Procardia XL Tablets (1% or less)
▲ Prograf (3% to 15%)
Proleukin for Injection (Less than 1%)
▲ Prometrium Capsules (Less than 5% to 19%)
ProSom Tablets (2%)
Protonix (Less than 1%)
Protopic Ointment (Greater than or equal to 1%)
Proventil HFA Inhalation Aerosol (Less than 3%)
Provera Tablets
▲ Provigil Tablets (4%)
Prozac (Less than 1%)
Pulmicort Respules (Less than 1%)
Pulmicort Turbuhaler Powder (Rare)
Quinaglute Dura-Tabs Tablets
Quinidex Extentabs (Occasional)
▲ Rapamune (3% to 20%)
▲ Rebetol Capsules (23% to 36%)
▲ Rebetron Combination Therapy (23% to 36%)
Reglan (Less frequent)
Relafen Tablets (Less than 1%)
Remeron (Frequent)
Remicade for IV Injection (Less than 2%)

▲ Reminyl (7%)
Requip Tablets (1% or more)
Retrovir Capsules, Tablets & Syrup
Retrovir IV Infusion
Rhinocort Nasal Inhaler (Rare)
▲ Rilutek Tablets (4.2% to 6.1%)
Risperdal (Infrequent)
Ritalin
▲ Rituxan (Among most frequent)
▲ Roferon-A Injection (16% to 28%)
Romazicon Injection (1% to 3%)
Rythmol Tablets (Less than 1%)
Salagen Tablets (Less than 1%)
Sandimmune (Rare)
Sandostatin Injection (1% to 4%)
▲ Sandostatin LAR Depot (5% to 15%)
Sectral Capsules (2%)
Sedapap Tablets (Infrequent)
Sensorcaine Injection
Sensorcaine with Epinephrine Injection
Sensorcaine-MPF Injection
Sensorcaine-MPF with Epinephrine Injection
Septra
Serophene Tablets (Less than 1 in 100 patients)
▲ Serostim for Injection (1% to 10%)
Serzone Tablets
▲ Simulect for Injection (3% to 10%)
Sinemet CR Tablets (2.2%)
Sinemet Tablets
Solu-Medrol Sterile Powder
Sonata Capsules (Frequent)
▲ Soriatane Capsules (1% to 10%)
Sporanox Capsules (Infrequent)
Sporanox Oral Solution (1.1% to 2.0%)
Stadol NS Nasal Spray (Less than 1%)
Sular Tablets (Less than or equal to 1%)
Sustiva Capsules (2% to 3%)
Symmetrel (1% to 5%)
▲ Synarel Nasal Solution for Endometriosis (3% of patients)
Tagamet
Talacen Caplets (Infrequent)
Talwin Nx Tablets
Tambocor Tablets (1% to 3%)
Tasmar Tablets (Frequent)
▲ Temodar Capsules (6%)
Tenex Tablets (3% or less)
▲ Tenoretic Tablets (0.6% to 12%)
▲ Tenormin (0.6% to 12%)
Tequin (Less than 0.1%)

Testoderm Transdermal Systems
Testopel Pellets
Testred Capsules
Teveten Tablets (1%)
Thalomid Capsules
Tiazac Capsules (Less than 2%)
Timolide Tablets
Timolol GFS
Timoptic (Less frequent)
Tolectin 200 Tablets (1% to 3%)
Tolectin 600 Tablets (1% to 3%)
Tolectin DS Capsules (1% to 3%)
Tonocard Tablets (Less than 1%)
▲ Topamax (8% to 13.4%)
▲ Toprol-XL Tablets (About 5 of 100 patients)
Toradol (1% or less)
Tranxene
Travatan Ophthalmic Solution (1% to 5%)
Trecator-SC Tablets
Trental Tablets (Less than 1%)
Tricor Tablets
Tri-Levlen
Tri-Norinyl
Triphasil
▲ Trisenox Injection (20%)
Trivora Tablets
▲ Trizivir Tablets (9%)
Trovan (Less than 1%)
Ultracet Tablets (Less than 1%)
Ultram Tablets (Less than 1%)
Uniretic Tablets (Less than 1%)
Valium Injectable
Valium Tablets (Infrequent)
▲ Valtrex Caplets (Less than 1% to 7%)
Vanceril Double Strength Inhalation Aerosol (Fewer than 2%)
Vascor Tablets (0.5% to 2.0%)
Vaseretic Tablets
Vasotec I.V. Injection
Vasotec Tablets (0.5% to 1%)
▲ Vesanoid Capsules (14%)
▲ Viadur Implant (5.3%)
Viagra Tablets (Less than 2%)
Vicoprofen Tablets (Less than 1%)
Vioxx (Greater than 0.1% to 1.9%)
Viracept
Vistide Injection
Vivelle Transdermal System
Vivelle-Dot Transdermal System
Voltaren (Less than 1%)
Wellbutrin Tablets (Frequent)
▲ Xanax Tablets (13.8% to 13.9%)

▲ Xenical Capsules (3.4%)
Yasmin 28 Tablets (Greater than 1%)
Zanaflex Tablets (Frequent)
Zantac Injection (Rare)
Zantac Tablets, Granules, & Syrup (Rare)
Zarontin (Rare)
Zaroxolyn Tablets
Zebeta Tablets (Up to 0.2%)
▲ Zenapax for Injection (2% to 5%)
Zestoretic Tablets (0.3% to 1%)
Zestril Tablets (Greater than 1%)
Ziac Tablets
Zocor Tablets
▲ Zoladex (1% to 54%)
Zoladex 3-month
Zoloft (Infrequent)
▲ Zometa for Intravenous Infusion (12%)
Zomig (Infrequent)
▲ Zonegran Capsules (6%)
Zosyn (1.0% or less)
Zovia
Zyban (Frequent)
Zyprexa
Zyrtec (Less than 2%)
Zyrtec-D (Less than 2%)

Depression, aggravation of

Bextra Tablets (0.1% to 1.9%)
Celexa (Frequent)
Coreg Tablets (0.1% to 1%)
Evoxac Capsules (Less than 1%)
Halcion Tablets
Intron A for Injection (Less than 5%)
Lupron Depot 3.75 mg (A possibility)
Lupron Depot—3 Month 11.25 mg (Possible)
Meridia Capsules
Nexium (Less than 1%)
Sustiva Capsules (Less than 2%)
Tegretol
Zoloft (Infrequent)

Depression, psychotic

8-MOP Capsules
Celexa (Infrequent)
Copaxone (Infrequent)
Effexor Tablets (Rare)
Effexor XR Capsules (Infrequent)
▲ Ifex for Injection (Among most common)
Paxil (Rare)
Remeron (Rare)
Rilutek Tablets (Rare)

Depressive reactions
▲ Combivir Tablets (9%)
▲ Epivir (9%)
Rescriptor Tablets (Less than 2%)
Soma Compound (Infrequent or rare)
Soma Compound w/Codeine
(Infrequent or rare)
Soma Tablets
Xanax Tablets

Disinhibition
Versed Syrup (Less than 1%)

Disordered sense of smell
Ambien Tablets (Rare)
Astelin Nasal Spray
Axert Tablets (Rare)
Betaseron
Cardura Tablets (Less than 0.5%)
Cerebyx Injection (Infrequent)
Colazal Capsules
Doxil Injection (Less than 1%)
Effexor Tablets (Infrequent)
Effexor XR Capsules (Infrequent)
Evoxac Capsules (Less than 1%)
Flumadine (Less than 0.3%)
Gabitril Tablets (Infrequent)
Hivid Tablets (Less than 1%)
Intron A for Injection (Less than 5%)
Iopidine 0.5% Ophthalmic Solution
(0.2%)
Lamictal (Rare)
Levaquin (Less than 0.5%)
Lipitor Tablets (Less than 2%)
Luvox Tablets (Infrequent)
Miacalcin Nasal Spray (Less than 1%)
Nexium (Less than 1%)
Norvasc Tablets (Less than or equal to
0.1%)
Norvir (Less than 2%)
Paxil (Rare)
Prevacid (Less than 1%)
Prevpac (Less than 1%)
Prozac (Rare)
Remeron (Rare)
Rescriptor Tablets
Sarafem Pulvules (Rare)
Sonata Capsules (Less than 1% to
2%)
Sustiva Capsules (Less than 2%)
Tasmar Tablets (Infrequent)
Tequin (Less than 0.1%)
Topamax (Infrequent)
Zomig (Infrequent)
Zonegran Capsules (Infrequent)

Zyrtec (Less than 2%)
Zyrtec-D (Less than 2%)

Disorientation
AcipHex Tablets
Actimmune (Rare)
Akineton
Alferon N Injection (1%)
Arthrotec Tablets (Rare)
Asacol Tablets
Ativan Tablets (Less frequent)
Biaxin
Botox
Cataflam Tablets (Rare)
Cosopt Ophthalmic Solution
Daranide Tablets
Demerol
Demser Capsules
Dilaudid Oral Liquid (Less frequent)
Dilaudid Tablets - 8 mg (Less
frequent)
Dilaudid-HP (Less frequent)
Dolobid Tablets (Less than 1 in 100)
Dolophine Tablets
Dopram Injectable
Eldepryl Capsules
Etrafon
Famvir Tablets (Infrequent)
Flexeril Tablets (Less than 1%)
Floxin
Halcion Tablets
Ifex for Injection (Less frequent)
INFeD Injection
Levbid
Levsin
Lodosyn Tablets
Maxalt (Infrequent)
Mepergan Injection
MS Contin Tablets (Less frequent)
MSIR (Less frequent)
Myambutol Tablets
Mylocel Tablets (Extremely rare)
Nebcin
Norpramin Tablets
Oncaspar
Oramorph SR Tablets (Less frequent)
Orthoclone OKT3
Parnate Tablets
Pediazole Suspension
Phenergan Suppositories
Phenergan Syrup
Phenergan VC Syrup
Phenergan VC with Codeine Syrup
Phenergan with Codeine Syrup

Phenergan with Dextromethorphan Syrup
Prevpac
Rescriptor Tablets (Less than 2%)
Roxanol
Roxanol 100
Roxanol-T
Sinemet CR Tablets
Sinemet Tablets
Sinequan (Infrequent)
Soma Compound (Very rare)
Soma Compound w/Codeine (Very rare)
Soma Tablets
Sterile FUDR (Remote possibility)
Surmontil Capsules
Tagamet
Talacen Caplets
Talwin Nx Tablets
Timolol GFS
Timoptic (Less frequent)
▲ Tonocard Tablets (2.1% to 11.2%)
Transderm Scop (Infrequent)
Vivactil Tablets
Voltaren (Rare)

Disorientation, place
Blocadren Tablets
Corgard Tablets
Corzide
Cosopt Ophthalmic Solution
Inderal
Inderide
Nadolol Tablets
Normodyne Tablets
Sectral Capsules
Tenoretic Tablets
Tenormin
Timolide Tablets
Timolol GFS
Timoptic
Toprol-XL Tablets
Zebeta Tablets
Ziac Tablets

Disorientation, time
Blocadren Tablets
Corgard Tablets
Corzide
Cosopt Ophthalmic Solution
Inderal
Inderide
Nadolol Tablets
Normodyne Tablets
Sectral Capsules

Tenoretic Tablets
Tenormin
Timolide Tablets
Timolol GFS
Timoptic
Toprol-XL Tablets
Zebeta Tablets
Ziac Tablets

Disorientation, spatial
Serophene Tablets

Double vision
Abelcet Injection
AcipHex Tablets
Adalat CC Tablets (Less than 1.0%)
Agrylin Capsules (1% to 5%)
Ambien Tablets (Frequent)
Arthrotec Tablets (Rare)
Ativan Injection (Occasional)
Axert Tablets (Rare)
Azactam for Injection (Less than 1%)
Azopt Ophthalmic Suspension (Less than 1%)
Benadryl Parenteral
Betagan
Betaseron
Betimol Ophthalmic Solution
Blocadren Tablets
Botox (Rare)
Brevicon 28-Day Tablets (Rare)
Buprenex Injectable (Less than 1%)
Carbatrol Capsules
Carteolol
Cataflam Tablets (Less than 1%)
Celexa (Rare)
▲ Cerebyx Injection (3.3%)
Chibroxin Ophthalmic Solution
Chirocaine Injection (2.5%)
Cipro (Less than 1%)
Cipro I.V. (1% or less)
Clomid Tablets (1.5%)
Cognex Capsules (Infrequent)
Copaxone (At least 2%)
Cosopt Ophthalmic Solution
Dantrium Capsules (Less frequent)
▲ Depacon Injection (16%)
▲ Depakene (16%)
Depakote ER Tablets (Greater than 1%)
▲ Depakote Sprinkle Capsules (16%)
▲ Depakote Tablets (1% to 16%)
Depen Titratable Tablets
Depo-Provera Contraceptive Injection
Dilaudid Oral Liquid (Less frequent)

Dilaudid Tablets - 8 mg (Less frequent)
Dilaudid-HP (Less frequent)
Diprivan (Less than 1%)
Duranest Injections
Effexor Tablets (Infrequent)
Effexor XR Capsules (Infrequent)
ELA-Max Cream
Eldepryl Capsules
EMLA (Unlikely)
Evoxac Capsules (Less than 1%)
Exelon (Infrequent)
Fareston Tablets
▲ Felbatol (3.4% to 6.1%)
femhrt Tablets
Flexeril Tablets (Less than 1%)
Floxin
Gabitril Tablets (1% or more)
Geodon Capsules (Frequent)
Gliadel Wafer (1%)
Indocin Capsules/Suspension/Suppositories (Less than 1%)
Intron A for Injection (Less than 5%)
Ismo Tablets (Fewer than 1%)
Kadian Capsules (Less than 3%)
Keppra Tablets (2%)
Klonopin Tablets (Infrequent)
▲ Lamictal (24% to 49%)
Levaquin (Less than 0.3%)
Levlen (Rare)
Levlite (Rare)
Levo-Dromoran
Lidoderm Patch
Lodosyn Tablets
Luvox Tablets (Infrequent)
Matulane Capsules
Mirapex Tablets (1% or more)
Modicon (Rare)
Motrin (Less than 1%)
MS Contin Tablets (Less frequent)
MSIR (Less frequent)
Naprelan Tablets (Less than 1%)
▲ Neurontin (5.9%)
Norinyl
Noroxin Tablets
Norvasc Tablets (More than 0.1% to 1%)
Norvir (Less than 2%)
Numorphan
Oramorph SR Tablets (Less frequent)
Ortho Tri-Cyclen (Rare)
Orthoclone OKT3
Ortho-Cyclen (Rare)

Ortho-Novum (Rare)
Ovcon
Paxil (Rare)
Periactin Tablets (No incidence data in labeling)
Permax Tablets (2.1%)
Phenergan Injection
Phenergan Suppositories
Phenergan Tablets
Photofrin for Injection
Pletal Tablets (Less than 2%)
Premphase Tablets
Prempro Tablets
Prevacid (Less than 1%)
Prevpac (Less than 1%)
Prinivil Tablets (0.3% to 1.0%)
Prinzide Tablets
ProSom Tablets (Rare)
Protonix (Less than 1%)
Protopam Chloride for Injection
Provera Tablets
Prozac (Rare)
Quinaglute Dura-Tabs Tablets
Quinidex Extentabs
Remeron (Rare)
ReoPro Vials (0.1%)
Requip Tablets (2%)
Rescriptor Tablets (Less than 2%)
Rescula Ophthalmic Solution (Less than 1%)
Rilutek Tablets (Rare)
Risperdal (Rare)
Robaxin Injectable
Robaxin Tablets
Romazicon Injection (1% to 3%)
Sarafem Pulvules (Rare)
Serophene Tablets
Serzone Tablets (Infrequent)
Sinemet CR Tablets
Sinemet Tablets
Soma Compound (Very rare)
Soma Compound w/Codeine (Very rare)
Soma Tablets
Sonata Capsules (Infrequent)
Soriatane Capsules (1% to 5%)
Sustiva Capsules (Less than 2%)
Tambocor Tablets (1% to 3%)
Tasmar Tablets (Infrequent)
Tegretol
▲ Temodar Capsules (5%)
Tensilon Injectable
Thalomid Capsules
Timolide Tablets

Timolol GFS
Timoptic (Less frequent)
Tonocard Tablets (Less than 1%)
▲ Topamax (14.2% to 14.6%)
Tranxene
Trecator-SC Tablets (Rare)
▲ Trileptal (5% to 40%)
Tri-Levlen (Rare)
Tri-Norinyl
Valium Injectable
Valium Tablets (Infrequent)
Versed Injection (Less than 1%)
Versed Syrup (Less than 1%)
Viagra Tablets
Vistide Injection
▲ Visudyne for Injection (1% to 10%)
Voltaren (Less than 1%)
Wellbutrin SR
Wellbutrin Tablets (Rare)
Xalatan (Less than 1%)
Xanax Tablets
Xylocaine Injection (Less than 1%)
Xylocaine with Epinephrine Injection
  (Less than 1%)
Zestoretic Tablets
Zestril Tablets (0.3% to 1.0%)
Zoloft (Rare)
Zomig (Rare)
▲ Zonegran Capsules (6%)
Zyban
Zyprexa (Infrequent)

Dreaming

Amerge Tablets (Rare)
Dilaudid Oral Liquid (Less frequent)
Dilaudid Tablets - 8 mg (Less
  frequent)
Limbitrol (Less common)
MS Contin Tablets (Less frequent)
MSIR (Less frequent)
Nicotrol Nasal Spray (Under 5%)
▲ Orudis Capsules (3% to 9%)
▲ Oruvail Capsules (3% to 9%)
Tenoretic Tablets (Up to 3%)
Tenormin (Up to 3%)
Versed Injection (Less than 1%)

Dreaming abnormalities

AcipHex Tablets
Actiq (Less than 1%)
Ambien Tablets (1%)
Anaprox (Less than 1%)
Anzemet (Infrequently)
▲ Aricept Tablets (3%)
Arthrotec Tablets (Rare)

Axert Tablets (Rare)
Axid Pulvules (1.9%)
Blocadren Tablets (Less than 1%)
Buprenex Injectable (Less than 1%)
Cardizem
Catapres Tablets
Catapres-TTS (0.5% or less)
Clorpres Tablets
Cognex Capsules (Infrequent)
Combipres Tablets
Copaxone (Frequent)
Cozaar Tablets (Less than 1%)
Crixivan Capsules (Less than 2%)
Cytovene (At least 3 subjects)
Depacon Injection (1% to 5%)
Depakene (1% to 5%)
Depakote ER Tablets (1% to 5%)
Depakote Sprinkle Capsules (1% to
  5%)
Depakote Tablets (1% to 5%)
Dilaudid-HP (Less frequent)
Diprivan (Less than 1%)
Duraclon Injection (Rare)
Duragesic Transdermal System (1% or
  greater)
EC-Naprosyn (Less than 1%)
▲ Effexor Tablets (4%)
▲ Effexor XR Capsules (4% to 7%)
▲ Eldepryl Capsules (2 of 49 patients)
Emadine Ophthalmic Solution (Less
  than 5%)
Enalaprilat Injection
Etrafon
Evoxac Capsules (Less than 1%)
Exelon (Infrequent)
Feldene Capsules (Occasional)
Flexeril Tablets (Less than 1%)
Floxin (Less than 1%)
Fortovase Capsules (Less than 2%)
Gabitril Tablets (Infrequent)
Halcion Tablets (Rare)
Hyzaar
Inderal
Intron A for Injection (Less than 5%)
Invirase Capsules (Less than 2%)
Iopidine Sterile Ophthalmic Solution
Kadian Capsules (Less than 3%)
Kaletra (Less than 2%)
Klonopin Tablets (Infrequent)
Lamictal (Infrequent)
Levaquin (Less than 0.3%)
Levo-Dromoran
Levorphanol Tartrate Tablets (1% to
  3%)

Lipitor Tablets (Less than 2%)
Lodine XL Extended-Release Tablets (Less than 1%)
Lodosyn Tablets
Lotensin HCT Tablets (0.3% or more)
Luvox Tablets
Maxalt (Infrequent)
Meridia Capsules
▲ Mirapex Tablets
Motrin (Less than 1%)
▲ Naprelan Tablets (3% to 9%)
Naprosyn (Less than 1%)
Neurontin (Infrequent)
Nipent for Injection (Less than 3%)
Norvasc Tablets (More than 0.1% to 1%)
Norvir (Less than 2%)
Nubain Injection (1% or less)
Oramorph SR Tablets (Less frequent)
Orap Tablets (2.7%)
OxyContin Tablets (Between 1% and 5%)
▲ Paxil (4%)
Permax Tablets (2.7%)
Ponstel Capsules (Occasional)
Prevacid (Less than 1%)
Prevpac (Less than 1%)
Prilosec (Less than 1%)
▲ Prograf (3% to 15%)
ProSom Tablets (2%)
Protonix (Less than 1%)
▲ Prozac (Less than 1% to 5%)
▲ Remeron (4%)
▲ Requip Tablets (11%)
Rescriptor Tablets (Less than 2%)
Rilutek Tablets (Rare)
Risperdal (Frequent)
Rythmol Tablets (Less than 1%)
Salagen Tablets (Less than 1%)
▲ Sarafem Pulvules (3%)
Sectral Capsules (2%)
Serentil
Seroquel Tablets (Infrequent)
▲ Serzone Tablets (3%)
Sinemet CR Tablets (1.8%)
Sinemet Tablets
Singulair (Very rare)
Sporanox Capsules (2%)
Stadol NS Nasal Spray (Less than 1%)
Sular Tablets (Less than or equal to 1%)
Sustiva Capsules (1% to 4%)
Symmetrel (1% to 5%)
Talacen Caplets (Infrequent)

Talwin Nx Tablets
Tambocor Tablets (Less than 1%)
▲ Tasmar Tablets (16% to 21%)
Tequin (0.1% to 3%)
Thioridazine Hydrochloride Tablets
Tiazac Capsules (Less than 2%)
Tonocard Tablets (Less than 1%)
Topamax (Infrequent)
Toradol (1% or less)
Trilafon
Trovan (Less than 1%)
Vantin (Less than 1%)
Vaseretic Tablets
Vasotec I.V. Injection
Vasotec Tablets (0.5% to 1.0%)
Viagra Tablets (Less than 2%)
Vicoprofen Tablets (Less than 1%)
Vistide Injection
Wellbutrin SR (At least 1%)
Wellbutrin Tablets
Xanax Tablets (1.8%)
Zanaflex Tablets (Infrequent)
Zebeta Tablets
Ziac Tablets
Zoloft (Infrequent)
Zonegran Capsules (Infrequent)
▲ Zyban (5%)
Zyprexa

Elation
▲ Marinol Capsules (8% to 24%)

Emotional disturbances
Accutane Capsules
Avalide Tablets
Avapro Tablets (Less than 1%)
Depacon Injection
Depakene
Depakote ER Tablets
Depakote Sprinkle Capsules
Depakote Tablets
Efudex (Infrequent)
Imitrex Nasal Spray (Rare)
Lariam Tablets (Less than 1%)
Paxil (Infrequent)
Plaquenil Tablets
Prelone Syrup

Emotional lability
Accutane Capsules
Actiq (Less than 1%)
Activella Tablets (0% to 6%)
▲ Adderall XR Capsules (1% to 9%)
Adenoscan (Less than 1%)
Ambien Tablets (Infrequent)

AndroGel (Up to 3%)
Aricept Tablets (Infrequent)
Asacol Tablets
Avonex
Betapace AF Tablets (Rare)
Betapace Tablets (Rare)
Blocadren Tablets
Cardura Tablets (Less than 0.5%)
Celexa (Infrequent)
▲ CellCept (3% to 10%)
Cerebyx Injection (Infrequent)
Claritin-D 12 Hour (Less frequent)
Claritin-D 24 Hour (Fewer than 2%)
Copaxone (At least 2%)
Coreg Tablets (0.1% to 1%)
Corgard Tablets
Corzide
Cosopt Ophthalmic Solution
▲ Crinone 4% Gel (23%)
▲ Crinone 8% Gel (22%)
DaunoXome Injection (Less than or
    equal to 5%)
▲ Depacon Injection (6%)
▲ Depakene (6%)
Depakote ER Tablets (Greater than
    1%)
▲ Depakote Sprinkle Capsules (6%)
▲ Depakote Tablets (1% to 6%)
Diprivan (Less than 1%)
Doxil Injection (1% to 5%)
Effexor Tablets (Frequent)
Effexor XR Capsules (Frequent)
Elmiron Capsules
Emcyt Capsules (2%)
▲ Esclim Transdermal System (2.1% to
    8.3%)
Evoxac Capsules (Less than 1%)
Exelon (Infrequent)
▲ Felbatol (6.5%)
Floxin
▲ Gabitril Tablets (3%)
Gengraf Capsules (1% to less than
    3%)
▲ Gonal-F for Injection (5.1%)
Hivid Tablets (Less than 1%)
Inderal
Inderide
▲ Infergen (6% to 12%)
Intron A for Injection (Less than 5%)
Kaletra (Less than 2%)
Keppra Tablets (2%)
Klonopin Tablets (1%)
Lamictal (1.3%)
Levaquin (Less than 0.3%)
Levoxyl Tablets

Lipitor Tablets (Less than 2%)
Lunelle Monthly Injection
▲ Lupron Depot 3.75 mg (10.8%)
▲ Lupron Depot—3 Month 11.25 mg
    (10.8% to 22%)
Lupron Depot-PED (Less than 2%)
Lupron Injection Pediatric (Less than
    2%)
Luvox Tablets (Infrequent)
Meridia Capsules (1.3%)
Motrin (Less than 1%)
Nadolol Tablets
Naprelan Tablets (Less than 1%)
Naropin Injection (Less than 1%)
Neoral (1% to less than 3%)
▲ Neurontin (4.2% to 6%)
▲ Nicotrol Nasal Spray (Over 5%)
Nipent for Injection (Less than 3%)
Normodyne Tablets
Norplant System (Less than 1%)
Norvir (Less than 2%)
Oncaspar (Less than 1%)
Ovidrel for Injection (Less than 2%)
OxyContin Tablets (Less than 1%)
Paxil (Frequent)
Pediapred Oral Solution
▲ PEG-Intron Powder for Injection
    (28%)
Permax Tablets (Infrequent)
Prevacid (Less than 1%)
Prevpac (Less than 1%)
▲ Prograf (3% to 15%)
▲ Prometrium Capsules (6%)
ProSom Tablets (Infrequent)
Protonix (Less than 1%)
Provigil Tablets (1%)
Prozac (Frequent)
Pulmicort Respules (1% to 3%)
▲ Rapamune (3% to 20%)
▲ Rebetol Capsules (7% to 12%)
▲ Rebetron Combination Therapy (7%
    to 12%)
Remeron (Infrequent)
Requip Tablets (Infrequent)
Rescriptor Tablets (Less than 2%)
Retrovir Capsules, Tablets & Syrup
Retrovir IV Infusion
Rilutek Tablets (Infrequent)
Risperdal (Rare)
Roferon-A Injection (Less than 3%)
Romazicon Injection (1% to 3%)
Salagen Tablets (Less than 1%)
Sarafem Pulvules (Frequent)
Sectral Capsules
Seroquel Tablets (Rare)

Serzone Tablets
Sonata Capsules (Frequent)
Sustiva Capsules (Less than 2%)
▲ Synarel Nasal Solution for Central Precocious Puberty (6%)
▲ Synarel Nasal Solution for Endometriosis (15% of patients)
Tasmar Tablets (Frequent)
Tenoretic Tablets
Tenormin
Thalomid Capsules
Timolide Tablets
Timolol GFS
Timoptic
Topamax (1.8% to 2.4%)
Toprol-XL Tablets
Trileptal (2% to 3%)
Trovan (Less than 1%)
Ultracet Tablets (Less than 1%)
▲ Ultram Tablets (7% to 14%)
Uniretic Tablets (Less than 1%)
Unithroid Tablets
Viracept
Wellbutrin SR (Infrequent)
Yasmin 28 Tablets
Zanaflex Tablets (Infrequent)
Zebeta Tablets
Ziac Tablets
▲ Zoladex (60%)
Zoladex 3-month
Zoloft (Infrequent to 2%)
Zomig (Infrequent)
Zyban (Infrequent)
Zyprexa
Zyrtec (Less than 2%)
Zyrtec-D (Less than 2%)

Euphoria

Actiq (Less than 1%)
Adderall Tablets
Adderall XR Capsules
Adipex-P
Akineton
Ambien Tablets (Frequent)
Artane
Axert Tablets (Rare)
Benadryl Parenteral
Betaseron
Bicillin C-R
Bicillin L-A
Celestone Soluspan
Celexa (Infrequent)
Claritin-D 12 Hour (Less frequent)
Claritin-D 24 Hour (Fewer than 2%)
Copaxone (At least 2%)

Cortone
Darvocet-N
Darvon Compound-65 Pulvules
Darvon Pulvules
Darvon-N Tablets
Decadron
Demerol
Depacon Injection (0.9%)
Desoxyn Tablets
Dexedrine
DextroStat Tablets
Dilaudid Oral Liquid
Dilaudid Tablets - 8 mg
Dilaudid-HP (Less frequent)
Diprivan (Less than 1%)
Dolophine Tablets
▲ Duragesic Transdermal System (3% to 10%)
Duramorph Injection
Duranest Injections
Effexor Tablets (Infrequent)
Effexor XR Capsules (Infrequent)
ELA-Max Cream
Eldepryl Capsules
EMLA (Unlikely)
Ergamisol Tablets
Felbatol (Infrequent)
Floxin (Less than 1%)
Flumadine (Less than 0.3%)
Fortovase Capsules (Less than 2%)
Gabitril Tablets (Frequent)
Halcion Tablets (0.5% to 0.9%)
Haldol
Haldol Decanoate
Hivid Tablets (Less than 1%)
Hydrocortone
Imitrex Injection (Infrequent)
Imitrex Nasal Spray (Infrequent)
Imitrex Tablets (Infrequent)
Infumorph
Invirase Capsules (Less than 2%)
Ionamin Capsules
Kadian Capsules (Less than 3%)
Lamictal (Infrequent)
Levbid
Levsin
Lidoderm Patch
Limbitrol
Lodosyn Tablets
Luvox Tablets (Infrequent)
▲ Marinol Capsules (3% to 10%)
Maxalt (Frequent)
Mepergan Injection
Migranal Nasal Spray (Infrequent)

Miltown Tablets
Moban (Less frequent)
Motofen Tablets
▲ MS Contin Tablets (Among most frequent)
▲ MSIR (Among most frequent)
Nardil Tablets (Less common)
Neurontin (Infrequent)
Norvir (Less than 2%)
Nubain Injection (1% or less)
Numorphan
▲ Oramorph SR Tablets (Among most frequent)
OxyContin Tablets (Between 1% and 5%)
OxyFast Oral Concentrate Solution
OxyIR Capsules
Paxil (Rare)
Percocet Tablets
Percodan Tablets
Percolone Tablets
Periactin Tablets (No incidence data in labeling)
Permax Tablets (Infrequent)
Phenergan Injection
Phenergan Suppositories
Phenergan Tablets
Phenergan VC with Codeine Syrup
Phenergan with Codeine Syrup
Phrenilin (Infrequent)
Prednisone
Prelone Syrup
ProSom Tablets (Infrequent)
Prozac (Infrequent)
Remeron (Infrequent)
Requip Tablets (Infrequent)
Rescriptor Tablets
Rilutek Tablets (Rare)
Risperdal (Infrequent)
Romazicon Injection (1% to 3%)
Roxanol
Roxanol 100
Roxanol-T
Roxicodone Intensol
Roxicodone Oral Solution
Roxicodone Tablets
Rynatan Tablets
Sarafem Pulvules (Infrequent)
Sedapap Tablets (Infrequent)
Seroquel Tablets (Rare)
Serzone Tablets (Infrequent)
Sinemet CR Tablets
Sinemet Tablets
Solu-Medrol Sterile Powder

Soma Compound (Very rare)
Soma Compound w/Codeine
Soma Tablets
Sonata Capsules (Frequent)
Stadol NS Nasal Spray (1% or greater)
Sterile FUDR (Remote possibility)
Sustiva Capsules (Less than 2%)
Symmetrel (0.1% to 1%)
Talacen Caplets
Talwin Nx Tablets
Tambocor Tablets (Less than 1%)
Tasmar Tablets (1%)
Tequin (Less than 0.1%)
Thalomid Capsules
Topamax (Frequent)
Toradol (1% or less)
Trileptal
Trovan (Less than 1%)
Tussionex
Tussi-Organidin NR Liquid
Tussi-Organidin-S NR Liquid
Tylenol with Codeine
Tylox Capsules
Ultracet Tablets (At least 1%)
▲ Ultram Tablets (1% to 14%)
Versed Injection (Less than 1%)
Vicoprofen Tablets (Less than 1%)
Wellbutrin SR
Wellbutrin Tablets (1.2%)
▲ Xylocaine Injection (Among most common)
▲ Xylocaine with Epinephrine Injection (Among most common)
Zanaflex Tablets (Infrequent)
Zarontin
Zoloft (Infrequent)
Zomig (Rare)
Zonegran Capsules (Infrequent)
Zyban
Zyprexa (2%)
Zyrtec (Less than 2%)
Zyrtec-D (Less than 2%)

Excitability
Actifed Cold & Allergy
Actifed Cold & Sinus
Alka-Seltzer Plus Cold & Cough Medicine Liqui-Gels
Alka-Seltzer Plus Cold Medicine Liqui-Gels
Alka-Seltzer Plus Night-Time Cold Medicine Liqui-Gels
Anadrol-50 Tablets
Astramorph/PF Injection

Benadryl Allergy
Benadryl Allergy & Sinus
Benadryl Parenteral
Bromfed
Children's Benadryl Allergy
Children's Benadryl Allergy & Sinus
Children's Tylenol Cold
Children's Tylenol Cold Plus Cough
Children's Vicks NyQuil Cold/Cough
Chlor-Trimeton Allergy Tablets
Claritin-D 12 Hour
Claritin-D 24 Hour
Cogentin
Comtrex Acute Head Cold
Comtrex Flu Therapy Day & Night
  (Nighttime)
Contac Severe Cold and Flu
Coricidin D Cold, Flu & Sinus
Coricidin HBP Cold & Flu
Crixivan Capsules (Less than 2%)
Dimetapp Elixir
Donnatal (In elderly patients)
Drixoral Allergy Sinus
Drixoral Cold & Allergy
Drixoral Cold & Flu
Duramorph Injection
Etrafon
Extendryl
Flexeril Tablets (Less than 1%)
Guaifed Capsules
Guaifed-PD Capsules
Infumorph
Klonopin Tablets (Infrequent)
Levbid
Levsin
Narcan Injection
Naropin Injection
Nesacaine
NuLev
Orap Tablets
Orudis Capsules (Greater than 1%)
Oruvail Capsules (Greater than 1%)
Oxandrin Tablets
PediaCare Multisymptom Cold Liquid
PediaCare NightRest Cough-Cold
  Liquid
Pediatric Vicks 44m Cough & Cold
  Relief
Periactin Tablets (No incidence data in
  labeling)
Phenergan Injection
Phenergan Suppositories
Phenergan Tablets
Phrenilin (Infrequent)

Polocaine
Polocaine-MPF
Protopam Chloride for Injection
  (Several cases)
Robinul Injectable
Robitussin Honey Flu Nighttime
  Liquid
Ryna-12 S Suspension
Rynatan Pediatric Suspension
Rynatan Tablets
Rynatuss
Sedapap Tablets (Infrequent)
Sensorcaine Injection
Sensorcaine with Epinephrine
  Injection
Sensorcaine-MPF Injection
Sensorcaine-MPF with Epinephrine
  Injection
Serentil
Serevent Inhalation Aerosol
Singlet Caplets
Sudafed Sinus & Allergy Tablets
Talacen Caplets (Rare)
Talwin Nx Tablets
TheraFlu Cold & Cough Night Time
  Hot Liquid
TheraFlu Cold & Sore Throat Night
  Time Hot Liquid
TheraFlu Severe Cold & Congestion
  Night Time Caplets
Triaminic Cold & Allergy Softchews
Triaminic Cold & Cough Softchews
Tylenol Allergy Sinus
Tylenol Cold Complete Formula
Tylenol Flu NightTime Gelcaps
Tylenol Flu NightTime Liquid
Vicks NyQuil LiquiCaps/Liquid
  Multi-Symptom Cold/Flu Relief
Zephrex
Zyrtec-D

Excitement, paradoxical

Etrafon
Halcion Tablets
Librium Capsules
Miltown Tablets
ProSom Tablets
Valium Injectable
Valium Tablets
Versed Syrup (Less than 1%)

Fear

Bicillin L-A
Claritin-D 12 Hour
Claritin-D 24 Hour

Dilaudid Injection
Dilaudid Powder
Dilaudid Rectal Suppositories
Dilaudid Tablets
Hycodan
Hycomine Compound Tablets
Hycotuss Expectorant Syrup
Lortab
Maxidone Tablets
Norco
Rynatan Tablets
Tussionex
Vicodin
Vicodin Tuss Expectorant
Xanax Tablets (1.4%)
Zydone Tablets
Zyrtec-D

Feeling, drugged
▲ Ambien Tablets (3%)
Neurontin (Infrequent)
Paxil (2%)

Feeling, high
Neurontin (Rare)

Feeling, intoxicated
Ambien Tablets (Rare)
Imitrex Injection (Rare)
▲ Phrenilin (Among most frequent)
▲ Sedapap Tablets (Among the most
frequent)
Trileptal

Feeling, strange
Ambien Tablets (Rare)
Amerge Tablets (Infrequent)
Imitrex Injection (2.2%)
Imitrex Nasal Spray (Infrequent)
Imitrex Tablets
MS Contin Tablets (Less frequent)
Neurontin (Rare)
Trileptal (1% to 2%)

Floating feeling
Dilaudid Oral Liquid (Less frequent)
Dilaudid Tablets - 8 mg (Less
frequent)
Dilaudid-HP (Less frequent)
Mintezol
MS Contin Tablets (Less frequent)
MSIR (Less frequent)
Nubain Injection (1% or less)
Oramorph SR Tablets (Less frequent)
Stadol NS Nasal Spray (1% or
greater)

Frigidity, unspecified
Wellbutrin Tablets (Infrequent)

Grogginess
Versed Injection (Less than 1%)

Hallucinations
Actimmune (Rare)
Actiq (1% to 2%)
Allegra-D
Ambien Tablets (Infrequent)
AmBisome for Injection (Less
common)
Amerge Tablets (Rare)
Amicar
Amphotec (1% to 5%)
Ancobon Capsules
Aricept Tablets
Artane (Rare)
Arthrotec Tablets (Rare)
Ativan Injection (1%)
Avelox Tablets (0.05% to 1%)
Azulfidine (Rare)
Bactrim
Betaseron
Biaxin
Blocadren Tablets (Less than 1%)
Brethine Tablets (Less than 1%)
Buprenex Injectable (Infrequent)
Campath Ampules
Cardizem
Catapres Tablets
Ceclor (Rare)
Celexa (Infrequent)
▲ CellCept (3% to 10%)
Celontin Capsules (Rare)
Chibroxin Ophthalmic Solution
Cipro (Less than 1%)
Cipro I.V. (1% or less)
Claritin-D 12 Hour
Claritin-D 24 Hour
Clozaril Tablets (Less than 1%)
Cogentin
Cognex Capsules (2%)
Comtan Tablets
Copaxone (Infrequent)
Corgard Tablets
Corzide
Cosopt Ophthalmic Solution
Cylert
Cytovene
D.H.E. 45 Injection
Darvocet-N
Darvon Compound-65 Pulvules
Darvon Pulvules

Darvon-N Tablets
DaunoXome Injection (Less than or equal to 5%)
Demerol
Demser Capsules
Depacon Injection
Depakene
Depakote ER Tablets (Greater than 1%)
Depakote Sprinkle Capsules
Depakote Tablets (1% to 5%)
Didronel Tablets
Digitek Tablets
Dilaudid Oral Liquid (Less frequent)
Dilaudid Tablets - 8 mg (Less frequent)
Dilaudid-HP (Less frequent)
Diprivan (Less than 1%)
Dolobid Tablets (Less than 1 in 100)
Dostinex Tablets
▲ Duraclon Injection (5.3%)
▲ Duragesic Transdermal System (3% to 10%)
Effexor Tablets (Infrequent)
Effexor XR Capsules (Infrequent)
▲ Eldepryl Capsules (3 of 49 patients)
Elspar for Injection (No incidence data in labeling)
Ergamisol Tablets (Less frequent)
Ery-Tab Tablets (Isolated reports)
Erythrocin Stearate (Isolated reports)
Erythromycin (Isolated reports)
Eskalith
Etrafon
Evoxac Capsules (Less than 1%)
▲ Exelon (4%)
Famotidine Injection (Infrequent)
Famvir Tablets (Infrequent)
Felbatol (Infrequent)
Feldene Capsules (Rare)
Flexeril Tablets (Less than 1%)
Floxin (Less than 1%)
Flumadine (Less than 0.3%)
Focalin Tablets
Fortovase Capsules (Less than 2%)
Foscavir Injection (Between 1% and 5%)
Gabitril Tablets (Frequent)
Gastrocrom Oral Concentrate (Less common)
Genoptic (Rare)
Halcion Tablets
Haldol
Haldol Decanoate

Hivid Tablets (Less than 1%)
▲ Ifex for Injection (Among most common)
Imitrex Injection
Imitrex Tablets (Rare)
Inderal
Inderide
Invirase Capsules (Less than 2%)
Kadian Capsules (Less than 3%)
Keflex
Klonopin Tablets
Lamictal (Infrequent)
Lanoxin/Lanoxicaps
Lariam Tablets
Leukeran Tablets (Rare)
Levaquin (Less than 0.3%)
Levbid
Levsin
Limbitrol
Lithobid Slow-Release Tablets
Lodine XL Extended-Release Tablets
Lodosyn Tablets
Luvox Tablets (Infrequent)
Marinol Capsules (Greater than 1%)
Matulane Capsules
Mepergan Injection
Merrem I.V. (0.1% to 1.0%)
Mexitil Capsules (About 3 in 1,000)
Minipress Capsules (Less than 1%)
Minizide Capsules (Rare)
▲ Mirapex Tablets (9% to 17%)
Motrin (Less than 1%)
MS Contin Tablets (Less frequent)
MSIR (Less frequent)
Myambutol Tablets
Mylocel Tablets (Extremely rare)
Nadolol Tablets
Naropin Injection (Less than 1%)
Nembutal (Less than 1%)
Neurontin (Infrequent)
Nipent for Injection (Less than 3%)
Norflex
Noroxin Tablets
Norpramin Tablets
Norvir (Less than 2%)
Nubain Injection (1% or less)
Numorphan
Oramorph SR Tablets (Less frequent)
Orudis Capsules (Rare)
Oruvail Capsules (Rare)
OxyContin Tablets (Less than 1%)
Paxil (Infrequent)
Pediazole Suspension
Pepcid (Infrequent)

Periactin Tablets (No incidence data in labeling)
▲ Permax Tablets (13.8%)
Phenergan Suppositories
Phenergan Tablets
Phenergan VC with Codeine Syrup
Phenergan with Codeine Syrup
Ponstel Capsules (Rare)
Prevacid (Less than 1%)
Prevpac (Less than 1%)
Prilosec (Less than 1%)
Primaxin
Procanbid Extended-Release Tablets (Occasional)
▲ Prograf (3% to 15%)
ProSom Tablets (Rare)
Protonix (Less than 1%)
Provigil Tablets (At least 1%)
Prozac (Infrequent)
Reglan (Rare)
Remeron (Infrequent)
Reminyl (Greater than or equal to 2%)
▲ Requip Tablets (5% to 10%)
Rescriptor Tablets (Less than 2%)
Rilutek Tablets (Infrequent)
Roferon-A Injection (Infrequent)
Rynatan Tablets
Sandostatin LAR Depot (1% to 4%)
Sarafem Pulvules (Infrequent)
Septra
Seroquel Tablets (Infrequent)
Serzone Tablets (Infrequent)
▲ Sinemet CR Tablets (3.9%)
Sinemet Tablets
Sinequan (Infrequent)
Singulair
Sonata Capsules (Less than 1%)
Stadol NS Nasal Spray (Less than 1%)
Surmontil Capsules
Sustiva Capsules (Less than 2%)
Symmetrel (1% to 5%)
Tagamet
Talacen Caplets
Talwin Nx Tablets
▲ Tasmar Tablets (8% to 10%)
Tenoretic Tablets
Tenormin
Tequin (Less than 0.1%)
Tiazac Capsules (Less than 2%)
Timolide Tablets
Timolol GFS
Timoptic (Less frequent)
▲ Tonocard Tablets (2.1% to 11.2%)
Topamax (Frequent)

Toradol (1% or less)
Transderm Scop (Infrequent)
Trilisate Liquid (Rare)
Trilisate Tablets (Rare)
Trovan (Less than 1%)
Ultracet Tablets (Less than 1%)
▲ Ultram Tablets (Less than 1% to 14%)
Valcyte Tablets (Less than 5%)
Valium Injectable
Valium Tablets
Vantin (Less than 1%)
Versed Injection (Less than 1%)
Versed Syrup (Less than 1%)
▲ Vesanoid Capsules (6%)
Vioxx (Less than 0.1%)
Vistide Injection
Vivactil Tablets
Wellbutrin SR
Wellbutrin Tablets (Frequent)
Xanax Tablets (Rare)
Zantac Injection
Zantac Tablets, Granules, & Syrup (Rare)
Zebeta Tablets
Ziac Tablets
Zoloft (Infrequent)
Zomig (Rare)
Zosyn (1.0% or less)
Zovirax Capsules, Tablets, & Suspension
Zovirax for Injection (Approximately 1%)
Zyban
Zyprexa
Zyrtec-D

Hallucinations, auditory

Bicillin C-R
Bicillin L-A
Catapres Tablets (Rare)
Catapres-TTS (0.5% or less)
Clorpres Tablets
Combipres Tablets
Orthoclone OKT3
Valtrex Caplets

Hallucinations, visual

Bicillin C-R
Bicillin L-A
Carbatrol Capsules
Catapres Tablets (Rare)
Catapres-TTS (0.5% or less)
Clorpres Tablets
Cogentin
Combipres Tablets

Orthoclone OKT3
Salagen Tablets (Rare)
Talwin Nx Tablets
Tegretol
Tessalon Capsules
Valtrex Caplets

Hangover
AcipHex Tablets (Rare)
Effexor Tablets (Infrequent)
Effexor XR Capsules (Infrequent)
Maxalt (Infrequent)
Neurontin (Rare)
Nipent for Injection (Less than 3%)
▲ ProSom Tablets (3%)
Serzone Tablets (Infrequent)
Sonata Capsules (Infrequent)
Thalomid Capsules
Zyprexa (Infrequent)

Hostility
Amerge Tablets (Rare)
Aricept Tablets (Infrequent)
Cerebyx Injection (Infrequent)
Cognex Capsules (2%)
Copaxone (Infrequent)
Depacon Injection
Depakene
Depakote ER Tablets
Depakote Sprinkle Capsules
Depakote Tablets
Duragesic Transdermal System (Less than 1%)
Effexor Tablets (Infrequent)
Effexor XR Capsules (Infrequent)
Floxin
Gabitril Tablets (2%)
Geodon Capsules (Frequent)
Keppra Tablets (2%)
Klonopin Tablets
Lamictal (Frequent)
Luvox Tablets (Infrequent)
Neurontin (5.2% to 7.6%)
Nipent for Injection (Less than 3%)
Nubain Injection (1% or less)
Paxil (Infrequent)
Permax Tablets (Infrequent)
Prevacid (Less than 1%)
Prevpac (Less than 1%)
ProSom Tablets (Infrequent)
Prozac (Infrequent)
Remeron (Infrequent)
Rilutek Tablets (Frequent)
Sarafem Pulvules (Infrequent)
Serzone Tablets (Infrequent)

Sonata Capsules (Rare)
Stadol NS Nasal Spray (Less than 1%)
Tasmar Tablets (Infrequent)
Tequin (Less than 0.1%)
Thalomid Capsules
Wellbutrin SR (Infrequent)
▲ Wellbutrin Tablets (5.6%)
Xanax Tablets (Rare)
Zyban (Infrequent)
▲ Zyprexa (15%)

Hyperactivity
Aerobid (1% to 3%)
Amerge Tablets (Rare)
Amoxil (Rare)
Augmentin (Rare)
Ceclor (Rare)
Ceclor CD
Ceftin for Oral Suspension (0.1% to 1%)
Cefzil (Less than 1%)
Depacon Injection
Depakene
Depakote ER Tablets
Depakote Sprinkle Capsules
Depakote Tablets
Dopram Injectable
Etrafon
▲ Geref for Injection (1 patient in 6)
Infumorph
Klonopin Tablets (Infrequent)
Levoxyl Tablets
Moban (Less frequent)
Neurontin
Roferon-A Injection (Infrequent)
Spectracef Tablets
Tasmar Tablets (1%)
Thioridazine Hydrochloride Tablets (Extremely rare)
Trilafon
Unithroid Tablets
Ventolin Inhalation Aerosol (1%)
Versed Injection (No incidence data in labeling)
Zarontin

Hyperexcitability
Lufyllin
Lufyllin-GG

Hyperexcitability, reflex
Theo-Dur Extended-Release Tablets
Uni-Dur Extended-Release Tablets

Hyperirritability
Mintezol

Hypnotic effects
Trilafon

Hypoactivity
Aerobid (1% to 3%)
Valium Injectable

Hysteria
Ambien Tablets (Rare)
Cognex Capsules (Rare)
Diprivan (Less than 1%)
Imitrex Injection (Rare)
Imitrex Tablets (Rare)
Klonopin Tablets
Luvox Tablets (Infrequent)
Neurontin (Rare)
Paxil (Rare)
Periactin Tablets (No incidence data in labeling)
Phenergan Injection
Phenergan Suppositories
Phenergan Tablets
Rynatan Tablets
Trileptal

Illusion, unspecified
Ambien Tablets (Infrequent)
Evoxac Capsules
Klonopin Tablets (Infrequent)
Zoloft (Rare)

Impairment of sensation
AmBisome for Injection (Less common)
▲ Astelin Nasal Spray (7.9%)
Cognex Capsules (Rare)
Copaxone (At least 2%)
Crixivan Capsules (Less than 2%)
Cytovene
Enalaprilat Injection
Evoxac Capsules (Less than 1%)
Floxin Otic Solution (Single report)
Fortovase Capsules (Less than 2%)
Halcion Tablets (Rare)
Hivid Tablets
Imitrex Injection (Rare)
Imitrex Nasal Spray (Rare)
Imitrex Tablets (Rare)
Invirase Capsules (Less than 2%)
Levulan Kerastick (Up to 2%)
Lexxel Tablets
Maxalt (Rare)
Neurontin (Infrequent)
Prinivil Tablets (0.3% to 1.0%)
Prinzide Tablets

▲ Taxotere for Injection Concentrate (7 of 134 patients)
Thalomid Capsules
Vaseretic Tablets
Vasotec I.V. Injection
Vasotec Tablets (0.5% to 1.0%)
Xeloda Tablets
Zestril Tablets (0.3% to 1.0%)

Impairment of sensation, one side of face
Prilosec (Less than 1%)

Inebriated feeling
Klonopin Tablets (Infrequent)

Insomnia
8-MOP Capsules
Accupril Tablets (0.5% to 1.0%)
Accuretic Tablets (1.2%)
Accutane Capsules
AcipHex Tablets
Actifed Cold & Allergy
Actiq (1% to 2%)
Activella Tablets (0% to 6%)
▲ Actonel Tablets (4.7%)
Adalat CC Tablets (Less than 1.0%)
Adderall Tablets
▲ Adderall XR Capsules (1.5% to 17%)
Adipex-P
Advil Cold and Sinus
Aerobid (1% to 3%)
Agrylin Capsules (1% to 5%)
Alferon N Injection (2%)
Allegra (Less than 1%)
▲ Allegra-D (12.6%)
Alphagan Ophthalmic Solution (Less than 3%)
Alphagan P Ophthalmic Solution (Less than 1%)
Altace Capsules (Less than 1%)
Ambien Tablets (Frequent)
Amoxil (Rare)
▲ Amphotec (5% or more)
Anadrol-50 Tablets
Anaprox (Less than 1%)
▲ Angiomax for Injection (7%)
Arava Tablets (1% to 3%)
▲ Aredia for Injection (22.2%)
▲ Aricept Tablets (9%)
Arimidex Tablets 2% to 5.9%
▲ Arixtra Injection (5%)
▲ Aromasin Tablets (11%)
Arthrotec Tablets (Rare)
Asacol Tablets (2%)

Atacand HCT Tablets (0.5% or greater)
Atrovent Inhalation Aerosol (Less than 1%)
Atrovent Inhalation Solution (0.9%)
Augmentin (Rare)
Avelox Tablets (0.05% to 1%)
Axert Tablets (Infrequent)
Axid Pulvules (2.7%)
Aygestin Tablets
Azactam for Injection (Less than 1%)
Azulfidine (Rare)
Bactrim
Benadryl Allergy & Sinus
Benadryl Allergy & Sinus Headache
Benadryl Parenteral
Betapace AF Tablets (2.6% to 4.1%)
Betoptic S Ophthalmic Suspension (Rare)
Bextra Tablets (0.1% to 1.9%)
Biaxin
Blocadren Tablets (Less than 1%)
Bontril
Brethine Tablets (1.5%)
Bromfed
▲ Campath Ampules (10%)
Captopril Tablets (About 0.5 to 2%)
Carafate (Less than 0.5%)
Cardizem
Cardura Tablets (1% to 1.2%)
Carnitor Injection (1% to 3%)
Carteolol (Occasional)
▲ Casodex Tablets (5%)
Cataflam Tablets (Less than 1%)
Catapres Tablets (About 5 in 1,000 patients)
Catapres-TTS (2 of 101 patients)
Ceclor (Rare)
Ceclor CD (0.1% to 1%)
Cedax Oral Suspension (0.1% to 1%)
Cefzil (Less than 1%)
Celebrex Capsules (2.3%)
Celestone Soluspan
▲ Celexa (15%)
▲ CellCept (8.9% to 40.8%)
Celontin Capsules
▲ Cenestin Tablets (42%)
Cerebyx Injection (Infrequent)
Children's Benadryl Allergy & Sinus
Children's Sudafed Cold & Cough
Children's Tylenol Cold
Children's Vicks NyQuil Cold/Cough
Cipro (Less than 1%)
Cipro I.V. (1% or less)

Claritin (At least one patient)
▲ Claritin-D 12 Hour (16%)
▲ Claritin-D 24 Hour (5%)
Clinoril Tablets (Less than 1%)
Clomid Tablets (Fewer than 1%)
Clorpres Tablets (About 5 in 1,000)
Clozaril Tablets (2%)
▲ Cognex Capsules (6%)
Colazal Capsules (2%)
Colestid Tablets (Infrequent)
▲ CombiPatch (8% to 6%)
Combipres Tablets (About 5 in 1,000)
Combivent Inhalation Aerosol (Less than 2%)
▲ Combivir Tablets (11%)
Compazine
▲ Concerta (4%)
Condylox Topical Solution (Less than 5%)
Contac 12 Hour Cold Caplets
Contac Severe Cold and Flu
Copaxone (At least 2%)
Cordarone Tablets (1% to 3%)
Coreg Tablets (Greater than 2%)
Coricidin D Cold, Flu & Sinus
Corlopam Injection (2%)
Cortifoam Rectal Foam
Cortone
Cosopt Ophthalmic Solution
Covera-HS Tablets (Less than 2%)
Cozaar Tablets (1.4%)
Crinone 4% Gel (Less than 5%)
Crinone 8% Gel (Less than 5%)
▲ Crixivan Capsules (3.1%)
▲ Cylert (Most frequent)
Cytovene (At least 3 subjects)
Dantrium Capsules (Less frequent)
Dapsone Tablets USP
▲ DaunoXome Injection (Up to 6%)
Decadron
Demadex (1.2%)
Demser Capsules
▲ Depacon Injection (9% to 15%)
▲ Depakene (15%)
Depakote ER Tablets (1% to 5%)
▲ Depakote Sprinkle Capsules (9% to 15%)
▲ Depakote Tablets (1% to 15%)
▲ Depo-Provera Contraceptive Injection (More than 5%)
Desoxyn Tablets
Dexedrine
DextroStat Tablets
Dilantin
Dilaudid Oral Liquid (Less frequent)

Dilaudid Tablets - 8 mg (Less frequent)
Dilaudid-HP (Less frequent)
Diovan Capsules
Diovan HCT Tablets (Greater than 0.2%)
Dipentum Capsules (Rare)
Diprivan (Less than 1%)
Ditropan XL (2% to 5%)
Dolobid Tablets (Greater than 1 in 100)
Dolophine Tablets
Donnatal
▲ Dostinex Tablets (1% to less than 10%)
Doxil Injection (Less than 1% to 5%)
Drixoral Cold & Allergy
Drixoral Cold & Flu
Duraclon Injection (0.5%)
Dynabac Tablets (0.9% to 1%)
DynaCirc (0.5% to 1%)
EC-Naprosyn (Less than 1%)
▲ Effexor Tablets (3% to 22.5%)
▲ Effexor XR Capsules (17% to 22%)
Efudex
Eldepryl Capsules (1 of 49 patients)
Eligard (Less than 2%)
Elmiron Capsules
▲ Emcyt Capsules (3%)
Enalaprilat Injection
Engerix-B Vaccine (Less than 1%)
▲ Epivir (11%)
▲ Epogen for Injection (13% to 16%)
Ergamisol Tablets (1%)
▲ Estring Vaginal Ring (4%)
Etrafon
▲ Evista Tablets (5.5%)
Evoxac Capsules (2.4%)
▲ Exelon (9%)
Famotidine Injection (Infrequent)
Famvir Tablets (1.5% to 2.5%)
▲ Felbatol (8.6% to 17.5%)
Feldene Capsules (Occasional)
▲ Femara Tablets (6%)
femhrt Tablets
Ferrlecit Injection (Greater than 1%)
Flexeril Tablets (Less than 1%)
▲ Flolan for Injection (4% to 9%)
Flomax Capsules (1.4% to 2.4%)
Florinef Acetate Tablets
▲ Flovent Inhalation Aerosol (3% to 13%)
Flovent Rotadisk
▲ Floxin (3% to 7%)
Floxin Otic Solution (Single report)

Flumadine (2.1% to 3.4%)
▲ Focalin Tablets (Among most common)
Foradil Aerolizer (1.5%)
▲ Fortovase Capsules (5.6%)
Foscavir Injection (Between 1% and 5%)
▲ Gabitril Tablets (6%)
Gastrocrom Oral Concentrate (Less common)
Gemzar for Injection (Infrequent)
Gengraf Capsules (1% to less than 3%)
Gliadel Wafer (2%)
Glucotrol XL (Less than 3%)
Grifulvin V (Occasional)
Gris-PEG Tablets (Occasional)
Halcion Tablets (Rare)
Haldol
Haldol Decanoate
Havrix Vaccine (Less than 1%)
▲ Herceptin I.V. (14%)
Hivid Tablets (Less than 1%)
Hydrocortone
Hytrin Capsules (At least 1%)
Hyzaar
Imdur Tablets (Less than or equal to 5%)
Indapamide Tablets (Less than 5%)
Inderal
Inderide
Indocin Capsules/Suspension/Suppositories (Less than 1%)
▲ Infergen (24% to 39%)
Innohep Injection (Greater than or equal to 1%)
▲ Intron A for Injection (Up to 12%)
Invirase Capsules (Less than 2%)
Ionamin Capsules
Iopidine 0.5% Ophthalmic Solution (Less than 3%)
Iopidine Sterile Ophthalmic Solution
Ismo Tablets (Fewer than 1%)
Isoptin SR Tablets (1% or less)
Kadian Capsules (Less than 3%)
Kaletra (1.1% to 2.4%)
Keppra Tablets (1% or more)
Klonopin Tablets (Infrequent)
Kytril Injection (Less than 2%)
▲ Kytril Tablets (3% to 5%)
▲ Lamictal (5.6%)
Lescol Capsules (2.7%)
Lescol XL Tablets (1.8%)

▲ Leukine (11%)
▲ Leustatin Injection (7%)
Levaquin (0.3% to 2.9%)
Levbid
Levlen
Levlite
Levo-Dromoran
Levoxyl Tablets
Levsin
Lexxel Tablets
Lipitor Tablets (Greater than or equal to 2%)
Lodine (Less than 1%)
Lodine XL Extended-Release Tablets (Less than 1%)
Lodosyn Tablets
Lorabid
Lotensin HCT Tablets (0.3% to 1%)
Lotensin Tablets (Less than 1%)
Lotrel Capsules
Loxitane Capsules
Lufyllin
Lufyllin-GG
Lupron Depot 3.75 mg (Less than 5%)
Lupron Depot 7.5 mg (Less than 5%)
Lupron Depot—3 Month 11.25 mg (Less than 5%)
▲ Lupron Depot—3 Month 22.5 mg (8.5%)
Lupron Depot—4 Month 30 mg (Less than 5%)
▲ Lupron Injection (5% or more)
▲ Luvox Tablets (4% to (21%)
Matulane Capsules
Mavik Tablets (0.3% to 1.0%)
Maxair (Less than 1%)
Maxalt (Infrequent)
Maxzide
▲ Megace Oral Suspension (Up to 6%)
▲ Mepron Suspension (10% to 19%)
▲ Meridia Capsules (10.7%)
Merrem I.V. (0.1% to 1.0%)
▲ Metadate (Among most common)
▲ Methylin (Among most common)
Mevacor Tablets (0.5% to 1.0%)
Miacalcin Nasal Spray (Less than 1%)
Micardis HCT Tablets
Micardis Tablets (More than 0.3%)
Midamor Tablets (Less than or equal to 1%)
Migranal Nasal Spray (Infrequent)
Minipress Capsules
▲ Mirapex Tablets (17% to 27%)
Mobic Tablets (0.4% to 3.6%)

Modicon
Moduretic Tablets (Less than or equal to 1%)
Monopril Tablets (1.0% or more)
Monurol Sachet (Less than 1%)
Motofen Tablets (1 in 200 to 1 in 600)
Motrin (Less than 1%)
Motrin Sinus Headache Caplets
MS Contin Tablets (Less frequent)
MSIR (Less frequent)
Mycobutin Capsules (1%)
Mykrox Tablets
▲ Mylotarg for Injection (14% to 22%)
Naprelan Tablets (Less than 3%)
Naprosyn (Less than 1%)
Nardil Tablets (Common)
Naropin Injection (Less than 1%)
Natrecor for Injection (2%)
Navane
Nembutal (Less than 1%)
Neoral (1% to less than 3%)
▲ Neulasta Injection (15% to 72%)
▲ Neumega for Injection (33%)
Nexium (Less than 1%)
Niaspan
Nicotrol Nasal Spray
▲ Nilandron Tablets (16.3%)
▲ Nipent for Injection (3% to 10%)
Noroxin Tablets (Less frequent)
Norpramin Tablets
Norvasc Tablets (More than 0.1% to 1%)
Norvir (1.3% to (2.6%)
NuLev
Omnicef (0.2%)
Oramorph SR Tablets (Less frequent)
▲ Orap Tablets (2 of 20 patients)
▲ Organ Injection (3.1%)
Ortho Tri-Cyclen
Ortho-Cyclen
Ortho-Novum
▲ Orudis Capsules (3% to 9%)
▲ Oruvail Capsules (3% to 9%)
Ovidrel for Injection (Less than 2%)
Oxandrin Tablets
Oxsoralen-Ultra Capsules
OxyContin Tablets (Between 1% and 5%)
Pacerone Tablets (1% to 3%)
Parnate Tablets
▲ Paxil (1.3 to 24%)
Pediatric Vicks 44m Cough & Cold Relief
Pediazole Suspension

▲ PEG-Intron Powder for Injection (23%)
Pentasa Capsules (Less than 1%)
Pepcid (Infrequent)
Periactin Tablets (No incidence data in labeling)
▲ Permax Tablets (7.9%)
Phenergan Injection
Phenergan Suppositories
Phenergan Tablets
Phenergan VC Syrup
Phenergan with Dextromethorphan Syrup
▲ Photofrin for Injection (14%)
Plavix Tablets (1% to 2.5%)
Plendil (0.5% to 1.5%)
Pletal Tablets (Less than 2%)
Ponstel Capsules (Occasional)
Pravachol Tablets
Prednisone
Prelone Syrup
Premphase Tablets
Prempro Tablets
Prevpac
Prilosec (Less than 1%)
Primatene Tablets
Prinivil Tablets (0.3% to 1.0%)
Prinzide Tablets
ProAmatine Tablets (Rare)
Procardia XL Tablets (Less than 3%)
▲ Procrit for Injection (13% to 21%)
▲ Prograf (32% to 64%)
Proleukin for Injection
Prometrium Capsules (Less than 5%)
Protonix (Greater than or equal to 1%)
Protopic Ointment (Up to 4%)
Proventil HFA Inhalation Aerosol
Proventil Inhalation Aerosol
Proventil Inhalation Solution 0.083% (1% to 3.1%)
▲ Proventil Repetabs Tablets (2% to 11%)
Proventil Solution for Inhalation 0.5% (1% to 3.1%)
Provera Tablets
▲ Provigil Tablets (3%)
▲ Prozac (1% to 33%)
Pulmicort Turbuhaler Powder (1% to 3%)
▲ Rapamune (13% to 22%)
▲ Rebetol Capsules (26% to 39%)
▲ Rebetron Combination Therapy (26% to 39%)
Recombivax HB (Less to greater than 1%)

ReFacto Vials
Reglan (Less frequent)
Relafen Tablets (1% to 3%)
▲ Reminyl (5%)
ReoPro Vials (0.3%)
Requip Tablets (1% or more)
Rescriptor Tablets (Less than 2%)
Rescula Ophthalmic Solution (1% to 5%)
▲ Retrovir Capsules, Tablets & Syrup (2.4% to 5%)
▲ Retrovir IV Infusion (3% to 5%)
Rifater Tablets
Rilutek Tablets (2.1% to 2.9%)
▲ Risperdal (23% to 26%)
▲ Ritalin (One of the two most common)
Rituxan (1% to 5%)
Robaxin Tablets
Robinul Injectable
Robinul Tablets
Robitussin Cough & Cold
Robitussin Pediatric Cough & Cold
Robitussin-CF Liquid
Robitussin-DAC Syrup
Robitussin-PE Liquid
▲ Roferon-A Injection (14%)
▲ Romazicon Injection (3% to 9%)
Rowasa Rectal Suspension Enema (0.12%)
Roxanol
Roxanol 100
Roxanol-T
▲ Roxicodone Tablets (Greater than or equal to 3%)
Rynatan Tablets
Rythmol Tablets (1.5%)
Salagen Tablets (Less than 1%)
▲ Sandostatin LAR Depot (5% to 15%)
▲ Sarafem Pulvules (9% to 24%)
▲ Sectral Capsules (3%)
▲ Semprex-D Capsules (4%)
Septra
Serevent Inhalation Aerosol (1% to 3%)
Serophene Tablets (Approximately 1 in 50 patients)
▲ Serostim for Injection 11.2%
▲ Serzone Tablets (11%)
▲ Simulect for Injection (Greater than or equal to 10%)
Sinemet CR Tablets (1.2%)
Sinemet Tablets
Singulair
Sinutab Non-Drying Liquid Caps

Skelid Tablets (More than or equal to 1%)
Solu-Medrol Sterile Powder
Soma Compound (Infrequent or rare)
Soma Compound w/Codeine (Infrequent or rare)
Soma Tablets
Sonata Capsules (Infrequent)
▲ Soriatane Capsules (1% to 10%)
Spectracef Tablets (0.1% to 1%)
Sporanox Capsules (Infrequent)
Sporanox Oral Solution (Less than 2%)
▲ Stadol NS Nasal Spray (11%)
Stelazine
Stimate Nasal Spray
Sudafed Tablets
Sudafed Nasal Decongestant Tablets
Sular Tablets (Less than or equal to 1%)
Surmontil Capsules
▲ Sustiva Capsules (1% to 7%)
▲ Symmetrel (5% to 10%)
▲ Synarel Nasal Solution for Endometriosis (8% of patients)
Synercid I.V. (Less than 1%)
Talacen Caplets (Infrequent)
Talwin Nx Tablets
Tambocor Tablets (1% to 3%)
Tamiflu (1.1% to 1.2%)
Tarka Tablets (Less frequent)
▲ Temodar Capsules (10%)
Tenex Tablets (Less than 3% to 4%)
Tequin (0.1% to 3%)
Teveten Tablets (Less than 1%)
Thalomid Capsules
Theo-Dur Extended-Release Tablets
TheraFlu Cold & Cough Night Time Hot Liquid
TheraFlu Cold & Sore Throat Night Time Hot Liquid
TheraFlu Severe Cold & Congestion Night Time Caplets
Thiothixene Capsules
Thorazine
Tiazac Capsules (Less than 2%)
▲ Tikosyn Capsules (4%)
Timolide Tablets (Less than 1%)
Timolol GFS
Timoptic (Less frequent)
Tonocard Tablets (Less than 1%)
Topamax (Frequent)
Toprol-XL Tablets
Toradol (1% or less)

Tranxene
▲ Trasylol Injection (3%)
Trental Tablets
Triaminic Allergy Congestion Liquid
Triaminic Chest Congestion Liquid
Triaminic Cold & Allergy Liquid
Triaminic Cold & Allergy Softchews
Triaminic Cold & Cough Liquid
Triaminic Cold & Night Time Cough Liquid
Triaminic Cough & Congestion Liquid
Triaminic Cough & Sore Throat Liquid
Triaminic Cough & Sore Throat Softchews
Triaminic Cough Liquid
Triaminic Flu, Cough & Fever
Tricor Tablets (1%)
Trilafon
Trileptal (2% to 4%)
Tri-Levlen
▲ Trisenox Injection (43%)
▲ Trizivir Tablets (7% to 13%)
Trovan (Less than 1%)
Twinrix Vaccine (Less than 1%)
Tylenol Cold Complete Formula
Tylenol Cold Non-Drowsy
Tylenol Flu NightTime Liquid
Tylenol Sinus NightTime Caplets
Tylenol Sinus Non-Drowsy
Ultracet Tablets (2%)
Uni-Dur Extended-Release Tablets
Uniphyl Tablets
Uniretic Tablets (Less than 1%)
Unithroid Tablets
▲ Vagifem Tablets (3% to 5%)
▲ Valcyte Tablets (16%)
Valium Injectable
Valium Tablets
Vanceril Double Strength Inhalation Aerosol (Fewer than 2%)
Vantin (Less than 1%)
Vascor Tablets (0.5 to 2.65%)
Vaseretic Tablets (0.5% to 2.0%)
Vasotec I.V. Injection
Vasotec Tablets (0.5% to 1.0%)
Ventolin HFA Inhalation Aerosol
Ventolin Inhalation Aerosol
Verelan Capsules (1% or less)
Verelan PM Capsules (2% or less)
Versed Injection (Less than 1%)
▲ Vesanoid Capsules (14%)
Viagra Tablets (Less than 2%)

Vicks 44D Cough & Head Congestion Relief Liquid
Vicks DayQuil LiquiCaps/Liquid Multi-Symptom Cold/Flu Relief
▲ Vicoprofen Tablets (3% to 9%)
Vioxx (Greater than 0.1% to 1.9%)
Viracept
Vistide Injection
Vivactil Tablets
Volmax Extended-Release Tablets (2.4%)
Voltaren (Less than 1%)
Voltaren Ophthalmic Solution (Less than 3%)
▲ Wellbutrin SR (11% to 16%)
▲ Wellbutrin Tablets (18.6%)
▲ Xanax Tablets (8.9% to 29.4%)
Xeloda Tablets
Xopenex Inhalation Solution
Zantac Injection
Zantac Tablets, Granules, & Syrup (Rare)
Zaroxolyn Tablets
Zebeta Tablets (1.5% to 2.5%)
▲ Zenapax for Injection (Greater than 5%)
Zephrex
▲ Zerit (29%)
Zestoretic Tablets
Zestril Tablets (0.3% to 1.0%)
Ziac Tablets (1.1% to 1.2%)
▲ Ziagen (7% to 13%)
Zithromax Capsules & Tablets (1% or less)
Zithromax for IV Infusion (1% or less)
Zithromax for Oral Suspension (1% or less)
Zocor Tablets
▲ Zoladex (5% to 11%)
Zoladex 3-month
▲ Zoloft (16% to 28%)
▲ Zometa for Intravenous Infusion (14% to 15.1%)
Zomig (Infrequent)
▲ Zonegran Capsules (6%)
▲ Zosyn (4.5% to 6.6%)
▲ Zyban (31% to 40%)
Zyflo Filmtab Tablets (Less common)
▲ Zyprexa (20%)
Zyrtec (Less than 2%)
Zyrtec-D (Less than 2%)
Zyvox (2.5%)

Intoxication, chronic
Miltown Tablets

Irritability
▲ Acel-Imune (25%)
▲ ActHIB Vaccine (10.1% to 77.9%)
▲ Aerobid (3% to 9%)
Aquasol A Parenteral
Aricept Tablets (Frequent)
Arthrotec Tablets (Rare)
Attenuvax
Benadryl Parenteral
Bromfed
Cafcit
Cataflam Tablets (Less than 1%)
Catapres-TTS (0.5% or less)
Cedax Oral Suspension (0.1% to 1%)
Ceftin for Oral Suspension (0.1% to 1%)
Celontin Capsules
Cipro (Less than 1%)
Cipro I.V. (1% or less)
Claritin (At least one patient)
Claritin-D 12 Hour (Less frequent)
Claritin-D 24 Hour (Fewer than 2%)
Clomid Tablets
Clozaril Tablets (Less than 1%)
▲ Comvax (32.2% to 57.0%)
Cylert
Cytovene
Dipentum Capsules (Rare)
Diphtheria & Tetanus Toxoids
Efudex
Eldepryl Capsules
Elspar for Injection (No incidence data in labeling)
Engerix-B Vaccine (Less than 1%)
Extendryl
Fortovase Capsules (Less than 2%)
▲ Gabitril Tablets (10%)
▲ Gamimune N (Among most common)
Gastrocrom Oral Concentrate (2 of 87 patients)
Guaifed Capsules
Guaifed-PD Capsules
Halcion Tablets
HibTITER (133 of 1,118 vaccinations)
▲ Indapamide Tablets (Greater than or equal to 5%)
▲ Infanrix Vaccine (28.8% to 36.3%)
▲ Intron A for Injection (Up to 16%)
Invirase Capsules (Less than 2%)
Iopidine Sterile Ophthalmic Solution
▲ IPOL Vaccine (6.7% to 64.5%)

▲ Lamictal (3.0%)
Levoxyl Tablets
Lexxel Tablets
Liquid PedvaxHIB
Lufyllin
Lufyllin-GG
Maxalt (Infrequent)
Meruvax II
M-M-R II
Mumpsvax
Narcan Injection
▲ Nicotrol Nasal Spray (Over 5%)
Novarel for Injection
▲ PEG-Intron Powder for Injection (28%)
Periactin Tablets (No incidence data in labeling)
Plaquenil Tablets
Plendil (0.5% to 1.5%)
Pregnyl for Injection
▲ Prevnar for Injection (68.9% to 72.8%)
Prinivil Tablets (0.3% to 1.0%)
Prinzide Tablets
Proleukin for Injection
▲ Prometrium Capsules (5% to 8%)
Proventil Repetabs Tablets (Less than 1%)
Pulmicort Respules (Less than 1%)
Pulmicort Turbuhaler Powder (Rare)
▲ Rebetol Capsules (23% to 32%)
▲ Rebetron Combination Therapy (23% to 32%)
Recombivax HB (Greater than 1%)
Retrovir Capsules, Tablets & Syrup (1.6%)
Retrovir IV Infusion (2%)
Rhinocort Nasal Inhaler (Rare)
▲ Roferon-A Injection (Less than 5% to 15%)
Rynatan Tablets
Serophene Tablets
Singulair (Very rare)
Skelaxin Tablets
Soma Compound (Infrequent or rare)
Soma Compound w/Codeine (Infrequent or rare)
Soma Tablets
Symmetrel (1% to 5%)
Talacen Caplets (Rare)
Talwin Nx Tablets
Tasmar Tablets (1%)
Tetanus & Diphtheria Toxoids Adsorbed for Adult Use
Theo-Dur Extended-Release Tablets

Tranxene
▲ Tripedia Vaccine (5% to 15%)
Twinrix Vaccine (Less than 1%)
Uni-Dur Extended-Release Tablets
Uniphyl Tablets
Unithroid Tablets
Varivax (Greater than or equal to 1%)
Volmax Extended-Release Tablets (Less frequent)
Voltaren (Less than 1%)
Wellbutrin SR (2% to 3%)
▲ Xanax Tablets (33.1%)
Zarontin
Zephrex
Zestoretic Tablets
Zestril Tablets (0.3% to 1.0%)
Zomig (Rare)
▲ Zonegran Capsules (9%)
Zyban (Frequent)

Jitteriness
Compazine
Etrafon
Nardil Tablets (Less common)
Procardia Capsules (2% or less)
Reglan
Stelazine
Thorazine

Language problems, unspecified
▲ Topamax (2.2% to 11.7%)

Laughing, easy
▲ Marinol Capsules (8% to 24%)

Libido decreased
AcipHex Tablets
Actiq (Less than 1%)
Adalat CC Tablets (Less than 1.0%)
Aldoclor Tablets
Aldomet Tablets
Aldoril Tablets
Ambien Tablets (Rare)
Amerge Tablets (Rare)
Anadrol-50 Tablets
Androderm (Less than 1%)
AndroGel (Up to 3%)
Aricept Tablets (Infrequent)
Asacol Tablets
Atromid-S Capsules
Axid Pulvules
Betaseron
Blocadren Tablets (0.6%)
Bontril
Calcijex Injection

Cardura Tablets (0.8%)
▲ Casodex Tablets (2% to 5%)
Celexa (2%)
Claritin (At least one patient)
Claritin-D 12 Hour (Less frequent)
Claritin-D 24 Hour
Clozaril Tablets (Less than 1%)
Copaxone (Infrequent)
Cordarone Tablets (1% to 3%)
Coreg Tablets (0.1% to 1%)
Corgard Tablets (1 to 5 per 1000
  patients)
Corzide (1 to 5 of 1000 patients)
Cosopt Ophthalmic Solution
Cozaar Tablets (Less than 1%)
▲ Crinone 8% Gel (10%)
Cytotec Tablets (Infrequent)
Delatestryl Injection
Depo-Provera Contraceptive Injection
  (1% to 5%)
Diovan HCT Tablets (Greater than
  0.2%)
Dolophine Tablets
▲ Duraclon Injection (3%)
DynaCirc (0.5% to 1%)
▲ Effexor Tablets (2% to 5.7%)
▲ Effexor XR Capsules (3% to 6%)
Eligard (Less than 2%)
Estring Vaginal Ring (At least 1
  report)
Exelon (Infrequent)
Famotidine Injection (Infrequent)
Flomax Capsules (1.0% to 2.0%)
Gabitril Tablets (Infrequent)
Gengraf Capsules (1% to less than
  3%)
Glucotrol XL (Less than 1%)
Hectorol
Hytrin Capsules (0.6%)
Hyzaar
Imdur Tablets (Less than or equal to
  5%)
Indapamide Tablets (Less than 5%)
▲ Infergen (5%)
Intron A for Injection (Up to 5%)
Inversine Tablets
Iopidine Sterile Ophthalmic Solution
Kadian Capsules (Less than 3%)
Kaletra (Less than 2%)
Klonopin Tablets (1%)
Lamictal (Rare)
Lexxel Tablets
Lipitor Tablets (Less than 2%)
Lopid Tablets

Lotensin HCT Tablets (0.3% to 1%)
Lotrel Capsules
Lupron Depot 3.75 mg (Less than
  5%)
▲ Lupron Depot 7.5 mg (5.4%)
▲ Lupron Depot—3 Month 11.25 mg
  (1.8% to 11%)
Lupron Depot—3 Month 22.5 mg
  (Less than 5%)
Lupron Depot—4 Month 30 mg (Less
  than 5%)
Lupron Injection (Less than 5%)
Luvox Tablets (2%)
Mavik Tablets (0.3% to 1.0%)
Megace Oral Suspension (Up to 5%)
Meridia Capsules
Mexitil Capsules (Less than 1% or
  about 4 in 1,000)
Midamor Tablets (Less than or equal
  to 1%)
Mirapex Tablets (1%)
▲ Mirena Intrauterine System (5% or
  more)
Moduretic Tablets
Monopril Tablets (0.2% to 1.0%)
MS Contin Tablets (Less frequent)
MSIR (Less frequent)
Nadolol Tablets (1 to 5 of 1000
  patients)
Neoral (1% to less than 3%)
▲ Nilandron Tablets (11%)
Norpramin Tablets
Norvir (Less than 2%)
Oramorph SR Tablets (Less frequent)
OxyContin Tablets
Pacerone Tablets (1% to 3%)
▲ Paxil (3% to 9%)
Pepcid (Infrequent)
Permax Tablets (Infrequent)
Plendil (0.5% to 1.5%)
Prevacid (Less than 1%)
Prevpac (Less than 1%)
Prinivil Tablets (0.4%)
Prinzide Tablets (0.3% to 1%)
Procardia XL Tablets (1% or less)
Propecia Tablets (1.8%)
▲ Proscar Tablets (3.3%)
ProSom Tablets (Rare)
Protonix (Less than 1%)
Provigil Tablets (At least 1%)
▲ Prozac (3% to 11%)
Requip Tablets (Infrequent)
Rescriptor Tablets (Less than 2%)
Rilutek Tablets (Infrequent)

Rocaltrol
Roxanol 100
Sandostatin Injection (Less than 1%)
Sandostatin LAR Depot (Rare)
▲ Sarafem Pulvules (4%)
Seroquel Tablets (Rare)
Serzone Tablets (1%)
Sonata Capsules (Infrequent)
Soriatane Capsules (Less than 1%)
Sporanox Capsules (0.2% to 1.2%)
Sular Tablets (Less than or equal to 1%)
Surmontil Capsules
Symmetrel (0.1% to 1%)
▲ Synarel Nasal Solution for Endometriosis (22% of patients)
Tambocor Tablets (Less than 1%)
Tarka Tablets
Tasmar Tablets (Infrequent)
Tenex Tablets (3% or less)
Testoderm Transdermal Systems
Testopel Pellets
Testred Capsules
Thalomid Capsules
Timolide Tablets (Less than 1%)
Timolol GFS
Timoptic
Topamax (Frequent)
Toprol-XL Tablets
Tricor Tablets (2%)
Trileptal
Trovan (Less than 1%)
Uniretic Tablets (Less than 1%)
Vaseretic Tablets (0.5% to 2.0%)
Vicoprofen Tablets (Less than 1%)
Wellbutrin SR (Infrequent)
▲ Wellbutrin Tablets (3.1%)
▲ Xanax Tablets (14.4%)
Zantac Injection
Zebeta Tablets
Zestoretic Tablets (0.3% to 1%)
Zestril Tablets (0.4%)
▲ Zoladex (61%)
▲ Zoloft (1% to 11%)
Zonegran Capsules (Infrequent)
Zyban (Infrequent)
Zyprexa (Infrequent)
Zyrtec (Less than 2%)
Zyrtec-D (Less than 2%)

Libido increased

Anadrol-50 Tablets
Androderm
AndroGel (One patient)
Aricept Tablets (Frequent)

Avonex
Bontril
Celexa (Infrequent)
Clozaril Tablets (Less than 1%)
Cognex Capsules (Infrequent)
Delatestryl Injection
Depo-Provera Contraceptive Injection (Fewer than 1%)
▲ Dostinex Tablets (Less than 10%)
Effexor Tablets (Infrequent)
Effexor XR Capsules (Infrequent)
Exelon (Infrequent)
Gabitril Tablets (Infrequent)
Gengraf Capsules (1% to less than 3%)
Haldol
Haldol Decanoate
Klonopin Tablets (Infrequent)
Lamictal (Rare)
Lodosyn Tablets
Lotensin Tablets (Less than 1%)
Lupron Injection
Luvox Tablets (Infrequent)
Meridia Capsules
Moban
Neoral (1% to less than 3%)
Neurontin (Rare)
Norpramin Tablets
Paxil (Rare)
Permax Tablets (Infrequent)
Prevacid (Less than 1%)
Prevpac (Less than 1%)
Prozac (Infrequent)
Remeron (Infrequent)
Reminyl (Infrequent)
Requip Tablets (Infrequent)
Rilutek Tablets (Infrequent)
Risperdal (Infrequent)
Sarafem Pulvules (Infrequent)
Seroquel Tablets (Infrequent)
Serzone Tablets (Infrequent)
Sinemet CR Tablets
Sinemet Tablets
Surmontil Capsules
Synarel Nasal Solution for Endometriosis (1% of patients)
Tasmar Tablets (Infrequent)
Testoderm Transdermal Systems (1%)
Testopel Pellets
Testred Capsules
Topamax (Rare)
Trileptal
Vistide Injection
Wellbutrin SR

Wellbutrin Tablets (Frequent)
▲ Xanax Tablets (7.7%)
Zarontin (Rare)
▲ Zoladex (12%)
Zoloft (Rare)
Zyban
Zyprexa

Libido, changes

Activella Tablets
Adderall Tablets
Adderall XR Capsules
Adipex-P
Alesse-21 Tablets
Alesse-28 Tablets
Alora Transdermal System
▲ Android Capsules (Among most
    common)
Avalide Tablets
Avapro Tablets (Less than 1%)
Brevicon 28-Day Tablets
Cenestin Tablets
Climara Transdermal System
Cyclessa Tablets
Desogen Tablets
Desoxyn Tablets
Dexedrine
DextroStat Tablets
Esclim Transdermal System
Estinyl Tablets
Estrace
Estratest
Estrostep 21 Tablets
Estrostep Fe Tablets
Etrafon
femhrt Tablets
Flexeril Tablets (Rare)
Fortovase Capsules (2.2%)
Halcion Tablets
Invirase Capsules (Less than 2%)
Ionamin Capsules
Levlen
Levlite
Levora Tablets
Librium Capsules (Isolated cases)
Librium for Injection (Isolated cases)
Limbitrol
Lo/Ovral
Loestrin
Low-Ogestrel-28 Tablets
Lunelle Monthly Injection
Menest Tablets
Microgestin Fe
Mircette Tablets
Modicon

Monopril HCT (Less than 2%)
Necon
Neurontin (Infrequent)
Nipent for Injection (Less than 3%)
Nordette-28 Tablets
Norinyl
▲ Novantrone for Injection (4%)
Ogen Tablets
Ogestrel Tablets
Ortho Dienestrol Cream
Ortho Tri-Cyclen
Ortho-Cept
Ortho-Cyclen
Ortho-Est Tablets
Ortho-Novum
Ortho-Prefest Tablets
Orudis Capsules (Rare)
Oruvail Capsules (Rare)
Ovcon
Ovral
Ovrette Tablets
Oxandrin Tablets
Premarin
Premphase Tablets
Prempro Tablets
Provera Tablets
Roferon-A Injection (Less than 4%)
Serentil
Sinequan
Thioridazine Hydrochloride Tablets
Trilafon
Tri-Levlen
Tri-Norinyl
Triphasil
Trivora Tablets
Valium Injectable
Valium Tablets (Infrequent)
Vivactil Tablets
Vivelle Transdermal System
Vivelle-Dot Transdermal System
▲ Xanax Tablets (7.1%)
Yasmin 28 Tablets
Zovia

Libido, loss

Catapres Tablets (About 3 in 100
    patients)
Catapres-TTS (0.5% or less)
Clorpres Tablets (About 3%)
Combipres Tablets (About 3%)
▲ Eulexin Capsules (36%)
Klonopin Tablets (Infrequent)
Lescol Capsules
Lescol XL Tablets

Mevacor Tablets (0.5% to 1.0%)
Nolvadex Tablets
Orap Tablets
Pravachol Tablets
Roferon-A Injection (Infrequent)
Vascor Tablets (0.5% to 2.0%)
Zantac Tablets, Granules, & Syrup
   (Occasional)
Ziac Tablets (0.4%)
Zocor Tablets

Listlessness

Aricept Tablets (Infrequent)
Indocin
   Capsules/Suspension/Suppositories
   (Greater than 1%)
Rum-K
Synvisc

Manic behavior

Ambien Tablets (Rare)
Betaseron
Bextra Tablets (Rare)
Celexa
Cipro (Less than 1%)
Cipro I.V. (1% or less)
Copaxone (Infrequent)
Effexor Tablets (0.5%)
Effexor XR Capsules (0.5%)
Evoxac Capsules (Less than 1%)
Felbatol
Floxin
Halcion Tablets
Herceptin I.V. (At least one of 958
   patients)
Hivid Tablets (Less than 1%)
Intron A for Injection (Less than 5%)
Lamictal (Rare)
Levaquin (Less than 0.3%)
Levbid
Levsin
Luvox Tablets (Approximately 1%)
Nardil Tablets (Less frequent)
Neurontin (Rare)
Orthoclone OKT3 (Less than 1%)
Parnate Tablets
Paxil (Infrequent)
Permax Tablets (Infrequent)
Protopam Chloride for Injection
   (Several cases)
Prozac (0.1% to 0.8%)
Remeron (Approximately 0.2%)
Requip Tablets (Infrequent)
Rescriptor Tablets (Less than 2%)
Retrovir IV Infusion

Rilutek Tablets (Infrequent)
Risperdal
Roferon-A Injection
Rythmol Tablets (Less than 1%)
Seroquel Tablets (Infrequent)
Serzone Tablets (0.3% to 1.6%)
Sustiva Capsules
Symmetrel
Tasmar Tablets (Infrequent)
Tenex Tablets
Topamax (Rare)
Trileptal
Valtrex Caplets
Wellbutrin SR
Wellbutrin Tablets (Frequent)
Xanax Tablets
Zoloft (0.4% to 2%)
Zyban

Manic behavior, mild

Celexa
Effexor Tablets (0.5%)
Effexor XR Capsules (0.3%)
Lamictal (Rare)
Limbitrol
Luvox Tablets (Approximately 1%)
▲ Nardil Tablets (Most common)
Norpramin Tablets
Paxil (Approximately 1.0%)
Prozac (0.1% to 0.8%)
Remeron (Approximately 0.2%)
Sarafem Pulvules
Serzone Tablets (0.3% to 1.6%)
Surmontil Capsules
Vivactil Tablets
Wellbutrin SR (Rare)
Wellbutrin Tablets (Frequent)
Xanax Tablets
Zoloft (Approximately 0.4%)
Zyban (Rare)

Melancholia

Celexa (Rare)

Memory impairment

Cataflam Tablets (Less than 1%)
Cogentin
Copaxone (Infrequent)
Cozaar Tablets (Less than 1%)
Eldepryl Capsules
Eskalith
Halcion Tablets (0.5% to 0.9%)
Hyzaar
Imitrex Nasal Spray (Rare)
Imitrex Tablets (Rare)

▲ Klonopin Tablets (4%)
Lamictal (2.4%)
Lithobid Slow-Release Tablets
Lodosyn Tablets
▲ Lupron Depot 3.75 mg (Among most
frequent)
Lupron Depot—3 Month 11.25 mg
(Less than 5%)
Lupron Injection (Less than 5%)
Maxalt (Infrequent)
Monopril HCT
Monopril Tablets (0.2% to 1.0%)
Prinivil Tablets (0.3% to 1.0%)
Prinzide Tablets
Rifamate Capsules (Uncommon)
Rifater Tablets (Uncommon)
Roferon-A Injection (Less than 4%)
▲ Serzone Tablets (4%)
Sinemet CR Tablets
Timolide Tablets
Tonocard Tablets (Less than 1%)
▲ Topamax (12.4% to 1(2.6%)
Transderm Scop (Infrequent)
▲ Vesanoid Capsules (3%)
Voltaren (Less than 1%)
Wellbutrin SR (Up to 3%)
Wellbutrin Tablets (Infrequent)
▲ Xanax Tablets (33.1%)
Zestoretic Tablets
Ziac Tablets
▲ Zonegran Capsules (6%)
Zyban (Infrequent)

Memory loss, short-term
Blocadren Tablets
Clozaril Tablets (Less than 1%)
Corgard Tablets
Corzide
Cosopt Ophthalmic Solution
Crinone 4% Gel (Less than 5%)
Crinone 8% Gel (Less than 5%)
Cytovene
Ergamisol Tablets (10 out of 463
patients)
Hivid Tablets (Less than 1%)
Inderal
Inderide
Lescol Capsules
Lescol XL Tablets
Levbid
Levsin
Meridia Capsules
Mevacor Tablets (0.5% to 1.0%)
Mexitil Capsules (Less than 1% to
about 9 in 1,000)

Nadolol Tablets
Normodyne Tablets
Parnate Tablets
Pravachol Tablets
Rythmol Tablets (Less than 1%)
Sectral Capsules
Tenoretic Tablets
Tenormin
Testoderm Transdermal Systems (1%)
Timolol GFS
Timoptic
Toprol-XL Tablets
Zocor Tablets

Mental acuity, loss of
Crixivan Capsules (Less than 2%)
Lodosyn Tablets
Retrovir Capsules, Tablets & Syrup
Retrovir IV Infusion
Sinemet CR Tablets
Sinemet Tablets
Tasmar Tablets (1%)

Mental clouding
Compazine
Dilaudid Powder
Dilaudid Rectal Suppositories
Dilaudid Tablets
Halcion Tablets
Hycodan
Hycomine Compound Tablets
Hycotuss Expectorant Syrup
Lortab
Maxidone Tablets
Norco
Numorphan
Tussionex
Vicodin
Vicodin Tuss Expectorant
Vioxx (Greater than 0.1% to 1.9%)
Zydone Tablets

Mental perception, altered
Mykrox Tablets

Mental performance, impairment
Aldoclor Tablets
Aldomet Tablets
Aldoril Tablets
Alferon N Injection (1%)
Ambien Tablets (Infrequent)
Amerge Tablets (Infrequent)
Anaprox (Less than 1%)
Arthrotec Tablets (Rare)

Ativan Injection
Cardura Tablets (Less than 0.5%)
Celexa (Frequent)
Claritin (At least one patient)
Claritin-D 12 Hour (Less frequent)
Claritin-D 24 Hour
Clozaril Tablets
Compazine
Copaxone (Infrequent)
Coreg Tablets (0.1% to 1%)
Cosopt Ophthalmic Solution
D.H.E. 45 Injection
Demerol
Dilaudid Injection
Dilaudid Powder
Dilaudid Rectal Suppositories
Dilaudid Tablets
Dostinex Tablets (1%)
EC-Naprosyn (Less than 1%)
Ergamisol Tablets (Less frequent)
Eskalith
Etrafon
Exelon (Infrequent)
Felbatol
Fludara for Injection (Up to 1%)
Flumadine (0.3% to 2.1%)
Fortovase Capsules (Less than 2%)
▲ Gabitril Tablets (6%)
Gengraf Capsules (1% to less than 3%)
Grifulvin V
Hivid Tablets (Less than 1%)
Hycodan
Hycomine Compound Tablets
Hycotuss Expectorant Syrup
Imdur Tablets (Less than or equal to 5%)
Imitrex Injection (Rare)
Imitrex Nasal Spray (Rare)
Imitrex Tablets (Infrequent)
▲ Intron A for Injection (Up to 14%)
Inversine Tablets
Invirase Capsules (Less than 2%)
Kadian Capsules (Less than 3%)
Klonopin Tablets (1% to 2%)
Lamictal (1.7%)
Levaquin (Less than 0.3%)
Levbid
Levsin
Limbitrol
Lithobid Slow-Release Tablets
Lortab
Loxitane Capsules
Maxalt (Frequent)

Maxidone Tablets
Meridia Capsules
Migranal Nasal Spray (Infrequent)
Miltown Tablets
MS Contin Tablets
▲ Naprelan Tablets (3% to 9%)
Naprosyn (Less than 1%)
Neoral (1% to less than 3%)
▲ Nicotrol Nasal Spray (Over 5%)
Norco
Norpramin Tablets
Orap Tablets
Paxil (Frequent)
Percocet Tablets
Percodan Tablets
Percolone Tablets
Phenergan Injection
Phenergan Suppositories
Phenergan Syrup
Phenergan Tablets
Phenergan VC Syrup
Phenergan VC with Codeine Syrup
Phenergan with Codeine Syrup
Phenergan with Dextromethorphan Syrup
Prometrium Capsules (Less than 5%)
ProSom Tablets
Prozac
▲ Rebetol Capsules (10% to 14%)
Rebetron Combination Therapy
Remeron
Requip Tablets (Infrequent)
Rescriptor Tablets (Less than 2%)
Rifadin
Rifamate Capsules
Rifater Tablets
Risperdal (Infrequent)
▲ Roferon-A Injection (4%)
Seroquel Tablets
▲ Serzone Tablets (3%)
Sinemet Tablets
Surmontil Capsules
▲ Sustiva Capsules (1% to 9%)
Tarka Tablets (Less frequent)
Timolide Tablets
Timolol GFS
Timoptic
▲ Topamax (6.7% to 15.4%)
Toradol (1% or less)
Trovan (Less than 1%)
Tussionex
Tylenol with Codeine
Tylox Capsules
Ultracet Tablets

Ultram Tablets (Less than 1%)
Vicodin
Vicodin Tuss Expectorant
Vistaril Intramuscular Solution
(Seldom)
Vivactil Tablets
Xanax Tablets
Zarontin
Zebeta Tablets
Zestril Tablets (0.3% to 1.0%)
Ziac Tablets
Zoloft (1.3% to 2%)
▲ Zonegran Capsules (6%)
▲ Zyban (9%)
Zydone Tablets
Zyrtec (Less than 2%)
Zyrtec-D (Less than 2%)

Mental slowness

Celontin Capsules
Tonocard Tablets (Less than 1%)
▲ Topamax (8% to 15.4%)
▲ Zonegran Capsules (4%)

Mental status, altered

Clozaril Tablets
Cuprimine Capsules
▲ Digitek Tablets (5%)
Eldepryl Capsules
Etrafon
Haldol Decanoate
▲ Idamycin PFS Injection (41%)
Lanoxin/Lanoxicaps
Levaquin (Less than 0.3%)
Moban
Navane
Oncaspar
Orap Tablets
Orthoclone OKT3 (Less than 1%)
▲ Prograf (Approximately 55%)
▲ Proleukin for Injection (73%)
Risperdal
▲ Roferon-A Injection (10% to 17%)
Serentil
Seroquel Tablets
Sinemet CR Tablets
Stelazine

Mood changes

Adalat CC Tablets (Rare)
Aerobid (1% to 3%)
Alesse-21 Tablets
Aygestin Tablets
Betapace Tablets (Less than 1% to
3%)
Celestone Soluspan

Clomid Tablets
Cortone
Decadron
Dilaudid Injection
Dilaudid Oral Liquid (Less frequent)
Dilaudid Powder
Dilaudid Rectal Suppositories
Dilaudid Tablets
Dilaudid Tablets - 8 mg (Less
frequent)
Dilaudid-HP (Less frequent)
Dipentum Capsules (Rare)
Eldepryl Capsules
Enbrel for Injection
Feldene Capsules (Rare)
Florinef Acetate Tablets
Hexalen Capsules
Hivid Tablets (Less than 1%)
Hycodan
Hycomine Compound Tablets
Hycotuss Expectorant Syrup
Hydrocortone
Levlen
Levlite
Levorphanol Tartrate Tablets
Lortab
Lupron Depot 3.75 mg
Lupron Injection (Less than 5%)
Marinol Capsules
Maxidone Tablets
Meridia Capsules
Modicon
Monopril HCT
Monopril Tablets (0.2% to 1.0%)
MS Contin Tablets (Less frequent)
MSIR (Less frequent)
Norco
Oncaspar
Oramorph SR Tablets (Less frequent)
Ortho Tri-Cyclen
Orthoclone OKT3
Ortho-Cyclen
Ortho-Novum
Prednisone
Prelone Syrup
▲ Procardia Capsules (7%)
▲ Procardia XL Tablets (7%)
Serophene Tablets
Solu-Medrol Sterile Powder
▲ Tonocard Tablets (1.5% to 11.0%)
▲ Topamax (3.5% to 10.1%)
Tri-Levlen
Tussionex
Univasc Tablets (Less than 1%)

Versed Syrup (Less than 1%)
Vicodin
Vicodin Tuss Expectorant
Vicoprofen Tablets (Less than 1%)
Wellbutrin Tablets (Infrequent)
Zydone Tablets

Nervousness
8-MOP Capsules
Accupril Tablets (0.5% to 1.0%)
Accuretic Tablets (0.5% to 1%)
Accutane Capsules
Aceon Tablets (1.1%)
AcipHex Tablets
Actifed Cold & Allergy
Actiq (1% to 2%)
Activella Tablets
Adalat CC Tablets (Rare)
▲ Adderall XR Capsules (6%)
Adenoscan (2%)
Advil Cold and Sinus
▲ Aerobid (3% to 9%)
Agrylin Capsules (1% to 5%)
Albalon Ophthalmic Solution
Alesse-21 Tablets
Alesse-28 Tablets
Alferon N Injection (1%)
Allegra (Less than 1%)
Allegra-D (1.4%)
Altace Capsules (Less than 1%)
▲ Alupent Inhalation Aerosol (6.8%)
▲ Alupent Inhalation Solution (14.1%)
Ambien Tablets (1%)
AmBisome for Injection (Less
    common)
Amphotec (1% to 5%)
AndroGel (Up to 3%)
▲ Angiomax for Injection (5%)
Aricept Tablets (Frequent)
Arimidex Tablets (2% to 5%)
▲ Artane (30% to 50%)
Arthrotec Tablets (Rare)
Asacol Tablets (2% or greater)
Astelin Nasal Spray (Infrequent)
▲ Atrovent Inhalation Aerosol (3.1%)
Atrovent Inhalation Solution (0.5%)
Avalide Tablets (1% or greater)
Avapro Tablets (1% or greater)
Avelox Tablets (0.05% to 1%)
Axert Tablets (Rare)
Axid Pulvules (1.1%)
Bactrim
Benadryl Allergy & Sinus
Benadryl Allergy & Sinus Headache
Benadryl Parenteral

▲ Betaseron (8%)
Bextra Tablets (0.1% to 1.9%)
Bicillin C-R
Bicillin L-A
Blocadren Tablets (Less than 1%)
▲ Brethine Ampuls (16.9% to 38.0%)
▲ Brethine Tablets (35%)
Brevicon 28-Day Tablets
Bromfed
Campath Ampules
Captopril Tablets
Cardizem
Cardura Tablets (2%)
▲ Casodex Tablets (2% to 5%)
▲ Catapres Tablets (About 3 in 100
    patients)
Catapres-TTS (1 of 101 patients)
Ceclor (Rare)
Ceclor CD (0.1% to 1%)
Cefzil (Less than 1%)
Celebrex Capsules (0.1% to 1.9%)
▲ CellCept (11.4%)
Celontin Capsules
▲ Cenestin Tablets (28%)
Cerebyx Injection (Frequent)
Children's Benadryl Allergy & Sinus
Children's Sudafed Cold & Cough
Children's Tylenol Cold
Children's Vicks NyQuil Cold/Cough
Cipro
Cipro I.V.
▲ Claritin (4%)
▲ Claritin-D 12 Hour (5%)
▲ Claritin-D 24 Hour (3%)
Clinoril Tablets (Greater than 1%)
▲ Clorpres Tablets (About 3%)
Cogentin
Cognex Capsules (Frequent)
Colazal Capsules
▲ CombiPatch (5% to 6%)
▲ Combipres Tablets (About 3%)
Combivent Inhalation Aerosol (Less
    than 2%)
Compazine
▲ Concerta (Amongst most common)
Contac 12 Hour Cold Caplets
Contac Severe Cold and Flu
Contac Severe Cold and Flu Non-
    Drowsy
Copaxone (2%)
Coreg Tablets (0.1% to 1%)
Coricidin D Cold, Flu & Sinus
Corlopam Injection (1% to 2%)
Cosopt Ophthalmic Solution
Cozaar Tablets (Less than 1%)

▲ Crinone 8% Gel (16%)
Crixivan Capsules (Less than 2%)
Cyclessa Tablets
Dantrium Capsules (Less frequent)
Daranide Tablets
Demadex (1.1%)
▲ Depacon Injection (0.9% to 11%)
▲ Depakene (11%)
Depakote ER Tablets (1% to 5%)
▲ Depakote Sprinkle Capsules (7% to 11%)
▲ Depakote Tablets (1% to 11%)
▲ Depo-Provera Contraceptive Injection (More than 5%)
Desogen Tablets
Detrol Tablets (1.1%)
Dilantin
Dilaudid Oral Liquid (Less frequent)
Dilaudid Tablets - 8 mg (Less frequent)
Dilaudid-HP
Ditropan XL (2% to 5%)
Dolobid Tablets (Less than 1 in 100)
Donnatal
▲ Dostinex Tablets (1% to less than 10%)
Doxil Injection (Less than 1%)
Drixoral Allergy Sinus
Drixoral Cold & Allergy
Drixoral Cold & Flu
▲ Duraclon Injection (3%)
▲ Duragesic Transdermal System (3% to 10%)
Duranest Injections
Dynabac Tablets (0.1% to 1%)
DynaCirc (0.5% to 1%)
▲ Effexor Tablets (2% to 21.3%)
▲ Effexor XR Capsules (10% to 12%)
ELA-Max Cream
Eldepryl Capsules
EMLA (Unlikely)
Enalaprilat Injection
EpiPen Jr. Auto-Injector
Ergamisol Tablets (1% to 2%)
Estring Vaginal Ring (At least 1 report)
Estrostep 21 Tablets
Estrostep Fe Tablets
Eulexin Capsules (1%)
Exelon (2% or more)
▲ Felbatol (7.0% to 16.1%)
Feldene Capsules (Occasional)
▲ femhrt Tablets (5.4%)
Ferrlecit Injection (Two or more patients)

Flexeril Tablets (1% to 3%)
▲ Flolan for Injection (7% to 21%)
Flovent Rotadisk (1% to 3%)
Floxin (1% to 3%)
Flumadine (1.3% to 2.1%)
▲ Focalin Tablets (Among most common)
Foradil Aerolizer
Foscavir Injection (Between 1% and 5%)
▲ Gabitril Tablets (10%)
Gastrocrom Oral Concentrate (Less common)
Gengraf Capsules (1% to less than 3%)
▲ Glucotrol XL (3.6%)
▲ Halcion Tablets (5.2%)
Hivid Tablets (Less than 1%)
Hytrin Capsules (2.3%)
Hyzaar
Imdur Tablets (Less than or equal to 5%)
Indapamide Tablets (Less than 5%)
Indocin Capsules/Suspension/Suppositories (Less than 1%)
▲ Infergen (16% to 31%)
Intron A for Injection (Up to 3%)
Iopidine 0.5% Ophthalmic Solution (Less than 3%)
Ismo Tablets (Fewer than 1%)
Kaletra (Less than 2%)
▲ Keppra Tablets (4%)
Klonopin Tablets (1% to 3%)
Lamictal (Frequent)
Levaquin (0.1% to less than 1.0%)
Levbid
Levlen
Levlite
Levo-Dromoran
Levora Tablets
Levorphanol Tartrate Tablets (1% to 3%)
Levoxyl Tablets
Levsin
Lexxel Tablets
Lidoderm Patch
Lo/Ovral
Lodine (1% to 3%)
Lodine XL Extended-Release Tablets (1% to 3%)
Lodosyn Tablets
Loestrin
Lorabid

Lotensin HCT Tablets (0.3% to 1%)
Lotensin Tablets (Less than 1%)
Lotrel Capsules
Low-Ogestrel-28 Tablets
Lunelle Monthly Injection
Lupron Depot 3.75 mg (Less than 5%)
▲ Lupron Depot—3 Month 11.25 mg (4.8% to 5%)
Lupron Depot—3 Month 22.5 mg (Less than 5%)
Lupron Depot-PED (Less than 2%)
Lupron Injection (Less than 5%)
Lupron Injection Pediatric (Less than 2%)
▲ Luvox Tablets (2% to 12%)
Marinol Capsules (Greater than 1%)
Matulane Capsules
▲ Maxair (4.5% to 6.9%)
Maxalt (Infrequent)
▲ Meridia Capsules (5.2%)
Merrem I.V. (0.1% to 1.0%)
▲ Metadate (Among most common)
▲ Methylin (Among most common)
▲ Mexitil Capsules (5% to 11.3%)
Micardis HCT Tablets
Microgestin Fe
Midamor Tablets (Less than or equal to 1%)
Migranal Nasal Spray (Infrequent)
Minipress Capsules (1% to 4%)
Minizide Capsules
Mirapex Tablets (1% or more)
Mircette Tablets
▲ Mirena Intrauterine System (5% or more)
Mobic Tablets (Less than 2%)
Modicon
Moduretic Tablets (Less than or equal to 1%)
Monurol Sachet (Less than 1%)
Motofen Tablets (1 in 200 to 1 in 600)
Motrin (1% to less than 3%)
Motrin Sinus Headache Caplets
MS Contin Tablets (Less frequent)
MSIR (Less frequent)
Mykrox Tablets (Less than 2%)
Naprelan Tablets (Less than 1%)
Narcan Injection
Naropin Injection (Less than 1%)
Nascobal Gel
Necon
Nembutal (Less than 1%)
Neoral (1% to less than 3%)

▲ Neumega for Injection (Greater than or equal to 10%)
Neurontin (2.4%)
Nexium (Less than 1%)
Nilandron Tablets (2%)
▲ Nipent for Injection (3% to 10%)
Nordette-28 Tablets
Norinyl
Norplant System
Norvasc Tablets (More than 0.1% to 1%)
Norvir (Less than 2%)
Nubain Injection (1% or less)
NuLev
Numorphan
Ogestrel Tablets
OptiPranolol (A small number of patients)
Oramorph SR Tablets (Less frequent)
▲ Orap Tablets (8.3%)
Ortho Tri-Cyclen
Ortho-Cept
Ortho-Cyclen
Ortho-Novum
▲ Orudis Capsules (3% to 9%)
▲ Oruvail Capsules (3% to 9%)
Ovcon
Ovral
Ovrette Tablets
Oxsoralen-Ultra Capsules
OxyContin Tablets (Between 1% and 5%)
▲ Paxil (4% to 9%)
Pediatric Vicks 44m Cough & Cold Relief
Periactin Tablets (No incidence data in labeling)
Permax Tablets (Frequent)
Phenergan Injection
Phenergan Suppositories
Phenergan Tablets
Phenergan VC Syrup
Phenergan VC with Codeine Syrup
Plaquenil Tablets
Plendil (0.5% to 1.5%)
Ponstel Capsules (Occasional)
Premphase Tablets
Prempro Tablets
Prevacid (Less than 1%)
Prevpac (Less than 1%)
Prilosec (Less than 1%)
Primatene Tablets
Prinivil Tablets (0.3% to 1.0%)
Prinzide Tablets

ProAmatine Tablets (Less frequent)
▲ Procardia Capsules (2% or less to 7%)
▲ Procardia XL Tablets (Less than 3% to 7%)
▲ Prograf (3%)
Prometrium Capsules
▲ ProSom Tablets (8%)
Protonix (Less than 1%)
▲ Proventil HFA Inhalation Aerosol (7%)
▲ Proventil Inhalation Aerosol (Less than 10%)
Proventil Inhalation Solution 0.083% (4%)
▲ Proventil Repetabs Tablets (2% to 20%)
▲ Proventil Solution for Inhalation 0.5% (4%)
Provera Tablets
▲ Provigil Tablets (8%)
▲ Prozac (11% to 16%)
Quinidex Extentabs (2%)
▲ Rebetol Capsules (4% to 5%)
▲ Rebetron Combination Therapy (4% to 5%)
Relafen Tablets (1% to 3%)
Requip Tablets (1% or more)
Rescriptor Tablets (Less than 2%)
Retrovir Capsules, Tablets & Syrup (1.6)%
Retrovir IV Infusion (2%)
Rhinocort Nasal Inhaler (Less than 1%)
Risperdal (Frequent)
▲ Ritalin (One of the two most common)
Rituxan (1% to 5%)
Robinul Injectable
Robinul Tablets
Robitussin Cough & Cold
Robitussin Pediatric Cough & Cold
Robitussin-CF Liquid
Robitussin-DAC Syrup
Robitussin-PE Liquid
Roferon-A Injection (Less than 3% to less than 5%)
▲ Romazicon Injection (3% to 9%)
Roxicodone Tablets (Less than 3%)
Rynatan Tablets
Salagen Tablets (Less than 1%)
Sandostatin LAR Depot (1% to 4%)
▲ Sarafem Pulvules (7% to 14%)
▲ Semprex-D Capsules (3%)
Septra
Serevent Inhalation Aerosol (1% to 3%)

Serophene Tablets (Approximately 1 in 50 patients)
▲ Serostim for Injection (1% to 10%)
Sinemet CR Tablets
Sinemet Tablets
Sinutab Non-Drying Liquid Caps
Skelaxin Tablets
Skelid Tablets (Greater than or equal to 1%)
Sonata Capsules (Frequent)
Spectracef Tablets (0.1% to 1%)
Stadol NS Nasal Spray (1% or greater)
Sudafed Tablets
Sudafed Nasal Decongestant Tablets
Sular Tablets (Less than or equal to 1%)
Sustiva Capsules (1% to 2%)
Symmetrel (1% to 5%)
Synagis Intramuscular (More than 1%)
Tasmar Tablets (Infrequent)
Tenex Tablets (Less frequent)
Tequin (Less than 0.1%)
Teveten Tablets (Less than 1%)
▲ Thalomid Capsules (2.8% to 9.4%)
TheraFlu Cold & Cough Night Time Hot Liquid
TheraFlu Cold & Sore Throat Night Time Hot Liquid
TheraFlu Severe Cold & Congestion Night Time Caplets
Tiazac Capsules (Less than 2%)
Timolide Tablets (Less than 1%)
Timolol GFS
Timoptic (Less frequent)
▲ Tonocard Tablets (0.4% to 11.5%)
▲ Topamax (13.3% to 20.6%)
Toradol (1% or less)
Tranxene (Less common)
Trental Tablets
Triaminic Allergy Congestion Liquid
Triaminic Chest Congestion Liquid
Triaminic Cold & Allergy Liquid
Triaminic Cold & Allergy Softchews
Triaminic Cold & Cough Liquid
Triaminic Cold & Night Time Cough Liquid
Triaminic Cough & Congestion Liquid
Triaminic Cough & Sore Throat Liquid
Triaminic Cough & Sore Throat Softchews

Triaminic Cough Liquid
Triaminic Flu, Cough & Fever
Tricor Tablets
Trileptal (2% to 4%)
Tri-Levlen
Tri-Norinyl
Triphasil
Trivora Tablets
Tylenol Cold Complete Formula
Tylenol Cold Non-Drowsy
Tylenol Flu NightTime Liquid
Tylenol Sinus NightTime Caplets
Tylenol Sinus Non-Drowsy
Ultracet Tablets (At least 1%)
▲ Ultram Tablets (1% to 14%)
Uniretic Tablets (Less than 1%)
Unithroid Tablets
Univasc Tablets (Less than 1%)
Vantin (Less than 1%)
Varivax (Greater than or equal to 1%)
▲ Vascor Tablets (7.37% to 11.63%)
Vaseretic Tablets (0.5% to 2.0%)
Vasotec I.V. Injection
Vasotec Tablets (0.5% to 1.0%)
▲ Ventolin Inhalation Aerosol (1% to 10%)
Versed Injection (Less than 1%)
Vicks 44D Cough & Head Congestion Relief Liquid
Vicks DayQuil LiquiCaps/Liquid Multi-Symptom Cold/Flu Relief
▲ Vicoprofen Tablets (3% to 9%)
Vistide Injection
▲ Volmax Extended-Release Tablets (8.5%)
▲ Wellbutrin SR (3% to 5%)
▲ Xanax Tablets 4.1%
▲ Xopenex Inhalation Solution (2.8% to 9.6%)
▲ Xylocaine Injection (Among most common)
▲ Xylocaine with Epinephrine Injection (Among most common)
Yasmin 28 Tablets (Greater than 1%)
Zanaflex Tablets (3%)
Zaroxolyn Tablets (Less than 2%)
Zephrex
Zestoretic Tablets
Zestril Tablets (0.3% to 1.0%)
Zithromax Capsules & Tablets (1% or less)
Zithromax for IV Infusion (1% or less)
Zithromax for Oral Suspension (1% or less)

▲ Zoladex (3% to 5%)
Zoladex 3-month
▲ Zoloft (6%)
Zonegran Capsules (2%)
Zovia
▲ Zyban (4%)
Zyflo Filmtab Tablets (Less common)
▲ Zyprexa (16%)
Zyrtec (Less than 2%)
Zyrtec-D (Less than 2%)

Neuropsychiatric disorders, life-threatening, aggravation of

Roferon-A Injection

Neuropsychometrics performance, decrease

Blocadren Tablets
Corgard Tablets
Corzide
Cosopt Ophthalmic Solution
Inderal
Inderide
Nadolol Tablets
Normodyne Tablets
Sectral Capsules
Tenoretic Tablets
Tenormin
Timolol GFS
Timoptic
Toprol-XL Tablets

Neurosis, unspecified

Ambien Tablets (Rare)
Avonex
Betaseron
Cerebyx Injection (Infrequent)
Cognex Capsules (Infrequent)
Evoxac Capsules
Exelon (Infrequent)
Gabitril Tablets (Infrequent)
Intron A for Injection (Less than 5%)
Lamictal (Rare)
Neurontin (Rare)
Nipent for Injection (Less than 3%)
Paxil (Infrequent)
Permax Tablets (Infrequent)
Prevacid (Less than 1%)
Prevpac (Less than 1%)
Prozac (Infrequent)
Remeron (Infrequent)
Requip Tablets (Infrequent)
Sarafem Pulvules (Infrequent)
Sustiva Capsules

Topamax (Infrequent)
Uniretic Tablets (Less than 1%)

Nightmares

Aldoclor Tablets
Aldomet Tablets
Aldoril Tablets
Allegra (Less than 1%)
Axert Tablets (Rare)
Biaxin
Blocadren Tablets
Cardura Tablets (Less than 0.5%)
Cataflam Tablets (Less than 1%)
Catapres Tablets
Catapres-TTS (0.5% or less)
Celexa (Infrequent)
Cipro (Less than 1%)
Cipro I.V. (1% or less)
Claritin (At least one patient)
Claritin-D 12 Hour (Less frequent)
Claritin-D 24 Hour (Fewer than 2%)
Clorpres Tablets
▲ Clozaril Tablets (4%)
Combipres Tablets
Coreg Tablets (0.1% to 1%)
Cosopt Ophthalmic Solution
Duraclon Injection (Rare)
▲ Effexor XR Capsules (4% to 7%)
Eldepryl Capsules
Etrafon
Evoxac Capsules (Less than 1%)
Floxin
Gengraf Capsules (1% to less than 3%)
Halcion Tablets (Rare)
Imdur Tablets (Less than or equal to 5%)
Intron A for Injection (Less than 5%)
Ismo Tablets (Fewer than 1%)
Klonopin Tablets (Infrequent)
Levaquin
Lodosyn Tablets
Marinol Capsules (Less than 1%)
Matulane Capsules
Meridia Capsules
Nardil Tablets (Infrequent)
Naropin Injection (Less than 1%)
Nembutal (Less than 1%)
Neoral (1% to less than 3%)
Norpramin Tablets
Orudis Capsules (Rare)
Oruvail Capsules (Rare)
Plaquenil Tablets
Prevpac

Procardia XL Tablets (1% or less)
Relafen Tablets (Less than 1%)
Reminyl (Infrequent)
Rescriptor Tablets (Less than 2%)
Risperdal (Rare)
Sinemet CR Tablets
Sinemet Tablets
Surmontil Capsules
Tequin
Timolide Tablets
Timolol GFS
Timoptic
Toprol-XL Tablets
Trovan
Vantin (Less than 1%)
Ventolin Inhalation Aerosol (1%)
Versed Injection (Less than 1%)
Vivactil Tablets
Voltaren (Less than 1%)
Zoloft (Infrequent)
Zyrtec (Less than 2%)
Zyrtec-D (Less than 2%)

Obsessive compulsive symptoms

Zyprexa (Infrequent)

Orgasmic dysfunction, female

▲ Effexor XR Capsules (4%)
Prozac
Sarafem Pulvules

Oversedation

Versed Injection (1.60)%

Overstimulation

Adderall Tablets
Adderall XR Capsules
Adipex-P
Bontril
Desoxyn Tablets
Dexedrine
DextroStat Tablets
Eldepryl Capsules
Halcion Tablets
Ionamin Capsules
Miltown Tablets
Parafon Forte DSC Caplets (Occasional)
Parnate Tablets

Panic

Ambien Tablets (Rare)
Amerge Tablets (Rare)
Celexa (Infrequent)
Cozaar Tablets (Less than 1%)

Effexor Tablets
Effexor XR Capsules
Hyzaar
Imitrex Injection
Imitrex Nasal Spray
Imitrex Tablets
Lamictal (Infrequent)
Tasmar Tablets (1%)
Trileptal

Paranoia

Adalat CC Tablets (Rare)
Allegra-D (Less than 1%)
Aricept Tablets (Infrequent)
Artane (One case)
Arthrotec Tablets (Rare)
Betaseron
Celexa (Infrequent)
Cipro
Cipro I.V. (1% or less)
Clozaril Tablets (Less than 1%)
Cognex Capsules (Infrequent)
Copaxone (Infrequent)
Duragesic Transdermal System (1% or greater)
Effexor Tablets (Infrequent)
Effexor XR Capsules (Infrequent)
Etrafon
Evoxac Capsules
Exelon (2% or more)
Felbatol
Flexeril Tablets
Floxin
Gabitril Tablets (Frequent)
Gliadel Wafer (1%)
Hivid Tablets (Less than 1%)
Lamictal (Infrequent)
Levaquin (Less than 0.3%)
Lodosyn Tablets
Luvox Tablets (Infrequent)
▲ Marinol Capsules (3% to 10%)
Mirapex Tablets (Less than 1%)
Neurontin (Infrequent)
Orthoclone OKT3 (Less than 1%)
Paxil (Infrequent)
Permax Tablets (Frequent)
Procardia Capsules (Less than 0.5%)
Prozac (Infrequent)
Remeron (Infrequent)
Reminyl (Infrequent)
Requip Tablets (Infrequent)
Rescriptor Tablets (Less than 2%)
Rilutek Tablets (Infrequent)
Romazicon Injection (1% to 3%)

Sandostatin Injection (Less than 1%)
Sandostatin LAR Depot (Rare)
Sarafem Pulvules (Infrequent)
Seroquel Tablets (Infrequent)
Serzone Tablets (Infrequent)
Sinemet CR Tablets
Sinemet Tablets
Sustiva Capsules
Symmetrel
Tasmar Tablets (Infrequent)
Tequin (Less than 0.1%)
Topamax (Infrequent)
Trilafon
Trileptal
Trovan (Less than 1%)
Ultracet Tablets (Less than 1%)
Wellbutrin SR
Wellbutrin Tablets (Infrequent)
Zoloft (Infrequent)
Zyban
Zyprexa

Personality changes

Ambien Tablets (Rare)
Cardizem
Celestone Soluspan
Cerebyx Injection (Infrequent)
Cortone
Decadron
Depacon Injection (1% to 5%)
Depakene (1% to 5%)
Depakote ER Tablets (1% to 5%)
Depakote Sprinkle Capsules (1% to 5%)
Depakote Tablets (1% to 5%)
Eldepryl Capsules
Enbrel for Injection
Evoxac Capsules
Exelon (Infrequent)
Florinef Acetate Tablets
Gabitril Tablets (Frequent)
Hydrocortone
Imitrex Tablets (Rare)
Intron A for Injection (Less than 5%)
Lamictal (Infrequent)
Levo-Dromoran
▲ Lupron Depot 3.75 mg (Among most frequent)
Lupron Depot—3 Month 11.25 mg (Less than 5%)
Lupron Depot-PED (Less than 2%)
Lupron Injection Pediatric (Less than 2%)
Neurontin (Rare)

Norvir (Less than 2%)
Orudis Capsules (Rare)
Oruvail Capsules (Rare)
Permax Tablets (2.1%)
Prednisone
Prelone Syrup
Prometrium Capsules (Less than 5%)
Prozac (Infrequent)
Requip Tablets (Infrequent)
Rilutek Tablets (Infrequent)
Roxicodone Tablets (Less than 3%)
Sarafem Pulvules (Infrequent)
Solu-Medrol Sterile Powder
Tiazac Capsules (Less than 2%)
Topamax (Frequent)
Trileptal
Vistide Injection
▲ Zyprexa (8%)

Phobia, unspecified
Imitrex Injection

Phobic disorder
Cipro (Less than 1%)
Cipro I.V. (1% or less)
Floxin
Imitrex Tablets (Rare)
Luvox Tablets (Infrequent)
Zyprexa (Infrequent)

Phonophobia
Imitrex Tablets (Frequent)
Accutane Capsules
▲ Alocril Ophthalmic Solution (1% to 10%)
▲ Alphagan Ophthalmic Solution (Approximately 3% to 9%)
Alphagan P Ophthalmic Solution (1% to 4%)
▲ Alrex Sterile Ophthalmic Suspension (5% to 15%)
Amerge Tablets (Frequent)
Betaseron
▲ Betimol Ophthalmic Solution (More than 5%)
Betoptic S Ophthalmic Suspension (Small number of patients)
Botox
Calcijex Injection
Cardura Tablets (Less than 0.5%)
Carteolol (Occasional)
Celexa (Infrequent)
Celontin Capsules
Cerebyx Injection (Infrequent)
Chibroxin Ophthalmic Solution
Ciloxan (Less than 1%)

Claritin-D 12 Hour (Less frequent)
Clomid Tablets (1.5%)
Copaxone (Infrequent)
▲ Cordarone Tablets (4% to 9%)
Cosopt Ophthalmic Solution (Less than 1%)
CytoGam Intravenous (Infrequent)
Depakote ER Tablets (Greater than 1%)
Effexor Tablets (Infrequent)
Effexor XR Capsules (Infrequent)
Ergamisol Tablets
Etrafon
Floxin (Less than 1%)
Gabitril Tablets (Infrequent)
Gamimune N (Infrequent)
Geodon Capsules (Infrequent)
Havrix Vaccine (Less than 1%)
Hectorol
Hivid Tablets (Less than 1%)
Imdur Tablets (Less than or equal to 5%)
Imitrex Injection (Infrequent)
Imitrex Tablets (Frequent)
Intron A for Injection (Less than 5%)
Iopidine 0.5% Ophthalmic Solution (Less than 3%)
Lacrisert Sterile Ophthalmic Insert
Lamictal (Infrequent)
Lodine (Less than 1%)
Lodine XL Extended-Release Tablets (Less than 1%)
▲ Lotemax Ophthalmic Suspension (5% to 15%)
Lumigan Ophthalmic Solution (1% to 3%)
Luvox Tablets (Infrequent)
Matulane Capsules
Maxalt (Rare)
Migranal Nasal Spray (Infrequent)
Neurontin (Infrequent)
Nilandron Tablets (2%)
Nipent for Injection (Less than 3%)
Nizoral Tablets (Less than 1%)
Norvir (Less than 2%)
Ocuflox Ophthalmic Solution
OptiPranolol (A small number of patients)
▲ Orthoclone OKT3 (10%)
▲ Pacerone Tablets (4% to 9%)
Paxil (Rare)
Permax Tablets (Infrequent)
Photofrin for Injection
Plaquenil Tablets (Fairly common)

Prevacid (Less than 1%)
Prevpac (Less than 1%)
Prinivil Tablets (0.3% to 1.0%)
Prinzide Tablets
ProSom Tablets (Infrequent)
Prozac (Infrequent)
Quinaglute Dura-Tabs Tablets
Quinidex Extentabs
Quixin Ophthalmic Solution (1% to 3%)
Requip Tablets (Infrequent)
Rescriptor Tablets (Less than 2%)
Rescula Ophthalmic Solution (1% to 5%)
Retrovir Capsules, Tablets & Syrup
Retrovir IV Infusion
▲ Rev-Eyes Eyedrops (10% to 40%)
Rilutek Tablets (Rare)
Risperdal (Rare)
Rocaltrol
Sandoglobulin I.V.
Sarafem Pulvules (Infrequent)
Serentil
Serophene Tablets
▲ Serostim for Injection (1% to 10%)
Serzone Tablets (Infrequent)
Sonata Capsules (Infrequent)
▲ Soriatane Capsules (1% to 10%)
Sterile FUDR (Remote possibility)
Tambocor Tablets (Less than 1%)
Topamax (Infrequent)
Travatan Ophthalmic Solution (1% to 4%)
Trilafon
Trileptal
Trovan (Less than 1%)
Trusopt Sterile Ophthalmic Solution (Approximately 1% to 5%)
Twinrix Vaccine (Less than 1%)
Vexol 1% Ophthalmic Suspension (Less than 1%)
Viagra Tablets (Less than 2%)
▲ Vitravene for Injection (5% to 20%)
Xalatan (1% to 4%)
Zaditor Ophthalmic Solution (Less than 5%)
Zaditor Ophthalmic Solution (Less than 5%)
Zestoretic Tablets
Zestril Tablets (0.3% to 1.0%)
Zoloft (Rare)
Zonegran Capsules (Rare)
Zosyn (1.0% or less)

Psychiatric disturbances

Accutane Capsules
Aldoclor Tablets
Aldomet Tablets
Aldoril Tablets
Aralen Tablets
Artane (Rare)
Arthrotec Tablets (Rare)
Chibroxin Ophthalmic Solution
Clinoril Tablets (Less than 1 in 100)
Cogentin
Cortone
Cosopt Ophthalmic Solution
Cuprimine Capsules
Decadron
Didronel Tablets
Famotidine Injection (Infrequent)
Florinef Acetate Tablets
Fortovase Capsules (Less than 2%)
▲ Gengraf Capsules (5.0%)
Hydrocortone
Indocin Capsules/Suspension/Suppositories (Less than 1%)
Infergen
Invirase Capsules (Less than 2%)
Lescol Capsules
Lescol XL Tablets
▲ Leukine (15%)
Mintezol
Nembutal (Less than 1%)
Neoral
Nizoral Tablets (Rare)
Noroxin Tablets
Pepcid (Infrequent)
Prednisone
Prilosec (Less than 1%)
Primaxin (Less than 0.2%)
Pulmicort Respules (Less than 1%)
Pulmicort Turbuhaler Powder (Rare)
Sandimmune
Solu-Medrol Sterile Powder
Thioridazine Hydrochloride Tablets (Extremely rare)
Timolol GFS
Timoptic (Less frequent)
Tonocard Tablets (Less than 1%)
Trecator-SC Tablets
Zarontin

Psychoses

Accutane Capsules
Adderall Tablets (Rare)
Adderall XR Capsules

Adipex-P
Aldoclor Tablets
Aldomet Tablets
Aldoril Tablets
Amphotec (1% to 5%)
Ancobon Capsules
Antabuse Tablets
Aralen Tablets (Rare)
Aredia for Injection (Up to 4%)
Avonex
Betaseron
Bextra Tablets (Rare)
Biaxin
Bicillin L-A
Bontril (Rare)
Buprenex Injectable (Less than 1%)
Calcijex Injection (Rare)
Cataflam Tablets (Rare)
Cedax Capsules
Cedax Oral Suspension
Celestone Soluspan
Celexa (Infrequent)
▲ CellCept (3% to 10%)
Celontin Capsules (Rare)
Cerebyx Injection (Infrequent)
Chibroxin Ophthalmic Solution
Clinoril Tablets (Less than 1 in 100)
Clomid Tablets
Cognex Capsules (Rare)
Cortone
Covera-HS Tablets (Less than 2%)
Dapsone Tablets USP
Decadron
Depacon Injection
Depakene
Depakote ER Tablets (Greater than 1%)
Depakote Sprinkle Capsules
Depakote Tablets
Desoxyn Tablets (Rare)
Dexedrine (Rare at recommended doses)
DextroStat Tablets (Rare)
Effexor Tablets (Rare)
Effexor XR Capsules (Infrequent)
Exelon (Infrequent)
Felbatol
Floxin
Fortovase Capsules (Less than 2%)
Gabitril Tablets (Infrequent)
Gastrocrom Oral Concentrate (Less common)
Hectorol
Hivid Tablets (Less than 1%)

Hydrocortone
Indocin Capsules/Suspension/Suppositories (Less than 1%)
Invirase Capsules (Less than 2%)
Ionamin Capsules (Rare)
Isoptin SR Tablets (1% or less)
Klonopin Tablets
Lamictal (Infrequent)
Lariam Tablets
Levbid
Levsin
Luvox Tablets (Infrequent to frequent)
Macrobid Capsules (Rare)
Macrodantin Capsules (Rare)
Mexitil Capsules (Less than 1% or about 2 in 1,000)
Mirapex Tablets (1% or more)
Nardil Tablets (Infrequent)
Neurontin (Infrequent)
Noroxin Tablets
Orthoclone OKT3
Paxil (Rare)
Pediapred Oral Solution
Pediazole Suspension
Permax Tablets (2.1%; frequent)
Plaquenil Tablets
Prednisone
Prelone Syrup
Prevpac
Procanbid Extended-Release Tablets (Occasional)
▲ Prograf (3% to 15%)
Prozac (Infrequent)
Pulmicort Respules (Less than 1%)
Pulmicort Turbuhaler Powder (Rare)
Quinaglute Dura-Tabs Tablets
Quinidex Extentabs
Rhinocort Nasal Inhaler (Rare)
Rifadin (Rare)
Rilutek Tablets (Rare)
Ritalin
Rocaltrol (Rare)
Roferon-A Injection
Rythmol Tablets (Less than 1%)
Sarafem Pulvules (Infrequent)
Serophene Tablets
Sinemet CR Tablets
Sinemet Tablets
Solu-Medrol Sterile Powder
Sustiva Capsules (Less than 2%)
Symmetrel (0.1% to 1%)
Tagamet
Tarka Tablets

Tasmar Tablets (Infrequent)
Tenoretic Tablets
Tenormin
Tequin (Less than 0.1%)
Thalomid Capsules
Tonocard Tablets (Less than 1%)
Topamax (Frequent)
Toradol
Trilafon
Valcyte Tablets (Less than 5%)
Valtrex Caplets
Verelan Capsules (1% or less)
Verelan PM Capsules (2% or less)
Voltaren (Rare)
Wellbutrin SR
Wellbutrin Tablets (Infrequent)
Zarontin
Zoloft
Zovirax Capsules, Tablets, & Suspension
Zovirax for Injection
Zyban

Psychoses, aggravation
Clozaril Tablets
Cortone
Decadron
Etrafon
Hydrocortone
Norpramin Tablets
Pediapred Oral Solution
Prednisone
Prelone Syrup
Serentil
Seroquel Tablets (Infrequent)
Solu-Medrol Sterile Powder
Surmontil Capsules
Thioridazine Hydrochloride Tablets
Vivactil Tablets

Psychoses, toxic
Astramorph/PF Injection
Chibroxin Ophthalmic Solution
Cipro
Cipro I.V. (1% or less)
Concerta
Duramorph Injection
Floxin
Focalin Tablets (Rare)
Infumorph
Levaquin
Metadate
Methylin
Rifamate Capsules (Uncommon)
Rifater Tablets (Uncommon)

Ritalin

Psychosis, activation
Carbatrol Capsules
Compazine
Stelazine
Tegretol
Wellbutrin SR
Zyban

Psychosis, paranoid
Zarontin (Rare)

Psychotic symptoms, paradoxical exacerbation
Haldol
Haldol Decanoate
Navane (Infrequent)
Thiothixene Capsules

Rage
Librium Capsules
Valium Tablets
Xanax Tablets (Rare)

Schizophrenia, precipitation
Nardil Tablets (Less frequent)
Zyprexa

Sedation
Aldoclor Tablets
Aldomet Tablets
Aldoril Tablets
Amerge Tablets (Rare)
Ancobon Capsules
Ativan Injection
▲ Ativan Tablets (15.9%)
▲ Benadryl Parenteral (Among most frequent)
▲ Buprenex Injectable (Most frequent)
▲ Catapres Tablets (About 10 in 100 patients)
Catapres-TTS (3 of 101 patients)
▲ Clorpres Tablets (About 10%)
▲ Clozaril Tablets (More than (5% to 39%)
▲ Combipres Tablets (About 10%)
Corgard Tablets (6 of 1000 patients)
Corzide (6 of 1000 patients)
▲ Darvocet-N (Among most frequent)
▲ Darvon Compound-65 Pulvules (Among most frequent)
▲ Darvon Pulvules (Among most frequent)
▲ Darvon-N Tablets (Among most frequent)
▲ Demerol (Among most frequent)

▲ Demser Capsules (Almost all patients)
Depacon Injection
Depakene
Depakote ER Tablets
Depakote Tablets
Dilaudid Injection
Dilaudid Oral Liquid
Dilaudid Powder
Dilaudid Rectal Suppositories
Dilaudid Tablets
Dilaudid Tablets - 8 mg
▲ Dilaudid-HP (Among most frequent)
▲ Dolophine Tablets (Among most
    frequent)
Duraclon Injection
Etrafon (Less frequent)
Halcion Tablets
Hycodan
Hycomine Compound Tablets
Hycotuss Expectorant Syrup
Imitrex Injection (2.7%)
Imitrex Nasal Spray (Infrequent)
Imitrex Tablets
Kadian Capsules (Less than 3%)
▲ Lortab (Among most frequent)
▲ Maxidone Tablets (Among most
    frequent)
▲ Mepergan Injection (Among most
    frequent)
Motofen Tablets
▲ MS Contin Tablets (Among most
    frequent)
▲ MSIR (Among most frequent)
Nadolol Tablets (6 of 1000 patients)
Navane
▲ Norco (Among most frequent)
▲ Nubain Injection (36%)
▲ Oramorph SR Tablets (Among most
    frequent)
▲ Orap Tablets (14 of 20 patients)
▲ OxyFast Oral Concentrate Solution
    (Among most frequent)
▲ OxyIR Capsules (Among most
    frequent)
▲ Percocet Tablets (Among most
    frequent)
▲ Percodan Tablets (Among most
    frequent)
▲ Percolone Tablets (Among most
    frequent)
Periactin Tablets (No incidence data in
    labeling)
Phenergan Suppositories
Phenergan Syrup
Phenergan VC Syrup

Phenergan VC with Codeine Syrup
Phenergan with Codeine Syrup
Phenergan with Dextromethorphan
    Syrup
▲ Phrenilin (Among most frequent)
Roferon-A Injection (Infrequent)
▲ Roxanol (Among most frequent)
▲ Roxanol 100 (Among most frequent)
▲ Roxanol-T (Among most frequent)
▲ Roxicodone Intensol (Among most
    frequent)
▲ Roxicodone Oral Solution (Among
    most frequent)
▲ Ryna-12 S Suspension (Among most
    common)
▲ Rynatan Pediatric Suspension (Among
    most common)
▲ Rynatan Tablets (Among most com-
    mon)
▲ Rynatuss (Among most common)
▲ Sedapap Tablets (Among the most
    frequent)
▲ Semprex-D Capsules (6% more
    common than with placebo)
Soma Compound w/Codeine
Talacen Caplets
Talwin Nx Tablets
▲ Tenex Tablets (5% to 39%)
Tessalon Capsules
Thiothixene Capsules
▲ Tussi-12
Tussionex
▲ Tylenol with Codeine (Among most
    frequent)
▲ Tylox Capsules (Among most
    frequent)
Valcyte Tablets
Versed Injection (1.6%)
Versed Syrup (Less than 1%)
▲ Vicodin (Among most frequent)
Vicodin Tuss Expectorant
▲ Wellbutrin Tablets (19.8%)
Xanax Tablets
▲ Zanaflex Tablets (48%)
▲ Zofran Injection (8%)
▲ Zofran Tablets & Oral Solution (20%)
▲ Zydone Tablets (Among most
    frequent)

Sensorium, clouded
Betapace AF Tablets (Rare)
Betapace Tablets (Rare)
Blocadren Tablets
Corgard Tablets
Corzide
Cosopt Ophthalmic Solution

Inderal
Inderide
Mexitil Capsules (1.9% to 2.6%)
Nadolol Tablets
Normodyne Tablets
Sectral Capsules
Tenoretic Tablets
Tenormin
Timolide Tablets
Timolol GFS
Timoptic
Toprol-XL Tablets
Xanax Tablets
Zebeta Tablets
Ziac Tablets

Sensory deficit, persistent
Duranest Injections
Nesacaine

Sensory disturbances
Foscavir Injection (Between 1% and 5%)
▲ Leukine (6%)
▲ Paraplatin for Injection (4% to 6%)
Paxil
▲ Prograf (Approximately 55%)
▲ Proleukin for Injection (10%)
▲ Wellbutrin Tablets (4.0%)
Xanax Tablets

Serotonin syndrome
Celexa (At least 3 patients)
Effexor Tablets
Effexor XR Capsules
Imitrex Injection
Imitrex Tablets
Luvox Tablets
Meridia Capsules
Paxil
Prozac
Zoloft

Sexual activity, decrease
▲ Catapres Tablets (About 3 in 100 patients)
Catapres-TTS (0.5% or less)
Clorpres Tablets (About 3%)
Combipres Tablets (About 3%)
▲ Duraclon Injection (3%)
Risperdal (Frequent)

Sexual dysfunction
Aceon Tablets (0.3% to 1.4%)
Avalide Tablets
Avapro Tablets (Less than 1%)

Betapace Tablets (Less than 1% to 2%)
Cardizem
Cardura Tablets (2%)
Catapres-TTS (2 of 101 patients)
Celexa
Copaxone (Infrequent)
Duranest Injections
Effexor Tablets (2%)
Effexor XR Capsules
Eldepryl Capsules
Eskalith
Evoxac Capsules (Less than 1%)
Geodon Capsules (Infrequent)
Hivid Tablets (Less than 1%)
Lithobid Slow-Release Tablets
Luvox Tablets
Maxzide
Monopril HCT (Less than 2%)
Monopril Tablets (Less than 1.0% to 1.0%)
Nardil Tablets (Common)
Naropin Injection
Nesacaine
Neurontin (Infrequent)
Norvasc Tablets (Less than 1% to 2%)
▲ Paxil (3.7% to 10.0%)
Polocaine
Polocaine-MPF
Procardia Capsules (2% or less)
Prozac
Risperdal (Frequent)
Roferon-A Injection (Infrequent)
Sarafem Pulvules
Sensorcaine Injection
Sensorcaine with Epinephrine Injection
Tiazac Capsules (Less than 2%)
Viracept
Wellbutrin Tablets (Frequent)
Xanax Tablets (7.4%)
Xylocaine Injection
Xylocaine with Epinephrine Injection
Ziac Tablets
▲ Zoladex (21%)
▲ Zoladex 3-month (One of the two most common)
Zoloft (Frequent)

Sleep disturbances
Aceon Tablets (2.5%)
Adalat CC Tablets (Rare)
Advair Diskus (1% to 3%)
Allegra-D (Less than 1%)
Ambien Tablets (Infrequent)

Amerge Tablets (Infrequent)
Anzemet (Infrequently)
Arava Tablets (1% to 3%)
Astelin Nasal Spray (Infrequent)
Ativan Tablets (Less frequent)
Avalide Tablets
Avapro Tablets (Less than 1%)
▲ Avonex (19%)
▲ Betapace Tablets (1% to 8%)
Celexa (At least 2%)
▲ Clozaril Tablets (4%)
▲ Combivir Tablets (11%)
Copaxone (At least 2%)
Cordarone Tablets (1% to 3%)
Coreg Tablets (0.1% to 1%)
Corgard Tablets
Corzide
Cozaar Tablets (Less than 1%)
▲ Crinone 4% Gel (18%)
▲ Crinone 8% Gel (18%)
Crixivan Capsules (Less than 2%)
Depakote ER Tablets (Greater than 1%)
Effexor Tablets (Infrequent)
Eldepryl Capsules
▲ Epivir (11%)
Flovent Diskus (1% to 3%)
Floxin (1% to 3%)
Fludara for Injection (1% to 3%)
Halcion Tablets
▲ Hectorol (3.3%)
HibTITER
Hyzaar
Imitrex Injection (Rare)
Imitrex Nasal Spray (Infrequent)
Imitrex Tablets (Rare to infrequent)
Klonopin Tablets (Infrequent)
Lamictal (1.4%)
Levaquin (0.1%)
Lithium
Lupron Depot 7.5 mg (Less than 5%)
Lupron Depot—3 Month 11.25 mg (Less than 5%)
▲ Lupron Depot—3 Month 22.5 mg (8.5%)
Lupron Depot—4 Month 30 mg (Less than 5%)
▲ Lupron Injection (5% or more)
Luvox Tablets (Infrequent)
▲ Mexitil Capsules (7.1% to 7.5%)
Mirapex Tablets (1%)
Monopril HCT
Monopril Tablets (0.2% to 1.0%)
Nadolol Tablets
Nardil Tablets (Common)

Nexium (Less than 1%)
Noroxin Tablets (Less frequent)
Numorphan
Pacerone Tablets (1% to 3%)
Prevacid (Less than 1%)
▲ Prevnar for Injection (18.1% to 33.3%)
Prevpac (Less than 1%)
Procardia Capsules (2% or less)
ProSom Tablets (Infrequent)
Protonix (Less than 1%)
Provigil Tablets (At least 1%)
Prozac (Frequent)
▲ Quinidex Extentabs (3%)
Recombivax HB (Less than 1%)
Rescriptor Tablets
Risperdal (Frequent)
▲ Roferon-A Injection (5% to 11%)
Sarafem Pulvules (Frequent)
Serevent Diskus (1% to 3%)
Sinemet CR Tablets
Sonata Capsules (Rare)
▲ Tasmar Tablets (24% to 25%)
Tonocard Tablets (Less than 1%)
Tricor Tablets (Less than 1%)
▲ Trizivir Tablets (7% to 11%)
Ultram Tablets (1% to 5%)
Univasc Tablets (Less than 1%)
Valium Tablets
Varivax (Greater than or equal to 1%)
Verelan Capsules (1.4%)
Versed Injection (Less than 1%)
Viracept
Visudyne for Injection (1% to 10%)
▲ Wellbutrin Tablets (4.0%)
Xanax Tablets (Rare)
▲ Xenical Capsules (3.9%)
Zarontin
Ziac Tablets
▲ Ziagen (7%)
Zyrtec (Less than 2%)
Zyrtec-D (Less than 2%)

Sleep talking
Sonata Capsules (Rare)

Sleep walking
Ambien Tablets (Rare)
Halcion Tablets
Neurontin
Requip Tablets (Infrequent)
Sonata Capsules (Rare)
Zoloft (Rare)

Sleep-inducing effects
Advair Diskus (1% to 3%)

Sleeping, excessive

Luvox Tablets (Infrequent)
Maxalt (Rare)
Nardil Tablets (Common)
Prinivil Tablets (0.3% to 1.0%)
Prinzide Tablets
Zestoretic Tablets
Zestril Tablets (0.3% to 1.0%)

Sluggishness

Phrenilin (Infrequent)
Sedapap Tablets (Infrequent)

Sociopathy

DextroStat Tablets
Neurontin (Rare)
Paxil (Rare)
Prozac (Rare)
Sarafem Pulvules (Rare)
Zyprexa (Infrequent)

Speech difficulties

Clozaril Tablets (Less than 1%)
▲ Demser Capsules (10%)
Marinol Capsules (Less than 1%)
Mexitil Capsules (2.6%)
Nubain Injection (1% or less)
Stadol NS Nasal Spray (Less than 1%)
Zyprexa (2%)

Speech disturbances

Accuretic Tablets
Actiq (Less than 1%)
Ambien Tablets (Infrequent)
Amphotec (1% to 5%)
▲ Avonex (3%)
▲ Betaseron (3%)
Brevibloc Injection (Less than 1%)
Carbatrol Capsules
Cerebyx Injection (Frequent)
Copaxone (2%)
Dantrium Capsules (Less frequent)
Depakote ER Tablets (1% to 5%)
Depakote Tablets (1% to 5%)
Duragesic Transdermal System (1% or greater)
Effexor Tablets (Infrequent)
Effexor XR Capsules (Infrequent)
Eldepryl Capsules
Ergamisol Tablets
Estrace
Evoxac Capsules (Less than 1%)
Fortovase Capsules (Less than 2%)
▲ Gabitril Tablets (4%)
Hivid Tablets (Less than 1%)
Imitrex Injection

Intron A for Injection (Less than 5%)
Invirase Capsules (Less than 2%)
Lamictal (2.5%)
Levaquin (Less than 0.3%)
Levbid
Levlen
Levlite
Levsin
Meridia Capsules
Migranal Nasal Spray (Rare)
Mirapex Tablets (1% or more)
Modicon
NuLev
▲ Orap Tablets (2 of 20 patients)
Ortho Tri-Cyclen
Ortho-Cyclen
Ortho-Est Tablets
Ortho-Novum
OxyContin Tablets (Less than 1%)
Permax Tablets (1.1%)
Prevacid (Less than 1%)
Prevpac
▲ Proleukin for Injection (7%)
Prometrium Capsules (Less than 5%)
Protonix
Romazicon Injection (Less than 1%)
Rythmol Tablets (Less than 1%)
Salagen Tablets (Less than 1%)
Tambocor Tablets (Less than 1%)
Tasmar Tablets (Frequent)
Tegretol
Tonocard Tablets (Less than 1%)
▲ Topamax (13.8% to 16.8%)
Trileptal (1% to 3%)
Tri-Levlen
Trovan (Less than 1%)
Ultram Tablets (Infrequent)
▲ Vesanoid Capsules (3%)
Vistide Injection
▲ Zanaflex Tablets (3%)
▲ Zonegran Capsules (5%)
Zyprexa (2%)

Speech, incoherent

Clozaril Tablets (Less than 1%)
Sensorcaine Injection
Sensorcaine with Epinephrine Injection
Sensorcaine-MPF Injection
Sensorcaine-MPF with Epinephrine Injection

Speech, slurring

Clozaril Tablets (1%)
Coly-Mycin M

Corgard Tablets (1 to 5 per 1000 patients)
Corzide (1 to 5 of 1000 patients)
▲ Dilantin (Among most common)
Eskalith
Etrafon
Halcion Tablets
Kadian Capsules (Less than 3%)
Klonopin Tablets
Lithium
Lithobid Slow-Release Tablets
Loxitane Capsules
Luvox Tablets (Rare)
Matulane Capsules
Miltown Tablets
Nadolol Tablets (1 to 5 of 1000 patients)
Serentil
Sonata Capsules (Rare)
Symmetrel (0.1% to 1%)
Tonocard Tablets (Less than 1%)
Tranxene
Trilafon
Valium Injectable
Valium Tablets (Infrequent)
Versed Injection (Less than 1%)
Vicoprofen Tablets (Less than 1%)
Xanax Tablets

Stimulation
Sinemet CR Tablets
Sinemet Tablets
Sonata Capsules (Rare)
Valium Injectable
Valium Tablets
Xanax Tablets (Rare)

Stupor
Ambien Tablets (Infrequent)
Amphotec (1% to 5%)
Ativan Injection (1.2%)
Betaseron
Celexa (Rare)
▲ Cerebyx Injection (7.7%)
Copaxone (Frequent)
Duragesic Transdermal System (Less than 1%)
Effexor Tablets (Infrequent)
Effexor XR Capsules (Infrequent)
Eskalith
Felbatol (2.6%)
Foscavir Injection (Between 1% and 5%)
Gabitril Tablets (Frequent)
▲ Gliadel Wafer (6%)

Hivid Tablets (Less than 1%)
Lamictal (Infrequent)
Levaquin (Less than 0.3%)
Lithium
Lithobid Slow-Release Tablets
Luvox Tablets (Infrequent)
Migranal Nasal Spray (Rare)
Moduretic Tablets (Less than or equal to 1%)
Naropin Injection (Less than 1%)
Neurontin (Infrequent)
Orthoclone OKT3
OxyContin Tablets (Less than 1%)
Paxil (Rare)
Permax Tablets (Rare)
PhosLo
ProSom Tablets (Infrequent)
Prozac (Rare)
Remeron (Rare)
Requip Tablets (Infrequent)
Rilutek Tablets (Infrequent)
Risperdal (Infrequent)
Romazicon Injection (Less than 1%)
Sarafem Pulvules (Rare)
Seroquel Tablets (Infrequent)
Sonata Capsules (Rare)
Streptomycin Sulfate Injection
Symmetrel
Tambocor Tablets (Less than 1%)
Topamax (Frequent)
Toradol (1% or less)
Trileptal
Ultracet Tablets (Less than 1%)
Zanaflex Tablets (Infrequent)
Zyprexa (Infrequent)

Stuttering
Seroquel Tablets (Rare)
Zyprexa (Infrequent)

Suicidal ideation
Accutane Capsules
Ambien Tablets
Avelox Tablets
▲ Avonex (4%)
Betaseron
Celontin Capsules (Rare)
Cognex Capsules (Rare)
Depakote Tablets
Effexor Tablets (Rare)
Effexor XR Capsules (Rare)
Exelon (Infrequent)
Floxin (Rare)
Halcion Tablets
Infergen

Intron A for Injection (Rare)
Klonopin Tablets (Infrequent)
Lamictal (Rare)
Levaquin (Rare)
Lodosyn Tablets
Lupron Depot 3.75 mg (Very rare)
Lupron Depot—3 Month 11.25 mg
(Very rare)
Miltown Tablets
Neurontin (Infrequent)
Nizoral Tablets (Rare)
PEG-Intron Powder for Injection
(Less than or equal to 1%)
Prozac (Less than 1%)
Rebetron Combination Therapy (Less
than 1%)
Reglan (Less frequent)
Remeron
Roferon-A Injection
Sarafem Pulvules
Serzone Tablets (Infrequent)
Sinemet CR Tablets
Sinemet Tablets
Symmetrel (Less than 0.1%)
Trilafon
Ultram Tablets (Infrequent)
Viracept
Wellbutrin SR (Infrequent)
Wellbutrin Tablets (Rare)
Xanax Tablets
Zarontin (Rare)
Zoloft (Rare)
Zyban (Infrequent)

Suicide, attempt of
Accutane Capsules
Ambien Tablets (Rare)
Avonex (One patient)
Betaseron
Celebrex Capsules
Celexa (Frequent)
Copaxone (Infrequent)
D.H.E. 45 Injection
Effexor Tablets (Infrequent)
Effexor XR Capsules (Infrequent)
Exelon (Infrequent)
Felbatol (Infrequent)
Floxin (Rare)
Fortovase Capsules (Rare)
Gabitril Tablets (Infrequent)
Hivid Tablets (Less than 1%)
Imitrex Tablets (Rare)
Infergen
Intron A for Injection

(Rare; less than 5%)
Invirase Capsules (Rare)
Klonopin Tablets (Infrequent)
Lamictal (Rare)
Levaquin (Rare)
Levo-Dromoran
Lupron Depot 3.75 mg (Very rare)
Lupron Depot—3 Month 11.25 mg
(Very rare)
Luvox Tablets (Infrequent)
Mirapex Tablets (Less than 1%)
Neurontin (Rare)
Paxil
PEG-Intron Powder for Injection
(Less than or equal to 1%)
Proleukin for Injection
Prozac (Frequent)
Rebetron Combination Therapy (Less
than 1%)
Remicade for IV Injection (Less than
2%)
Requip Tablets (Rare)
Rilutek Tablets (Infrequent)
Risperdal (1.2%)
Roferon-A Injection
Sandostatin LAR Depot (Rare)
Sarafem Pulvules (Infrequent)
Seroquel Tablets (Infrequent)
Serzone Tablets (Infrequent)
Sustiva Capsules
Symmetrel (Less than 0.1%)
Thalomid Capsules
Topamax (Frequent)
Vivactil Tablets
Xanax Tablets
Zanaflex Tablets (Rare)
Zoloft
Zyprexa (Frequent)

Talkativeness
Carbatrol Capsules
Tegretol
Xanax Tablets (2.2%)

Tenseness
Allegra-D
Claritin-D 12 Hour
Claritin-D 24 Hour
Clomid Tablets (Fewer than 1%)
▲ Indapamide Tablets (Greater than or
equal to 5%)
Loxitane Capsules
Prostin E2 Suppositories
Zyrtec-D

Thinking abnormality

Actiq (1% to 2%)
Ambien Tablets (Rare)
AmBisome for Injection (Less common)
▲ Amphotec (5% or more)
Androderm (Less than 1%)
Astelin Nasal Spray (Infrequent)
Ativan Injection (Less than 1%)
Brevibloc Injection (Less than 1%)
Campath Ampules
Cardura Tablets (Less than 0.5%)
▲ CellCept (3% to 10%)
Cerebyx Injection (Frequent)
▲ Cognex Capsules (3%)
Coreg Tablets (0.1% to 1%)
Cytovene (At least 3 subjects)
DaunoXome Injection (Less than or equal to 5%)
DDAVP Tablets
▲ Depacon Injection (6%)
▲ Depakene (6%)
Depakote ER Tablets (1% to 5%)
▲ Depakote Sprinkle Capsules (6%)
▲ Depakote Tablets (1% to 6%)
Diprivan (Less than 1%)
Doxil Injection (Less than 1%)
Duragesic Transdermal System (1% or greater)
Effexor Tablets (2%)
Effexor XR Capsules
Evoxac Capsules (Less than 1%)
▲ Felbatol (6.5%)
Flexeril Tablets (Less than 1%)
▲ Gabitril Tablets (6%)
Gliadel Wafer (2%)
Halcion Tablets
Hivid Tablets (Less than 1%)
▲ Infergen (8% to 10%)
Intron A for Injection (Less than 5%)
Kadian Capsules (Less than 3%)
Kaletra (Less than 2%)
Keppra Tablets (1% or more)
Lamictal (Frequent)
Levo-Dromoran
Levorphanol Tartrate Tablets (1% to 3%)
Lithobid Slow-Release Tablets
Lupron Depot—4 Month 30 mg (Less than 5%)
Luvox Tablets

▲ Marinol Capsules (3% to 10%)
Megace Oral Suspension (1% to 3%)
Meridia Capsules (Greater than or equal to 1%)
Mirapex Tablets (2% to 3%)
Nembutal (Less than 1%)
Neurontin (1.7%)
Nipent for Injection (Less than 3%)
Norvir (Up to 0.7%)
OxyContin Tablets (Between 1% and 5%)
Paxil (Infrequent)
Permax Tablets (Frequent)
Prevacid (Less than 1%)
Prevpac (Less than 1%)
ProAmatine Tablets (Less frequent)
▲ Prograf (3% to 15%)
ProSom Tablets (2%)
Protonix (Less than 1%)
Provigil Tablets (At least 1%)
Prozac (Less than 1%)
▲ Remeron (3%)
ReoPro Vials (2.1%)
Rilutek Tablets (Infrequent)
Salagen Tablets (Less than 1%)
▲ Sarafem Pulvules (3% to 6%)
Seroquel Tablets (Infrequent)
▲ Serostim for Injection (1% to 10%)
Serzone Tablets (Infrequent)
Sonata Capsules (Frequent)
Sular Tablets (Less than or equal to 1%)
Symmetrel (0.1% to 1%)
Tasmar Tablets (Infrequent)
Tequin (Less than 0.1%)
Thalomid Capsules
Toradol (1% or less)
Trileptal (2%)
Trovan (Less than 1%)
Ultracet Tablets (Less than 1%)
Vicoprofen Tablets (Less than 3%)
Wellbutrin SR
Wellbutrin Tablets (Infrequent)
Zanaflex Tablets (Infrequent)
Zoladex (1% or greater)
Zoladex 3-month
Zoloft (2%)
Zyban (1%)
Zyprexa
Zyrtec (Less than 2%)
Zyrtec-D (Less than 2%)

Part 2.
Side Effects by Brand

8-MOP Capsules
Depression
Depression, psychotic
Insomnia
Nervousness

Abelcet Injection
Double vision

Accupril Tablets
Depression (0.5% to 1.0%)
Insomnia (0.5% to 1.0%)
Nervousness (0.5% to 1.0%)

Accuretic Tablets
Depression (Greater than 0.5%)
Insomnia (1.2%)
Nervousness (0.5% to 1%)
Speech disturbances

Accutane Capsules
Depression
Emotional disturbances
Emotional lability
Insomnia
Nervousness
Photophobia
Psychiatric disturbances
Psychoses
Suicidal ideation
Suicide, attempt of

Acel-Imune
▲ Anxiety (9% to 18%)
▲ Irritability (25%)

Aceon Tablets
Anxiety (0.3% to 1%)
Depression (2.0%)
Nervousness (1.1%)
Sexual dysfunction (0.3% to 1.4%)
Sleep disturbances (2.5%)

AcipHex Tablets
Agitation (Rare)
Anxiety
Coma
Confusion (Rare)
Delirium
Depression
Disorientation
Double vision

Dreaming abnormalities
Hangover (Rare)
Insomnia
Libido decreased
Nervousness

ActHIB Vaccine
▲ Irritability (10.1% to 77.9%)

Actifed Cold & Allergy
Excitability
Insomnia
Nervousness

Actifed Cold & Sinus
Excitability

Actimmune
Confusion (Rare)
▲ Depression (3%)
Disorientation (Rare)
Hallucinations (Rare)

Actiq
Agitation (Less than 1%)
▲ Confusion (1% to 6%)
Dreaming abnormalities
 (Less than 1%)
Emotional lability (Less than 1%)
Euphoria (Less than 1%)
Hallucinations (1% to 2%)
Insomnia (1% to 2%)
Libido decreased (Less than 1%)
Nervousness (1% to 2%)
Speech disturbances (Less than 1%)
Thinking abnormality (1% to 2%)

Activella Tablets
Depression
Emotional lability (0% to 6%)
Insomnia (0% to 6%)
Libido, changes
Nervousness

Actonel Tablets
▲ Anxiety (4.3%)
▲ Depression (6.8%)
▲ Insomnia (4.7%)

Adalat CC Tablets
Anxiety (Less than 1.0%)
Confusion (Less than 1.0%)
Depression (Less than 1.0%)

Double vision (Less than 1.0%)
Insomnia (Less than 1.0%)
Libido decreased (Less than 1.0%)
Mood changes (Rare)
Nervousness (Rare)
Paranoia (Rare)
Sleep disturbances (Rare)

Adderall Tablets
Euphoria
Insomnia
Libido, changes
Overstimulation
Psychoses (Rare)

Adderall XR Capsules
Depression (0.7%)
▲ Emotional lability (1% to 9%)
Euphoria
▲ Insomnia (1.5% to 17%)
Libido, changes
▲ Nervousness (6%)
Overstimulation
Psychoses

Adenoscan
Emotional lability (Less than 1%)
Nervousness (2%)

Adipex-P
Central nervous system stimulation
Euphoria
Insomnia
Libido, changes
Overstimulation
Psychoses

Advair Diskus
Aggression
Agitation
Depression
Sleep disturbances (1% to 3%)
Sleep-inducing effects (1% to 3%)

Advil Cold and Sinus
Insomnia
Nervousness

Aerobid
Anxiety (1% to 3%)
Depression (1% to 3%)
Hyperactivity (1% to 3%)
Hypoactivity (1% to 3%)
Insomnia (1% to 3%)
▲ Irritability (3% to 9%)
Mood changes (1% to 3%)
▲ Nervousness (3% to 9%)

Agenerase
▲ Depression (9% to 16%)

Aggrenox Capsules
Agitation (Less than 1%)
Coma (Less than 1%)
Confusion (1.1%)

Agrylin Capsules
Confusion (1% to 5%)
Depression (1% to 5%)
Double vision (1% to 5%)
Insomnia (1% to 5%)
Nervousness (1% to 5%)

Akineton
Agitation
Behavioral changes
Disorientation
Euphoria

Albalon Ophthalmic Solution
Nervousness

Aldoclor Tablets
Confusion
Depression
Libido decreased
Mental performance, impairment
Nightmares
Psychiatric disturbances
Psychoses
Sedation

Aldomet Tablets
Confusion
Depression
Libido decreased
Mental performance, impairment
Nightmares
Psychiatric disturbances
Psychoses
Sedation

Aldoril Tablets
Confusion
Depression
Libido decreased
Mental performance, impairment
Nightmares
Psychiatric disturbances
Psychoses
Sedation

Alesse-21 Tablets
Depression
Libido, changes

Mood changes
Nervousness

Alesse-28 Tablets
Depression
Libido, changes
Nervousness

Alferon N Injection
Confusion (One patient to 3%)
Depression (One patient to 3%)
Disorientation (1%)
Insomnia (2%)
Mental performance, impairment (1%)
Nervousness (1%)

Alka-Seltzer Plus Cold & Cough Medicine Liqui-Gels
Excitability

Alka-Seltzer Plus Cold Medicine Liqui-Gels
Excitability

Alka-Seltzer Plus Night-Time Cold Medicine Liqui-Gels
Excitability

Allegra
Insomnia (Less than 1%)
Nervousness (Less than 1%)
Nightmares (Less than 1%)

Allegra-D
Agitation (1.9%)
Anxiety (1.4%)
Hallucinations
▲ Insomnia (12.6%)
Nervousness (1.4%)
Paranoia (Less than 1%)
Sleep disturbances (Less than 1%)
Tenseness

Alocril Ophthalmic Solution
▲ Photophobia (1% to 10%)

Aloprim for Injection
Agitation (Less than 1%)
Coma (Less than 1%)

Alora Transdermal System
Depression
Libido, changes

Alphagan Ophthalmic Solution
Anxiety (Less than 3%)
Depression (Less than 3%)
Insomnia (Less than 3%)

▲ Photophobia (Approximately 3% to 9%)

Alphagan P Ophthalmic Solution
Insomnia (Less than 1%)
Photophobia (1% to 4%)

Alrex Sterile Ophthalmic Suspension
▲ Photophobia (5% to 15%)

Altace Capsules
Anxiety (Less than 1%)
Depression (Less than 1%)
Insomnia (Less than 1%)
Nervousness (Less than 1%)

Alupent Inhalation Aerosol
▲ Nervousness (6.8%)

Alupent Inhalation Solution
▲ Nervousness (14.1%)

Ambien Tablets
Aggression (Rare)
Agitation (Infrequent)
Anxiety (1%)
Apathy (Rare)
Behavioral changes
Cognitive dysfunction (Infrequent)
Confusion (Frequent)
Delusions (Rare)
Dementia (Rare)
Depersonalization (Rare)
Depression (2%)
Disordered sense of smell (Rare)
Double vision (Frequent)
Dreaming abnormalities (1%)
Emotional lability (Infrequent)
Euphoria (Frequent)
▲ Feeling, drugged (3%)
Feeling, intoxicated (Rare)
Feeling, strange (Rare)
Hallucinations (Infrequent)
Hysteria (Rare)
Illusion, unspecified (Infrequent)
Insomnia (Frequent)
Libido decreased (Rare)
Manic behavior (Rare)
Mental performance, impairment (Infrequent)
Nervousness (1%)
Neurosis, unspecified (Rare)
Panic (Rare)
Personality changes (Rare)

Sleep disturbances (Infrequent)
Sleep walking (Rare)
Speech disturbances (Infrequent)
Stupor (Infrequent)
Suicidal ideation
Suicide, attempt of (Rare)
Thinking abnormality (Rare)

AmBisome for Injection
Agitation (Less common)
▲ Anxiety (7.4% to 13.7%)
Coma (Less common)
▲ Confusion (8.6% to 12.9%)
Depression (Less common)
Hallucinations (Less common)
Impairment of sensation (Less common)
Nervousness (Less common)
Thinking abnormality (Less common)

Amerge Tablets
Aggression (Rare)
Agitation (Rare)
Anxiety (Infrequent)
Cognitive dysfunction (Infrequent)
Confusion (Rare)
Consciousness, disorders of (Rare)
Depression (Infrequent)
Dreaming (Rare)
Feeling, strange (Infrequent)
Hallucinations (Rare)
Hostility (Rare)
Hyperactivity (Rare)
Libido decreased (Rare)
Mental performance, impairment (Infrequent)
Panic (Rare)
Photophobia (Frequent)
Sedation (Rare)
Sleep disturbances (Infrequent)

Amicar
Confusion
Delirium
Hallucinations

Amoxil
Agitation (Rare)
Anxiety (Rare)
Behavioral changes (Rare)
Confusion (Rare)
Hyperactivity (Rare)
Insomnia (Rare)

Amphotec
Agitation (1% to 5%)

▲ Confusion (5% or more)
Depression (1% to 5%)
Hallucinations (1% to 5%)
▲ Insomnia (5% or more)
Nervousness (1% to 5%)
Psychoses (1% to 5%)
Speech disturbances (1% to 5%)
Stupor (1% to 5%)
▲ Thinking abnormality (5% or more)

Anadrol-50 Tablets
Excitability
Insomnia
Libido decreased
Libido increased

Anaprox
Central nervous system depression (Less than 1%)
Cognitive dysfunction (Less than 1%)
Dreaming abnormalities (Less than 1%)
Insomnia (Less than 1%)
Mental performance, impairment (Less than 1%)

Ancobon Capsules
Confusion
Hallucinations
Psychoses
Sedation

Androderm
Anxiety (Less than 1%)
Confusion (Less than 1%)
▲ Depression (3%)
Libido decreased (Less than 1%)
Libido increased
Thinking abnormality (Less than 1%)

AndroGel
Anxiety (Fewer than 1%)
Depression (Up to 1%)
Emotional lability (Up to 3%)
Libido decreased (Up to 3%)
Libido increased (One patient)
Nervousness (Up to 3%)

Android Capsules
▲ Anxiety (Among most common)
▲ Depression (Among most common)
▲ Libido, changes (Among most common)

Angiomax for Injection
▲ Anxiety (6%)
Confusion (Rare)

▲ Insomnia (7%)
▲ Nervousness (5%)

Antabuse Tablets
Psychoses

Anzemet
Agitation (Infrequently)
Anxiety (Infrequently)
Confusion (Infrequently)
Depersonalization (Infrequently)
Dreaming abnormalities (Infrequently)
Sleep disturbances (Infrequently)

Apligraf
Confusion (1.8%)

Aquasol A Parenteral
Irritability

Aralen Tablets
Auditory disturbances
Psychiatric disturbances
Psychoses (Rare)

Arava Tablets
Anxiety (1% to 3%)
Depression (1% to 3%)
Insomnia (1% to 3%)
Sleep disturbances (1% to 3%)

Aredia for Injection
▲ Anxiety (14.3%)
▲ Insomnia (22.2%)
Psychoses (Up to 4%)

Aricept Tablets
Aggression (Frequent)
Agitation
Confusion
Delusions (Frequent)
▲ Depression (3%)
▲ Dreaming abnormalities (3%)
Emotional lability (Infrequent)
Hallucinations
Hostility (Infrequent)
▲ Insomnia (9%)
Irritability (Frequent)
Libido decreased (Infrequent)
Libido increased (Frequent)
Listlessness (Infrequent)
Nervousness (Frequent)
Paranoia (Infrequent)

Arimidex Tablets
▲ Anxiety (2% to 5%)
Confusion (2% to 5%)
▲ Depression (2.4% to 5.3%)

Insomnia (2% to 5.9%)
Nervousness (2% to 5%)

Arixtra Injection
▲ Confusion (3.1%)
▲ Insomnia (5%)

Aromasin Tablets
▲ Anxiety (10%)
▲ Confusion (2% to 5%)
▲ Depression (13%)
▲ Insomnia (11%)

Artane
Agitation
Behavior, inappropriate
Confusion
Delusions (Rare)
Euphoria
Hallucinations (Rare)
▲ Nervousness (30% to 50%)
Paranoia (One case)
Psychiatric disturbances (Rare)

Arthrotec Tablets
Anxiety (Rare)
Coma (Rare)
Confusion (Rare)
Depression (Rare)
Disorientation (Rare)
Double vision (Rare)
Dreaming abnormalities (Rare)
Hallucinations (Rare)
Insomnia (Rare)
Irritability (Rare)
Mental performance, impairment
  (Rare)
Nervousness (Rare)
Paranoia (Rare)
Psychiatric disturbances (Rare)

Asacol Tablets
Anxiety (2% or greater)
Confusion
Depression
Disorientation
Emotional lability
Insomnia (2%)
Libido decreased
Nervousness (2% or greater)

Astelin Nasal Spray
Anxiety (Infrequent)
Confusion
Depersonalization (Infrequent)
Depression (Infrequent)
Disordered sense of smell

▲ Impairment of sensation (7.9%)
Nervousness (Infrequent)
Sleep disturbances (Infrequent)
Thinking abnormality (Infrequent)

Astramorph/PF Injection
Anxiety
Excitability
Psychoses, toxic

Atacand HCT Tablets
Anxiety (0.5% or greater)
Depression (0.5% or greater)
Insomnia (0.5% or greater)

Atacand Tablets
Anxiety (0.5% or greater)
Depression (0.5% or greater)

Ativan Injection
Agitation (Infrequent)
Behavior, inappropriate (Occasional)
Central nervous system depression
Coma (Less than 1%)
Confusion (1.3%)
Delirium (1.3%)
Depression (1.3%)
Double vision (Occasional)
Hallucinations (1%)
Mental performance, impairment
Sedation
Stupor (1.2%)
Thinking abnormality (Less than 1%)
Agitation (Less frequent)
Depression (Less frequent)
Disorientation (Less frequent)
▲ Sedation (15.9%)
Sleep disturbances (Less frequent)

Atromid-S Capsules
Libido decreased

Atrovent Inhalation Aerosol
Insomnia (Less than 1%)
▲ Nervousness (3.1%)

Atrovent Inhalation Solution
Insomnia (0.9%)
Nervousness (0.5%)

Attenuvax
Central nervous system reactions
Irritability

Augmentin
Agitation (Rare)
Anxiety (Rare)
Behavioral changes (Rare)

Confusion (Rare)
Hyperactivity (Rare)
Insomnia (Rare)

Avalide Tablets
Anxiety (1% or greater)
Confusion
Depression
Emotional disturbances
Libido, changes
Nervousness (1% or greater)
Sexual dysfunction
Sleep disturbances

Avapro Tablets
Anxiety (Less than 1%)
Depression (Less than 1%)
Emotional disturbances
  (Less than 1%)
Libido, changes (Less than 1%)
Nervousness (1% or greater)
Sexual dysfunction (Less than 1%)
Sleep disturbances (Less than 1%)

Avelox Tablets
Anxiety (0.05% to 1%)
Central nervous system stimulation
Confusion (0.05% to 1%)
Depersonalization (0.05% to 1%)
Depression
Hallucinations (0.05% to 1%)
Insomnia (0.05% to 1%)
Nervousness (0.05% to 1%)
Suicidal ideation

Avonex
Anxiety
Confusion
Depersonalization
Depression
Emotional lability
Libido increased
Neurosis, unspecified
Psychoses
▲ Sleep disturbances (19%)
▲ Speech disturbances (3%)
▲ Suicidal ideation (4%)
Suicide, attempt of (One patient)

Axert Tablets
Anxiety (Infrequent)
Central nervous system stimulation
  (Infrequent)
Depression (Rare)
Disordered sense of smell (Rare)
Double vision (Rare)

Dreaming abnormalities (Rare)
Euphoria (Rare)
Insomnia (Infrequent)
Nervousness (Rare)
Nightmares (Rare)

Axid Pulvules

Anxiety (1.6%)
Confusion (Rare)
Dreaming abnormalities (1.9%)
Insomnia (2.7%)
Libido decreased
Nervousness (1.1%)

Aygestin Tablets

Depression
Insomnia
Mood changes

Azactam for Injection

Confusion (Less than 1%)
Double vision (Less than 1%)
Insomnia (Less than 1%)

Azmacort Inhalation Aerosol

Depression

Azopt Ophthalmic Suspension

Double vision (Less than 1%)

Azulfidine

Central nervous system reactions
Depression (Rare)
Hallucinations (Rare)
Insomnia (Rare)

Bactrim

Apathy
Depression
Hallucinations
Insomnia
Nervousness

Beconase AQ Nasal Spray

Depression

Beconase Inhalation Aerosol

Depression

Benadryl Allergy

Excitability

Benadryl Allergy & Sinus

Excitability
Insomnia
Nervousness

Benadryl Allergy & Sinus Headache

Insomnia
Nervousness

Benadryl Parenteral

Confusion
Double vision
Euphoria
Excitability
Insomnia
Irritability
Nervousness
▲ Sedation (Among most frequent)

Betagan

Confusion
Depression
Double vision

Betapace AF Tablets

Emotional lability (Rare)
Insomnia (2.6% to 4.1%)
Sensorium, clouded (Rare)

Betapace Tablets

▲ Anxiety (2% to 4%)
▲ Consciousness, disorders of (2% to 4%)
Depression (1% to 4%)
Emotional lability (Rare)
Mood changes (Less than 1% to 3%)
Sensorium, clouded (Rare)
Sexual dysfunction (Less than 1% to 2%)
▲ Sleep disturbances (1% to 8%)

Betaseron

Agitation
▲ Anxiety (15%)
Apathy
Coma
▲ Confusion (4%)
Delirium
Delusions
Dementia
Depersonalization
Depression
Disordered sense of smell
Double vision
Euphoria
Hallucinations
Libido decreased
Manic behavior
▲ Nervousness (8%)
Neurosis, unspecified
Paranoia
Photophobia

Psychoses
▲ Speech disturbances (3%)
Stupor
Suicidal ideation
Suicide, attempt of

Betaxon Ophthalmic Suspension

Anxiety (Less than 2%)

Betimol Ophthalmic Solution

Depression
Double vision
▲ Photophobia (More than 5%)

Betoptic S Ophthalmic Suspension

Depression (Rare)
Insomnia (Rare)
Photophobia (Small number of patients)

Bextra Tablets

Anxiety (0.1% to 1.9%)
Confusion (0.1% to 1.9%)
Depression (0.1% to 1.9%)
Depression, aggravation of (0.1% to 1.9%)
Insomnia (0.1% to 1.9%)
Manic behavior (Rare)
Nervousness (0.1% to 1.9%)
Psychoses (Rare)

Biaxin

Anxiety
Behavioral changes
Confusion
Depersonalization
Disorientation
Hallucinations
Insomnia
Nightmares
Psychoses

Bicillin C-R

Anxiety
Apathy
Coma
Confusion
Euphoria
Hallucinations, auditory
Hallucinations, visual
Nervousness

Bicillin L-A

Agitation
Anxiety
Coma

Confusion
Euphoria
Fear
Hallucinations, auditory
Hallucinations, visual
Nervousness
Psychoses

Blocadren Tablets

Catatonia
Depression
Disorientation, place
Disorientation, time
Double vision
Dreaming abnormalities (Less than 1%)
Emotional lability
Hallucinations (Less than 1%)
Insomnia (Less than 1%)
Libido decreased (0.6%)
Memory loss, short-term
Nervousness (Less than 1%)
Neuropsychometrics performance, decrease
Nightmares
Sensorium, clouded

Bontril

Agitation
Insomnia
Libido decreased
Libido increased
Overstimulation
Psychoses (Rare)

Botox

Disorientation
Double vision (Rare)
Photophobia

Brethine Ampuls

Anxiety (Less than 0.5%)
▲ Nervousness (16.9% to 38.0%)

Brethine Tablets

Anxiety (1%)
Hallucinations (Less than 1%)
Insomnia (1.5%)
▲ Nervousness (35%)

Brevibloc Injection

Agitation (About 2%)
Anxiety (Less than 1%)
Confusion (About 2%)
Depression (Less than 1%)
Speech disturbances (Less than 1%)

Thinking abnormality (Less than 1%)

Brevicon 28-Day Tablets
Depression
Double vision (Rare)
Libido, changes
Nervousness

Brevital
Anxiety
Delirium

Bromfed
Excitability
Insomnia
Irritability
Nervousness

Buprenex Injectable
Agitation (Rare)
Coma (Infrequent)
Depersonalization (Infrequent)
Double vision (Less than 1%)
Dreaming abnormalities
  (Less than 1%)
Hallucinations (Infrequent)
Psychoses (Less than 1%)
▲ Sedation (Most frequent)

Cafcit
Central nervous system stimulation
Irritability

Calcijex Injection
Libido decreased
Photophobia
Psychoses (Rare)

Campath Ampules
Apathy
Coma
Confusion
▲ Depression (1% to 7%)
Hallucinations
▲ Insomnia (10%)
Nervousness
Thinking abnormality

Captopril Tablets
Confusion
Depression
Insomnia (About 0.5 to 2%)
Nervousness

Carafate
Insomnia (Less than 0.5%)

Carbatrol Capsules
Agitation
Confusion
Depression
Double vision
Hallucinations, visual
Psychosis, activation
Speech disturbances
Talkativeness

Cardene I.V.
Confusion (Rare)

Cardizem
Depression
Dreaming abnormalities
Hallucinations
Insomnia
Nervousness
Personality changes
Sexual dysfunction

Cardura Tablets
Agitation (0.5% to 1%)
Anxiety (1.1%)
Confusion (Less than 0.5%)
Depersonalization (Less than 0.5%)
Depression (1%)
Disordered sense of smell (Less than
  0.5%)
Emotional lability (Less than 0.5%)
Insomnia (1% to 1.2%)
Libido decreased (0.8%)
Mental performance, impairment
  (Less than 0.5%)
Nervousness (2%)
Nightmares (Less than 0.5%)
Photophobia (Less than 0.5%)
Sexual dysfunction (2%)
Thinking abnormality (Less than
  0.5%)

Carnitor Injection
Anxiety (1% to 2%)
▲ Depression (5% to 6%)
Insomnia (1% to 3%)

Carteolol
Depression
Double vision
Insomnia (Occasional)
Photophobia (Occasional)

Casodex Tablets
▲ Anxiety (2% to 5%)
▲ Confusion (2% to 5%)
▲ Depression (4%)

▲ Insomnia (5%)
▲ Libido decreased (2% to 5%)
▲ Nervousness (2% to 5%)

Cataflam Tablets
Anxiety (Less than 1%)
Coma (Rare)
Depression (Less than 1%)
Disorientation (Rare)
Double vision (Less than 1%)
Insomnia (Less than 1%)
Irritability (Less than 1%)
Memory impairment (Less than 1%)
Nightmares (Less than 1%)
Psychoses (Rare)

Catapres Tablets
Agitation (About 3 in 100 patients)
Anxiety
Behavioral changes
Delirium
Depression (About 1 in 100 patients)
Dreaming abnormalities
Hallucinations
Hallucinations, auditory (Rare)
Hallucinations, visual (Rare)
Insomnia (About 5 in 1,000 patients)
Libido, loss (About 3 in 100 patients)
▲ Nervousness (About 3 in 100 patients)
Nightmares
▲ Sedation (About 10 in 100 patients)
▲ Sexual activity, decrease (About 3 in 100 patients)

Catapres-TTS
Agitation (0.5% or less)
Anxiety (0.5% or less)
Behavioral changes (0.5% or less)
Delirium (0.5% or less)
Depression (0.5% or less)
Dreaming abnormalities
    (0.5% or less)
Hallucinations, auditory (0.5% or less)
Hallucinations, visual (0.5% or less)
Insomnia (2 of 101 patients)
Irritability (0.5% or less)
Libido, loss (0.5% or less)
Nervousness (1 of 101 patients)
Nightmares (0.5% or less)
Sedation (3 of 101 patients)
Sexual activity, decrease (0.5% or less)
Sexual dysfunction (2 of 101 patients)

Ceclor
Confusion (Rare)

Hallucinations (Rare)
Hyperactivity (Rare)
Insomnia (Rare)
Nervousness (Rare)

Ceclor CD
Anxiety (0.1% to 1%)
Confusion
Hyperactivity
Insomnia (0.1% to 1%)
Nervousness (0.1% to 1%)

Cedax Capsules
Psychoses

Cedax Oral Suspension
Agitation (0.1% to 1%)
Insomnia (0.1% to 1%)
Irritability (0.1% to 1%)
Psychoses

Ceftin for Oral Suspension
Hyperactivity (0.1% to 1%)
Irritability (0.1% to 1%)

Cefzil
Confusion (Less than 1%)
Hyperactivity (Less than 1%)
Insomnia (Less than 1%)
Nervousness (Less than 1%)

Celebrex Capsules
Anxiety (0.1% to 1.9%)
Depression (0.1% to 1.9%)
Insomnia (2.3%)
Nervousness (0.1% to 1.9%)
Suicide, attempt of

Celestone Soluspan
Euphoria
Insomnia
Mood changes
Personality changes
Psychoses

Celestone Soluspan Injectable Suspension
Depression

Celexa
Aggression (Infrequent)
▲ Agitation (3%)
▲ Anxiety (4%)
Apathy (Infrequent)
Catatonia (Rare)
Confusion (Frequent)
Delusions (Rare)
Depersonalization (Infrequent)

Depression (Frequent)
Depression, aggravation of (Frequent)
Depression, psychotic (Infrequent)
Double vision (Rare)
Emotional lability (Infrequent)
Euphoria (Infrequent)
Hallucinations (Infrequent)
▲ Insomnia (15%)
Libido decreased (2%)
Libido increased (Infrequent)
Manic behavior
Manic behavior, mild
Melancholia (Rare)
Mental performance, impairment
  (Frequent)
Nightmares (Infrequent)
Panic (Infrequent)
Paranoia (Infrequent)
Photophobia (Infrequent)
Psychoses (Infrequent)
Serotonin syndrome (At least 3
  patients)
Sexual dysfunction
Sleep disturbances (At least 2%)
Stupor (Rare)
Suicide, attempt of (Frequent)

CellCept
▲ Agitation (3% to 10%)
▲ Anxiety (3% to 28.4%)
▲ Confusion (13.5%)
▲ Delirium (3% to 10%)
▲ Depression (3% to 15.6%)
▲ Emotional lability (3% to 10%)
▲ Hallucinations (3% to 10%)
▲ Insomnia (8.9% to 40.8%)
▲ Nervousness (11.4%)
▲ Psychoses (3% to 10%)
▲ Thinking abnormality (3% to 10%)

Celontin Capsules
Aggression
Behavior, hypochondriacal
Confusion
Depression
Hallucinations (Rare)
Insomnia
Irritability
Mental slowness
Nervousness
Photophobia
Psychoses (Rare)
Suicidal ideation (Rare)

Cenestin Tablets
▲ Depression (28%)

▲ Insomnia (42%)
Libido, changes
▲ Nervousness (28%)

Cerebyx Injection
▲ Agitation (3.3% to 9.5%)
Central nervous system depression
  (Infrequent)
Coma (Infrequent)
Confusion (Infrequent)
Delirium
Depersonalization (Infrequent)
Depression (Infrequent)
Disordered sense of smell (Infrequent)
▲ Double vision (3.3%)
Emotional lability (Infrequent)
Hostility (Infrequent)
Insomnia (Infrequent)
Nervousness (Frequent)
Neurosis, unspecified (Infrequent)
Personality changes (Infrequent)
Photophobia (Infrequent)
Psychoses (Infrequent)
Speech disturbances (Frequent)
▲ Stupor (7.7%)
Thinking abnormality (Frequent)

Chibroxin Ophthalmic Solution
Central nervous system reactions
Central nervous system stimulation
Confusion
Depression
Double vision
Hallucinations
Photophobia
Psychiatric disturbances
Psychoses
Psychoses, toxic

Children's Benadryl Allergy
Excitability

**Children's Benadryl Allergy &
Sinus**
Excitability
Insomnia
Nervousness

**Children's Sudafed Cold &
Cough**
Insomnia
Nervousness

Children's Tylenol Cold
Excitability

Insomnia
Nervousness

Children's Tylenol Cold Plus Cough
Excitability

Children's Vicks NyQuil Cold/Cough
Excitability
Insomnia
Nervousness

Chirocaine Injection
Anxiety (1%)
Confusion (Less than 1%)
Double vision (2.5%)

Chlor-Trimeton Allergy Tablets
Excitability

Ciloxan
Photophobia (Less than 1%)

Cipro
Agitation
Anxiety
Central nervous system stimulation
Confusion
Delirium
Depersonalization (Less than 1%)
Depression (Less than 1%)
Double vision (Less than 1%)
Hallucinations (Less than 1%)
Insomnia (Less than 1%)
Irritability (Less than 1%)
Manic behavior (Less than 1%)
Nervousness
Nightmares (Less than 1%)
Paranoia
Phobic disorder (Less than 1%)
Psychoses, toxic

Cipro I.V.
Agitation
Anxiety (1% or less)
Central nervous system stimulation
Confusion (1% or less)
Delirium
Depersonalization (1% or less)
Depression (1% or less)
Double vision (1% or less)
Hallucinations (1% or less)
Insomnia (1% or less)
Irritability (1% or less)
Manic behavior (1% or less)

Nervousness
Nightmares (1% or less)
Paranoia (1% or less)
Phobic disorder (1% or less)
Psychoses, toxic (1% or less)

Claritin
Agitation (At least one patient)
Anxiety (At least one patient)
Confusion (At least one patient)
Depression (At least one patient)
Insomnia (At least one patient)
Irritability (At least one patient)
Libido decreased
 (At least one patient)
Mental performance, impairment
 (At least one patient)
▲ Nervousness (4%)
Nightmares (At least one patient)

Claritin-D 12 Hour
Aggression (Less frequent)
Agitation (Less frequent)
Anxiety (Less frequent)
Apathy (Less frequent)
Central nervous system stimulation
Confusion (Less frequent)
Depression (Less frequent)
Emotional lability (Less frequent)
Euphoria (Less frequent)
Excitability
Fear
Hallucinations
▲ Insomnia (16%)
Irritability (Less frequent)
Libido decreased (Less frequent)
Mental performance, impairment
 (Less frequent)
▲ Nervousness (5%)
Nightmares (Less frequent)
Photophobia (Less frequent)
Tenseness

Claritin-D 24 Hour
Aggression (Fewer than 2%)
Agitation (Fewer than 2%)
Anxiety (Fewer than 2%)
Apathy (Fewer than 2%)
Central nervous system stimulation
Confusion (Fewer than 2%)
Depression (Fewer than 2%)
Emotional lability (Fewer than 2%)
Euphoria (Fewer than 2%)
Excitability
Fear

Hallucinations
▲ Insomnia (5%)
Irritability (Fewer than 2%)
Libido decreased
Mental performance, impairment
▲ Nervousness (3%)
Nightmares (Fewer than 2%)
Tenseness

Climara Transdermal System
Depression
Libido, changes

Clinoril Tablets
Depression (Less than 1%)
Insomnia (Less than 1%)
Nervousness (Greater than 1%)
Psychiatric disturbances
 (Less than 1 in 100)
Psychoses (Less than 1 in 100)

Clomid Tablets
Anxiety
Depression (Fewer than 1%)
Double vision (1.5%)
Insomnia (Fewer than 1%)
Irritability
Mood changes
Photophobia (1.5%)
Psychoses
Tenseness (Fewer than 1%)

Clorpres Tablets
Agitation (About 3%)
Anxiety
Behavioral changes
Delirium
Depression (About 1%)
Dreaming abnormalities
Hallucinations, auditory
Hallucinations, visual
Insomnia (About 5 in 1,000)
Libido, loss (About 3%)
▲ Nervousness (About 3%)
Nightmares
▲ Sedation (About 10%)
Sexual activity, decrease (About 3%)

Clozaril Tablets
▲ Agitation (4%)
Anxiety (1%)
Central nervous system reactions
▲ Confusion (3%)
Delirium
Delusions (Less than 1%)
Depression (1%)

Hallucinations (Less than 1%)
Insomnia (2%)
Irritability (Less than 1%)
Libido decreased (Less than 1%)
Libido increased (Less than 1%)
Memory loss, short-term (Less than 1%)
Mental performance, impairment
Mental status, altered
▲ Nightmares (4%)
Paranoia (Less than 1%)
Psychoses, aggravation
▲ Sedation (More than 5% to 39%)
▲ Sleep disturbances (4%)
Speech difficulties (Less than 1%)
Speech, incoherent (Less than 1%)
Speech, slurring (1%)

Cogentin
Depression
Excitability
Hallucinations
Hallucinations, visual
Memory impairment
Nervousness
Psychiatric disturbances

Cogentin Tablets
Confusion

Cognex Capsules
▲ Agitation (7%)
▲ Anxiety (3%)
Apathy (Infrequent)
Coma (Rare)
▲ Confusion (7%)
Delirium (Infrequent)
▲ Depression (4%)
Double vision (Infrequent)
Dreaming abnormalities (Infrequent)
Hallucinations (2%)
Hostility (2%)
Hysteria (Rare)
Impairment of sensation (Rare)
▲ Insomnia (6%)
Libido increased (Infrequent)
Nervousness (Frequent)
Neurosis, unspecified (Infrequent)
Paranoia (Infrequent)
Psychoses (Rare)
Suicidal ideation (Rare)
▲ Thinking abnormality (3%)

Colazal Capsules
Anxiety
Depression

Disordered sense of smell
Insomnia (2%)
Nervousness

Colestid Tablets
Insomnia (Infrequent)

Coly-Mycin M
Speech, slurring

CombiPatch
▲ Depression (8% to 9%)
▲ Insomnia (8% to 6%)
▲ Nervousness (5% to 6%)

Combipres Tablets
Agitation (About 3%)
Anxiety
Behavioral changes
Delirium
Depression (About 1%)
Dreaming abnormalities
Hallucinations, auditory
Hallucinations, visual
Insomnia (About 5 in 1,000)
Libido, loss (About 3%)
▲ Nervousness (About 3%)
Nightmares
▲ Sedation (About 10%)
Sexual activity, decrease (About 3%)

Combivent Inhalation Aerosol
Central nervous system stimulation
Insomnia (Less than 2%)
Nervousness (Less than 2%)

Combivir Tablets
▲ Depressive reactions (9%)
▲ Insomnia (11%)
▲ Sleep disturbances (11%)

Compazine
Agitation
Catatonia
Central nervous system reactions
Coma
Insomnia
Jitteriness
Mental clouding
Mental performance, impairment
Nervousness
Psychosis, activation

Comtan Tablets
Agitation (1%)
Anxiety (2%)
Consciousness, disorders of

Hallucinations

Comtrex Acute Head Cold
Excitability

Comtrex Flu Therapy Day & Night (Nighttime)
Excitability

Comvax
Agitation
▲ Irritability (32.2% to 57.0%)

Concerta
Depression
▲ Insomnia (4%)
▲ Nervousness (Among most common)
Psychoses, toxic

Condylox Topical Solution
Insomnia (Less than 5%)

Contac 12 Hour Cold Caplets
Insomnia
Nervousness

Contac Severe Cold and Flu
Excitability
Insomnia
Nervousness

Contac Severe Cold and Flu Non-Drowsy
Nervousness

Copaxone
▲ Agitation (4%)
▲ Anxiety (23%)
Coma (Infrequent)
Confusion (2%)
Depersonalization (Infrequent)
Depression (At least 2%)
Depression, psychotic (Infrequent)
Double vision (At least 2%)
Dreaming abnormalities (Frequent)
Emotional lability (At least 2%)
Euphoria (At least 2%)
Hallucinations (Infrequent)
Hostility (Infrequent)
Impairment of sensation (At least 2%)
Insomnia (At least 2%)
Libido decreased (Infrequent)
Manic behavior (Infrequent)
Memory impairment (Infrequent)
Mental performance, impairment (Infrequent)
Nervousness (2%)

Paranoia (Infrequent)
Photophobia (Infrequent)
Sexual dysfunction (Infrequent)
Sleep disturbances (At least 2%)
Speech disturbances (2%)
Stupor (Frequent)
Suicide, attempt of (Infrequent)

Cordarone Tablets

Insomnia (1% to 3%)
Libido decreased (1% to 3%)
▲ Photophobia (4% to 9%)
Sleep disturbances (1% to 3%)

Coreg Tablets

Depression (Greater than 2%)
Depression, aggravation of (0.1% to 1%)
Emotional lability (0.1% to 1%)
Insomnia (Greater than 2%)
Libido decreased (0.1% to 1%)
Mental performance, impairment (0.1% to 1%)
Nervousness (0.1% to 1%)
Nightmares (0.1% to 1%)
Sleep disturbances (0.1% to 1%)
Thinking abnormality (0.1% to 1%)

Corgard Tablets

Behavioral changes (6 of 1000 patients)
Catatonia
Depression
Disorientation, place
Disorientation, time
Emotional lability
Hallucinations
Libido decreased (1 to 5 per 1000 patients)
Memory loss, short-term
Neuropsychometrics performance, decrease
Sedation (6 of 1000 patients)
Sensorium, clouded
Sleep disturbances
Speech, slurring (1 to 5 per 1000 patients)

Coricidin D Cold, Flu & Sinus

Excitability
Insomnia
Nervousness

Coricidin HBP Cold & Flu

Excitability

Corlopam Injection

Anxiety (1% to 2%)
Insomnia (2%)
Nervousness (1% to 2%)

Cortifoam Rectal Foam

Insomnia

Cortone

Depression
Euphoria
Insomnia
Mood changes
Personality changes
Psychiatric disturbances
Psychoses
Psychoses, aggravation

Corzide

Catatonia
Depression
Disorientation, place
Disorientation, time
Emotional lability
Hallucinations
Libido decreased (1 to 5 of 1000 patients)
Memory loss, short-term
Neuropsychometrics performance, decrease
Sedation (6 of 1000 patients)
Sensorium, clouded
Sleep disturbances
Speech, slurring (1 to 5 of 1000 patients)

Cosopt Ophthalmic Solution

Anxiety
Behavioral changes
Catatonia
Confusion
Depression (Less than 1%)
Disorientation
Disorientation, place
Disorientation, time
Double vision
Emotional lability
Hallucinations
Insomnia
Libido decreased
Memory loss, short-term
Mental performance, impairment
Nervousness
Neuropsychometrics performance, decrease

Nightmares
Photophobia (Less than 1%)
Psychiatric disturbances
Sensorium, clouded

Covera-HS Tablets
Confusion (Less than 2%)
Insomnia (Less than 2%)
Psychoses (Less than 2%)

Cozaar Tablets
Anxiety (Less than 1%)
Confusion (Less than 1%)
Depression (Less than 1%)
Dreaming abnormalities
(Less than 1%)
Insomnia (1.4%)
Libido decreased (Less than 1%)
Memory impairment (Less than 1%)
Nervousness (Less than 1%)
Panic (Less than 1%)
Sleep disturbances (Less than 1%)

Crinone 4% Gel
Aggression (Less than 5%)
▲ Depression (19%)
▲ Emotional lability (23%)
Insomnia (Less than 5%)
Memory loss, short-term (Less than
5%)
▲ Sleep disturbances (18%)

Crinone 8% Gel
Aggression (Less than 5%)
▲ Depression (11% to 15%)
▲ Emotional lability (22%)
Insomnia (Less than 5%)
▲ Libido decreased (10%)
Memory loss, short-term (Less than
5%)
▲ Nervousness (16%)
▲ Sleep disturbances (18%)

Crixivan Capsules
Agitation (Less than 2%)
Anxiety (Less than 2%)
Depression (Less than 2%)
Dreaming abnormalities (Less than
2%)
Excitability (Less than 2%)
Impairment of sensation (Less than
2%)
▲ Insomnia (3.1%)
Mental acuity, loss of (Less than 2%)
Nervousness (Less than 2%)
Sleep disturbances (Less than 2%)

Cuprimine Capsules
Agitation
Anxiety
Mental status, altered
Psychiatric disturbances

Cyclessa Tablets
Depression
Libido, changes
Nervousness

Cylert
Depression
Hallucinations
▲ Insomnia (Most frequent)
Irritability

CytoGam Intravenous
Photophobia (Infrequent)

Cytotec Tablets
Anxiety (Infrequent)
Behavioral changes (Infrequent)
Confusion
Libido decreased (Infrequent)

Cytovene
Anxiety (At least 3 subjects)
Confusion (At least 3 subjects)
Depression (At least 3 subjects)
Dreaming abnormalities
(At least 3 subjects)
Hallucinations
Impairment of sensation
Insomnia (At least 3 subjects)
Irritability
Memory loss, short-term
Thinking abnormality
(At least 3 subjects)

D.H.E. 45 Injection
Anxiety (Occasional)
Apathy
Confusion
Hallucinations
Mental performance, impairment
Suicide, attempt of

Dantrium Capsules
Confusion (Less frequent)
Depression (Less frequent)
Double vision (Less frequent)
Insomnia (Less frequent)
Nervousness (Less frequent)
Speech disturbances (Less frequent)

Dapsone Tablets USP
Insomnia

Psychoses

Daranide Tablets
Confusion
Depression
Disorientation
Nervousness

Darvocet-N
Euphoria
Hallucinations
▲ Sedation (Among most frequent)

Darvon Compound-65 Pulvules
Euphoria
Hallucinations
▲ Sedation (Among most frequent)

Darvon Pulvules
Euphoria
Hallucinations
▲ Sedation (Among most frequent)

Darvon-N Tablets
Euphoria
Hallucinations
▲ Sedation (Among most frequent)

DaunoXome Injection
Anxiety (Less than or equal to 5%)
Confusion (Less than or equal to 5%)
▲ Depression (3% to 7%)
Emotional lability (Less than or equal to 5%)
Hallucinations (Less than or equal to 5%)
▲ Insomnia (Up to 6%)
Thinking abnormality (Less than or equal to 5%)

DDAVP Injection
Coma (Rare)

DDAVP Nasal Spray
Coma (Rare)
Depression

DDAVP Rhinal Tube
Coma (Rare)
Depression

DDAVP Tablets
Thinking abnormality

Decadron
Depression
Euphoria
Insomnia
Mood changes

Personality changes
Psychiatric disturbances
Psychoses
Psychoses, aggravation

Delatestryl Injection
Anxiety
Depression
Libido decreased
Libido increased

Demadex
Insomnia (1.2%)
Nervousness (1.1%)

Demerol
Agitation
Disorientation
Euphoria
Hallucinations
Mental performance, impairment
▲ Sedation (Among most frequent)

Demser Capsules
Anxiety
Awareness, heightened
Confusion
Depression
Disorientation
Hallucinations
Insomnia
▲ Sedation (Almost all patients)
▲ Speech difficulties (10%)

Depacon Injection
Aggression
Agitation (1% or more)
Anxiety (1% to 5%)
Behavioral deterioration
Catatonia (1% or more)
Central nervous system depression
Coma (Rare)
Confusion (1% to 5%)
Dementia (Several reports)
▲ Depression (4% to 5%)
▲ Double vision (16%)
Dreaming abnormalities (1% to 5%)
Emotional disturbances
▲ Emotional lability (6%)
Euphoria (0.9%)
Hallucinations
Hostility
Hyperactivity
▲ Insomnia (9% to 15%)
▲ Nervousness (0.9% to 11%)

Personality changes (1% to 5%)
Psychoses
Sedation
▲ Thinking abnormality (6%)

Depakene
Aggression
Agitation (1% or more)
Anxiety (1% to 5%)
Behavioral deterioration
Catatonia (1% or more)
Central nervous system depression
Coma (Rare)
Confusion (1% to 5%)
Dementia (Several reports)
▲ Depression (5%)
▲ Double vision (16%)
Dreaming abnormalities (1% to 5%)
Emotional disturbances
▲ Emotional lability (6%)
Hallucinations
Hostility
Hyperactivity
▲ Insomnia (15%)
▲ Nervousness (11%)
Personality changes (1% to 5%)
Psychoses
Sedation
▲ Thinking abnormality (6%)

Depakote ER Tablets
Aggression
Agitation (Greater than 1%)
Anxiety (1% to 5%)
Behavioral deterioration
Catatonia (Greater than 1%)
Central nervous system depression
Coma (Rare)
Confusion (1% to 5%)
Dementia (Several reports)
Depression (Greater than 1%)
Double vision (Greater than 1%)
Dreaming abnormalities (1% to 5%)
Emotional disturbances
Emotional lability (Greater than 1%)
Hallucinations (Greater than 1%)
Hostility
Hyperactivity
Insomnia (1% to 5%)
Nervousness (1% to 5%)
Personality changes (1% to 5%)
Photophobia (Greater than 1%)
Psychoses (Greater than 1%)
Sedation
Sleep disturbances (Greater than 1%)

Speech disturbances (1% to 5%)
Thinking abnormality (1% to 5%)

Depakote Sprinkle Capsules
Aggression
Agitation
Anxiety (1% to 5%)
Behavioral deterioration
Catatonia
Coma (Rare)
Confusion (1% to 5%)
Dementia (Several reports)
▲ Depression (4% to 5%)
▲ Double vision (16%)
Dreaming abnormalities (1% to 5%)
Emotional disturbances
▲ Emotional lability (6%)
Hallucinations
Hostility
Hyperactivity
▲ Insomnia (9% to 15%)
▲ Nervousness (7% to 11%)
Personality changes (1% to 5%)
Psychoses
▲ Thinking abnormality (6%)

Depakote Tablets
Aggression
Agitation (1% to 5%)
Anxiety (1% to 5%)
Behavioral deterioration
Catatonia (1% to 5%)
Central nervous system depression
Coma (Rare)
Confusion (1% to 5%)
Dementia (Several reports)
Depression (1% to 5%)
▲ Double vision (1% to 16%)
Dreaming abnormalities (1% to 5%)
Emotional disturbances
▲ Emotional lability (1% to 6%)
Hallucinations (1% to 5%)
Hostility
Hyperactivity
▲ Insomnia (1% to 15%)
▲ Nervousness (1% to 11%)
Personality changes (1% to 5%)
Psychoses
Sedation
Speech disturbances (1% to 5%)
Suicidal ideation
▲ Thinking abnormality (1% to 6%)

Depen Titratable Tablets
Double vision

DepoCyt Injection
▲ Confusion (4% to 14%)

Depo-Provera Contraceptive Injection
Depression (1% to 5%)
Double vision
▲ Insomnia (More than 5%)
Libido decreased (1% to 5%)
Libido increased (Fewer than 1%)
▲ Nervousness (More than 5%)

Desmopressin Acetate Injection
Coma (Rare)

Desmopressin Acetate Rhinal Tube
Depression

Desogen Tablets
Depression
Libido, changes
Nervousness

Desoxyn Tablets
Euphoria
Insomnia
Libido, changes
Overstimulation
Psychoses (Rare)

Detrol LA Capsules
Anxiety (1%)

Detrol Tablets
Nervousness (1.1%)

Dexedrine
Agitation
Euphoria
Insomnia
Libido, changes
Overstimulation
Psychoses (Rare at recommended doses)

DextroStat Tablets
Euphoria
Insomnia
Libido, changes
Overstimulation
Psychoses (Rare)
Sociopathy

Diamox
Confusion (Occasional)

Didronel Tablets
Confusion
Depression
Hallucinations
Psychiatric disturbances

Digitek Tablets
Anxiety
Apathy
Central nervous system reactions
Confusion
Delirium
Depression
Hallucinations
▲ Mental status, altered (5%)

Dilantin
▲ Confusion (Among most common)
Insomnia
Nervousness
▲ Speech, slurring (Among most common)

Dilaudid Injection
Anxiety
Fear
Mental performance, impairment
Mood changes
Sedation

Dilaudid Oral Liquid
Agitation (Less frequent)
Depression (Less frequent)
Disorientation (Less frequent)
Double vision (Less frequent)
Dreaming (Less frequent)
Euphoria
Floating feeling (Less frequent)
Hallucinations (Less frequent)
Insomnia (Less frequent)
Mood changes (Less frequent)
Nervousness (Less frequent)
Sedation

Dilaudid Powder
Anxiety
Fear
Mental clouding
Mental performance, impairment
Mood changes
Sedation

Dilaudid Rectal Suppositories
Anxiety
Fear
Mental clouding

Mental performance, impairment
Mood changes
Sedation

Dilaudid Tablets
Anxiety
Fear
Mental clouding
Mental performance, impairment
Mood changes
Sedation

Dilaudid Tablets - 8 mg
Agitation (Less frequent)
Depression (Less frequent)
Disorientation (Less frequent)
Double vision (Less frequent)
Dreaming (Less frequent)
Euphoria
Floating feeling (Less frequent)
Hallucinations (Less frequent)
Insomnia (Less frequent)
Mood changes (Less frequent)
Nervousness (Less frequent)
Sedation

Dilaudid-HP
Agitation (Less frequent)
Depression (Less frequent)
Disorientation (Less frequent)
Double vision (Less frequent)
Dreaming abnormalities
  (Less frequent)
Euphoria (Less frequent)
Floating feeling (Less frequent)
Hallucinations (Less frequent)
Insomnia (Less frequent)
Mood changes (Less frequent)
Nervousness
▲ Sedation (Among most frequent)

Dimetapp Elixir
Excitability

Diovan Capsules
Anxiety
Insomnia

Diovan HCT Tablets
Anxiety (Greater than 0.2%)
Confusion
Depression (Greater than 0.2%)
Insomnia (Greater than 0.2%)
Libido decreased (Greater than 0.2%)

Dipentum Capsules
Depression (1.5%)

Insomnia (Rare)
Irritability (Rare)
Mood changes (Rare)

Diphtheria & Tetanus Toxoids
▲ Anxiety (22.6%)
Irritability

Diprivan
Agitation (Less than 1%)
Anxiety (Less than 1%)
Awareness, altered (Less than 1%)
Behavior, inappropriate (Less than
  1%)
Combativeness (Less than 1%)
Confusion (Less than 1%)
Delirium (Less than 1%)
Depression (Less than 1%)
Double vision (Less than 1%)
Dreaming abnormalities
  (Less than 1%)
Emotional lability (Less than 1%)
Euphoria (Less than 1%)
Hallucinations (Less than 1%)
Hysteria (Less than 1%)
Insomnia (Less than 1%)
Thinking abnormality (Less than 1%)

Ditropan XL
Confusion (2% to 5%)
Insomnia (2% to 5%)
Nervousness (2% to 5%)

Diuril
Confusion

Dolobid Tablets
Confusion (Less than 1 in 100)
Depression (Less than 1 in 100)
Disorientation (Less than 1 in 100)
Hallucinations (Less than 1 in 100)
Insomnia (Greater than 1 in 100)
Nervousness (Less than 1 in 100)

Dolophine Tablets
Agitation
Disorientation
Euphoria
Insomnia
Libido decreased
▲ Sedation (Among most frequent)

Donnatal
Agitation (In elderly patients)
Excitability (In elderly patients)
Insomnia
Nervousness

Dopram Injectable
Disorientation
Hyperactivity

Dostinex Tablets
▲ Anxiety (1% to less than 10%)
Confusion
▲ Depression (3%)
Hallucinations
▲ Insomnia (1% to less than 10%)
▲ Libido increased (Less than 10%)
Mental performance, impairment (1%)
▲ Nervousness (1% to less than 10%)

Doxil Injection
Anxiety (Less than 1% to 5%)
Confusion (Less than 1%)
Depression (Less than 1% to 5%)
Disordered sense of smell (Less than 1%)
Emotional lability (1% to 5%)
Insomnia (Less than 1% to 5%)
Nervousness (Less than 1%)
Thinking abnormality (Less than 1%)

Drixoral Allergy Sinus
Excitability
Nervousness

Drixoral Cold & Allergy
Excitability
Insomnia
Nervousness

Drixoral Cold & Flu
Excitability
Insomnia
Nervousness

Duraclon Injection
▲ Agitation (3%)
▲ Anxiety (38%)
Behavioral changes (Rare)
▲ Confusion (13.2% to 38%)
Delirium (Rare)
Depression (1%)
Dreaming abnormalities (Rare)
▲ Hallucinations (5.3%)
Insomnia (0.5%)
▲ Libido decreased (3%)
▲ Nervousness (3%)
Nightmares (Rare)
Sedation
▲ Sexual activity, decrease (3%)

Duragesic Transdermal System
Agitation (1% or greater)

▲ Anxiety (3% to 10%)
▲ Confusion (10% or more)
Depersonalization (Less than 1%)
▲ Depression (3% to 10%)
Dreaming abnormalities (1% or greater)
▲ Euphoria (3% to 10%)
▲ Hallucinations (3% to 10%)
Hostility (Less than 1%)
▲ Nervousness (3% to 10%)
Paranoia (1% or greater)
Speech disturbances (1% or greater)
Stupor (Less than 1%)
Thinking abnormality (1% or greater)

Duramorph Injection
Anxiety
Euphoria
Excitability
Psychoses, toxic

Duranest Injections
Central nervous system depression
Central nervous system stimulation
Confusion
Depression
Double vision
Euphoria
Nervousness
Sensory deficit, persistent
Sexual dysfunction

Dyazide Capsules
Confusion

Dynabac Tablets
Anxiety (0.1% to 1%)
Depression (0.1% to 1%)
Insomnia (0.9% to 1%)
Nervousness (0.1% to 1%)

DynaCirc
Depression (0.5% to 1%)
Insomnia (0.5% to 1%)
Libido decreased (0.5% to 1%)
Nervousness (0.5% to 1%)

EC-Naprosyn
Central nervous system depression (Less than 1%)
Cognitive dysfunction (Rare)
Dreaming abnormalities (Less than 1%)
Insomnia (Less than 1%)
Mental performance, impairment (Less than 1%)

Ecotrin Enteric Coated Aspirin
Agitation
Coma
Confusion

Edecrin
Confusion

Effexor Tablets
▲ Agitation (2% to 4.5%)
Alcohol abuse (Rare)
▲ Anxiety (2% to 11.2%)
Apathy (Infrequent)
Catatonia
Central nervous system stimulation
(Infrequent)
Confusion (2%)
Delirium
Delusions (Rare)
Dementia (Rare)
Depersonalization (1%)
Depression (1%)
Depression, psychotic (Rare)
Disordered sense of smell (Infrequent)
Double vision (Infrequent)
▲ Dreaming abnormalities (4%)
Emotional lability (Frequent)
Euphoria (Infrequent)
Hallucinations (Infrequent)
Hangover (Infrequent)
Hostility (Infrequent)
▲ Insomnia (3% to 22.5%)
▲ Libido decreased (2% to 5.7%)
Libido increased (Infrequent)
Manic behavior (0.5%)
Manic behavior, mild (0.5%)
▲ Nervousness (2% to 21.3%)
Panic
Paranoia (Infrequent)
Photophobia (Infrequent)
Psychoses (Rare)
Serotonin syndrome
Sexual dysfunction (2%)
Sleep disturbances (Infrequent)
Speech disturbances (Infrequent)
Stupor (Infrequent)
Suicidal ideation (Rare)
Suicide, attempt of (Infrequent)
Thinking abnormality (2%)

Effexor XR Capsules
▲ Agitation (3%)
Alcohol abuse (Rare)
Anxiety
Apathy (Infrequent)
Catatonia
Central nervous system stimulation
(Infrequent)
Confusion (Frequent)
Delirium
Delusions (Rare)
Dementia (Rare)
Depersonalization (Frequent)
▲ Depression (3%)
Depression, psychotic (Infrequent)
Disordered sense of smell (Infrequent)
Double vision (Infrequent)
▲ Dreaming abnormalities (4% to 7%)
Emotional lability (Frequent)
Euphoria (Infrequent)
Hallucinations (Infrequent)
Hangover (Infrequent)
Hostility (Infrequent)
▲ Insomnia (17% to 22%)
▲ Libido decreased (3% to 6%)
Libido increased (Infrequent)
Manic behavior (0.5%)
Manic behavior, mild (0.3%)
▲ Nervousness (10% to 12%)
▲ Nightmares (4% to 7%)
▲ Orgasmic dysfunction, female (4%)
Panic
Paranoia (Infrequent)
Photophobia (Infrequent)
Psychoses (Infrequent)
Serotonin syndrome
Sexual dysfunction
Speech disturbances (Infrequent)
Stupor (Infrequent)
Suicidal ideation (Rare)
Suicide, attempt of (Infrequent)
Thinking abnormality

Efudex
Emotional disturbances (Infrequent)
Insomnia
Irritability

ELA-Max Cream
Central nervous system depression
Central nervous system stimulation
Confusion
Double vision
Euphoria
Nervousness

Eldepryl Capsules
Agitation
Anxiety (1 of 49 patients)
Apathy

Behavioral changes
Confusion (3 of 49 patients)
Delusions
Depression
Disorientation
Double vision
▲ Dreaming abnormalities (2 of 49 patients)
Euphoria
▲ Hallucinations (3 of 49 patients)
Insomnia (1 of 49 patients)
Irritability
Memory impairment
Mental status, altered
Mood changes
Nervousness
Nightmares
Overstimulation
Personality changes
Sexual dysfunction
Sleep disturbances
Speech disturbances

Eligard
Depression (Less than 2%)
Insomnia (Less than 2%)
Libido decreased (Less than 2%)

Elmiron Capsules
Depression
Emotional lability
Insomnia

Elspar for Injection
Agitation (No incidence data in labeling)
Coma (No incidence data in labeling)
Confusion (No incidence data in labeling)
Depression (No incidence data in labeling)
Hallucinations (No incidence data in labeling)
Irritability (No incidence data in labeling)

Emadine Ophthalmic Solution
Dreaming abnormalities (Less than 5%)

Emcyt Capsules
Anxiety (1%)
Emotional lability (2%)
Insomnia (3%)

EMLA
Central nervous system depression (Unlikely)
Central nervous system stimulation (Unlikely)
Confusion (Unlikely)
Double vision (Unlikely)
Euphoria (Unlikely)
Nervousness (Unlikely)

Enalaprilat Injection
Confusion
Depression
Dreaming abnormalities
Impairment of sensation
Insomnia
Nervousness
Depression (Infrequent)
Mood changes
Personality changes

Engerix-B Vaccine
Agitation (Less than 1%)
Insomnia (Less than 1%)
Irritability (Less than 1%)

EpiPen Auto-Injector
Anxiety

EpiPen Jr. Auto-Injector
Anxiety
Nervousness

Epivir
▲ Depressive reactions (9%)
▲ Insomnia (11%)
▲ Sleep disturbances (11%)

Epogen for Injection
▲ Anxiety (2% to 7%)
▲ Insomnia (13% to 16%)

Ergamisol Tablets
Anxiety (1%)
Coma
Confusion (Less frequent)
Depression (1% to 2%)
Euphoria
Hallucinations (Less frequent)
Insomnia (1%)
Memory loss, short-term (10 out of 463 patients)
Mental performance, impairment (Less frequent)
Nervousness (1% to 2%)
Photophobia
Speech disturbances

Ery-Tab Tablets
Confusion (Isolated reports)
Hallucinations (Isolated reports)

Erythrocin Stearate
Confusion (Isolated reports)
Hallucinations (Isolated reports)

Erythromycin
Confusion (Isolated reports)
Hallucinations (Isolated reports)

Esclim Transdermal System
▲ Anxiety (Up to 8.3%)
Depression
▲ Emotional lability (2.1% to 8.3%)
Libido, changes

Eskalith
Coma
Confusion
Hallucinations
Memory impairment
Mental performance, impairment
Sexual dysfunction
Speech, slurring
Stupor

Estinyl Tablets
Depression
Libido, changes

Estrace
Depression
Libido, changes
Speech disturbances

Estratest
Anxiety
Depression
Libido, changes

Estring Vaginal Ring
Anxiety (1% to 3%)
Depression (At least 1 report)
▲ Insomnia (4%)
Libido decreased (At least 1 report)
Nervousness (At least 1 report)

Estrostep 21 Tablets
Depression
Libido, changes
Nervousness

Estrostep Fe Tablets
Depression
Libido, changes
Nervousness

Etrafon
Anxiety
Catatonia
Confusion
Confusion, nocturnal
Delusions
Disorientation
Dreaming abnormalities
Excitability
Excitement, paradoxical
Hallucinations
Hyperactivity
Insomnia
Jitteriness
Libido, changes
Mental performance, impairment
Mental status, altered
Nightmares
Paranoia
Photophobia
Psychoses, aggravation
Sedation (Less frequent)
Speech, slurring

Eulexin Capsules
Anxiety (1%)
Confusion (1%)
Depression (1%)
▲ Libido, loss (36%)
Nervousness (1%)

Evista Tablets
▲ Depression (6.4%)
▲ Insomnia (5.5%)

Evoxac Capsules
Aggression
Agitation (Less than 1%)
Anxiety (1.3%)
Apathy
Coma (Less than 1%)
Confusion (Less than 1%)
Delirium
Delusions
Dementia
Depersonalization (Less than 1%)
Depression (1% to 3%)
Depression, aggravation of
  (Less than 1%)
Disordered sense of smell
  (Less than 1%)
Double vision (Less than 1%)
Dreaming abnormalities
  (Less than 1%)
Emotional lability (Less than 1%)

Hallucinations (Less than 1%)
Illusion, unspecified
Impairment of sensation
  (Less than 1%)
Insomnia (2.4%)
Manic behavior (Less than 1%)
Neurosis, unspecified
Nightmares (Less than 1%)
Paranoia
Personality changes
Sexual dysfunction (Less than 1%)
Speech disturbances (Less than 1%)
Thinking abnormality (Less than 1%)

Exelon
▲ Aggression (3%)
  Agitation (2% or more)
▲ Anxiety (5%)
  Apathy (Infrequent)
▲ Confusion (8%)
  Delirium (Infrequent)
  Delusions (2% or more)
  Dementia (Infrequent)
  Depersonalization (Infrequent)
▲ Depression (6%)
  Double vision (Infrequent)
  Dreaming abnormalities (Infrequent)
  Emotional lability (Infrequent)
▲ Hallucinations (4%)
▲ Insomnia (9%)
  Libido decreased (Infrequent)
  Libido increased (Infrequent)
  Mental performance, impairment
    (Infrequent)
  Nervousness (2% or more)
  Neurosis, unspecified (Infrequent)
  Paranoia (2% or more)
  Personality changes (Infrequent)
  Psychoses (Infrequent)
' Suicidal ideation (Infrequent)
  Suicide, attempt of (Infrequent)

Extendryl
  Excitability
  Irritability

Famotidine Injection
  Agitation (Infrequent)
  Anxiety (Infrequent)
  Confusion (Infrequent)
  Depression (Infrequent)
  Hallucinations (Infrequent)
  Insomnia (Infrequent)
  Libido decreased (Infrequent)
  Psychiatric disturbances (Infrequent)

Famvir Tablets
  Confusion (Infrequent)
  Delirium (Infrequent)
  Disorientation (Infrequent)
  Hallucinations (Infrequent)
  Insomnia (1.5% to 2.5%)

Fareston Tablets
  Depression
  Double vision

Felbatol
  Aggression (Frequent)
  Agitation (Frequent)
▲ Anxiety (5.2% to 5.3%)
  Apathy
  Coma
  Confusion
  Delusions
▲ Depression (5.3%)
▲ Double vision (3.4% to 6.1%)
▲ Emotional lability (6.5%)
  Euphoria (Infrequent)
  Hallucinations (Infrequent)
▲ Insomnia (8.6% to 17.5%)
  Manic behavior
  Mental performance, impairment
▲ Nervousness (7.0% to 16.1%)
  Paranoia
  Psychoses
  Stupor (2.6%)
  Suicide, attempt of (Infrequent)
▲ Thinking abnormality (6.5%)

Feldene Capsules
  Anxiety (Occasional)
  Coma (Rare)
  Confusion (Occasional)
  Depression (Occasional)
  Dreaming abnormalities (Occasional)
  Hallucinations (Rare)
  Insomnia (Occasional)
  Mood changes (Rare)
  Nervousness (Occasional)

Femara Tablets
  Anxiety (Less frequent)
  Depression (Less frequent)
▲ Insomnia (6%)

femhrt Tablets
▲ Depression (5.8%)
  Double vision
  Insomnia
  Libido, changes
▲ Nervousness (5.4%)

Ferrlecit Injection

Agitation (Greater than 1%)
Insomnia (Greater than 1%)
Nervousness (Two or more patients)

Flexeril Tablets

Aggression
Agitation (Less than 1%)
Anxiety (Less than 1%)
Delusions (Rare)
Depression (Less than 1%)
Disorientation (Less than 1%)
Double vision (Less than 1%)
Dreaming abnormalities (Less than 1%)
Excitability (Less than 1%)
Hallucinations (Less than 1%)
Insomnia (Less than 1%)
Libido, changes (Rare)
Nervousness (1% to 3%)
Paranoia
Thinking abnormality (Less than 1%)

Flolan for Injection

▲ Agitation (11%)
▲ Anxiety (7% to 21%)
▲ Confusion (6%)
▲ Depression (13% to 37%)
▲ Insomnia (4% to 9%)
▲ Nervousness (7% to 21%)

Flomax Capsules

Insomnia (1.4% to 2.4%)
Libido decreased (1.0% to 2.0%)

Florinef Acetate Tablets

Depression
Insomnia
Mood changes
Personality changes
Psychiatric disturbances

Flovent Diskus

Aggression
Agitation
Depression
Sleep disturbances (1% to 3%)

Flovent Inhalation Aerosol

Aggression
Agitation
Depression
▲ Insomnia (3% to 13%)

Flovent Rotadisk

Aggression
Agitation

Depression
Insomnia
Nervousness (1% to 3%)

Floxin

Aggression
Agitation
Anxiety (Less than 1%)
Central nervous system stimulation
Cognitive dysfunction (Less than 1%)
Confusion (Less than 1%)
Depression (Less than 1%)
Disorientation
Double vision
Dreaming abnormalities (Less than 1%)
Emotional lability
Euphoria (Less than 1%)
Hallucinations (Less than 1%)
Hostility
▲ Insomnia (3% to 7%)
Manic behavior
Nervousness (1% to 3%)
Nightmares
Paranoia
Phobic disorder
Photophobia (Less than 1%)
Psychoses
Psychoses, toxic
Sleep disturbances (1% to 3%)
Suicidal ideation (Rare)
Suicide, attempt of (Rare)

Floxin Otic Solution

Impairment of sensation (Single report)
Insomnia (Single report)

Fludara for Injection

Agitation
Coma
Confusion
Depression (Up to 1%)
Mental performance, impairment (Up to 1%)
Sleep disturbances (1% to 3%)

Flumadine

Agitation (0.3% to 1%)
Confusion (Less than 0.3%)
Depression (0.3% to 1%)
Disordered sense of smell (Less than 0.3%)
Euphoria (Less than 0.3%)
Hallucinations (Less than 0.3%)
Insomnia (2.1% to 3.4%)

Mental performance, impairment (0.3% to 2.1%)
Nervousness (1.3% to 2.1%)

Focalin Tablets

Depression
Hallucinations
▲ Insomnia (Among most common)
▲ Nervousness (Among most common)
Psychoses, toxic (Rare)

Foradil Aerolizer

Insomnia (1.5%)
Nervousness

Fortovase Capsules

Agitation (Less than 2%)
Anxiety (2.2%)
Behavioral changes (Less than 2%)
Confusion (Less than 2%)
Depression (2.7%)
Dreaming abnormalities (Less than 2%)
Euphoria (Less than 2%)
Hallucinations (Less than 2%)
Impairment of sensation (Less than 2%)
▲ Insomnia
Irritability (Less than 2%)
Libido, changes (2.2%)
Mental performance, impairment (Less than 2%)
Psychiatric disturbances (Less than 2%)
Psychoses (Less than 2%)
Speech disturbances (Less than 2%)
Suicide, attempt of (Rare)

Foscavir Injection

Aggression (Between 1% and 5%)
Agitation (Between 1% and 5%)
▲ Anxiety (5% or greater)
Coma (Less than 1%)
▲ Confusion (5% or greater)
Dementia (Between 1% and 5%)
▲ Depression (5% or greater)
Hallucinations (Between 1% and 5%)
Insomnia (Between 1% and 5%)
Nervousness (Between 1% and 5%)
Sensory disturbances (Between 1% and 5%)
Stupor (Between 1% and 5%)

Gabitril Tablets

Agitation (1%)
Anxiety (1% or more)

Apathy (Infrequent)
Coma (Infrequent)
▲ Confusion (5%)
Delusions (Infrequent)
Depersonalization (Frequent)
▲ Depression (3%)
Disordered sense of smell (Infrequent)
Double vision (1% or more)
Dreaming abnormalities (Infrequent)
▲ Emotional lability (3%)
Euphoria (Frequent)
Hallucinations (Frequent)
Hostility (2%)
▲ Insomnia (6%)
▲ Irritability (10%)
Libido decreased (Infrequent)
Libido increased (Infrequent)
▲ Mental performance, impairment (6%)
▲ Nervousness (10%)
Neurosis, unspecified (Infrequent)
Paranoia (Frequent)
Personality changes (Frequent)
Photophobia (Infrequent)
Psychoses (Infrequent)
▲ Speech disturbances (4%)
Stupor (Frequent)
Suicide, attempt of (Infrequent)
▲ Thinking abnormality (6%)

Gamimune N

Anxiety
▲ Irritability (Among most common)
Photophobia (Infrequent)

Gammar-P I.V.

Anxiety

Gastrocrom Oral Concentrate

Anxiety (Less common)
Behavioral changes (Less common)
Depression (Less common)
Hallucinations (Less common)
Insomnia (Less common)
Irritability (2 of 87 patients)
Nervousness (Less common)
Psychoses (Less common)

Gemzar for Injection

Insomnia (Infrequent)

Gengraf Capsules

Anxiety (1% to less than 3%)
Confusion (1% to less than 3%)
Depression (Rare)
Emotional lability (1% to less than 3%)

Insomnia (1% to less than 3%)
Libido decreased (1% to less than 3%)
Libido increased (1% to less than 3%)
Mental performance, impairment (1% to less than 3%)
Nervousness (1% to less than 3%)
Nightmares (1% to less than 3%)
▲ Psychiatric disturbances (5.0%)

Genoptic
Hallucinations (Rare)

Genotropin Lyophilized Powder
Aggression

Geodon Capsules
Agitation (Frequent)
Anxiety
Confusion (Frequent)
Delirium (Frequent)
Double vision (Frequent)
Hostility (Frequent)
Photophobia (Infrequent)
Sexual dysfunction (Infrequent)

Geref for Injection
▲ Hyperactivity (1 patient in 6)

Gliadel Wafer
Coma (1%)
▲ Confusion (10%)
▲ Depression (3%)
Double vision (1%)
Insomnia (2%)
Paranoia (1%)
▲ Stupor (6%)
Thinking abnormality (2%)

Glucotrol XL
Anxiety (Less than 3%)
Confusion (Less than 1%)
Depression (Less than 3%)
Insomnia (Less than 3%)
Libido decreased (Less than 1%)
▲ Nervousness (3.6%)

Gonal-F for Injection
Anxiety
▲ Emotional lability (5.1%)

Grifulvin V
Confusion (Occasional)
Insomnia (Occasional)
Mental performance, impairment

Gris-PEG Tablets
Confusion (Occasional)

Insomnia (Occasional)

Guaifed Capsules
Excitability
Irritability

Guaifed-PD Capsules
Excitability
Irritability

Halcion Tablets
Aggression
Agitation
Anxiety, paradoxical
Awareness, altered
Behavior, inappropriate
Central nervous system depression, neonatal
Central nervous system stimulation, paradoxical
Confusion (0.5% to 0.9%)
Delusions
Depersonalization
Depression (0.5% to 0.9%)
Depression, aggravation of
Disorientation
Dreaming abnormalities (Rare)
Euphoria (0.5% to 0.9%)
Excitement, paradoxical
Hallucinations
Impairment of sensation (Rare)
Insomnia (Rare)
Irritability
Libido, changes
Manic behavior
Memory impairment (0.5% to 0.9%)
Mental clouding
▲ Nervousness (5.2%)
Nightmares (Rare)
Overstimulation
Sedation
Sleep disturbances
Sleep walking
Speech, slurring
Suicidal ideation
Thinking abnormality

Haldol
Agitation
Anxiety
Catatonia
Confusion
Depression
Euphoria
Hallucinations
Insomnia

Libido increased
Psychotic symptoms, paradoxical
  exacerbation

Haldol Decanoate

Agitation
Anxiety
Catatonia
Confusion
Depression
Euphoria
Hallucinations
Insomnia
Libido increased
Mental status, altered
Psychotic symptoms, paradoxical
  exacerbation

Havrix Vaccine

Insomnia (Less than 1%)
Photophobia (Less than 1%)

Hectorol

Libido decreased
Photophobia
Psychoses
▲ Sleep disturbances (3.3%)

Helixate Concentrate

Depersonalization

Herceptin I.V.

Confusion (At least one of 958
  patients)
▲ Depression (6%)
▲ Insomnia (14%)
Manic behavior
  (At least one of 958 patients)

Hexalen Capsules

Central nervous system reactions
Consciousness, disorders of
Mood changes

HibTITER

Irritability (133 of 1,118 vaccinations)
Sleep disturbances

Hivid Tablets

Agitation (Less than 1%)
Anxiety (Less than 1%)
Confusion (Less than 1%)
Dementia (Less than 1%)
Depersonalization (Less than 1%)
Depression (0.4%)
Disordered sense of smell
  (Less than 1%)

Emotional lability (Less than 1%)
Euphoria (Less than 1%)
Hallucinations (Less than 1%)
Impairment of sensation
Insomnia (Less than 1%)
Manic behavior (Less than 1%)
Memory loss, short-term
  (Less than 1%)
Mental performance, impairment
  (Less than 1%)
Mood changes (Less than 1%)
Nervousness (Less than 1%)
Paranoia (Less than 1%)
Photophobia (Less than 1%)
Psychoses (Less than 1%)
Sexual dysfunction (Less than 1%)
Speech disturbances (Less than 1%)
Stupor (Less than 1%)
Suicide, attempt of (Less than 1%)
Thinking abnormality (Less than 1%)

Hycodan

Anxiety
Fear
Mental clouding
Mental performance, impairment
Mood changes
Sedation

Hycomine Compound Tablets

Anxiety
Fear
Mental clouding
Mental performance, impairment
Mood changes
Sedation

Hycotuss Expectorant Syrup

Anxiety
Fear
Mental clouding
Mental performance, impairment
Mood changes
Sedation

Hydrocortone

Depression
Euphoria
Insomnia
Mood changes
Personality changes
Psychiatric disturbances
Psychoses
Psychoses, aggravation

HydroDIURIL Tablets
Confusion

Hytrin Capsules
Anxiety (At least 1%)
Depression (0.3%)
Insomnia (At least 1%)
Libido decreased (0.6%)
Nervousness (2.3%)

Hyzaar
Anxiety
Confusion
Depression
Dreaming abnormalities
Insomnia
Libido decreased
Memory impairment
Nervousness
Panic
Sleep disturbances

Idamycin PFS Injection
▲ Mental status, altered (41%)

Ifex for Injection
Coma (Occasional)
▲ Confusion (Among most common)
▲ Depression, psychotic (Among most common)
Disorientation (Less frequent)
▲ Hallucinations (Among most common)

Imdur Tablets
Anxiety (Less than or equal to 5%)
Confusion (Less than or equal to 5%)
Depression (Less than or equal to 5%)
Insomnia (Less than or equal to 5%)
Libido decreased (Less than or equal to 5%)
Mental performance, impairment (Less than or equal to 5%)
Nervousness (Less than or equal to 5%)
Nightmares (Less than or equal to 5%)
Photophobia (Less than or equal to 5%)

Imitrex Injection
Aggression
Agitation (Infrequent)
Anxiety (1.1%)
Apathy
Confusion (Infrequent)
Depression (Rare)

Euphoria (Infrequent)
Feeling, intoxicated (Rare)
Feeling, strange (2.2%)
Hallucinations
Hysteria (Rare)
Impairment of sensation (Rare)
Mental performance, impairment (Rare)
Panic
Phobia, unspecified
Photophobia (Infrequent)
Sedation (2.7%)
Serotonin syndrome
Sleep disturbances (Rare)
Speech disturbances

Imitrex Nasal Spray
Agitation (Infrequent)
Anxiety (Infrequent)
Apathy (Rare)
Confusion (Infrequent)
Depression (Infrequent)
Emotional disturbances (Rare)
Euphoria (Infrequent)
Feeling, strange (Infrequent)
Impairment of sensation (Rare)
Memory impairment (Rare)
Mental performance, impairment (Rare)
Panic
Sedation (Infrequent)
Sleep disturbances (Infrequent)

Imitrex Tablets
Aggression (Rare)
Agitation (Up to 2%)
Anxiety
Apathy (Rare)
Awareness, heightened (Rare)
Confusion (Infrequent)
Depression (Infrequent)
Euphoria (Infrequent)
Feeling, strange
Hallucinations (Rare)
Hysteria (Rare)
Impairment of sensation (Rare)
Memory impairment (Rare)
Mental performance, impairment (Infrequent)
Panic
Personality changes (Rare)
Phobic disorder (Rare)
Phonophobia (Frequent)
Photophobia (Frequent)
Sedation

Serotonin syndrome
Sleep disturbances (Rare to
  infrequent)
Suicide, attempt of (Rare)

Indapamide Tablets
▲ Agitation (Greater than or equal to
  5%)
▲ Anxiety (Greater than or equal to 5%)
  Depression (Less than 5%)
  Insomnia (Less than 5%)
▲ Irritability (Greater than or equal to
  5%)
  Libido decreased (Less than 5%)
  Nervousness (Less than 5%)
▲ Tenseness (Greater than or equal to
  5%)

Inderal
  Depression
  Disorientation, place
  Disorientation, time
  Dreaming abnormalities
  Emotional lability
  Hallucinations
  Insomnia
  Memory loss, short-term
  Neuropsychometrics performance,
    decrease
  Sensorium, clouded

Inderal Injectable
  Catatonia

Inderide
  Catatonia
  Depression
  Disorientation, place
  Disorientation, time
  Emotional lability
  Hallucinations
  Insomnia
  Memory loss, short-term
  Neuropsychometrics performance,
    decrease
  Sensorium, clouded

Indocin Capsules/Suspension/ Suppositories
  Anxiety (Less than 1%)
  Coma (Less than 1%)
  Confusion (Less than 1%)
  Depersonalization (Less than 1%)
  Depression (Greater than 1%)
  Double vision (Less than 1%)
  Insomnia (Less than 1%)

Listlessness (Greater than 1%)
Nervousness (Less than 1%)
Psychiatric disturbances (Less than
  1%)
Psychoses (Less than 1%)

Indocin I.V.
  Coma (Less than 1%)

Infanrix Vaccine
▲ Anxiety (3.3% to 9.2%)
▲ Irritability (28.8% to 36.3%)

INFeD Injection
  Disorientation

Infergen
▲ Agitation (4% to 6%)
▲ Anxiety (10% to 19%)
▲ Confusion (4%)
▲ Depression (18% to 26%)
▲ Emotional lability (6% to 12%)
▲ Insomnia (24% to 39%)
▲ Libido decreased (5%)
▲ Nervousness (16% to 31%)
  Psychiatric disturbances
  Suicidal ideation
  Suicide, attempt of
▲ Thinking abnormality (8% to 10%)

Infumorph
  Anxiety
  Euphoria
  Excitability
  Hyperactivity
  Psychoses, toxic

Innohep Injection
  Confusion (Greater than or equal to
    1%)
  Insomnia (Greater than or equal to
    1%)

Intron A for Injection
  Aggression (Less than 5%)
  Agitation (Less than 5%)
▲ Anxiety (Up to 5%)
  Apathy (Less than 5%)
  Central nervous system reactions
    (Less than 5%)
  Coma (Less than 5%)
▲ Confusion (Up to 12%)
  Consciousness, disorders of (Less
    than 5%)
▲ Depression (2% to 40%)
  Depression, aggravation of (Less than
    5%)

Disordered sense of smell (Less than 5%)

Double vision (Less than 5%)

Dreaming abnormalities (Less than 5%)

Emotional lability (Less than 5%)

▲ Insomnia (Up to 12%)

▲ Irritability (Up to 16%)

Libido decreased (Up to 5%)

Manic behavior (Less than 5%)

▲ Mental performance, impairment (Up to 14%)

Nervousness (Up to 3%)

Neurosis, unspecified (Less than 5%)

Nightmares (Less than 5%)

Personality changes (Less than 5%)

Photophobia (Less than 5%)

Speech disturbances (Less than 5%)

Suicidal ideation (Rare)

Suicide, attempt of (Rare; less than 5%)

Thinking abnormality (Less than 5%)

Inversine Tablets

Libido decreased

Mental performance, impairment

Invirase Capsules

Agitation (Less than 2%)

Anxiety (Less than 2%)

Confusion (Less than 2%)

Depression (Less than 2%)

Dreaming abnormalities (Less than 2%)

Euphoria (Less than 2%)

Hallucinations (Less than 2%)

Impairment of sensation (Less than 2%)

Insomnia (Less than 2%)

Irritability (Less than 2%)

Libido, changes (Less than 2%)

Mental performance, impairment (Less than 2%)

Psychiatric disturbances (Less than 2%)

Psychoses (Less than 2%)

Speech disturbances (Less than 2%)

Suicide, attempt of (Rare)

Ionamin Capsules

Euphoria

Insomnia

Libido, changes

Overstimulation

Psychoses (Rare)

Iopidine 0.5% Ophthalmic Solution

Depression (Less than 3%)

Disordered sense of smell (0.2%)

Insomnia (Less than 3%)

Nervousness (Less than 3%)

Photophobia (Less than 3%)

Iopidine Sterile Ophthalmic Solution

Dreaming abnormalities

Insomnia

Irritability

Libido decreased

IPOL Vaccine

Anxiety

▲ Irritability (6.7% to 64.5%)

Ismo Tablets

Agitation (Fewer than 1%)

Anxiety (Fewer than 1%)

Confusion (Fewer than 1%)

Double vision (Fewer than 1%)

Insomnia (Fewer than 1%)

Nervousness (Fewer than 1%)

Nightmares (Fewer than 1%)

Isoptin SR Tablets

Confusion (1% or less)

Insomnia (1% or less)

Psychoses (1% or less)

JE-VAX Vaccine

Behavioral changes (One case)

Kadian Capsules

Agitation (Less than 3%)

▲ Anxiety (Less than 3% to 6%)

Apathy (Less than 3%)

Confusion (Less than 3%)

Depression (Less than 3%)

Double vision (Less than 3%)

Dreaming abnormalities (Less than 3%)

Euphoria (Less than 3%)

Hallucinations (Less than 3%)

Insomnia (Less than 3%)

Libido decreased (Less than 3%)

Mental performance, impairment (Less than 3%)

Sedation (Less than 3%)

Speech, slurring (Less than 3%)

Thinking abnormality (Less than 3%)

Kaletra

Agitation (Less than 2%)
Anxiety (Less than 2%)
Confusion (Less than 2%)
Depression (Less than 2%)
Dreaming abnormalities (Less than 2%)
Emotional lability (Less than 2%)
Insomnia (1.1% to 2.4%)
Libido decreased (Less than 2%)
Nervousness (Less than 2%)
Thinking abnormality (Less than 2%)

Keflex

Agitation
Confusion
Hallucinations

Keppra Tablets

Anxiety (2%)
Confusion (1% or more)
▲ Depression (4%)
Double vision (2%)
Emotional lability (2%)
Hostility (2%)
Insomnia (1% or more)
▲ Nervousness (4%)
Thinking abnormality (1% or more)

Klonopin Tablets

Aggression (Infrequent)
Agitation
Anxiety (Infrequent)
Apathy (Infrequent)
▲ Behavioral changes (5% to 25%)
▲ Central nervous system depression (Most frequent)
Coma
Confusion (1%)
Depersonalization (Infrequent)
▲ Depression (4% to 7%)
Double vision (Infrequent)
Dreaming abnormalities (Infrequent)
Emotional lability (1%)
Excitability (Infrequent)
Hallucinations
Hostility
Hyperactivity (Infrequent)
Hysteria
Illusion, unspecified (Infrequent)
Inebriated feeling (Infrequent)
Insomnia (Infrequent)
Libido decreased (1%)
Libido increased (Infrequent)
Libido, loss (Infrequent)

▲ Memory impairment (4%)
Mental performance, impairment (1% to 2%)
Nervousness (1% to 3%)
Nightmares (Infrequent)
Psychoses
Sleep disturbances (Infrequent)
Speech, slurring
Suicidal ideation (Infrequent)
Suicide, attempt of (Infrequent)

Kogenate FS

Depersonalization

K-Phos

Confusion

Kytril Injection

Agitation (Less than 2%)
Anxiety (Less than 2%)
Central nervous system stimulation (Less than 2%)
Insomnia (Less than 2%)

Kytril Tablets

Anxiety (2%)
▲ Insomnia (3% to 5%)

Lacrisert Sterile Ophthalmic Insert

Photophobia

Lamictal

Agitation (Infrequent)
▲ Anxiety (3.8%)
Apathy (Infrequent)
Central nervous system depression (Infrequent)
Central nervous system stimulation (Rare)
Confusion (1.8%)
Delirium (Rare)
Delusions (Rare)
Depersonalization (Infrequent)
▲ Depression (4.2%)
Disordered sense of smell (Rare)
▲ Double vision (24% to 49%)
Dreaming abnormalities (Infrequent)
Emotional lability (1.3%)
Euphoria (Infrequent)
Hallucinations (Infrequent)
Hostility (Frequent)
▲ Insomnia (5.6%)
▲ Irritability (3.0%)
Libido decreased (Rare)
Libido increased (Rare)

Manic behavior (Rare)
Manic behavior, mild (Rare)
Memory impairment (2.4%)
Mental performance, impairment (1.7%)
Nervousness (Frequent)
Neurosis, unspecified (Rare)
Panic (Infrequent)
Paranoia (Infrequent)
Personality changes (Infrequent)
Photophobia (Infrequent)
Psychoses (Infrequent)
Sleep disturbances (1.4%)
Speech disturbances (2.5%)
Stupor (Infrequent)
Suicidal ideation (Rare)
Suicide, attempt of (Rare)
Thinking abnormality (Frequent)

Lanoxin/Lanoxicaps

Anxiety
Apathy
Central nervous system reactions
Confusion
Delirium
Depression
Hallucinations
Mental status, altered

Lariam Tablets

Anxiety
Central nervous system reactions
Confusion
Depression
Emotional disturbances (Less than 1%)
Hallucinations
Psychoses

Lescol Capsules

Anxiety
Depression
Insomnia (2.7%)
Libido, loss
Memory loss, short-term
Psychiatric disturbances

Lescol XL Tablets

Anxiety
Depression
Insomnia (1.8%)
Libido, loss
Memory loss, short-term
Psychiatric disturbances

Leukeran Tablets

Agitation (Rare)
Confusion (Rare)
Hallucinations (Rare)

Leukine

▲ Anxiety (11%)
▲ Central nervous system reactions (11%)
▲ Insomnia (11%)
▲ Psychiatric disturbances (15%)
▲ Sensory disturbances (6%)

Leustatin Injection

▲ Insomnia (7%)

Levaquin

Aggression (Less than 0.5%)
Agitation (0.5% to less than 1.0%)
Anxiety (0.1% to less than 1.0%)
Central nervous system stimulation
Coma (Less than 0.3%)
Confusion (Less than 0.3%)
Delirium (Less than 0.3%)
Depression (Less than 0.3%)
Disordered sense of smell (Less than 0.5%)
Double vision (Less than 0.3%)
Dreaming abnormalities (Less than 0.3%)
Emotional lability (Less than 0.3%)
Hallucinations (Less than 0.3%)
Insomnia (0.3% to 2.9%)
Manic behavior (Less than 0.3%)
Mental performance, impairment (Less than 0.3%)
Mental status, altered (Less than 0.3%)
Nervousness (0.1% to less than 1.0%)
Nightmares
Paranoia (Less than 0.3%)
Psychoses, toxic
Sleep disturbances (0.1%)
Speech disturbances (Less than 0.3%)
Stupor (Less than 0.3%)
Suicidal ideation (Rare)
Suicide, attempt of (Rare)

Levbid

Agitation
Anxiety
Central nervous system reactions
Coma
Confusion
Disorientation
Euphoria

Excitability
Hallucinations
Insomnia
Manic behavior
Memory loss, short-term
Mental performance, impairment
Nervousness
Psychoses
Speech disturbances
Depression
Double vision (Rare)
Insomnia
Libido, changes
Mood changes
Nervousness
Speech disturbances

Levlite

Depression
Double vision (Rare)
Insomnia
Libido, changes
Mood changes
Nervousness
Speech disturbances

Levo-Dromoran

Central nervous system stimulation
Coma
Confusion
Depression
Double vision
Dreaming abnormalities
Insomnia
Nervousness
Personality changes
Suicide, attempt of
Thinking abnormality

Levora Tablets

Depression
Libido, changes
Nervousness

Levorphanol Tartrate Tablets

▲ Confusion (3% to 9%)
Dreaming abnormalities (1% to 3%)
Mood changes
Nervousness (1% to 3%)
Thinking abnormality (1% to 3%)

Levoxyl Tablets

Anxiety
Emotional lability
Hyperactivity
Insomnia

Irritability
Nervousness

Levsin

Anxiety
Central nervous system reactions
Coma
Confusion
Disorientation
Euphoria
Excitability
Hallucinations
Insomnia
Manic behavior
Memory loss, short-term
Mental performance, impairment
Nervousness
Psychoses
Speech disturbances

Levsin/Levsinex

Agitation

Levulan Kerastick

Impairment of sensation (Up to 2%)

Lexxel Tablets

Agitation
Anxiety
Confusion
Depression
Impairment of sensation
Insomnia
Irritability
Libido decreased
Nervousness

Librium Capsules

Central nervous system stimulation,
  paradoxical
Confusion (Some patients)
Excitement, paradoxical
Libido, changes (Isolated cases)
Rage

Librium for Injection

Confusion
Libido, changes (Isolated cases)

Lidoderm Patch

Central nervous system stimulation
Confusion
Depression
Double vision
Euphoria
Nervousness

Limbitrol

Confusion (Less common)
Delusions
Dreaming (Less common)
Euphoria
Hallucinations
Libido, changes
Manic behavior, mild
Mental performance, impairment

Lindane

Central nervous system stimulation

Lipitor Tablets

Depression (Less than 2%)
Disordered sense of smell (Less than 2%)
Dreaming abnormalities (Less than 2%)
Emotional lability (Less than 2%)
Insomnia (Greater than or equal to 2%)
Libido decreased (Less than 2%)

Liquid PedvaxHIB

Irritability

Lithium

Coma
Confusion
Sleep disturbances
Speech, slurring
Stupor

Lithobid Slow-Release Tablets

Coma
Confusion
Hallucinations
Memory impairment
Mental performance, impairment
Sexual dysfunction
Speech, slurring
Stupor
Thinking abnormality

Lo/Ovral

Depression
Libido, changes
Nervousness

Lodine

Confusion (Less than 1%)
Depression (1% to 3%)
Insomnia (Less than 1%)
Nervousness (1% to 3%)
Photophobia (Less than 1%)

Lodine XL Extended-Release Tablets

Anxiety (Less than 1%)
Coma
Confusion (Less than 1%)
Depression (1% to 3%)
Dreaming abnormalities (Less than 1%)
Hallucinations
Insomnia (Less than 1%)
Nervousness (1% to 3%)
Photophobia (Less than 1%)

Lodosyn Tablets

Agitation
Anxiety
Confusion
Delusions
Dementia
Disorientation
Double vision
Dreaming abnormalities
Euphoria
Hallucinations
Insomnia
Libido increased
Memory impairment
Mental acuity, loss of
Nervousness
Nightmares
Paranoia
Suicidal ideation

Loestrin

Depression
Libido, changes
Nervousness

Lopid Tablets

Confusion
Depression
Libido decreased

Lorabid

Insomnia
Nervousness

Lortab

Anxiety
Fear
Mental clouding
Mental performance, impairment
Mood changes
▲ Sedation (Among most frequent)

Lotemax Ophthalmic Suspension
▲ Photophobia (5% to 15%)

Lotensin HCT Tablets
Dreaming abnormalities (0.3% or more)
Insomnia (0.3% to 1%)
Libido decreased (0.3% to 1%)
Nervousness (0.3% to 1%)

Lotensin Tablets
Anxiety (Less than 1%)
Insomnia (Less than 1%)
Libido increased (Less than 1%)
Nervousness (Less than 1%)

Lotrel Capsules
Anxiety
Insomnia
Libido decreased
Nervousness

Lovenox Injection
Confusion (2.2%)

Low-Ogestrel-28 Tablets
Depression
Libido, changes
Nervousness

Loxitane Capsules
Agitation
Confusion
Insomnia
Mental performance, impairment
Speech, slurring
Tenseness

Lufyllin
Agitation
Hyperexcitability
Insomnia
Irritability

Lufyllin-GG
Agitation
Central nervous system stimulation
Hyperexcitability
Insomnia
Irritability

Lumigan Ophthalmic Solution
Photophobia (1% to 3%)

Lunelle Monthly Injection
Depression
Emotional lability
Libido, changes
Nervousness

Lupron Depot 3.75 mg
Anxiety (Less than 5%)
Confusion
▲ Delusions (Among most frequent)
▲ Depression (10.8%)
Depression, aggravation of (A possibility)
▲ Emotional lability (10.8%)
Insomnia (Less than 5%)
Libido decreased (Less than 5%)
▲ Memory impairment (Among most frequent)
Mood changes
Nervousness (Less than 5%)
▲ Personality changes (Among most frequent)
Suicidal ideation (Very rare)
Suicide, attempt of (Very rare)

Lupron Depot 7.5 mg
Agitation (Less than 5%)
Insomnia (Less than 5%)
▲ Libido decreased (5.4%)
Sleep disturbances (Less than 5%)

Lupron Depot–3 Month 11.25 mg
Agitation
Anxiety (Less than 5%)
Delusions (Less than 5%)
▲ Depression (10.8% to 22%)
Depression, aggravation of (Possible)
▲ Emotional lability (10.8% to 22%)
Insomnia (Less than 5%)
▲ Libido decreased (1.8% to 11%)
Memory impairment (Less than 5%)
▲ Nervousness (4.8% to 5%)
Personality changes (Less than 5%)
Sleep disturbances (Less than 5%)
Suicidal ideation (Very rare)
Suicide, attempt of (Very rare)

Lupron Depot–3 Month 22.5 mg
Anxiety (Less than 5%)
Delusions (Less than 5%)
Depression (Less than 5%)
▲ Insomnia (8.5%)
Libido decreased (Less than 5%)
Nervousness (Less than 5%)
▲ Sleep disturbances (8.5%)

Lupron Depot–4 Month 30 mg
Confusion (Less than 5%)
Dementia (Less than 5%)
Depression (Less than 5%)
Insomnia (Less than 5%)
Libido decreased (Less than 5%)
Sleep disturbances (Less than 5%)
Thinking abnormality (Less than 5%)

Lupron Depot-PED
Emotional lability (Less than 2%)
Nervousness (Less than 2%)
Personality changes (Less than 2%)

Lupron Injection
Anxiety (Less than 5%)
Depression (Less than 5%)
▲ Insomnia (5% or more)
Libido decreased (Less than 5%)
Libido increased
Memory impairment (Less than 5%)
Mood changes (Less than 5%)
Nervousness (Less than 5%)
▲ Sleep disturbances (5% or more)

Lupron Injection Pediatric
Emotional lability (Less than 2%)
Nervousness (Less than 2%)
Personality changes (Less than 2%)

Luvox Tablets
Agitation (2%)
Agoraphobia (Infrequent)
Anxiety (1% to 5%)
Apathy (Frequent)
Central nervous system depression
(Infrequent)
Central nervous system stimulation
(2%)
Coma (Rare)
Confusion
Delirium (Infrequent)
Delusions (Infrequent)
Depersonalization (Infrequent)
Depression (2%)
Disordered sense of smell (Infrequent)
Double vision (Infrequent)
Dreaming abnormalities
Emotional lability (Infrequent)
Euphoria (Infrequent)
Hallucinations (Infrequent)
Hostility (Infrequent)
Hysteria (Infrequent)
▲ Insomnia (4% to 21%)
Libido decreased (2%)
Libido increased (Infrequent)

Manic behavior (Approximately 1%)
Manic behavior, mild (Approximately
1%)
▲ Nervousness (2% to 12%)
Paranoia (Infrequent)
Phobic disorder (Infrequent)
Photophobia (Infrequent)
Psychoses (Infrequent to frequent)
Serotonin syndrome
Sexual dysfunction
Sleep disturbances (Infrequent)
Sleeping, excessive (Infrequent)
Speech, slurring (Rare)
Stupor (Infrequent)
Suicide, attempt of (Infrequent)
Thinking abnormality

LYMErix Vaccine
Coma (Greater than 1%)
Depression (1.02%)

Macrobid Capsules
Confusion (Rare)
Depression (Rare)
Psychoses (Rare)

Macrodantin Capsules
Confusion (Rare)
Depression (Rare)
Psychoses (Rare)

Marinol Capsules
Anxiety (Greater than 1%)
▲ Awareness, heightened (8% to 24%)
Confusion (Greater than 1%)
Depersonalization (Greater than 1%)
Depression (Less than 1%)
▲ Elation (8% to 24%)
▲ Euphoria (3% to 10%)
Hallucinations (Greater than 1%)
▲ Laughing, easy (8% to 24%)
Mood changes
Nervousness (Greater than 1%)
Nightmares (Less than 1%)
▲ Paranoia (3% to 10%)
Speech difficulties (Less than 1%)
▲ Thinking abnormality (3% to 10%)

Matulane Capsules
Coma
Confusion
Depression
Double vision
Hallucinations
Insomnia
Nervousness

Nightmares
Photophobia
Speech, slurring

Mavik Tablets
Anxiety (0.3% to 1.0%)
Insomnia (0.3% to 1.0%)
Libido decreased (0.3% to 1.0%)

Maxair
Anxiety (Less than 1%)
Confusion (Less than 1%)
Depression (Less than 1%)
Insomnia (Less than 1%)
▲ Nervousness (4.5% to 6.9%)
Agitation (Infrequent)
Anxiety (Infrequent)
Confusion (Infrequent)
Depersonalization (Rare)
Depression (Infrequent)
Disorientation (Infrequent)
Dreaming abnormalities (Infrequent)
Euphoria (Frequent)
Hangover (Infrequent)
Impairment of sensation (Rare)
Insomnia (Infrequent)
Irritability (Infrequent)
Memory impairment (Infrequent)
Mental performance, impairment
  (Frequent)
Nervousness (Infrequent)
Photophobia (Rare)
Sleeping, excessive (Rare)

Maxidone Tablets
Anxiety
Fear
Mental clouding
Mental performance, impairment
Mood changes
▲ Sedation (Among most frequent)

Maxzide
Anxiety
Depression
Insomnia
Sexual dysfunction

Megace Oral Suspension
Confusion (1% to 3%)
Depression (1% to 3%)
▲ Insomnia (Up to 6%)
Libido decreased (Up to 5%)
Thinking abnormality (1% to 3%)

Menest Tablets
Depression
Libido, changes

Mepergan Injection
Agitation
Disorientation
Euphoria
Hallucinations
▲ Sedation (Among most frequent)

Mepron Suspension
▲Anxiety (7%)
▲ Insomnia (10% to 19%)

Meridia Capsules
Agitation (Greater than or equal to
  1%)
Anger
▲ Anxiety (4.5%)
Central nervous system stimulation
  (1.5%)
Confusion
▲ Depression (4.3%)
Depression, aggravation of
Dreaming abnormalities
Emotional lability (1.3%)
▲ Insomnia (10.7%)
Libido decreased
Libido increased
Memory loss, short-term
Mental performance, impairment
Mood changes
▲ Nervousness (5.2%)
Nightmares
Serotonin syndrome
Speech disturbances
Thinking abnormality (Greater than or
  equal to 1%)

Merrem I.V.
Agitation (0.1% to 1.0%)
Anxiety (0.1% to 1.0%)
Confusion (0.1% to 1.0%)
Delirium (0.1% to 1.0%)
Depression (0.1% to 1.0%)
Hallucinations (0.1% to 1.0%)
Insomnia (0.1% to 1.0%)
Nervousness (0.1% to 1.0%)

Meruvax II
Irritability

Metadate
Depression
▲ Insomnia (Among most common)

▲ Nervousness (Among most common)
Psychoses, toxic

Methylin
Depression
▲ Insomnia (Among most common)
▲ Nervousness (Among most common)
Psychoses, toxic

MetroGel-Vaginal Gel
Depression (Less than 1%)

Mevacor Tablets
Anxiety (0.5% to 1.0%)
Depression (0.5% to 1.0%)
Insomnia (0.5% to 1.0%)
Libido, loss (0.5% to 1.0%)
Memory loss, short-term (0.5% to
1.0%)

Mexitil Capsules
Confusion (1.9% to 2.6%)
Depression (2.4%)
Hallucinations (About 3 in 1,000)
Libido decreased (Less than 1% or
about 4 in 1,000)
Memory loss, short-term (Less than
1% to about 9 in 1,000)
▲ Nervousness (5% to 11.3%)
Psychoses (Less than 1% or about 2 in
1,000)
Sensorium, clouded (1.9% to 2.6%)
▲ Sleep disturbances (7.1% to 7.5%)
Speech difficulties (2.6%)

Miacalcin Nasal Spray
Agitation (Less than 1%)
Anxiety (Less than 1%)
Depression (1% to 3%)
Disordered sense of smell
(Less than 1%)
Insomnia (Less than 1%)

Micardis HCT Tablets
Anxiety
Depression
Insomnia
Nervousness

Micardis Tablets
Anxiety (More than 0.3%)
Depression (More than 0.3%)
Insomnia (More than 0.3%)

Microgestin Fe
Depression
Libido, changes
Nervousness

Midamor Tablets
Confusion (Less than or equal to 1%)
Depression (Less than or equal to 1%)
Insomnia (Less than or equal to 1%)
Libido decreased (Less than or equal
to 1%)
Nervousness (Less than or equal to
1%)

Migranal Nasal Spray
Anxiety (Rare)
Confusion (Infrequent)
Depression (Rare)
Euphoria (Infrequent)
Insomnia (Infrequent)
Mental performance, impairment
(Infrequent)
Nervousness (Infrequent)
Photophobia (Infrequent)
Speech disturbances (Rare)
Stupor (Rare)

Miltown Tablets
Euphoria
Excitement, paradoxical
Intoxication, chronic
Mental performance, impairment
Overstimulation
Speech, slurring
Suicidal ideation

Minipress Capsules
Depression (1% to 4%)
Hallucinations (Less than 1%)
Insomnia
Nervousness (1% to 4%)

Minizide Capsules
Depression (Rare)
Hallucinations (Rare)
Nervousness

Mintezol
Confusion
Depression
Floating feeling
Hyperirritability
Psychiatric disturbances

Mirapex Tablets
Agitation (1.1%)
Anxiety (1% or more)
Apathy (1% or more)
▲ Confusion (4% to 10%)
Delusions (1%)
Depression (1% or more)

Double vision (1% or more)
▲ Dreaming abnormalities (11%)
▲ Hallucinations (9% to 17%)
▲ Insomnia (17% to 27%)
Libido decreased (1%)
Nervousness (1% or more)
Paranoia (Less than 1%)
Psychoses (1% or more)
Sleep disturbances (1%)
Speech disturbances (1% or more)
Suicide, attempt of (Less than 1%)
Thinking abnormality (2% to 3%)
Libido, changes
Nervousness

Mirena Intrauterine System

▲ Depression (5% or more)
▲ Libido decreased (5% or more)
▲ Nervousness (5% or more)

Mithracin

Depression

M-M-R II

Irritability

Moban

Depression (Less frequent)
Euphoria (Less frequent)
Hyperactivity (Less frequent)
Libido increased
Mental status, altered

Mobic Tablets

Anxiety (Less than 2%)
Confusion (Less than 2%)
Depression (Less than 2%)
Insomnia (0.4% to 3.6%)
Nervousness (Less than 2%)

Modicon

Depression
Double vision (Rare)
Insomnia
Libido, changes
Mood changes
Nervousness
Speech disturbances

Moduretic Tablets

Confusion (Less than or equal to 1%)
Depression (Less than or equal to 1%)
Insomnia (Less than or equal to 1%)
Libido decreased
Nervousness (Less than or equal to 1%)
Stupor (Less than or equal to 1%)

Monopril HCT

Confusion
Depression (Less than 2%)
Libido, changes (Less than 2%)
Memory impairment
Mood changes
Sexual dysfunction (Less than 2%)
Sleep disturbances

Monopril Tablets

Behavioral changes (0.4% to 1.0%)
Confusion (0.2% to 1.0%)
Depression (0.4% to 1.0%)
Insomnia (1.0% or more)
Libido decreased (0.2% to 1.0%)
Memory impairment (0.2% to 1.0%)
Mood changes (0.2% to 1.0%)
Sexual dysfunction (Less than 1.0% to 1.0%)
Sleep disturbances (0.2% to 1.0%)

Monurol Sachet

Insomnia (Less than 1%)
Nervousness (Less than 1%)

Motofen Tablets

Confusion (1 in 200 to 1 in 600)
Depression
Euphoria
Insomnia (1 in 200 to 1 in 600)
Nervousness (1 in 200 to 1 in 600)
Sedation

Motrin

Coma (Rare; less than 1%)
Confusion (Less than 1%)
Depression (Less than 1%)
Double vision (Less than 1%)
Dreaming abnormalities (Less than 1%)
Emotional lability (Less than 1%)
Hallucinations (Less than 1%)
Insomnia (Less than 1%)
Nervousness (1% to less than 3%)

Motrin Sinus Headache Caplets

Insomnia
Nervousness

MS Contin Tablets

Agitation (Less frequent)
Depression (Less frequent)
Disorientation (Less frequent)
Double vision (Less frequent)
Dreaming (Less frequent)

▲ Euphoria (Among most frequent)
Feeling, strange (Less frequent)
Floating feeling (Less frequent)
Hallucinations (Less frequent)
Insomnia (Less frequent)
Libido decreased (Less frequent)
Mental performance, impairment
Mood changes (Less frequent)
Nervousness (Less frequent)
▲ Sedation (Among most frequent)

MSIR
Agitation (Less frequent)
Depression (Less frequent)
Disorientation (Less frequent)
Double vision (Less frequent)
Dreaming (Less frequent)
▲ Euphoria (Among most frequent)
Floating feeling (Less frequent)
Hallucinations (Less frequent)
Insomnia (Less frequent)
Libido decreased (Less frequent)
Mood changes (Less frequent)
Nervousness (Less frequent)
▲ Sedation (Among most frequent)

Mumpsvax
Irritability

Myambutol Tablets
Confusion
Disorientation
Hallucinations

Mycobutin Capsules
Confusion (More than one patient)
Insomnia (1%)

Mykrox Tablets
Anxiety (Less than 2%)
Depression (Less than 2%)
Insomnia
Mental perception, altered
Nervousness (Less than 2%)

Mylocel Tablets
Disorientation (Extremely rare)
Hallucinations (Extremely rare)

Mylotarg for Injection
▲ Depression (8% to 13%)
▲ Insomnia (14% to 22%)

Myobloc Injectable Solution
Anxiety (2% or greater)
Confusion (2% or greater)

Nadolol Tablets
Behavioral changes (6 of 1000 patients)
Catatonia
Depression
Disorientation, place
Disorientation, time
Emotional lability
Hallucinations
Libido decreased (1 to 5 of 1000 patients)
Memory loss, short-term
Neuropsychometrics performance, decrease
Sedation (6 of 1000 patients)
Sensorium, clouded
Sleep disturbances
Speech, slurring (1 to 5 of 1000 patients)

Naprelan Tablets
Anxiety (Less than 1%)
▲ Cognitive dysfunction (3% to 9%)
Confusion (Less than 1%)
Depression (Less than 1%)
Double vision (Less than 1%)
▲ Dreaming abnormalities (3% to 9%)
Emotional lability (Less than 1%)
Insomnia (Less than 3%)
▲ Mental performance, impairment (3% to 9%)
Nervousness (Less than 1%)

Naprosyn
Central nervous system depression (Less than 1%)
Cognitive dysfunction (Less than 1%)
Dreaming abnormalities (Less than 1%)
Insomnia (Less than 1%)
Mental performance, impairment (Less than 1%)

Narcan Injection
Agitation (Infrequent)
Excitability
Irritability
Nervousness

Nardil Tablets
Agitation (Uncommon)
Anxiety (Less frequent)
Coma (Less frequent)
Delirium (Less frequent)
Euphoria (Less common)
Insomnia (Common)

Jitteriness (Less common)
Manic behavior (Less frequent)
▲ Manic behavior, mild (Most common)
Nightmares (Infrequent)
Psychoses (Infrequent)
Schizophrenia, precipitation (Less frequent)
Sexual dysfunction (Common)
Sleep disturbances (Common)
Sleeping, excessive (Common)

Naropin Injection
Agitation (Less than 1%)
Anxiety (1% to 5%)
Coma (Less than 1%)
Confusion (Less than 1%)
Depression
Emotional lability (Less than 1%)
Excitability
Hallucinations (Less than 1%)
Insomnia (Less than 1%)
Nervousness (Less than 1%)
Nightmares (Less than 1%)
Sexual dysfunction
Stupor (Less than 1%)

Nasacort Nasal Inhaler
Depression

Nascobal Gel
Anxiety
Nervousness

Natrecor for Injection
▲ Anxiety (3%)
Confusion (At least 1%)
Insomnia (2%)

Navane
Agitation
Insomnia
Mental status, altered
Psychotic symptoms, paradoxical exacerbation (Infrequent)
Sedation

Navelbine Injection
Auditory disturbances

Nebcin
Confusion
Disorientation

Necon
Depression
Libido, changes
Nervousness

Nembutal
Agitation (Less than 1%)
Anxiety (Less than 1%)
Central nervous system depression (Less than 1%)
Confusion (Less than 1%)
Hallucinations (Less than 1%)
Insomnia (Less than 1%)
Nervousness (Less than 1%)
Nightmares (Less than 1%)
Psychiatric disturbances (Less than 1%)
Thinking abnormality (Less than 1%)

Neoral
Anxiety (1% to less than 3%)
Confusion (1% to less than 3%)
Consciousness, disorders of
Depression (Rare)
Emotional lability (1% to less than 3%)
Insomnia (1% to less than 3%)
Libido decreased (1% to less than 3%)
Libido increased (1% to less than 3%)
Mental performance, impairment (1% to less than 3%)
Nervousness (1% to less than 3%)
Nightmares (1% to less than 3%)
Psychiatric disturbances

Neptazane Tablets
Confusion (Occasional)

Nesacaine
Anxiety
Depression
Excitability
Sensory deficit, persistent
Sexual dysfunction

Neulasta Injection
▲ Insomnia (15% to 72%)

Neumega for Injection
▲ Insomnia (33%)
▲ Nervousness (Greater than or equal to 10%)

Neurontin
Aggression
Agitation (Infrequent)
Anxiety (Frequent)
Apathy (Infrequent)
Behavioral changes
Central nervous system depression
Confusion

Depersonalization (Infrequent)
Depression (1.8%)
▲ Double vision (5.9%)
Dreaming abnormalities (Infrequent)
▲ Emotional lability (4.2% to 6%)
Euphoria (Infrequent)
Feeling, drugged (Infrequent)
Feeling, high (Rare)
Feeling, strange (Rare)
Hallucinations (Infrequent)
Hangover (Rare)
▲ Hostility (5.2% to 7.6%)
Hyperactivity
Hysteria (Rare)
Impairment of sensation (Infrequent)
Libido increased (Rare)
Libido, changes (Infrequent)
Manic behavior (Rare)
Nervousness (2.4%)
Neurosis, unspecified (Rare)
Paranoia (Infrequent)
Personality changes (Rare)
Photophobia (Infrequent)
Psychoses (Infrequent)
Sexual dysfunction (Infrequent)
Sleep walking
Sociopathy (Rare)
Stupor (Infrequent)
Suicidal ideation (Infrequent)
Suicide, attempt of (Rare)
Thinking abnormality (1.7%)

Nexium
Apathy (Less than 1%)
Confusion (Less than 1%)
Depression, aggravation of (Less than 1%)
Disordered sense of smell (Less than 1%)
Insomnia (Less than 1%)
Nervousness (Less than 1%)
Sleep disturbances (Less than 1%)

Niaspan
Insomnia

Nicotrol Nasal Spray
▲ Anxiety (Over 5%)
Apathy (Under 5%)
▲ Confusion (3%)
Depression (Under 5%)
Dreaming (Under 5%)
▲ Emotional lability (Over 5%)
Insomnia
▲ Irritability (Over 5%)

▲ Mental performance, impairment (Over 5%)

Nilandron Tablets
▲ Depression (8.6%)
▲ Insomnia (16.3%)
▲ Libido decreased (11%)
Nervousness (2%)
Photophobia (2%)

Nimotop Capsules
Depression (Up to 1.4%)

Nipent for Injection
▲ Anxiety (3% to 10%)
▲ Central nervous system reactions (1% to 11%)
▲ Depression (3% to 10%)
Dreaming abnormalities (Less than 3%)
Emotional lability (Less than 3%)
Hallucinations (Less than 3%)
Hangover (Less than 3%)
Hostility (Less than 3%)
▲ Insomnia (3% to 10%)
Libido, changes (Less than 3%)
▲ Nervousness (3% to 10%)
Neurosis, unspecified (Less than 3%)
Photophobia (Less than 3%)
Thinking abnormality (Less than 3%)

Nizoral Tablets
Depression (Rare)
Photophobia (Less than 1%)
Psychiatric disturbances (Rare)
Suicidal ideation (Rare)

Nolvadex Tablets
Depression (Infrequent)
Libido, loss

Norco
Anxiety
Fear
Mental clouding
Mental performance, impairment
Mood changes
▲ Sedation (Among most frequent)

Nordette-28 Tablets
Depression
Libido, changes
Nervousness

Norflex
Agitation
Confusion (Infrequent)
Hallucinations

Norinyl
Depression
Double vision
Libido, changes
Nervousness

Normodyne Tablets
Catatonia
Depression
Disorientation, place
Disorientation, time
Emotional lability
Memory loss, short-term
Neuropsychometrics performance,
  decrease
Sensorium, clouded

Noroxin Tablets
Anxiety (Less frequent)
Central nervous system reactions
Central nervous system stimulation
Confusion
Depression (Less frequent)
Double vision
Hallucinations
Insomnia (Less frequent)
Psychiatric disturbances
Psychoses
Sleep disturbances (Less frequent)

Norplant System
Anxiety
Emotional lability (Less than 1%)
Nervousness

Norpramin Tablets
Agitation
Anxiety
Confusion
Delusions
Disorientation
Hallucinations
Insomnia
Libido decreased
Libido increased
Manic behavior, mild
Mental performance, impairment
Nightmares
Psychoses, aggravation

Norvasc Tablets
Agitation (Less than or equal to 0.1%)
Anxiety (More than 0.1% to 1%)
Apathy (Less than or equal to 0.1%)
Depersonalization (More than 0.1% to
  1%)
Depression (More than 0.1% to 1%)
Disordered sense of smell (Less than
  or equal to 0.1%)
Double vision (More than 0.1% to
  1%)
Dreaming abnormalities (More than
  0.1% to 1%)
Insomnia (More than 0.1% to 1%)
Nervousness (More than 0.1% to 1%)
Sexual dysfunction (Less than 1% to
  2%)

Norvir
Agitation (Less than 2%)
Anxiety (Less than 2%)
Confusion (Less than 2%)
Depression (Less than 2%)
Disordered sense of smell (Less than
  2%)
Double vision (Less than 2%)
Dreaming abnormalities (Less than
  2%)
Emotional lability (Less than 2%)
Euphoria (Less than 2%)
Hallucinations (Less than 2%)
Insomnia (1.3% to 2.6%)
Libido decreased (Less than 2%)
Nervousness (Less than 2%)
Personality changes (Less than 2%)
Photophobia (Less than 2%)
Thinking abnormality (Up to 0.7%)

Novantrone for Injection
▲ Anxiety (5%)
▲ Central nervous system reactions
  (30% to 34%)
▲ Libido, changes (4%)

Novarel for Injection
Depression
Irritability

Nubain Injection
Agitation
Confusion (1% or less)
Delusions (1% or less)
Depersonalization (1% or less)
Depression (1% or less)
Dreaming abnormalities (1% or less)
Euphoria (1% or less)
Floating feeling (1% or less)
Hallucinations (1% or less)
Hostility (1% or less)
Nervousness (1% or less)
▲ Sedation (36%)
Speech difficulties (1% or less)

NuLev
Confusion
Excitability
Insomnia
Nervousness
Speech disturbances

Numorphan
Central nervous system stimulation,
paradoxical
Confusion
Depression
Double vision
Euphoria
Hallucinations
Mental clouding
Nervousness
Sleep disturbances

Ocuflox Ophthalmic Solution
Photophobia

Ogen Tablets
Depression
Libido, changes

Ogestrel Tablets
Depression
Libido, changes
Nervousness

Omnicef
Insomnia (0.2%)

Oncaspar
Coma
Confusion (Less than 1%)
Disorientation
Emotional lability (Less than 1%)
Mental status, altered
Mood changes

OptiPranolol
Anxiety(A small number of patients)
Depression (A small number of
patients)
Nervousness (A small number of
patients)
Photophobia (A small number of
patients)

Oramorph SR Tablets
Agitation (Less frequent)
Confusion
Depression (Less frequent)
Disorientation (Less frequent)
Double vision (Less frequent)

Dreaming abnormalities
(Less frequent)
▲ Euphoria (Among most frequent)
Floating feeling (Less frequent)
Hallucinations (Less frequent)
Insomnia (Less frequent)
Libido decreased (Less frequent)
Mood changes (Less frequent)
Nervousness (Less frequent)
▲ Sedation (Among most frequent)

Orap Tablets
▲ Behavioral changes (27.7%)
Central nervous system reactions
▲ Depression (2 of 20 patients)
Dreaming abnormalities (2.7%)
Excitability
▲ Insomnia (2 of 20 patients)
Libido, loss
Mental performance, impairment
Mental status, altered
▲ Nervousness (8.3%)
▲ Sedation (14 of 20 patients)
▲ Speech disturbances (2 of 20 patients)

Orgaran Injection
▲ Insomnia (3.1%)

Ortho Dienestrol Cream
Depression
Libido, changes

Ortho Tri-Cyclen
Depression
Double vision (Rare)
Insomnia
Libido, changes
Mood changes
Nervousness
Speech disturbances

Ortho-Cept
Depression
Libido, changes
Nervousness

Orthoclone OKT3
Agitation
Central nervous system reactions
Cognitive dysfunction
Coma
Combativeness
Confusion
Delirium (Less than 1%)
Disorientation
Double vision
Hallucinations, auditory

Hallucinations, visual
Manic behavior (Less than 1%)
Mental status, altered (Less than 1%)
Mood changes
Paranoia (Less than 1%)
▲ Photophobia (10%)
Psychoses
Stupor

Ortho-Cyclen
Depression
Double vision (Rare)
Insomnia
Libido, changes
Mood changes
Nervousness
Speech disturbances

Ortho-Est Tablets
Depression
Libido, changes
Speech disturbances

Ortho-Novum
Depression
Double vision (Rare)
Insomnia
Libido, changes
Mood changes
Nervousness
Speech disturbances

Ortho-Prefest Tablets
▲ Depression (5%)
Libido, changes

Orudis Capsules
Central nervous system reactions
  (Less than 1%)
Confusion (Less than 1%)
Depression (Greater than 1%)
▲ Dreaming (3% to 9%)
Excitability (Greater than 1%)
Hallucinations (Rare)
▲ Insomnia (3% to 9%)
Libido, changes (Rare)
▲ Nervousness (3% to 9%)
Nightmares (Rare)
Personality changes (Rare)

Oruvail Capsules
Central nervous system reactions
  (Less than 1%)
Confusion (Less than 1%)
Depression (Greater than 1%)
▲ Dreaming (3% to 9%)
Excitability (Greater than 1%)

Hallucinations (Rare)
▲ Insomnia (3% to 9%)
Libido, changes (Rare)
▲ Nervousness (3% to 9%)
Nightmares (Rare)
Personality changes (Rare)

Ovcon
Depression
Double vision
Libido, changes
Nervousness

Ovidrel for Injection
Emotional lability (Less than 2%)
Insomnia (Less than 2%)

Ovral
Depression
Libido, changes
Nervousness

Ovrette Tablets
Depression
Libido, changes
Nervousness

Oxandrin Tablets
Depression
Excitability
Insomnia
Libido, changes

Oxsoralen-Ultra Capsules
Depression
Insomnia
Nervousness

OxyContin Tablets
Agitation (Less than 1%)
Anxiety (Between 1% and 5%)
Confusion (Between 1% and 5%)
Depersonalization (Less than 1%)
Depression (Less than 1%)
Dreaming abnormalities
  (Between 1% and 5%)
Emotional lability (Less than 1%)
Euphoria Between (1% and 5%)
Hallucinations (Less than 1%)
Insomnia (Between 1% and 5%)
Libido decreased
Nervousness (Between 1% and 5%)
Speech disturbances (Less than 1%)
Stupor (Less than 1%)
Thinking abnormality
  (Between 1% and 5%)

OxyFast Oral Concentrate Solution

Euphoria
▲ Sedation (Among most frequent)

OxyIR Capsules

Euphoria
▲ Sedation (Among most frequent)

Pacerone Tablets

Insomnia (1% to 3%)
Libido decreased (1% to 3%)
▲ Photophobia (4% to 9%)
Sleep disturbances (1% to 3%)

Parafon Forte DSC Caplets

Overstimulation (Occasional)

Paraplatin for Injection

▲ Central nervous system reactions (5%)
▲ Sensory disturbances (4% to 6%)

Parnate Tablets

Agitation
Anxiety
Confusion
Disorientation
Insomnia
Manic behavior
Memory loss, short-term
Overstimulation

Paxil

Agitation (1.1% to 5%)
Alcohol abuse (Infrequent)
▲ Anxiety (5% to 5.9%)
Bulimia (Rare)
Central nervous system stimulation
   (Frequent)
Confusion (1%)
Delirium (Rare)
Delusions (Rare)
Depersonalization (Infrequent)
Depression (Frequent)
Depression, psychotic (Rare)
Disordered sense of smell (Rare)
Double vision (Rare)
▲ Dreaming abnormalities (4%)
Emotional disturbances (Infrequent)
Emotional lability (Frequent)
Euphoria (Rare)
Feeling, drugged (2%)
Hallucinations (Infrequent)
Hostility (Infrequent)
Hysteria (Rare)
▲ Insomnia (1.3% to 24%)
▲ Libido decreased (3% to 9%)

Libido increased (Rare)
Manic behavior (Infrequent)
Manic behavior, mild
   (Approximately 1.0%)
Mental performance, impairment
   (Frequent)
▲ Nervousness (4% to 9%)
Neurosis, unspecified (Infrequent)
Paranoia (Infrequent)
Photophobia (Rare)
Psychoses (Rare)
Sensory disturbances
Serotonin syndrome
▲ Sexual dysfunction (3.7% to 10.0%)
Sociopathy (Rare)
Stupor (Rare)
Suicide, attempt of
Thinking abnormality (Infrequent)

PediaCare Multisymptom Cold Liquid

Excitability

PediaCare NightRest Cough-Cold Liquid

Excitability

Pediapred Oral Solution

Emotional lability
Psychoses
Psychoses, aggravation

Pediatric Vicks 44m Cough & Cold Relief

Excitability
Insomnia
Nervousness

Pediazole Suspension

Anxiety
Depression
Disorientation
Hallucinations
Insomnia
Psychoses

PEG-Intron Powder for Injection

▲ Anxiety (28%)
▲ Depression (29%)
▲ Emotional lability (28%)
▲ Insomnia (23%)
▲ Irritability (28%)
Suicidal ideation
   (Less than or equal to 1%)
Suicide, attempt of

(Less than or equal to 1%)

Pentasa Capsules
Depression (Less than 1%)
Insomnia (Less than 1%)

Pepcid
Agitation (Infrequent)
Anxiety (Infrequent)
Confusion (Infrequent)
Depression (Infrequent)
Hallucinations (Infrequent)
Insomnia (Infrequent)
Libido decreased (Infrequent)
Psychiatric disturbances (Infrequent)

Percocet Tablets
Euphoria
Mental performance, impairment
▲ Sedation (Among most frequent)

Percodan Tablets
Euphoria
Mental performance, impairment
▲ Sedation (Among most frequent)

Percolone Tablets
Euphoria
Mental performance, impairment
▲ Sedation (Among most frequent)

Periactin Tablets
Confusion (No incidence data in labeling)
Double vision (No incidence data in labeling)
Euphoria (No incidence data in labeling)
Excitability (No incidence data in labeling)
Hallucinations (No incidence data in labeling)
Hysteria (No incidence data in labeling)
Insomnia (No incidence data in labeling)
Irritability (No incidence data in labeling)
Nervousness (No incidence data in labeling)
Sedation (No incidence data in labeling)

Permax Tablets
Agitation (Infrequent)
▲ Anxiety (6.4%)
Apathy (Infrequent)

Coma (Infrequent)
▲ Confusion (11.1%)
Consciousness, disorders of
Delusions (Infrequent)
▲ Depression (3.2%)
Double vision (2.1%)
Dreaming abnormalities (2.7%)
Emotional lability (Infrequent)
Euphoria (Infrequent)
▲ Hallucinations (13.8%)
Hostility (Infrequent)
▲ Insomnia (7.9%)
Libido decreased (Infrequent)
Libido increased (Infrequent)
Manic behavior (Infrequent)
Nervousness (Frequent)
Neurosis, unspecified (Infrequent)
Paranoia (Frequent)
Personality changes (2.1%)
Photophobia (Infrequent)
Psychoses (2.1%; frequent)
Speech disturbances (1.1%)
Stupor (Rare)
Thinking abnormality (Frequent)

Pfizerpen for Injection
Coma

Phenergan Injection
Catatonia
Double vision
Euphoria
Excitability
Hysteria
Insomnia
Mental performance, impairment
Nervousness

Phenergan Suppositories
Catatonia
Confusion
Disorientation
Double vision
Euphoria
Excitability
Hallucinations
Hysteria
Insomnia
Mental performance, impairment
Nervousness
Sedation

Phenergan Syrup
Confusion (Rare)
Disorientation
Mental performance, impairment

Sedation

Phenergan Tablets
Catatonia
Double vision
Euphoria
Excitability
Hallucinations
Hysteria
Insomnia
Mental performance, impairment
Nervousness

Phenergan VC Syrup
Anxiety
Confusion (Rare)
Disorientation
Insomnia
Mental performance, impairment
Nervousness
Sedation

Phenergan VC with Codeine Syrup
Anxiety
Central nervous system depression
Confusion (Rare)
Disorientation
Euphoria
Hallucinations
Mental performance, impairment
Nervousness
Sedation

Phenergan with Codeine Syrup
Central nervous system depression
Confusion (Rare)
Disorientation
Euphoria
Hallucinations
Mental performance, impairment
Sedation

Phenergan with Dextromethorphan Syrup
Confusion (Rare)
Disorientation
Insomnia
Mental performance, impairment
Sedation

PhosLo
Coma
Confusion
Delirium

Stupor

Photofrin for Injection
▲ Anxiety (7%)
▲ Confusion (8%)
Double vision
▲ Insomnia (14%)
Photophobia

Phrenilin
Agitation (Infrequent)
Confusion
Depression
Euphoria (Infrequent)
Excitability (Infrequent)
▲ Feeling, intoxicated (Among most frequent)
▲ Sedation (Among most frequent)
Sluggishness (Infrequent)

Plaquenil Tablets
Emotional disturbances
Irritability
Nervousness
Nightmares
Photophobia (Fairly common)
Psychoses

Plavix Tablets
Anxiety (1% to 2.5%)
▲ Depression (3.6%)
Insomnia (1% to 2.5%)

Plendil
Anxiety (0.5% to 1.5%)
Depression (0.5% to 1.5%)
Insomnia (0.5% to 1.5%)
Irritability (0.5% to 1.5%)
Libido decreased (0.5% to 1.5%)
Nervousness (0.5% to 1.5%)

Pletal Tablets
Anxiety (Less than 2%)
Double vision (Less than 2%)
Insomnia (Less than 2%)

Podocon-25 Liquid
Coma

Polocaine
Anxiety
Depression
Excitability
Sexual dysfunction

Polocaine-MPF
Anxiety
Depression

Excitability
Sexual dysfunction

Ponstel Capsules
Coma (Rare)
Confusion (Occasional)
Depression (Occasional)
Dreaming abnormalities (Occasional)
Hallucinations (Rare)
Insomnia (Occasional)
Nervousness (Occasional)

Pravachol Tablets
Anxiety
Depression
Insomnia
Libido, loss
Memory loss, short-term

Prednisone
Depression
Euphoria
Insomnia
Mood changes
Personality changes
Psychiatric disturbances
Psychoses
Psychoses, aggravation

Pregnyl for Injection
Depression
Irritability

Prelone Syrup
Depression
Emotional disturbances
Euphoria
Insomnia
Mood changes
Personality changes
Psychoses
Psychoses, aggravation

Premarin
Depression
Libido, changes

Premphase Tablets
Depression
Double vision
Insomnia
Libido, changes
Nervousness

Prempro Tablets
▲ Depression (6% to 11%)
Double vision

Insomnia
Libido, changes
Nervousness

Prevacid
Agitation (Less than 1%)
Anxiety (Less than 1%)
Apathy (Less than 1%)
Confusion (Less than 1%)
Depersonalization (Less than 1%)
Depression (Less than 1%)
Disordered sense of smell (Less than 1%)
Double vision (Less than 1%)
Dreaming abnormalities (Less than 1%)
Emotional lability (Less than 1%)
Hallucinations (Less than 1%)
Hostility (Less than 1%)
Libido decreased (Less than 1%)
Libido increased (Less than 1%)
Nervousness (Less than 1%)
Neurosis, unspecified (Less than 1%)
Photophobia (Less than 1%)
Sleep disturbances (Less than 1%)
Speech disturbances (Less than 1%)
Thinking abnormality (Less than 1%)

Prevnar for Injection
▲ Irritability (68.9% to 72.8%)
▲ Sleep disturbances (18.1% to 33.3%)

Prevpac
Agitation (Less than 1%)
Anxiety (Less than 1%)
Apathy (Less than 1%)
Behavioral changes
Confusion (Less than 1% to 3%)
Depersonalization
Depression (Less than 1%)
Disordered sense of smell (Less than 1%)
Disorientation
Double vision (Less than 1%)
Dreaming abnormalities (Less than 1%)
Emotional lability (Less than 1%)
Hallucinations (Less than 1%)
Hostility (Less than 1%)
Insomnia
Libido decreased (Less than 1%)
Libido increased (Less than 1%)
Nervousness (Less than 1%)
Neurosis, unspecified (Less than 1%)
Nightmares

Photophobia (Less than 1%)
Psychoses
Sleep disturbances (Less than 1%)
Speech disturbances
Thinking abnormality (Less than 1%)

Priftin Tablets
Aggression (Less than 1%)
Behavioral changes

Prilosec
Aggression (Less than 1%)
Anxiety (Less than 1%)
Apathy (Less than 1%)
Confusion (Less than 1%)
Depression (Less than 1%)
Dreaming abnormalities (Less than 1%)
Hallucinations (Less than 1%)
Impairment of sensation, one side of face (Less than 1%)
Insomnia (Less than 1%)
Nervousness (Less than 1%)
Psychiatric disturbances (Less than 1%)

Primatene Tablets
Insomnia
Nervousness

Primaxin
Confusion (Less than 0.2%)
Hallucinations
Psychiatric disturbances (Less than 0.2%)

Prinivil Tablets
Confusion (0.3% to 1.0%)
Depression (Greater than 1%)
Double vision (0.3% to 1.0%)
Impairment of sensation (0.3% to 1.0%)
Insomnia (0.3% to 1.0%)
Irritability (0.3% to 1.0%)
Libido decreased (0.4%)
Memory impairment (0.3% to 1.0%)
Nervousness (0.3% to 1.0%)
Photophobia (0.3% to 1.0%)
Sleeping, excessive (0.3% to 1.0%)

Prinzide Tablets
Confusion
Depression (0.3% to 1%)
Double vision
Impairment of sensation
Insomnia

Irritability
Libido decreased (0.3% to 1%)
Memory impairment
Nervousness
Photophobia
Sleeping, excessive

ProAmatine Tablets
Anxiety (Less frequent)
Confusion (Less frequent)
Insomnia (Rare)
Nervousness (Less frequent)
Thinking abnormality (Less frequent)

Procanbid Extended-Release Tablets
Depression (Occasional)
Hallucinations (Occasional)
Psychoses (Occasional)

Procardia Capsules
Depression (Less than 0.5%)
Jitteriness (2% or less)
▲ Mood changes (7%)
▲ Nervousness (2% or less to 7%)
Paranoia (Less than 0.5%)
Sexual dysfunction (2% or less)
Sleep disturbances (2% or less)

Procardia XL Tablets
Anxiety (1% or less)
Depression (1% or less)
Insomnia (Less than 3%)
Libido decreased (1% or less)
▲ Mood changes (7%)
▲ Nervousness (Less than 3% to 7%)
Nightmares (1% or less)

Procrit for Injection
▲ Anxiety (2% to 11%)
▲ Insomnia (13% to 21%)

Prograf
▲ Agitation (3% to 15%)
▲ Anxiety (3% to 15%)
Coma
▲ Confusion (3% to 15%)
Delirium
▲ Depression (3% to 15%)
▲ Dreaming abnormalities (3% to 15%)
▲ Emotional lability (3% to 15%)
▲ Hallucinations (3% to 15%)
▲ Insomnia (32% to 64%)
▲ Mental status, altered (Approximately 55%)
▲ Nervousness (3%)
▲ Psychoses (3% to 15%)

▲ Sensory disturbances (Approximately 55%)
▲ Thinking abnormality (3% to 15%)

Proleukin for Injection
Agitation
▲ Anxiety (12%)
Coma (1%)
▲ Confusion (34%)
Depression (Less than 1%)
Insomnia
Irritability
▲ Mental status, altered (73%)
▲ Sensory disturbances (10%)
▲ Speech disturbances (7%)
Suicide, attempt of

Prometrium Capsules
Anxiety (Less than 5%)
Confusion (Less than 5%)
▲ Depression (Less than 5% to 19%)
▲ Emotional lability (6%)
Insomnia (Less than 5%)
▲ Irritability (5% to 8%)
Mental performance, impairment (Less than 5%)
Nervousness
Personality changes (Less than 5%)
Speech disturbances (Less than 5%)

Propecia Tablets
Libido decreased (1.8%)

Proscar Tablets
▲ Libido decreased (3.3%)

ProSom Tablets
Agitation (Infrequent)
Anxiety (Frequent)
Apathy (Infrequent)
Behavior, inappropriate
Confusion (2%)
Depression (2%)
Double vision (Rare)
Dreaming abnormalities (2%)
Emotional lability (Infrequent)
Euphoria (Infrequent)
Excitement, paradoxical
Hallucinations (Rare)
▲ Hangover (3%)
Hostility (Infrequent)
Libido decreased (Rare)
Mental performance, impairment
▲ Nervousness (8%)
Photophobia (Infrequent)
Sleep disturbances (Infrequent)
Stupor (Infrequent)

Thinking abnormality (2%)

Prostin E2 Suppositories
Tenseness

Protonix
Anxiety (Greater than or equal to 1%)
Confusion (Less than 1%)
Depression (Less than 1%)
Double vision (Less than 1%)
Dreaming abnormalities (Less than 1%)
Emotional lability (Less than 1%)
Hallucinations (Less than 1%)
Insomnia (Greater than or equal to 1%)
Libido decreased (Less than 1%)
Nervousness (Less than 1%)
Sleep disturbances (Less than 1%)
Speech disturbances
Thinking abnormality (Less than 1%)

Protopam Chloride for Injection
Double vision
Excitability (Several cases)
Manic behavior (Several cases)

Protopic Ointment
Depression (Greater than or equal to 1%)
Insomnia (Up to 4%)

Proventil HFA Inhalation Aerosol
Anxiety (Less than 3%)
Central nervous system stimulation
Depression (Less than 3%)
Insomnia
▲ Nervousness (7%)

Proventil Inhalation Aerosol
Central nervous system stimulation
Insomnia
▲ Nervousness (Less than 10%)

Proventil Inhalation Solution 0.083%
Insomnia (1% to 3.1%)
▲ Nervousness (4%)

Proventil Repetabs Tablets
Central nervous system stimulation
▲ Insomnia (2% to 11%)
Irritability (Less than 1%)
▲ Nervousness (2% to 20%)

Proventil Solution for Inhalation 0.5%
Insomnia (1% to 3.1%)
▲ Nervousness (4%)

Provera Tablets
Depression
Double vision
Insomnia
Libido, changes
Nervousness

Provigil Tablets
▲ Anxiety (4%)
Confusion (1%)
▲ Depression (4%)
Emotional lability (1%)
Hallucinations (At least 1%)
▲ Insomnia (3%)
Libido decreased (At least 1%)
▲ Nervousness (8%)
Sleep disturbances (At least 1%)
Thinking abnormality (At least 1%)

Prozac
Agitation (Frequent)
▲ Anxiety (2% to 28%)
Apathy (Infrequent)
Behavior, violent
Central nervous system depression (Infrequent)
Central nervous system stimulation (Infrequent)
Coma (Rare)
Confusion (Frequent)
Delusions (Rare)
Depersonalization (Infrequent)
Depression (Less than 1%)
Disordered sense of smell (Rare)
Double vision (Rare)
▲ Dreaming abnormalities (Less than 1% to 5%)
Emotional lability (Frequent)
Euphoria (Infrequent)
Hallucinations (Infrequent)
Hostility (Infrequent)
▲ Insomnia (1% to 33%)
▲ Libido decreased (3% to 11%)
Libido increased (Infrequent)
Manic behavior (0.1% to 0.8%)
Manic behavior, mild (0.1% to 0.8%)
Mental performance, impairment
▲ Nervousness (11% to 16%)
Neurosis, unspecified (Infrequent)
Orgasmic dysfunction, female
Paranoia (Infrequent)
Personality changes (Infrequent)
Photophobia (Infrequent)
Psychoses (Infrequent)
Serotonin syndrome
Sexual dysfunction
Sleep disturbances (Frequent)
Sociopathy (Rare)
Stupor (Rare)
Suicidal ideation (Less than 1%)
Suicide, attempt of (Frequent)
Thinking abnormality (Less than 1%)

Pulmicort Respules
Aggression (Less than 1%)
Anxiety (Less than 1%)
Depression (Less than 1%)
Emotional lability (1% to 3%)
Irritability (Less than 1%)
Psychiatric disturbances (Less than 1%)
Psychoses (Less than 1%)

Pulmicort Turbuhaler Powder
Aggression (Rare)
Anxiety (Rare)
Depression (Rare)
Insomnia (1% to 3%)
Irritability (Rare)
Psychiatric disturbances (Rare)
Psychoses (Rare)

Quinaglute Dura-Tabs Tablets
Confusion
Delirium
Depression
Double vision
Photophobia
Psychoses

Quinidex Extentabs
Confusion
Delirium
Depression (Occasional)
Double vision
Nervousness (2%)
Photophobia
Psychoses
▲ Sleep disturbances (3%)

Quixin Ophthalmic Solution
Photophobia (1% to 3%)

Rapamune
▲ Anxiety (3% to 20%)
▲ Confusion (3% to 20%)
▲ Depression (3% to 20%)

▲ Emotional lability (3% to 20%)
▲ Insomnia (13% to 22%)

Rebetol Capsules
▲ Depression (23% to 36%)
▲ Emotional lability (7% to 12%)
▲ Insomnia (26% to 39%)
▲ Irritability (23% to 32%)
▲ Mental performance, impairment (10% to 14%)
▲ Nervousness (4% to 5%)

Rebetron Combination Therapy
▲ Depression (23% to 36%)
▲ Emotional lability (7% to 12%)
▲ Insomnia (26% to 39%)
▲ Irritability (23% to 32%)
  Mental performance, impairment
▲ Nervousness (4% to 5%)
  Suicidal ideation (Less than 1%)
  Suicide, attempt of (Less than 1%)

Recombivax HB
  Agitation
  Insomnia (Less to greater than 1%)
  Irritability (Greater than 1%)
  Sleep disturbances (Less than 1%)

ReFacto Vials
  Insomnia

Reglan
  Agitation
  Anxiety
  Confusion (Less frequent)
  Consciousness, disorders of
  Depression (Less frequent)
  Hallucinations (Rare)
  Insomnia (Less frequent)
  Jitteriness
  Suicidal ideation (Less frequent)

Relafen Tablets
  Agitation (1%)
  Anxiety (Less than 1%)
  Confusion (Less than 1%)
  Depression (Less than 1%)
  Insomnia (1% to 3%)
  Nervousness (1% to 3%)
  Nightmares (Less than 1%)

Remeron
  Agitation (Frequent)
  Anxiety (Frequent)
  Apathy (Frequent)
  Confusion (2%)

  Delirium (Infrequent)
  Delusions (Infrequent)
  Dementia (Rare)
  Depersonalization (Infrequent)
  Depression (Frequent)
  Depression, psychotic (Rare)
  Disordered sense of smell (Rare)
  Double vision (Rare)
▲ Dreaming abnormalities (4%)
  Emotional lability (Infrequent)
  Euphoria (Infrequent)
  Hallucinations (Infrequent)
  Hostility (Infrequent)
  Libido increased (Infrequent)
  Manic behavior (Approximately 0.2%)
  Manic behavior, mild (Approximately 0.2%)
  Mental performance, impairment
  Neurosis, unspecified (Infrequent)
  Paranoia (Infrequent)
  Stupor (Rare)
  Suicidal ideation
▲ Thinking abnormality (3%)

Remicade for IV Injection
  Anxiety (Less than 2%)
  Confusion (Less than 2%)
  Delirium (Less than 2%)
  Depression (Less than 2%)
  Suicide, attempt of (Less than 2%)

Reminyl
  Agitation (Greater than or equal to 2%)
  Anxiety (Greater than or equal to 2%)
  Apathy (Infrequent)
  Confusion (Greater than or equal to 2%)
  Delirium (Infrequent)
▲ Depression (7%)
  Hallucinations (Greater than or equal to 2%)
▲ Insomnia (5%)
  Libido increased (Infrequent)
  Nightmares (Infrequent)
  Paranoia (Infrequent)

ReoPro Vials
  Agitation (0.7%)
  Anxiety (1.7%)
  Coma (0.4%)
  Confusion (0.6%)
  Double vision (0.1%)
  Insomnia (0.3%)
  Thinking abnormality (2.1%)

Requip Tablets

Aggression (Infrequent)
Agitation (Infrequent)
Anxiety (1% or more)
Apathy (Infrequent)
Coma (Infrequent)
▲ Confusion (5%)
Delirium (Infrequent)
Delusions (Infrequent)
Dementia (Infrequent)
Depersonalization (Infrequent)
Depression (1% or more)
Double vision (2%)
▲ Dreaming abnormalities (11%)
Emotional lability (Infrequent)
Euphoria (Infrequent)
▲ Hallucinations (5% to 10%)
Insomnia (1% or more)
Libido decreased (Infrequent)
Libido increased (Infrequent)
Manic behavior (Infrequent)
Mental performance, impairment (Infrequent)
Nervousness (1% or more)
Neurosis, unspecified (Infrequent)
Paranoia (Infrequent)
Personality changes (Infrequent)
Photophobia (Infrequent)
Sleep walking (Infrequent)
Stupor (Infrequent)
Suicide, attempt of (Rare)

Rescriptor Tablets

Agitation (Less than 2%)
Cognitive dysfunction (Less than 2%)
Confusion (Less than 2%)
Depressive reactions (Less than 2%)
Disordered sense of smell
Disorientation (Less than 2%)
Double vision (Less than 2%)
Dreaming abnormalities (Less than 2%)
Emotional lability (Less than 2%)
Euphoria
Hallucinations (Less than 2%)
Insomnia (Less than 2%)
Libido decreased (Less than 2%)
Manic behavior (Less than 2%)
Mental performance, impairment (Less than 2%)
Nervousness (Less than 2%)
Nightmares (Less than 2%)
Paranoia (Less than 2%)
Photophobia (Less than 2%)

Sleep disturbances

Rescula Ophthalmic Solution

Double vision (Less than 1%)
Insomnia (1% to 5%)
Photophobia (1% to 5%)

Retrovir Capsules, Tablets & Syrup

Anxiety
Confusion
Depression
Emotional lability
▲ Insomnia (2.4% to 5%)
Irritability (1.6%)
Mental acuity, loss of
Nervousness (1.6%)
Photophobia

Retrovir IV Infusion

Anxiety
Confusion
Depression
Emotional lability
▲ Insomnia (3% to 5%)
Irritability (2%)
Manic behavior
Mental acuity, loss of
Nervousness (2%)
Photophobia

Rev-Eyes Eyedrops

▲ Photophobia (10% to 40%)

Rhinocort Nasal Inhaler

Aggression (Rare)
Anxiety (Rare)
Depression (Rare)
Irritability (Rare)
Nervousness (Less than 1%)
Psychoses (Rare)

Rifadin

Behavioral changes
Confusion
Mental performance, impairment
Psychoses (Rare)

Rifamate Capsules

Confusion
Memory impairment (Uncommon)
Mental performance, impairment
Psychoses, toxic (Uncommon)

Rifater Tablets

Anxiety
Behavioral changes

Confusion
Insomnia
Memory impairment (Uncommon)
Mental performance, impairment
Psychoses, toxic (Uncommon)

Rilutek Tablets
Agitation (Frequent)
Apathy (Infrequent)
Central nervous system depression
   (Rare)
Coma (Infrequent)
Confusion (Infrequent)
Delirium (Infrequent)
Delusions (Infrequent)
Dementia (Rare)
Depersonalization (Infrequent)
▲ Depression (4.2% to 6.1%)
Depression, psychotic (Rare)
Double vision (Rare)
Dreaming abnormalities (Rare)
Emotional lability (Infrequent)
Euphoria (Rare)
Hallucinations (Infrequent)
Hostility (Frequent)
Insomnia (2.1% to 2.9%)
Libido decreased (Infrequent)
Libido increased (Infrequent)
Manic behavior (Infrequent)
Paranoia (Infrequent)
Personality changes (Infrequent)
Photophobia (Rare)
Psychoses (Rare)
Stupor (Infrequent)
Suicide, attempt of (Infrequent)
Thinking abnormality (Infrequent)

Risperdal
Aggression (1% to 3%)
▲ Agitation (22% to 26%)
▲ Anxiety (12% to 20%)
Apathy (Infrequent)
Catatonia (Infrequent)
Cognitive dysfunction
Coma (Rare)
Confusion (Infrequent)
Delirium (Rare)
Depression (Infrequent)
Double vision (Rare)
Dreaming abnormalities (Frequent)
Emotional lability (Rare)
Euphoria (Infrequent)
▲ Insomnia (23% to 26%)
Libido increased (Infrequent)
Manic behavior

Mental performance, impairment
   (Infrequent)
Mental status, altered
Nervousness (Frequent)
Nightmares (Rare)
Photophobia (Rare)
Sexual activity, decrease (Frequent)
Sexual dysfunction (Frequent)
Sleep disturbances (Frequent)
Stupor (Infrequent)
Suicide, attempt of (1.2%)

Ritalin
Behavior, inappropriate
Depression
▲ Insomnia (One of the two most
   common)
▲ Nervousness (One of the two most
   common)
Psychoses
Psychoses, toxic

Rituxan
Agitation (1% to 5%)
▲ Depression (Among most frequent)
Insomnia (1% to 5%)
Nervousness (1% to 5%)

Robaxin Injectable
Confusion
Double vision

Robaxin Tablets
Confusion
Double vision
Insomnia

Robinul Injectable
Confusion
Excitability
Insomnia
Nervousness

Robinul Tablets
Confusion
Insomnia
Nervousness

Robitussin Cough & Cold
Insomnia
Nervousness

Robitussin Honey Flu Nighttime Liquid
Excitability

Robitussin Pediatric Cough & Cold
Insomnia
Nervousness

Robitussin-CF Liquid
Insomnia
Nervousness

Robitussin-DAC Syrup
Insomnia
Nervousness

Robitussin-PE Liquid
Insomnia
Nervousness

Rocaltrol
Libido decreased
Photophobia
Psychoses (Rare)

Roferon-A Injection
Agitation
▲ Anxiety (5% to 6%)
Apathy (Infrequent)
▲ Behavioral changes (3%)
Central nervous system reactions
(Less than 5%)
Coma (Rare to infrequent)
▲ Confusion (Less than 4% to 8%)
▲ Depression (16% to 28%)
Emotional lability (Less than 3%)
Hallucinations (Infrequent)
Hyperactivity (Infrequent)
▲ Insomnia (14%)
▲ Irritability (Less than 5% to 15%)
Libido, changes (Less than 4%)
Libido, loss (Infrequent)
Manic behavior
Memory impairment (Less than 4%)
▲ Mental performance, impairment (4%)
▲ Mental status, altered (10% to 17%)
Nervousness (Less than 3% to less
than 5%)
Neuropsychiatric disorders, life-
threatening, aggravation of
Psychoses
Sedation (Infrequent)
Sexual dysfunction (Infrequent)
▲ Sleep disturbances (5% to 11%)
Suicidal ideation
Suicide, attempt of

Romazicon Injection
▲ Agitation (3% to 9%)
▲ Anxiety (3% to 9%)

Confusion (Less than 1%)
Delirium (Less than 1%)
Depersonalization (1% to 3%)
Depression (1% to 3%)
Double vision (1% to 3%)
Emotional lability (1% to 3%)
Euphoria (1% to 3%)
▲ Insomnia (3% to 9%)
▲ Nervousness (3% to 9%)
Paranoia (1% to 3%)
Speech disturbances (Less than 1%)
Stupor (Less than 1%)

Rowasa Rectal Suspension Enema
Insomnia (0.12%)

Roxanol
Agitation
Confusion
Disorientation
Euphoria
Insomnia
▲ Sedation (Among most frequent)

Roxanol 100
Agitation
Confusion
Disorientation
Euphoria
Insomnia
Libido decreased
▲ Sedation (Among most frequent)

Roxanol-T
Agitation
Confusion
Disorientation
Euphoria
Insomnia
▲ Sedation (Among most frequent)

Roxicodone Intensol
Confusion
Euphoria
▲ Sedation (Among most frequent)

Roxicodone Oral Solution
Confusion
Euphoria
▲ Sedation (Among most frequent)

Roxicodone Tablets
Agitation (Less than 3%)
Anxiety (Less than 3%)
Confusion (Less than 3%)
Euphoria

▲ Insomnia (Greater than or equal to 3%)
Nervousness (Less than 3%)
Personality changes (Less than 3%)

Rum-K
Listlessness

Ryna-12 S Suspension
Excitability
▲ Sedation (Among most common)

Rynatan Pediatric Suspension
Excitability
▲ Sedation (Among most common)

Rynatan Tablets
Anxiety
Central nervous system depression
Confusion
Euphoria
Excitability
Fear
Hallucinations
Hysteria
Insomnia
Irritability
Nervousness
▲ Sedation (Among most common)

Rynatuss
Excitability
▲ Sedation (Among most common)

Rythmol Tablets
Anxiety (1.5% to 2.0%)
Coma (Less than 1%)
Confusion (Less than 1%)
Depression (Less than 1%)
Dreaming abnormalities
(Less than 1%)
Insomnia (1.5%)
Manic behavior (Less than 1%)
Memory loss, short-term
(Less than 1%)
Psychoses (Less than 1%)
Speech disturbances (Less than 1%)

Salagen Tablets
Agitation (Rare)
Anxiety (Less than 1%)
Confusion (Less than 1%)
Delusions (Rare)
Depression (Less than 1%)
Dreaming abnormalities (Less than 1%)
Emotional lability (Less than 1%)

Hallucinations, visual (Rare)
Insomnia (Less than 1%)
Nervousness (Less than 1%)
Speech disturbances (Less than 1%)
Thinking abnormality (Less than 1%)

Sandimmune
Anxiety (Rare)
Confusion (2% or less)
Consciousness, disorders of
Depression (Rare)
Psychiatric disturbances

Sandoglobulin I.V
Photophobia

Sandostatin Injection
Anxiety (Less than 1%)
Depression (1% to 4%)
Libido decreased (Less than 1%)
Paranoia (Less than 1%)

Sandostatin LAR Depot
▲ Anxiety (5% to 15%)
▲ Confusion (5% to 15%)
▲ Depression (5% to 15%)
Hallucinations (1% to 4%)
▲ Insomnia (5% to 15%)
Libido decreased (Rare)
Nervousness (1% to 4%)
Paranoia (Rare)
Suicide, attempt of (Rare)

Sarafem Pulvules
Agitation (Frequent)
▲ Anxiety (13%)
Apathy (Infrequent)
Behavior, violent
Central nervous system depression
(Infrequent)
Central nervous system stimulation
(Infrequent)
Coma (Rare)
Confusion (Frequent)
Delusions (Rare)
Depersonalization (Infrequent)
Disordered sense of smell (Rare)
Double vision (Rare)
▲ Dreaming abnormalities (3%)
Emotional lability (Frequent)
Euphoria (Infrequent)
Hallucinations (Infrequent)
Hostility (Infrequent)
▲ Insomnia (9% to 24%)
▲ Libido decreased (4%)

Libido increased (Infrequent)
Manic behavior, mild
▲ Nervousness (7% to 14%)
Neurosis, unspecified (Infrequent)
Orgasmic dysfunction, female
Paranoia (Infrequent)
Personality changes (Infrequent)
Photophobia (Infrequent)
Psychoses (Infrequent)
Sexual dysfunction
Sleep disturbances (Frequent)
Sociopathy (Rare)
Stupor (Rare)
Suicidal ideation
Suicide, attempt of (Infrequent)
▲ Thinking abnormality (3% to 6%)

Sectral Capsules
Anxiety (Up to 2%)
Catatonia
Depression (2%)
Disorientation, place
Disorientation, time
Dreaming abnormalities (2%)
Emotional lability
▲ Insomnia (3%)
Memory loss, short-term
Neuropsychometrics performance, decrease
Sensorium, clouded

Sedapap Tablets
Agitation (Infrequent)
Confusion (Infrequent)
Depression (Infrequent)
Euphoria (Infrequent)
Excitability (Infrequent)
▲ Feeling, intoxicated (Among the most frequent)
▲ Sedation (Among the most frequent)
Sluggishness (Infrequent)

Semprex-D Capsules
▲ Insomnia (4%)
▲ Nervousness (3%)
▲ Sedation (6% more common vs. placebo)

Sensorcaine Injection
Anxiety
Confusion
Depression
Excitability
Sexual dysfunction
Speech, incoherent

Sensorcaine with Epinephrine Injection
Anxiety
Depression
Excitability
Sexual dysfunction
Speech, incoherent

Sensorcaine-MPF Injection
Anxiety
Confusion
Depression
Excitability
Speech, incoherent

Sensorcaine-MPF with Epinephrine Injection
Anxiety
Confusion
Depression
Excitability
Speech, incoherent

Septra
Apathy
Depression
Hallucinations
Insomnia
Nervousness

Serentil
Agitation
Behavior, inappropriate
Central nervous system reactions
Confusion
Dreaming abnormalities
Excitability
Libido, changes
Mental status, altered
Photophobia
Psychoses, aggravation
Speech, slurring

Serevent Diskus
Sleep disturbances (1% to 3%)

Serevent Inhalation Aerosol
Excitability
Insomnia (1% to 3%)
Nervousness (1% to 3%)

Serophene Tablets
Anxiety
Depression (Less than 1 in 100 patients)
Disorientation, spatial
Double vision

Insomnia (Approximately 1 in 50
patients)
Irritability
Mood changes
Nervousness
(Approximately 1 in 50 patients)
Photophobia
Psychoses

Seroquel Tablets
Apathy (Infrequent)
Catatonia (Infrequent)
Confusion (Infrequent)
Delirium (Rare)
Delusions (Infrequent)
Depersonalization (Infrequent)
Dreaming abnormalities (Infrequent)
Emotional lability (Rare)
Euphoria (Rare)
Hallucinations (Infrequent)
Libido decreased (Rare)
Libido increased (Infrequent)
Manic behavior (Infrequent)
Mental performance, impairment
Mental status, altered
Paranoia (Infrequent)
Psychoses, aggravation (Infrequent)
Stupor (Infrequent)
Stuttering (Rare)
Suicide, attempt of (Infrequent)
Thinking abnormality (Infrequent)

Serostim for Injection
▲ Anxiety (1% to 10%)
▲ Depression (1% to 10%)
▲ Insomnia (11.2%)
▲ Nervousness (1% to 10%)
▲ Photophobia (1% to 10%)
▲ Thinking abnormality (1% to 10%)

Serzone Tablets
Agitation
Anxiety
Apathy (Infrequent)
Central nervous system stimulation
▲ Confusion (7% to 8%)
Depersonalization (Infrequent)
Depression
Double vision (Infrequent)
▲ Dreaming abnormalities (3%)
Emotional lability
Euphoria (Infrequent)
Hallucinations (Infrequent)
Hangover (Infrequent)
Hostility (Infrequent)
▲ Insomnia (11%)

Libido decreased (1%)
Libido increased (Infrequent)
Manic behavior (0.3% to 1.6%)
Manic behavior, mild (0.3% to 1.6%)
▲ Memory impairment (4%)
▲ Mental performance, impairment (3%)
Paranoia (Infrequent)
Photophobia (Infrequent)
Suicidal ideation (Infrequent)
Suicide, attempt of (Infrequent)
Thinking abnormality (Infrequent)

Silvadene Cream 1%
Central nervous system reactions

Simulect for Injection
▲ Agitation (3% to 10%)
▲ Anxiety (3% to 10%)
▲ Depression (3% to 10%)
▲ Insomnia (Greater than or equal to
10%)

Sinemet CR Tablets
Agitation
Anxiety
▲ Confusion (3.7%)
Delusions
Dementia
Depression (2.2%)
Disorientation
Double vision
Dreaming abnormalities (1.8%)
Euphoria
▲ Hallucinations (3.9%)
Insomnia (1.2%)
Libido increased
Memory impairment
Mental acuity, loss of
Mental status, altered
Nervousness
Nightmares
Paranoia
Psychoses
Sleep disturbances
Stimulation
Suicidal ideation

Sinemet Tablets
Agitation
Anxiety
Confusion
Delusions
Dementia
Depression
Disorientation
Double vision

Dreaming abnormalities
Euphoria
Hallucinations
Insomnia
Libido increased
Mental acuity, loss of
Mental performance, impairment
Nervousness
Nightmares
Paranoia
Psychoses
Stimulation
Suicidal ideation

Sinequan
Confusion (Infrequent)
Disorientation (Infrequent)
Hallucinations (Infrequent)
Libido, changes

Singlet Caplets
Excitability

Singulair
Dreaming abnormalities (Very rare)
Hallucinations
Insomnia
Irritability (Very rare)

Sinutab Non-Drying Liquid Caps
Insomnia
Nervousness

Skelaxin Tablets
Irritability
Nervousness

Skelid Tablets
Anxiety (Greater than or equal to 1%)
Insomnia (More than or equal to 1%)
Nervousness (Greater than or equal to 1%)

Solu-Medrol Sterile Powder
Depression
Euphoria
Insomnia
Mood changes
Personality changes
Psychiatric disturbances
Psychoses
Psychoses, aggravation

Soma Compound
Agitation (Very rare to infrequent)
Confusion (Very rare)

Depressive reactions (Infrequent or rare)
Disorientation (Very rare)
Double vision (Very rare)
Euphoria (Very rare)
Insomnia (Infrequent or rare)
Irritability (Infrequent or rare)

Soma Compound w/Codeine
Agitation (Infrequent or rare)
Confusion (Very rare)
Depressive reactions (Infrequent or rare)
Disorientation (Very rare)
Double vision (Very rare)
Euphoria
Insomnia (Infrequent or rare)
Irritability (Infrequent or rare)
Sedation

Soma Tablets
Agitation
Confusion
Depressive reactions
Disorientation
Double vision
Euphoria
Insomnia
Irritability

Sonata Capsules
Agitation (Infrequent)
Anxiety (Less than 1% to 3%)
Apathy (Frequent)
Confusion (Infrequent)
Delusions (Rare)
Depersonalization (Less than 1% to 2%)
Depression (Frequent)
Disordered sense of smell (Less than 1% to 2%)
Double vision (Infrequent)
Emotional lability (Frequent)
Euphoria (Frequent)
Hallucinations (Less than 1%)
Hangover (Infrequent)
Hostility (Rare)
Insomnia (Infrequent)
Libido decreased (Infrequent)
Nervousness (Frequent)
Photophobia (Infrequent)
Sleep disturbances (Rare)
Sleep talking (Rare)
Sleep walking (Rare)
Speech, slurring (Rare)

Stimulation (Rare)
Stupor (Rare)
Thinking abnormality (Frequent)

Soriatane Capsules

Anxiety (Less than 1%)
▲ Depression (1% to 10%)
Double vision (1% to 5%)
▲ Insomnia (1% to 10%)
Libido decreased (Less than 1%)
▲ Photophobia (1% to 10%)

Spectracef Tablets

Hyperactivity
Insomnia (0.1% to 1%)
Nervousness (0.1% to 1%)

Sporanox Capsules

▲ Anxiety (3%)
Depression (Infrequent)
Dreaming abnormalities (2%)
Insomnia (Infrequent)
Libido decreased (0.2% to 1.2%)

Sporanox Oral Solution

Depression (1.1% to 2.0%)
Insomnia (Less than 2%)

Stadol NS Nasal Spray

Agitation (Less than 1%)
Anxiety (1% or greater)
▲ Confusion (3% to 9%)
Delusions (Less than 1%)
Depression (Less than 1%)
Dreaming abnormalities (Less than 1%)
Euphoria (1% or greater)
Floating feeling (1% or greater)
Hallucinations (Less than 1%)
Hostility (Less than 1%)
▲ Insomnia (11%)
Nervousness (1% or greater)
Speech difficulties (Less than 1%)

Stelazine

Agitation
Catatonia
Central nervous system reactions
Insomnia
Jitteriness
Mental status, altered
Psychosis, activation

Sterile FUDR

Confusion (Remote possibility)
Disorientation (Remote possibility)
Euphoria (Remote possibility)

Photophobia (Remote possibility)

Stimate Nasal Spray

Agitation
Coma
Insomnia

Streptomycin Sulfate Injection

Central nervous system depression, neonatal
Coma (Occasional)
Stupor

Sudafed Tablets

Insomnia
Nervousness

Sudafed Nasal Decongestant Tablets

Insomnia
Nervousness

Sudafed Sinus & Allergy Tablets

Excitability

Sular Tablets

Anxiety (Less than or equal to 1%)
Confusion (Less than or equal to 1%)
Depression (Less than or equal to 1%)
Dreaming abnormalities (Less than or equal to 1%)
Insomnia (Less than or equal to 1%)
Libido decreased (Less than or equal to 1%)
Nervousness (Less than or equal to 1%)
Thinking abnormality (Less than or equal to 1%)

Suprane Liquid for Inhalation

Agitation (Less than 1%)

Surmontil Capsules

Agitation
Anxiety
Confusion
Delusions
Disorientation
Hallucinations
Insomnia
Libido decreased
Libido increased
Manic behavior, mild
Mental performance, impairment
Nightmares

Psychoses, aggravation

Sustiva Capsules

Agitation (Less than 2%)
Anxiety (Less than 2%)
Apathy (Less than 2%)
Confusion (Less than 2%)
Delusions
Depression (2% to 3%)
Depression, aggravation of (Less than 2%)
Disordered sense of smell (Less than 2%)
Double vision (Less than 2%)
Dreaming abnormalities (1% to 4%)
Emotional lability (Less than 2%)
Euphoria (Less than 2%)
Hallucinations (Less than 2%)
▲ Insomnia (1% to 7%)
Manic behavior
▲ Mental performance, impairment (1% to 9%)
Nervousness (1% to 2%)
Neurosis, unspecified
Paranoia
Psychoses (Less than 2%)
Suicide, attempt of

Symmetrel

Aggression
Agitation (1% to 5%)
Anxiety (1% to 5%)
Behavior, inappropriate
Coma
Confusion (0.1% to 5%)
Consciousness, disorders of (Uncommon)
Delirium
Delusions
Depression (1% to 5%)
Dreaming abnormalities (1% to 5%)
Euphoria (0.1% to 1%)
Hallucinations (1% to 5%)
▲ Insomnia (5% to 10%)
Irritability (1% to 5%)
Libido decreased (0.1% to 1%)
Manic behavior
Nervousness (1% to 5%)
Paranoia
Psychoses (0.1% to 1%)
Speech, slurring (0.1% to 1%)
Stupor
Suicidal ideation (Less than 0.1%)
Suicide, attempt of (Less than 0.1%)
Thinking abnormality (0.1% to 1%)

Synagis Intramuscular

Nervousness (More than 1%)

Synarel Nasal Solution for Central Precocious Puberty

▲ Emotional lability (6%)

Synarel Nasal Solution for Endometriosis

▲ Depression (3% of patients)
▲ Emotional lability (15% of patients)
▲ Insomnia (8% of patients)
▲ Libido decreased (22% of patients)
Libido increased (1% of patients)

Synercid I.V.

Anxiety (Less than 1%)
Confusion (Less then 1%)
Insomnia (Less than 1%)

Synvisc

Anxiety
Listlessness

Tagamet

Agitation
Anxiety
Confusion (Occasional)
Depression
Disorientation
Hallucinations
Psychoses

Talacen Caplets

Confusion
Depression (Infrequent)
Disorientation
Dreaming abnormalities (Infrequent)
Euphoria
Excitability (Rare)
Hallucinations
Insomnia (Infrequent)
Irritability (Rare)
Sedation

Talwin Nx Tablets

Confusion
Depression
Disorientation
Dreaming abnormalities
Euphoria
Excitability
Hallucinations
Hallucinations, visual
Insomnia
Irritability
Sedation

Tambocor Tablets
Anxiety (1% to 3%)
Apathy (Less than 1%)
Confusion (Less than 1%)
Depersonalization (Less than 1%)
Depression (1% to 3%)
Double vision (1% to 3%)
Dreaming abnormalities (Less than 1%)
Euphoria (Less than 1%)
Insomnia (1% to 3%)
Libido decreased (Less than 1%)
Photophobia (Less than 1%)
Speech disturbances (Less than 1%)
Stupor (Less than 1%)

Tamiflu
Confusion
Insomnia (1.1% to 1.2%)

Tarka Tablets
Anxiety (0.3% or more)
Confusion
Insomnia (Less frequent)
Libido decreased
Mental performance, impairment (Less frequent)
Psychoses

Tasmar Tablets
Agitation (1%)
Anxiety (1% or more)
Apathy (Infrequent)
▲ Confusion (10% to 11%)
Consciousness, disorders of (Four cases)
Delirium (Rare)
Delusions (Infrequent)
Depression (Frequent)
Disordered sense of smell (Infrequent)
Double vision (Infrequent)
▲ Dreaming abnormalities (16% to 21%)
Emotional lability (Frequent)
Euphoria (1%)
▲ Hallucinations (8% to 10%)
Hostility (Infrequent)
Hyperactivity (1%)
Irritability (1%)
Libido decreased (Infrequent)
Libido increased (Infrequent)
Manic behavior (Infrequent)
Mental acuity, loss of (1%)
Nervousness (Infrequent)
Panic (1%)

Paranoia (Infrequent)
Psychoses (Infrequent)
▲ Sleep disturbances (24% to 25%)
Speech disturbances (Frequent)
Thinking abnormality (Infrequent)

Taxotere for Injection Concentrate
Confusion
▲ Impairment of sensation (7 of 134 patients)

Tegretol
Agitation
Confusion
Depression, aggravation of
Double vision
Hallucinations, visual
Psychosis, activation
Speech disturbances
Talkativeness

Temodar Capsules
▲ Anxiety (7%)
▲ Confusion (5%)
▲ Depression (6%)
▲ Double vision (5%)
▲ Insomnia (10%)

Tenex Tablets
Agitation (Less frequent)
Anxiety (Less frequent)
Behavior, violent
Confusion (3% or less)
Depression (3% or less)
Insomnia (Less than 3% to 4%)
Libido decreased (3% or less)
Manic behavior
Nervousness (Less frequent)
▲ Sedation (5% to 39%)

Tenoretic Tablets
Catatonia
▲ Depression (0.6% to 12%)
Disorientation, place
Disorientation, time
Dreaming (Up to 3%)
Emotional lability
Hallucinations
Memory loss, short-term
Neuropsychometrics performance, decrease
Psychoses
Sensorium, clouded

Tenormin
Catatonia

▲ Depression (0.6% to 12%)
Disorientation, place
Disorientation, time
Dreaming (Up to 3%)
Emotional lability
Hallucinations
Memory loss, short-term
Neuropsychometrics performance,
  decrease
Psychoses
Sensorium, clouded

Tensilon Injectable
Double vision

Tequin
Agitation (Less than 0.1%)
Anxiety (Less than 0.1%)
Central nervous system stimulation
Confusion (Less than 0.1%)
Depersonalization (Less than 0.1%)
Depression (Less than 0.1%)
Disordered sense of smell
  (Less than 0.1%)
Dreaming abnormalities (0.1% to 3%)
Euphoria (Less than 0.1%)
Hallucinations (Less than 0.1%)
Hostility (Less than 0.1%)
Insomnia (0.1% to 3%)
Nervousness (Less than 0.1%)
Nightmares
Paranoia (Less than 0.1%)
Psychoses (Less than 0.1%)
Thinking abnormality (Less than
  0.1%)

Tessalon Capsules
Behavior, inappropriate (Isolated
  instances)
Confusion
Hallucinations, visual
Sedation

Testoderm Transdermal Systems
Anxiety
Depression
Libido decreased
Libido increased (1%)
Memory loss, short-term (1%)

Testopel Pellets
Anxiety
Depression
Libido decreased
Libido increased

Testred Capsules
Anxiety
Depression
Libido decreased
Libido increased

Tetanus & Diphtheria Toxoids Adsorbed for Adult Use
Irritability

Teveten Tablets
Anxiety (Less than 1%)
Depression (1%)
Insomnia (Less than 1%)
Nervousness (Less than 1%)

Thalomid Capsules
Agitation
Anxiety
Confusion
Depression
Double vision
Emotional lability
Euphoria
Hangover
Hostility
Impairment of sensation
Insomnia
Libido decreased
▲ Nervousness (2.8% to 9.4%)
Psychoses
Suicide, attempt of
Thinking abnormality

Theo-Dur Extended-Release Tablets
Hyperexcitability, reflex
Insomnia
Irritability

TheraFlu Cold & Cough Night Time Hot Liquid
Excitability
Insomnia
Nervousness

TheraFlu Cold & Sore Throat Night Time Hot Liquid
Excitability
Insomnia
Nervousness

TheraFlu Severe Cold & Congestion Night Time Caplets
Excitability

Insomnia
Nervousness

Thioridazine Hydrochloride Tablets

Agitation
Behavioral changes
Confusion, nocturnal (Extremely rare)
Dreaming abnormalities
Hyperactivity (Extremely rare)
Libido, changes
Psychiatric disturbances (Extremely rare)
Psychoses, aggravation

Thiothixene Capsules

Agitation
Insomnia
Psychotic symptoms, paradoxical exacerbation
Sedation

Thorazine

Agitation
Catatonia (Rare)
Insomnia
Jitteriness

Thyrel TRH for Injection

Anxiety (Less frequent)

Tiazac Capsules

Depression (Less than 2%)
Dreaming abnormalities (Less than 2%)
Hallucinations (Less than 2%)
Insomnia (Less than 2%)
Nervousness (Less than 2%)
Personality changes (Less than 2%)
Sexual dysfunction (Less than 2%)

Tikosyn Capsules

Anxiety (Greater than 2%)
▲ Insomnia (4%)

Timolide Tablets

Catatonia
Confusion (Less than 1%)
Depression
Disorientation, place
Disorientation, time
Double vision
Emotional lability
Hallucinations
Insomnia (Less than 1%)
Libido decreased (Less than 1%)
Memory impairment

Mental performance, impairment
Nervousness (Less than 1%)
Nightmares
Sensorium, clouded

Timolol GFS

Anxiety
Behavioral changes
Catatonia
Confusion
Depression
Disorientation
Disorientation, place
Disorientation, time
Double vision
Emotional lability
Hallucinations
Insomnia
Libido decreased
Memory loss, short-term
Mental performance, impairment
Nervousness
Neuropsychometrics performance, decrease
Nightmares
Psychiatric disturbances
Sensorium, clouded

Timoptic

Anxiety (Less frequent)
Behavioral changes (Less frequent)
Catatonia
Confusion (Less frequent)
Depression (Less frequent)
Disorientation (Less frequent)
Disorientation, place
Disorientation, time
Double vision (Less frequent)
Emotional lability
Hallucinations (Less frequent)
Insomnia (Less frequent)
Libido decreased
Memory loss, short-term
Mental performance, impairment
Nervousness (Less frequent)
Neuropsychometrics performance, decrease
Nightmares
Psychiatric disturbances (Less frequent)
Sensorium, clouded

Tolectin 200 Tablets

Depression (1% to 3%)

Tolectin 600 Tablets
Depression (1% to 3%)

Tolectin DS Capsules
Depression (1% to 3%)

Tonocard Tablets
Agitation (Less than 1%)
Anxiety (1.1% to 1.5%)
▲ Awareness, altered (1.5% to 11.0%)
Coma (Less than 1%)
▲ Confusion (2.1% to 11.2%)
Depression (Less than 1%)
▲ Disorientation (2.1% to 11.2%)
Double vision (Less than 1%)
Dreaming abnormalities (Less than 1%)
▲ Hallucinations (2.1% to 11.2%)
Insomnia (Less than 1%)
Memory impairment (Less than 1%)
Mental slowness (Less than 1%)
▲ Mood changes (1.5% to 11.0%)
▲ Nervousness (0.4% to 11.5%)
Psychiatric disturbances (Less than 1%)
Psychoses (Less than 1%)
Sleep disturbances (Less than 1%)
Speech disturbances (Less than 1%)
Speech, slurring (Less than 1%)

Topamax
Aggression (2.7% to 4%)
▲ Agitation (4% to 4.4%)
▲ Anxiety (2.2% to 9.3%)
Apathy (1.8% to 4.5%)
▲ Confusion (8.9% to 15%)
Delirium (Infrequent)
Delusions (Infrequent)
Depersonalization (1.6% to 1.8%)
▲ Depression (8% to 13.4%)
Disordered sense of smell (Infrequent)
▲ Double vision (14.2% to 14.6%)
Dreaming abnormalities (Infrequent)
Emotional lability (1.8% to 2.4%)
Euphoria (Frequent)
Hallucinations (Frequent)
Insomnia (Frequent)
▲ Language problems, unspecified (2.2% to 11.7%)
Libido decreased (Frequent)
Libido increased (Rare)
Manic behavior (Rare)
▲ Memory impairment (12.4% to 12.6%)
▲ Mental performance, impairment (6.7% to 15.4%)

▲ Mental slowness (8% to 15.4%)
▲ Mood changes (3.5% to 10.1%)
▲ Nervousness (13.3% to 20.6%)
Neurosis, unspecified (Infrequent)
Paranoia (Infrequent)
Personality changes (Frequent)
Photophobia (Infrequent)
Psychoses (Frequent)
▲ Speech disturbances (13.8% to 16.8%)
Stupor (Frequent)
Suicide, attempt of (Frequent)

Toprol-XL Tablets
Catatonia
Confusion
▲ Depression (About 5 of 100 patients)
Disorientation, place
Disorientation, time
Emotional lability
Insomnia
Libido decreased
Memory loss, short-term
Neuropsychometrics performance, decrease
Nightmares
Sensorium, clouded

Toradol
Dreaming abnormalities (1% or less)
Euphoria (1% or less)
Hallucinations (1% or less)
Insomnia (1% or less)
Mental performance, impairment (1% or less)
Nervousness (1% or less)
Psychoses
Stupor (1% or less)
Thinking abnormality (1% or less)
Depression (1% or less)

Transderm Scop
Confusion (Infrequent)
Disorientation (Infrequent)
Hallucinations (Infrequent)
Memory impairment (Infrequent)

Tranxene
Confusion (Less common)
Depression
Double vision
Insomnia
Irritability
Nervousness (Less common)
Speech, slurring

Trasylol Injection
Agitation (1% to 2%)
Anxiety (1% to 2%)
▲ Confusion (4%)
▲ Insomnia (3%)

Travatan Ophthalmic Solution
Anxiety (1% to 5%)
Depression (1% to 5%)
Photophobia (1% to 4%)

Trecator-SC Tablets
Depression
Double vision (Rare)
Psychiatric disturbances

Trental Tablets
Agitation
Anxiety (Less than 1%)
Confusion (Less than 1%)
Depression (Less than 1%)
Insomnia
Nervousness

Triaminic Allergy Congestion Liquid
Insomnia
Nervousness

Triaminic Chest Congestion Liquid
Insomnia
Nervousness

Triaminic Cold & Allergy Liquid
Insomnia
Nervousness

Triaminic Cold & Allergy Softchews
Excitability
Insomnia
Nervousness

Triaminic Cold & Cough Liquid
Insomnia
Nervousness

Triaminic Cold & Cough Softchews
Excitability

Triaminic Cold & Night Time Cough Liquid
Insomnia
Nervousness

Triaminic Cough & Congestion Liquid
Insomnia
Nervousness

Triaminic Cough & Sore Throat Liquid
Insomnia
Nervousness

Triaminic Cough & Sore Throat Softchews
Insomnia
Nervousness

Triaminic Cough Liquid
Insomnia
Nervousness

Triaminic Flu, Cough & Fever
Insomnia
Nervousness

Tricor Tablets
Anxiety (Less than 1%)
Confusion (Less than 1%)
Depression
Insomnia (1%)
Libido decreased (2%)
Nervousness
Sleep disturbances (Less than 1%)

Trilafon
Catatonia
Confusion, nocturnal
Dreaming abnormalities
Hyperactivity
Hypnotic effects
Insomnia
Libido, changes
Paranoia
Photophobia
Psychoses
Speech, slurring
Suicidal ideation

Trileptal
Aggression
Agitation (1% to 2%)
▲ Anxiety (5% to 7%)
Apathy
Confusion (1% to 2%)
Delirium
Delusions
▲ Double vision (5% to 40%)
Emotional lability (2% to 3%)

Euphoria
Feeling, intoxicated
Feeling, strange (1% to 2%)
Hysteria
Insomnia (2% to 4%)
Libido decreased
Libido increased
Manic behavior
Nervousness (2% to 4%)
Panic
Paranoia
Personality changes
Photophobia
Speech disturbances (1% to 3%)
Stupor
Thinking abnormality (2%)

Tri-Levlen
Depression
Double vision (Rare)
Insomnia
Libido, changes
Mood changes
Nervousness
Speech disturbances

Trilisate Liquid
Confusion (Rare)
Hallucinations (Rare)

Trilisate Tablets
Confusion (Rare)
Hallucinations (Rare)

Tri-Norinyl
Depression
Double vision
Libido, changes
Nervousness

Tripedia Vaccine
Anxiety
▲ Irritability (5% to 15%)

Triphasil
Depression
Libido, changes
Nervousness

Trisenox Injection
▲ Agitation (5%)
▲ Anxiety (30%)
▲ Coma (5%)
▲ Confusion (5%)
▲ Depression (20%)
▲ Insomnia (43%)

Trivora Tablets
Depression
Libido, changes
Nervousness

Trizivir Tablets
▲ Depression (9%)
▲ Insomnia (7% to 13%)
▲ Sleep disturbances (7% to 11%)

Trovan
Agitation (Less than 1%)
Anxiety (Less than 1%)
Central nervous system stimulation
Confusion (Less than 1%)
Depersonalization (Less than 1%)
Depression (Less than 1%)
Dreaming abnormalities
 (Less than 1%)
Emotional lability (Less than 1%)
Euphoria (Less than 1%)
Hallucinations (Less than 1%)
Insomnia (Less than 1%)
Libido decreased (Less than 1%)
Mental performance, impairment
 (Less than 1%)
Nightmares
Paranoia (Less than 1%)
Photophobia (Less than 1%)
Speech disturbances (Less than 1%)
Thinking abnormality (Less than 1%)

Trusopt Sterile Ophthalmic Solution
Photophobia (Approximately 1% to
 5%)

Tussi-12
▲ Sedation

Tussionex
Anxiety
Euphoria
Fear
Mental clouding
Mental performance, impairment
Mood changes
Sedation

Tussi-Organidin NR Liquid
Euphoria

Tussi-Organidin-S NR Liquid
Euphoria

Twinrix Vaccine
Agitation (Less than 1%)

Insomnia (Less than 1%)
Irritability (Less than 1%)
Photophobia (Less than 1%)

Tylenol Allergy Sinus
Excitability

Tylenol Cold Complete Formula
Excitability
Insomnia
Nervousness

Tylenol Cold Non-Drowsy
Insomnia
Nervousness

Tylenol Flu NightTime Gelcaps
Excitability

Tylenol Flu NightTime Liquid
Excitability
Insomnia
Nervousness

Tylenol Sinus NightTime Caplets
Insomnia
Nervousness

Tylenol Sinus Non-Drowsy
Insomnia
Nervousness

Tylenol with Codeine
Euphoria
Mental performance, impairment
▲ Sedation (Among most frequent)

Tylox Capsules
Euphoria
Mental performance, impairment
▲ Sedation (Among most frequent)

Ultracet Tablets
Anxiety (At least 1%)
Cognitive dysfunction
Confusion (At least 1%)
Depersonalization (Less than 1%)
Depression (Less than 1%)
Emotional lability (Less than 1%)
Euphoria (At least 1%)
Hallucinations (Less than 1%)
Insomnia (2%)
Mental performance, impairment
Nervousness (At least 1%)
Paranoia (Less than 1%)
Stupor (Less than 1%)

Thinking abnormality (Less than 1%)

Ultram Tablets
▲ Agitation (1% to 14%)
▲ Anxiety (1% to 14%)
▲ Central nervous system stimulation (7% to 14%)
Cognitive dysfunction (Less than 1%)
Confusion (1% to 5%)
Depression (Less than 1%)
▲ Emotional lability (7% to 14%)
▲ Euphoria (1% to 14%)
▲ Hallucinations (Less than 1% to 14%)
Mental performance, impairment (Less than 1%)
▲ Nervousness (1% to 14%)
Sleep disturbances (1% to 5%)
Speech disturbances (Infrequent)
Suicidal ideation (Infrequent)

Uni-Dur Extended-Release Tablets
Hyperexcitability, reflex
Insomnia
Irritability

Uniphyl Tablets
Behavioral changes
Insomnia
Irritability

Uniretic Tablets
Anxiety (Less than 1%)
Depression (Less than 1%)
Emotional lability (Less than 1%)
Insomnia (Less than 1%)
Libido decreased (Less than 1%)
Nervousness (Less than 1%)
Neurosis, unspecified (Less than 1%)

Unithroid Tablets
Anxiety
Emotional lability
Hyperactivity
Insomnia
Irritability
Nervousness

Univasc Tablets
Anxiety (Less than 1%)
Mood changes (Less than 1%)
Nervousness (Less than 1%)
Sleep disturbances (Less than 1%)

Uroqid-Acid No. 2 Tablets
Confusion

Vagifem Tablets
▲ Insomnia (3% to 5%)

Valcyte Tablets
Agitation (Less than 5%)
Confusion (Less than 5%)
Hallucinations (Less than 5%)
▲ Insomnia (16%)
Psychoses (Less than 5%)
Sedation

Valium Injectable
Anger
Anxiety, paradoxical
Confusion
Depression
Double vision
Excitement, paradoxical
Hallucinations
Hypoactivity
Insomnia
Libido, changes
Speech, slurring
Stimulation

Valium Tablets
Anxiety, paradoxical
Confusion (Infrequent)
Depression (Infrequent)
Double vision (Infrequent)
Excitement, paradoxical
Hallucinations
Insomnia
Libido, changes (Infrequent)
Rage
Sleep disturbances
Speech, slurring (Infrequent)
Stimulation

Valtrex Caplets
Agitation
Behavioral changes
Coma
Confusion
Consciousness, disorders of
▲ Depression (Less than 1% to 7%)
Hallucinations, auditory
Hallucinations, visual
Manic behavior
Psychoses

Vanceril Double Strength Inhalation Aerosol
Depression (Fewer than 2%)
Insomnia (Fewer than 2%)

Vantin
Anxiety (Less than 1%)
Confusion (Less than 1%)
Dreaming abnormalities (Less than 1%)
Hallucinations (Less than 1%)
Insomnia (Less than 1%)
Nervousness (Less than 1%)
Nightmares (Less than 1%)

Varivax
Irritability (Greater than or equal to 1%)
Nervousness (Greater than or equal to 1%)
Sleep disturbances (Greater than or equal to 1%)

Vascor Tablets
Anxiety (0.5% to 2.0%)
Behavioral changes (0.5% to 2.0%)
Depression (0.5% to 2.0%)
Insomnia (0.5 to 2.65%)
Libido, loss (0.5% to 2.0%)
▲ Nervousness (7.37% to 11.63%)

Vaseretic Tablets
Confusion
Depression
Dreaming abnormalities
Impairment of sensation
Insomnia (0.5% to 2.0%)
Libido decreased (0.5% to 2.0%)
Nervousness (0.5% to 2.0%)

Vasotec I.V. Injection
Confusion
Depression
Dreaming abnormalities
Impairment of sensation
Insomnia
Nervousness

Vasotec Tablets
Confusion (0.5% to 1%)
Depression (0.5% to 1%)
Dreaming abnormalities (0.5% to 1.0%)
Impairment of sensation (0.5% to 1.0%)
Insomnia (0.5% to 1.0%)
Nervousness (0.5% to 1.0%)

Ventolin HFA Inhalation Aerosol
Central nervous system stimulation

Insomnia

Ventolin Inhalation Aerosol
Aggression (1%)
Agitation (1%)
Behavioral changes (1%)
Central nervous system stimulation
  (No incidence data in labeling)
Hyperactivity (1%)
Insomnia
▲ Nervousness (1% to 10%)
Nightmares (1%)

Verelan Capsules
Confusion (1% or less)
Insomnia (1% or less)
Psychoses (1% or less)
Sleep disturbances (1.4%)

Verelan PM Capsules
Confusion (2% or less)
Insomnia (2% or less)
Psychoses (2% or less)

Versed Injection
Agitation (Less than 1%)
Anxiety (Less than 1%)
Argumentativeness (Less than 1%)
Central nervous system depression,
  neonatal
Combativeness
Confusion (Less than 1%)
Double vision (Less than 1%)
Dreaming (Less than 1%)
Euphoria (Less than 1%)
Grogginess (Less than 1%)
Hallucinations (Less than 1%)
Hyperactivity
  (No incidence data in labeling)
Insomnia (Less than 1%)
Nervousness (Less than 1%)
Nightmares (Less than 1%)
Oversedation (1.6%)
Sedation (1.6%)
Sleep disturbances (Less than 1%)
Speech, slurring (Less than 1%)

Versed Syrup
Aggression (Less than 1%)
Agitation (2%)
Behavioral changes (Less than 1%)
Confusion (Less than 1%)
Disinhibition (Less than 1%)
Double vision (Less than 1%)
Excitement, paradoxical
  (Less than 1%)

Hallucinations (Less than 1%)
Mood changes (Less than 1%)
Sedation (Less than 1%)

Vesanoid Capsules
▲ Agitation (9%)
▲ Anxiety (17%)
▲ Central nervous system depression
  (3%)
▲ Coma (3%)
▲ Confusion (14%)
▲ Dementia (3%)
▲ Depression (14%)
▲ Hallucinations (6%)
▲ Insomnia (14%)
▲ Memory impairment (3%)
▲ Speech disturbances (3%)

Vexol 1% Ophthalmic Suspension
Photophobia (Less than 1%)

Viadur Implant
Anxiety (Less than 2%)
▲ Depression (5.3%)

Viagra Tablets
Anxiety
Depression (Less than 2%)
Double vision
Dreaming abnormalities
  (Less than 2%)
Insomnia (Less than 2%)
Photophobia (Less than 2%)

Vicks 44D Cough & Head Congestion Relief Liquid
Insomnia
Nervousness

Vicks DayQuil LiquiCaps/Liquid Multi-Symptom Cold/Flu Relief
Excitability
Insomnia
Nervousness

Vicodin
Anxiety
Fear
Mental clouding
Mental performance, impairment
Mood changes
▲ Sedation (Among most frequent)

Vicodin Tuss Expectorant
Anxiety

Fear
Mental clouding
Mental performance, impairment
Mood changes
Sedation

Vicoprofen Tablets
Agitation (Less than 1%)
▲ Anxiety (3% to 9%)
Confusion (Less than 3%)
Depression (Less than 1%)
Dreaming abnormalities (Less than 1%)
Euphoria (Less than 1%)
▲ Insomnia (3% to 9%)
Libido decreased (Less than 1%)
Mood changes (Less than 1%)
▲ Nervousness (3% to 9%)
Speech, slurring (Less than 1%)
Thinking abnormality (Less than 3%)

Vioxx
Anxiety (Greater than 0.1% to 1.9%)
Confusion
Depression (Greater than 0.1% to 1.9%)
Hallucinations (Less than 0.1%)
Insomnia (Greater than 0.1% to 1.9%)
Mental clouding (Greater than 0.1% to 1.9%)

Viracept
Anxiety
Depression
Emotional lability
Insomnia
Sexual dysfunction
Sleep disturbances
Suicidal ideation

Vistaril Intramuscular Solution
Mental performance, impairment (Seldom)

Vistide Injection
Agitation
Anxiety
Confusion
Delirium
Dementia
Depression
Double vision
Dreaming abnormalities
Hallucinations
Insomnia

Libido increased
Nervousness
Personality changes
Speech disturbances

Visudyne for Injection
▲ Double vision (1% to 10%)
▲ Sleep disturbances (1% to 10%)
▲ Photophobia (5% to 20%)

Vivactil Tablets
Agitation
Anxiety
Anxiety, paradoxical
Confusion
Delusions
Disorientation
Hallucinations
Insomnia
Libido, changes
Manic behavior, mild
Mental performance, impairment
Nightmares
Psychoses, aggravation
Suicide, attempt of

Vivelle Transdermal System
Depression
Libido, changes

Vivelle-Dot Transdermal System
Depression
Libido, changes

Volmax Extended-Release Tablets
Central nervous system stimulation
Insomnia (2.4%)
Irritability (Less frequent)
▲ Nervousness (8.5%)

Voltaren
Anxiety (Less than 1%)
Coma (Rare)
Depression (Less than 1%)
Disorientation (Rare)
Double vision (Less than 1%)
Insomnia (Less than 1%)
Irritability (Less than 1%)
Memory impairment (Less than 1%)
Nightmares (Less than 1%)
Psychoses (Rare)

Voltaren Ophthalmic Solution
Insomnia (Less than 3%)

Wellbutrin SR
▲ Agitation (0.3% to 9%)
▲ Anxiety (5% to 6%)
Awareness, altered (Rare)
Central nervous system stimulation (1% to 2%)
Coma
Confusion
Delirium
Delusions
Depersonalization (Infrequent)
Double vision
Dreaming abnormalities (At least 1%)
Emotional lability (Infrequent)
Euphoria
Hallucinations
Hostility (Infrequent)
▲ Insomnia (11% to 16%)
Irritability (2% to 3%)
Libido decreased (Infrequent)
Libido increased
Manic behavior
Manic behavior, mild (Rare)
Memory impairment (Up to 3%)
▲ Nervousness (3% to 5%)
Paranoia
Psychoses
Psychosis, activation
Suicidal ideation (Infrequent)
Thinking abnormality

Wellbutrin Tablets
▲ Agitation (31.9%)
▲ Anxiety (3.1%)
▲ Auditory disturbances (5.3%)
Coma
▲ Confusion (8.4%)
Delirium
Delusions (1.2%)
Depersonalization (Infrequent)
Depression (Frequent)
Double vision (Rare)
Dreaming abnormalities
Euphoria (1.2%)
Frigidity, unspecified (Infrequent)
Hallucinations (Frequent)
▲ Hostility (5.6%)
▲ Insomnia (18.6%)
▲ Libido decreased (3.1%)
Libido increased (Frequent)
Manic behavior (Frequent)
Manic behavior, mild (Frequent)
Memory impairment (Infrequent)
Mood changes (Infrequent)
Paranoia (Infrequent)

Psychoses (Infrequent)
▲ Sedation (19.8%)
▲ Sensory disturbances (4.0%)
Sexual dysfunction (Frequent)
▲ Sleep disturbances (4.0%)
Suicidal ideation (Rare)
Thinking abnormality (Infrequent)

Xalatan
Double vision (Less than 1%)
Photophobia (1% to 4%)

Xanax Tablets
Aggression (Rare)
Agitation (Rare; 2.9%)
▲ Anxiety (16.6%)
Behavior, inappropriate (Rare)
▲ Central nervous system depression (13.8% to 13.9%)
▲ Cognitive dysfunction (28.8%)
▲ Confusion (9.9% to 10.4%)
Depersonalization
▲ Depression (13.8% to 13.9%)
Depressive reactions
Double vision
Dreaming abnormalities (1.8%)
Fear (1.4%)
Hallucinations (Rare)
Hostility (Rare)
▲ Insomnia (8.9% to 29.4%)
▲ Irritability (33.1%)
▲ Libido decreased (14.4%)
▲ Libido increased (7.7%)
▲ Libido, changes (7.1%)
Manic behavior
Manic behavior, mild
▲ Memory impairment (33.1%)
Mental performance, impairment
▲ Nervousness (4.1%)
Rage (Rare)
Sedation
Sensorium, clouded
Sensory disturbances
▲ Sexual dysfunction (7.4%)
Sleep disturbances (Rare)
Speech, slurring
Stimulation (Rare)
Suicidal ideation
Suicide, attempt of
Talkativeness (2.2%)

Xeloda Tablets
Confusion (Less than 5%)
Impairment of sensation
Insomnia

Xenical Capsules
▲ Anxiety (2.8% to 4.4%)
▲ Depression (3.4%)
▲ Sleep disturbances (3.9%)

Xopenex Inhalation Solution
Anxiety (2.7%)
Insomnia
▲ Nervousness (2.8% to 9.6%)

Xylocaine Injection
Anxiety
▲ Central nervous system depression (Among most common)
▲ Central nervous system stimulation (Among most common)
▲ Confusion (Among most common)
Double vision (Less than 1%)
▲ Euphoria (Among most common)
▲ Nervousness (Among most common)
Sexual dysfunction

Xylocaine with Epinephrine Injection
Anxiety
▲ Central nervous system depression (Among most common)
▲ Central nervous system stimulation (Among most common)
▲ Confusion (Among most common)
Double vision (Less than 1%)
▲ Euphoria (Among most common)
▲ Nervousness (Among most common)
Sexual dysfunction

Yasmin 28 Tablets
Depression (Greater than 1%)
Emotional lability
Libido, changes
Nervousness (Greater than 1%)

Zaditor Ophthalmic Solution
Photophobia (Less than 5%)

Zanaflex Tablets
Agitation (Infrequent)
Anxiety (Frequent)
Dementia (Rare)
Depersonalization (Infrequent)
Depression (Frequent)
Dreaming abnormalities (Infrequent)
Emotional lability (Infrequent)
Euphoria (Infrequent)
▲ Nervousness (3%)
▲ Sedation (48%)
▲ Speech disturbances (3%)
Stupor (Infrequent)

Suicide, attempt of (Rare)
Thinking abnormality (Infrequent)

Zantac Injection
Agitation
Confusion (Rare)
Depression (Rare)
Hallucinations
Insomnia
Libido decreased

Zantac Tablets, Granules, & Syrup
Agitation (Rare)
Confusion (Rare)
Depression (Rare)
Hallucinations (Rare)
Insomnia (Rare)
Libido, loss (Occasional)

Zarontin
Aggression
Depression (Rare)
Euphoria
Hyperactivity
Irritability
Libido increased (Rare)
Mental performance, impairment
Psychiatric disturbances
Psychoses
Psychosis, paranoid (Rare)
Sleep disturbances
Suicidal ideation (Rare)

Zaroxolyn Tablets
Depression
Insomnia
Nervousness (Less than 2%)

Zebeta Tablets
Anxiety
Catatonia
Depression (Up to 0.2%)
Disorientation, place
Disorientation, time
Dreaming abnormalities
Emotional lability
Hallucinations
Insomnia (1.5% to 2.5%)
Libido decreased
Mental performance, impairment
Sensorium, clouded

Zenapax for Injection
▲ Anxiety (2% to 5%)
▲ Depression (2% to 5%)

▲ Insomnia (Greater than 5%)

Zephrex
 Excitability
 Insomnia
 Irritability
 Nervousness

Zerit
▲ Insomnia (29%)

Zestoretic Tablets
 Confusion
 Depression (0.3% to 1%)
 Double vision
 Insomnia
 Irritability
 Libido decreased (0.3% to 1%)
 Memory impairment
 Nervousness
 Photophobia
 Sleeping, excessive

Zestril Tablets
 Confusion (0.3% to 1.0%)
 Depression (Greater than 1%)
 Double vision (0.3% to 1.0%)
 Impairment of sensation
  (0.3% to 1.0%)
 Insomnia (0.3% to 1.0%)
 Irritability (0.3% to 1.0%)
 Libido decreased (0.4%)
 Mental performance, impairment
  (0.3% to 1.0%)
 Nervousness (0.3% to 1.0%)
 Photophobia (0.3% to 1.0%)
 Sleeping, excessive (0.3% to 1.0%)

Ziac Tablets
 Anxiety
 Catatonia
 Depression
 Disorientation, place
 Disorientation, time
 Dreaming abnormalities
 Emotional lability
 Hallucinations
 Insomnia (1.1% to 1.2%)
 Libido, loss (0.4%)
 Memory impairment
 Mental performance, impairment
 Sensorium, clouded
 Sexual dysfunction
 Sleep disturbances

Ziagen
▲ Insomnia (7% to 13%)
▲ Sleep disturbances (7%)

Zithromax Capsules & Tablets
 Agitation (1% or less)
 Insomnia (1% or less)
 Nervousness (1% or less)

Zithromax for IV Infusion
 Insomnia (1% or less)
 Nervousness (1% or less)

**Zithromax for Oral
Suspension**
 Agitation (1% or less)
 Insomnia (1% or less)
 Nervousness (1% or less)

Zocor Tablets
 Anxiety
 Depression
 Insomnia
 Libido, loss
 Memory loss, short-term

Zofran Injection
▲ Agitation (2% to 6%)
▲ Anxiety (2% to 6%)
▲ Sedation (8%)

Zofran Tablets & Oral Solution
▲ Agitation (6%)
▲ Anxiety (6%)
▲ Sedation (20%)

Zoladex
 Anxiety (1% to 5%)
▲ Depression (1% to 54%)
▲ Emotional lability (60%)
▲ Insomnia (5% to 11%)
▲ Libido decreased (61%)
▲ Libido increased (12%)
▲ Nervousness (3% to 5%)
▲ Sexual dysfunction (21%)
 Thinking abnormality (1% or greater)

Zoladex 3-month
 Anxiety
 Depression
 Emotional lability
 Insomnia
 Nervousness
▲ Sexual dysfunction (One of the two
  most common)
 Thinking abnormality

Zoloft

Aggression (Infrequent)
▲ Agitation (6%)
▲ Anxiety (4%)
Apathy (Infrequent)
Coma (Rare)
Confusion (Infrequent)
Delusions (Infrequent)
Depersonalization (Infrequent)
Depression (Infrequent)
Depression, aggravation of
(Infrequent)
Double vision (Rare)
Dreaming abnormalities (Infrequent)
Emotional lability (Infrequent to 2%)
Euphoria (Infrequent)
Hallucinations (Infrequent)
Illusion, unspecified (Rare)
▲ Insomnia (16% to 28%)
▲ Libido decreased (1% to 11%)
Libido increased (Rare)
Manic behavior (0.4% to 2%)
Manic behavior, mild
(Approximately 0.4%)
Mental performance, impairment
(1.3% to 2%)
▲ Nervousness (6%)
Nightmares (Infrequent)
Paranoia (Infrequent)
Photophobia (Rare)
Psychoses
Serotonin syndrome
Sexual dysfunction (Frequent)
Sleep walking (Rare)
Suicidal ideation (Rare)
Suicide, attempt of
Thinking abnormality (2%)

Zometa for Intravenous Infusion

▲ Agitation (12.8%)
▲ Anxiety (9% to 14%)
▲ Confusion (12.8%)
▲ Depression (12%)
▲ Insomnia (14% to 15.1%)

Zomig

Agitation (Infrequent)
Anxiety (Infrequent)
Apathy (Rare)
Depression (Infrequent)
Disordered sense of smell (Infrequent)
Double vision (Rare)
Emotional lability (Infrequent)
Euphoria (Rare)

Hallucinations (Rare)
Insomnia (Infrequent)
Irritability (Rare)

Zonegran Capsules

▲ Agitation (9%)
▲ Anxiety (3%)
Behavior, schizophrenic (2%)
▲ Confusion (6%)
▲ Depression (6%)
Disordered sense of smell (Infrequent)
▲ Double vision (6%)
Dreaming abnormalities (Infrequent)
Euphoria (Infrequent)
▲ Insomnia (6%)
▲ Irritability (9%)
Libido decreased (Infrequent)
▲ Memory impairment (6%)
▲ Mental performance, impairment (6%)
▲ Mental slowness (4%)
Nervousness (2%)
Photophobia (Rare)
▲ Speech disturbances (5%)

Zosyn

Aggression (1.0% or less)
▲ Agitation (2.1% to 7.1%)
Anxiety (1.2% to 3.2%)
Combativeness (1.0% or less)
Confusion (1.0% or less)
Depression (1.0% or less)
Hallucinations (1.0% or less)
▲ Insomnia (4.5% to 6.6%)
Photophobia (1.0% or less)

Zovia

Depression
Libido, changes
Nervousness

Zovirax Capsules, Tablets, & Suspension

Agitation
Behavior, violent
Coma
Confusion
Consciousness, disorders of
Delirium
Hallucinations
Psychoses

Zovirax for Injection

Agitation (Approximately 1%)
Behavior, inappropriate
Coma (Approximately 1%)
Confusion (Approximately 1%)

Delirium
Hallucinations (Approximately 1%)
Psychoses

Zyban
Agitation (Frequent)
▲ Anxiety (8%)
Central nervous system stimulation
  (Infrequent)
Coma
Confusion (Infrequent)
Delirium
Delusions
Depersonalization (Infrequent)
Depression (Frequent)
Double vision
▲ Dreaming abnormalities (5%)
Emotional lability (Infrequent)
Euphoria
Hallucinations
Hostility (Infrequent)
▲ Insomnia (31% to 40%)
Irritability (Frequent)
Libido decreased (Infrequent)
Libido increased
Manic behavior
Manic behavior, mild (Rare)
Memory impairment (Infrequent)
▲ Mental performance, impairment (9%)
▲ Nervousness (4%)
Paranoia
Psychoses
Psychosis, activation
Suicidal ideation (Infrequent)
Thinking abnormality (1%)

Zydone Tablets
Anxiety
Fear
Mental clouding
Mental performance, impairment
Mood changes
▲ Sedation (Among most frequent)

Zyflo Filmtab Tablets
Insomnia (Less common)
Nervousness (Less common)

Zyprexa
▲ Agitation (23%)
Alcohol abuse (Infrequent)
Antisocial reaction (Infrequent)
▲ Anxiety (9%)
Apathy
Behavioral changes
Central nervous system stimulation

(Infrequent)
Coma (Infrequent)
Confusion
Delirium (Infrequent)
Depersonalization (Infrequent)
Depression
Double vision (Infrequent)
Dreaming abnormalities
Emotional lability
Euphoria (2%)
Hallucinations
Hangover (Infrequent)
▲ Hostility (15%)
▲ Insomnia (20%)
Libido decreased (Infrequent)
Libido increased
▲ Nervousness (16%)
Obsessive compulsive symptoms
  (Infrequent)
Paranoia
▲ Personality changes (8%)
Phobic disorder (Infrequent)
Schizophrenia, precipitation
Sociopathy (Infrequent)
Speech difficulties (2%)
Speech disturbances (2%)
Stupor (Infrequent)
Stuttering (Infrequent)
Suicide, attempt of (Frequent)
Thinking abnormality

Zyrtec
Agitation (Less than 2%)
Anxiety (Less than 2%)
Confusion (Less than 2%)
Depersonalization (Less than 2%)
Depression (Less than 2%)
Disordered sense of smell
  (Less than 2%)
Emotional lability (Less than 2%)
Euphoria (Less than 2%)
Insomnia (Less than 2%)
Libido decreased (Less than 2%)
Mental performance, impairment
  (Less than 2%)
Nervousness (Less than 2%)
Nightmares (Less than 2%)
Sleep disturbances (Less than 2%)
Thinking abnormality (Less than 2%)

Zyrtec-D
Agitation (Less than 2%)
Anxiety (Less than 2%)
Central nervous system stimulation
Confusion (Less than 2%)

Depression (Less than 2%)
Disordered sense of smell
  (Less than 2%)
Emotional lability (Less than 2%)
Euphoria (Less than 2%)
Excitability
Fear
Hallucinations
Insomnia (Less than 2%)
Libido decreased (Less than 2%)

Mental performance, impairment
  (Less than 2%)
Nervousness (Less than 2%)
Nightmares (Less than 2%)
Sleep disturbances (Less than 2%)
Tenseness
Thinking abnormality (Less than 2%)

Zyvox
Insomnia (2.5%)

Psychotropic Herbs and Supplements

Some 35 herbs and nutritional supplements are currently being used to relieve a variety of mental and emotional problems, ranging from memory loss to nervousness and depression. The profiles in this section describe the verified effects of these products, as well as other claims made by their proponents. Also included is a brief discussion of their proposed mechanism of action and the contraindications, precautions, and potential interactions associated with their use. Information on use in pregnancy, typical dosage, and the effects of overdosage can be found as well. The profiles are organized alphabetically by the substance's most commonly used name.

The information in these profiles is drawn from in-depth monographs in two alternative medicine handbooks published by *Physicians' Desk Reference®—PDR® for Herbal Medicines*™ and *PDR® for Nutritional Supplements*™.

5-HTP

Why people take it

5-HTP (5-hydroxytryptophan) is valued primarily for its effect on depression. In one carefully designed study, it was found to work slightly better than the serotonin-boosting drug Luvox. Other trials, however, have been less encouraging.

5-HTP is also an effective weight-loss aid. In one carefully controlled clinical trial—and again in a follow-up study—it trimmed 5 percent off the subjects' body weight in a matter of weeks.

Although more research is needed, 5-HTP also seems to act as a mild painkiller. Clinical studies have shown it to be helpful for treating insomnia, fibromyalgia, and chronic tension headache.

What it is; how it works

As the name suggests, 5-HTP is a chemical cousin of the amino acid tryptophan. In fact, the body needs tryptophan to make 5-HTP, which is then converted to serotonin in the brain. Scientists believe it is this conversion that accounts for the antidepressant effects of 5-HTP.

5-HTP is commercially derived from the seeds of an African plant. Small amounts are also found in food, including bananas, tomatoes, plums, avocados, eggplant, walnuts, and pineapples.

Avoid if...

5-HTP should be strictly avoided by anyone with carcinoid tumors (small growths usually found in the intestinal tract). It is not recommended for people with heart disease, chest pain, or high blood pressure, as well as those who have suffered heart attacks. It should not be taken by patients who show signs of an allergic reaction to any component of the supplement. It should also be avoided during treatment with, or within 2 weeks of stopping, a drug classified as an MAO inhibitor, such as the antidepressants Nardil and Parnate.

Special cautions

A severe, life-threatening condition known as eosinophilia-myalgia syndrome (EMS) has been reported in a few people taking 5-HTP. Marked by muscle pain and excessive white blood cell counts, the syndrome has been linked to contaminants in the 5-HTP preparation, rather than 5-HTP itself. Switching preparations in one group of patients resolved the problem.

Supplemental 5-HTP has been know to cause side effects such as nausea, diarrhea, loss of appetite, vomiting, difficulty breathing, and irregular heartbeat. In high doses it can also cause neurological problems such as dilated pupils, abnormally sensitive reflexes, loss of muscle coordination, and blurred vision.

Possible drug interactions

Remember that 5-HTP should never be used while taking a prescription MAO inhibitor such as Nardil or Parnate, or within 2 weeks of stopping an MAO inhibitor. At least in theory, a dangerous interaction is possible.

It's also best to avoid combining 5-HTP with serotonin-boosting drugs such as Luvox and the antidepressant medications Paxil, Prozac, Serzone, and Zoloft. The excessive levels of serotonin that may result can trigger sweating, tremors, flushing, confusion, and agitation. Likewise, 5-HTP should not be combined with tricyclic antidepressants such as Elavil and Tofranil or with the antidepressant herb St. John's wort.

Similarly, patients should not use 5-HTP while taking migraine drugs such as Amerge, Imitrex, and Zomig, since the combination could increase the risk of adverse reactions. In addition, combining 5-HTP with the migraine remedy Sansert reduces its effectiveness; and 5-HTP can also decrease the effectiveness of the antihistamine Periactin.

Patients should also be aware that certain drugs, such as the blood pressure drugs Aldomet and Dibenzyline, inhibit 5-HTP's effect, while Carbidopa enhances its delivery to the brain.

Special information about pregnancy and breastfeeding

Pregnant women and nursing mothers should not take 5-HTP.

Available preparations and dosage

Because of its potential side effects, experts advise against taking 5-HTP by itself. In Europe, doctors prescribe 5-HTP along with carbidopa, which suppresses the conversion of 5-HTP to serotonin outside the brain, reducing serotonin-induced side effects in the body. High daily doses of 100 milligrams to 2 grams of 5-HTP are needed to gain the desired effects; and only when taken with carbidopa are such doses considered reasonably safe. The lower doses of 5-HTP found in dietary supplements are not likely to have any effect.

Overdosage

No overdoses have been reported. However, the first symptoms of overdose would likely be those of excessive serotonin levels, such as sweating, tremors, flushing, confusion, agitation, and rapid heartbeat. Untreated, the patient's condition could progress to coma, seizures, and death. If an overdose is suspected, seek medical help immediately.

Acetylcysteine

Why people take it

Acetylcysteine—also known as N-acetylcysteine or NAC—is available as a supplement and as a prescription drug. Doctors use it to treat acetaminophen overdose. They also prescribe it to thin the excess mucus that occurs with certain lung disorders, such as acute and chronic bronchitis.

As a nutritional supplement, acetylcysteine shows potential as a treatment for age-related memory loss, and may be helpful for a broad range of disorders. The evidence so far shows that it is an effective treatment for chronic obstructive pulmonary disease. Preliminary studies suggest supplemental acetylcysteine may be helpful for treating, and possibly preventing, heart disease. It also shows promise in treating diabetes, certain cancers, and immune system disorders, although more studies are needed.

Because of its liver-protecting abilities, some researchers suggest that acetylcysteine could help treat infectious liver diseases such as hepatitis C, although this remains to be seen.

What it is; how it works

Acetylcysteine is derived from the amino acid L-cysteine. It is preferred over L-cysteine because it is more stable and possibly better absorbed. As a drug, acetylcysteine is well known for its ability to increase liver stores of the antioxidant glutathione, which is why it's routinely given to treat liver damage due to acetaminophen poisoning. This versatile drug is also available as an inhalant called Mucomyst, which binds to mucus proteins, making the gluey substance more watery.

When given as a supplement, acetylcysteine may protect certain cells from damage and even death by increasing levels of L-cysteine and glutathione. Researchers believe this is why it may be helpful for diabetes, heart disease, and cancer, among other things. One study, however, suggested that acetylcysteine might have actually caused DNA damage in certain cells, leading the researchers to believe that the supplement may promote some cancers while inhibiting others.

Avoid if...

There are no known reasons to avoid acetylcysteine at recommended dosages.

Special cautions

Acetylcysteine may be harmful if given early in the treatment of critically ill patients and should therefore be used cautiously, if at all. Caution is also advised for patients with a history of peptic ulcers, since the supplement's mucus-thinning properties could disrupt the stomach's protective mucosal lining. In addition, acetylcysteine metabolism is reduced in patients with chronic liver disease as well as in preterm newborns.

Potential side effects of acetylcysteine include nausea, vomiting, diarrhea, headaches, and rashes. It could also interfere with certain tests for diabetes.

There is a small possibility that acetylcysteine could cause kidney stones. Patients who tend to form kidney stones, especially those caused by excess cystine, should not take this supplement.

Possible drug interactions

Acetylcysteine can cause headaches in those taking nitrates for the treatment of chest pain. It could also decrease blood levels of certain anti-seizure drugs such as Tegretol and Carbatrol.

Special information about pregnancy and breastfeeding

Pregnant women should use acetylcysteine only if prescribed by a doctor, and nursing mothers should avoid the supplement entirely.

Available preparations and dosage

When taking a prescription form of acetylcysteine such as Mucomyst, patients should follow their doctor's instructions.

As a dietary supplement, the usual dose is 600 milligrams, taken anywhere from once daily to 3 times a day. It is available in capsule and tablet form. Common brands include NAC Fuel by TwinLab and N-A-C Sustain by Jarrow Formulas. Various generic brands are also available. Patients should follow the manufacturer's labeling whenever possible.

An important note: Patients should be sure to drink at least 6 to 8 glasses of water a day to prevent the formation of kidney stones.

Overdosage

No information on overdosage with oral supplements is available. When given intravenously for acetaminophen poisoning, high doses can produce symptoms similar to those of a severe allergic reaction, including swelling of the face and throat and heart and blood pressure irregularities.

Acetyl-L-Carnitine

Why people take it

Acetyl-L-carnitine may help slow the progression of Alzheimer's disease in some patients, especially younger ones. In one of its larger clinical trials, researchers found that acetyl-L-carnitine provided the most benefit for patients less than 62 years old. Other, smaller studies showed benefits for patients with mild to moderate symptoms. None of the studies, however, found that the supplement could reverse Alzheimer's disease.

Acetyl-L-carnitine also shows some promise in treating stroke, diabetes-related nerve disorders, and Down's syndrome. Although more research is needed, preliminary evidence suggests it may also help slow the aging process, improve depression in the elderly, treat the mental decline associated with alcoholism, and improve sperm motility.

What it is; how it works

Acetyl-L-carnitine is a close chemical relative of the amino acid compound L-carnitine. The body makes acetyl-L-carnitine in the brain, liver, and kidneys. It also occurs naturally in meat and dairy products.

Acetyl-L-carnitine helps the body's cells produce energy. It also promotes production of acetylcholine, a chemical messenger that plays a role in memory and learning. In lab studies, acetyl-L-carnitine also appears to protect cells from the damage that often occurs during aging.

Researchers aren't sure how acetyl-L-carnitine helps improve memory and nerve disorders. Some speculate it may boost brain levels of acetylcholine, which is deficient in patients with age-related dementias like Alzheimer's. Others suggest it may slow the death of nerve cells in the brain and other parts of the body.

Avoid if...

There are no known reasons to avoid acetyl-L-carnitine at recommended dosages.

Special cautions

People with seizure disorders should take acetyl-L-carnitine only under a doctor's supervision. Although the incidence is rare, a few patients have experienced an increase in the number or severity of their seizures while taking this supplement.

Caregivers of patients with Alzheimer's should be aware that acetyl-L-carnitine has caused increased agitation in some patients.

Acetyl-L-carnitine may also cause stomach upsets, including nausea, vomiting, diarrhea, and cramping.

Possible drug interactions

Certain drugs may cause a decrease in the body's acetyl-L-carnitine levels. These include the anti-HIV drugs Videx, Hivid, and Zerit, and anti-seizure drugs such as Depakote. Antibiotics that contain pivalic acid, such as Spectracef, may also decrease acetyl-L-carnitine levels, although this shouldn't pose a problem if treatment is only for a short period.

Special information about pregnancy and breastfeeding

Because the safety of acetyl-L-carnitine supplements during pregnancy hasn't been tested, women who are pregnant or breastfeeding should not take this substance.

Available preparations and dosage

Typical dosages range from 500 milligrams to 2 grams daily, given in several smaller doses. Some studies, including those for Alzheimer's, used 3 grams a day. There is no consensus on how long treatment must continue before results are observed. Patients should follow the manufacturer's labeling whenever available.

Acetyl-L-carnitine is available in tablets and capsules from various companies, including TwinLab, Now Foods, and Jarrow Formulas. It is also a common ingredient in "brain boosting" supplements.

Overdosage
There are no reports of overdosage.

Alpha-GPC

Why people take it
Alpha-GPC (L-alpha-glycerylphosphorylcholine) is promoted as a "cognitive enhancer" that helps treat age-related memory disorders, including Alzheimer's disease and the aftereffects of stroke. It is also popular among athletes and bodybuilders because of its reputed ability to boost levels of human growth hormone. Although some preliminary research does support these claims, more convincing evidence is needed before this supplement can be considered effective.

What it is; how it works
Alpha-GPC is made from a naturally occurring soybean fat known as lecithin. It is closely related to phosphatidylcholine and serves a similar purpose, acting as a source of the essential nutrient choline. (Alpha-GPC is 40 percent choline.) In theory, the body could use this to make acetylcholine, a chemical messenger that plays a role in memory and learning and also encourages the body to secrete human growth hormone.

Whether alpha-GPC does indeed get converted into acetylcholine, and how much of it actually reaches the brain, is unknown. Animal studies suggest that the conversion does occur, but researchers aren't certain whether this would have any therapeutic effect on the body. Further clinical studies, as well as safety data, are needed to confirm any potential benefits of using this supplement.

Avoid if...
Unless patients have an allergic reaction, there are no known reasons to avoid alpha-GPC supplements.

Special cautions
There are no reported precautions for alpha-GPC, although it should probably not be given to children due to the lack of safety data.

Possible drug interactions
There are no known drug interactions.

Special information about pregnancy and breastfeeding
Due to the lack of safety data, pregnant and breastfeeding women should not take alpha-GPC.

Available preparations and dosage

Typical daily dosages range from 500 milligrams to 1 gram. No information is available on how long treatment should last. Patients should follow the manufacturer's labeling whenever available.

Overdosage

No information on overdosage is available.

Arginine Pyroglutamate

Why people take it

Preliminary research suggests that arginine pyroglutamate may help improve verbal memory in the elderly. One study also found that it may be useful for treating the memory problems associated with chronic alcohol abuse. Definitive evidence for both claims, however, is still lacking.

This supplement is also used by some bodybuilders because the arginine it contains tends to promote the production of human growth hormone. Enthusiasts believe this hormone builds muscle mass and promotes endurance. Many experts, however, warn against adult use of human growth hormone—or substances that promote its release.

What it is; how it works

Arginine pyroglutamate is a water-soluble molecule made from the naturally occurring acids L-arginine and pyroglutamate. The supplement is absorbed by the small intestine, where its two acids are split and sent to various metabolic pathways in the body. Some of the pyroglutamate appears to enter the brain, although more studies are needed to confirm this.

Scientists aren't sure how arginine pyroglutamate may help memory problems, but it appears to be structurally related to the experimental drug piracetam. Piracetam has been studied in Europe as a possible "cognitive enhancer," although clinical trials give mixed results on its effectiveness. Piracetam seems to enhance membrane fluidity in the brain and also appears to interact with glutamate receptors in the brain. Some researchers speculate that arginine pyroglutamate may work in a similar fashion.

In addition to stimulating the production of human growth hormone, the arginine in this compound serves as raw material for nitric oxide, one of the factors that promotes the dilation of blood vessels.

Avoid if...

Unless patients have an allergic reaction, there are no known reasons to completely avoid arginine pyroglutamate. However, due to its impact on the production of human growth hormone, it is not recommended for children, pregnant women, or nursing mothers.

Special cautions
Arginine pyroglutamate may cause minor stomach upsets. Because the arginine it contains affects insulin secretion, people with diabetes should take this compound with care. Arginine may also aggravate schizophrenia. Patients with this problem would be wise to avoid the substance.

Possible drug interactions
Because arginine tends to dilate blood vessels, it's best to avoid combining this supplement with Viagra, heart medicines such as nitroglycerin, and some blood pressure medicines. Patients should also check with their doctor before combining arginine pyroglutamate with any psychotropic medication.

Special information about pregnancy and breastfeeding
Due to its impact on human growth hormone, pregnant and breastfeeding women should not take arginine pyroglutamate.

Available preparations and dosage
Typical dosages range from 500 milligrams to 1,000 milligrams a day. A 500-milligram dose delivers about 150 milligrams of L-arginine and 350 milligrams of pyroglutamate. Patients should follow the manufacturer's labeling whenever available.

Overdosage
No information on overdosage is available.

Bugleweed

Latin name: Lycopus virginicus
Other names: Gypsywort, Sweet Bugle, Water Bugle, Virginia Water Horehound

Why people take it
Bugleweed is used in cases of mildly overactive thyroid, a condition which often leads to nervousness and insomnia. Bugleweed also relieves tension and pain in the breast.

What it is; how it works
Bugleweed does its work by inhibiting the action of thyroid hormones and the reproductive hormones associated with the menstrual cycle. It also reduces levels of prolactin, the hormone that triggers breast milk production.

The herb is a creeping perennial that grows to about 2 feet in height and has a mint-like smell. It was discovered on the banks of streams in

Virginia, but now grows throughout North America. A closely related plant called Gypsywort is found in Europe. Bugleweed's medicinal value lies in its fresh or dried above-ground parts collected during the flowering season.

Avoid if...
Bugleweed should not be used by people with thyroid insufficiency, those taking a thyroid medication, or anyone who will be undergoing a diagnostic test that employs radioactive isotopes.

Special cautions
Warn patients against stopping use of this herb abruptly. This could lead to excessive thyroid activity and symptoms such as breast pain.

Possible drug interactions
Do not use bugleweed if you are taking any thyroid medications.

Special information about pregnancy and breastfeeding
No harmful effects are known.

Available preparations and dosage
Bugleweed is available as a crushed dry herb, as a freshly pressed juice, and in liquid extract form. The dried herb may be used to make tea.

The best dosage of bugleweed varies according to the patient's age and weight. The daily dosage for an adult usually lies between 1 and 2 grams of bugleweed for tea. Liquid extracts should supply approximately 20 milligrams of the active ingredient.

Overdosage
Extremely high doses of bugleweed can cause enlargement of the thyroid gland. Suddenly stopping use of the herb can make the problem worse.

CDP-Choline

Why people take it
Touted as a stronger type of choline (see separate entry), CDP-choline is said to offer many of the same benefits. Like choline, it may sharpen the memory and boost learning, two traits that might help stall aging in the brain. Also like choline, it promises to alleviate some movement disorders. It has been tested in people who have trouble carrying out voluntary movements such as walking—people with Parkinson's disease, for example. And it has also been studied as a treatment for involuntary movements such as the continual chewing or writhing motions (called *tardive dyskinesia*) occasionally triggered by long-term use of antipsy-

chotic drugs. In addition, some evidence hints that it may be useful for treating stroke, brain injury, and vision problems.

Unfortunately, results to date have been less than spectacular. A number of studies have detected small improvements when people with Alzheimer's disease, head injury, or tardive dyskinesia were treated with large doses of the substance. Minor benefits have also been observed in studies of people with multi-infarct dementia or stroke. Likewise, some people with Parkinson's disease have enjoyed small improvements in their symptoms when CDP-choline was added to their regular drug regimen. On balance, though, experts agree that bigger and better studies are needed before CDP-choline can win a passing grade.

(Note, however, that although CDP-choline may still be considered experimental in the U.S., it's sold widely under a variety of brand names in Europe and Japan for treatment of all the disorders discussed above.)

What it is; how it works

Routinely present throughout the body, CDP-choline is a necessary ingredient in the production of compounds known as phospholipids, especially the phospholipid known as phosphatidylcholine. (See separate entry for more on the use of this compound as a dietary supplement.) In turn, phosphatidylcholine and other phospholipids are used to manufacture cell membranes, the barriers protecting the intricate machinery that allows cells to function properly.

Some research suggests that CDP-choline, like other forms of choline, boosts production of acetylcholine, a chemical messenger (neurotransmitter) that's deficient in the brains of people with Alzheimer's disease. Other studies indicate that the drug promotes formation and repair of cell membranes, thereby limiting nerve damage and aiding in recovery from stroke and head injury. To some degree, CDP-choline may also increase the circulation in the brain. At this point, however, all of these possible effects need further verification.

Avoid if...

Because of its potential impact on neurotransmitters, patients who suffer from bipolar disorder or Parkinson's disease should check with their doctor before using CDP-choline. The product should not be used by patients who are allergic to choline. It is also unwise to give it to children due to the lack of safety data.

Special cautions

People in research studies have taken as much as 1,000 milligrams of CDP-choline per day with few ill effects. The most common complaints have been gastrointestinal reactions (nausea, vomiting, diarrhea, stomach pain), dizziness, rash, headache, and fatigue. A small number of people have suffered low blood pressure and changes in heart rate after taking CDP-choline.

Possible drug interactions

CDP-choline could theoretically interfere with the action of drugs that work by blocking the effect of acetylcholine (for example, the antinausea medication scopolamine). Patients who are taking such drugs should check with their doctor before using CDP-choline.

Special information about pregnancy and breastfeeding

Because the safety of CDP-choline supplements during pregnancy hasn't been evaluated, it's best for pregnant and breastfeeding women to avoid them.

Available preparations and dosage

Typically, CDP-choline is sold in capsule form in strengths of 200 to 250 milligrams. Daily dosages of 500 to 2,000 milligrams are typical. Patients should follow the manufacturer's labeling whenever available.

Overdosage

No information on overdosage is available.

Choline

Why people take it

Choline is a vitamin-like compound that has recently gained acceptance as an essential nutrient. It is so important, in fact, that the National Academy of Sciences has increased the recommended intake for pregnant and nursing women in order to ensure normal brain development in the baby. Although the body can produce a certain amount of choline on its own, we also need to get an adequate supply from food. Studies have found that a dietary deficiency can lead to liver and kidney disorders, high blood pressure, and heart disease.

Choline is one of the building blocks of acetylcholine, a key chemical messenger in the nervous system. This fact has led researchers to study it for a wide variety of neurologic disorders, including the tremors and rigidity of Parkinson's disease, the memory loss of Alzheimer's disease, and the involuntary movements of tardive dyskinesia and Huntington's disease.

Choline shows promise as a way to control mood swings and reduce memory loss. Increases in acetylcholine in the brain seem to improve mood, alertness, and mental energy, while low levels are linked to depression and lack of concentration. Many people who use choline notice an improvement in overall disposition. Athletes who take choline-based supplements report greater energy and less fatigue. And researchers have also found that choline boosts the mood of at least some Alzheimer's patients. (Choline will not, however, cure Alzheimer's, though it might play a role in staving it off.)

Choline is also reported to help prevent or treat liver disorders such as cirrhosis, fatty liver, hepatitis, and damage due to drugs or toxic substances. In addition, it may confer some benefit to those with eczema, kidney and gallbladder disorders, and manic depression. It also appears to have some positive impact on cholesterol levels, although not to the extent of two related compounds, phosphatidylcholine and lecithin.

What it is; how it works

Closely related to the B-complex family of vitamins, choline is found in all living cells, where it supports the integrity of cell membranes. In addition to its role in the production of acetylcholine, it aids in the transport of fats into the body's cells. An adequate supply of choline is essential for proper liver function. It is also needed to hold down levels of the amino acid homocysteine—which plays a role in heart disease.

Avoid if...

People suffering from ulcers should avoid choline supplements, since they can increase stomach acid. And because of its potential impact on neurotransmitters, patients who have manic depression or Parkinson's disease should check with their doctor before using choline.

Special cautions

Choline is generally safe and nontoxic even at high levels, although megadoses are usually reserved for treating manic depression and other serious psychiatric disorders. High doses (more than 3.5 grams a day) can be counterproductive, actually causing depression in some people, and can lead to a fishy body odor and other side effects such as dizziness, low blood pressure, excessive sweating, nausea, diarrhea, and abdominal cramps. Excess consumption can also overstimulate muscles, leading to tightening in the shoulders and neck and, ultimately, a tension headache.

Certain patients should be particularly cautious of high doses, including those with liver or kidney disease, depression, Parkinson's disease, and trimethylaminuria (a rare genetic disorder that interferes with choline metabolism).

Possible drug interactions

Choline could theoretically interfere with the action of drugs that work by blocking the effect of acetylcholine (for example, the antinausea medication scopolamine). It's best to check with the doctor before combining choline with such drugs.

On the other hand, the anticancer drug methotrexate could interfere with choline metabolism and possibly block its beneficial effects. Animal studies show that choline supplementation may help offset this problem.

Special information about pregnancy and breastfeeding

For healthy women who eat a balanced diet, choline supplements are usually unnecessary during pregnancy and breastfeeding.

Available preparations and dosage

The new RDI for choline ranges from 425 to 550 milligrams per day for adults. Few people suffer an outright deficiency, since Americans' average dietary intake ranges from 500 to 1,000 milligrams daily. However, since many of the foods richest in choline, such as egg yolks and liver, are also high in cholesterol, intake may be falling among people who watch their cholesterol levels.

Choline is available as tablets, capsules, softgels, powder, and liquids. The different forms of Choline (bitartrate, chloride, and dihydrogencitate) vary in potency from 36 to 75 percent choline. The optimal daily supplemental dose of choline is often pegged at 250 to 350 milligrams, although some studies have used as much as 1,200 milligrams. To lower homocysteine levels, choline requires the vitamins B_6, B_{12}, and folic acid. Aside from eggs and liver, good dietary sources of choline are wheat germ, lentils, peanuts, soybeans, iceberg lettuce, cabbage, and cauliflower. Supplements such as lecithin and phosphatidylcholine supply significant amounts of basic choline. It's also found in brewer's yeast, and is often included in B-complex and multinutrient vitamins or sold in combination with vitamin B_6 or inositol. It should be taken with meals.

Overdosage

A dose of 200 grams or more (100 times the typical dose) could prove dangerous. Sustained megadoses of 3,500 milligrams daily or more tend to cause muscle stiffness and digestive upsets.

DHA

Why people take it

DHA (docosahexaenoic acid) is an essential fatty acid that has piqued interest in the medical community due to its abundant presence in fish oil (see separate entry). Researchers suspect that DHA supplements could prove useful for treating certain brain and mood disorders. DHA deficiencies have been noted in people with attention deficit disorder, dyslexia, depression, age-related mental decline, and Alzheimer's disease. DHA levels are also inadequate in those suffering from postpartum depression or the cognitive decline associated with alcoholism. In addition, DHA has gained a reputation as a "brain booster." Japanese students, for example, take DHA supplements to improve their performance on exams.

Researchers are also studying DHA as a potential treatment for vision disorders such as age-related macular degeneration, and for certain serious congenital disorders such as cystic fibrosis. Like the fish oil in which it's found, DHA is also used to reduce triglyceride levels and protect against heart disease

What it is; how it works

One of the two omega-3 fatty acids found in fish oil, DHA is essential for proper brain and eye development in infants. DHA is abundant in breast milk, and many studies have linked breast-feeding to better vision and higher IQ in children, particularly those born prematurely. Scientists in the U.S. are still debating whether adding DHA to commercial infant formulas confers similar benefits, but the World Health Organization already recommends it. In fact, DHA-enriched formulas are widely available in Japan and countries throughout Europe, and were finally approved for use in the U.S. in 2001.

The science backing DHA supplementation for children and adults is far more questionable. While most nutritionists agree that it's important to get enough omega-3 fats from the diet, the value of supplements is unknown. In theory, DHA could be helpful for various psychiatric disorders because it's one of the main fatty acids in brain and eye tissue, and it appears to be necessary for proper brain-cell signaling. However, most of the research is preliminary, and many of the findings contradict each other. Although some studies, for example, have revealed low DHA levels in people with attention deficit disorders and Alzheimer's disease, clinical trials of DHA supplements failed to improve these conditions.

Avoid if...

Because of possible blood-thinning effects, DHA supplements should not be used by patients who have a bleeding disorder such as hemophilia or a tendency to hemorrhage.

Special cautions

There have been no reports of serious reactions, even in those taking up to 6 grams of DHA a day for 3 months. Potential minor side effects include a fishy odor or taste, belching, upset stomach, nausea, and diarrhea. Infants and children should not take DHA supplements unless monitored by a physician.

Because DHA supplements may slightly increase the risk of hemorrhage, patients should stop taking them before any type of surgery. It is also advisable to check the Special Cautions in the entry on Fish Oil. In theory, the same warnings could apply to DHA supplements.

Possible drug interactions

There have been no reported interactions to date. But patients who are taking a blood-thinning drug such as aspirin or Coumadin should still check with their doctor before taking DHA supplements, which could further thin the blood. Increased bleeding could also occur if DHA is taken with supplemental garlic or the herb ginkgo. Possible signs of an interaction could include increased bruising and nosebleeds.

Special information about pregnancy and breastfeeding
Pregnant and breastfeeding women should check with their doctor before using DHA supplements.

Available preparations and dosage
DHA supplements are made from fish or algae and are available in capsule form; a common brand is Neuromins. Typical dosages for pregnant and nursing women are 100 to 200 milligrams a day. The dosages needed to lower triglyceride levels are higher, ranging from 1 to 4 grams a day. DHA is also found in certain infant formulas and in specially raised eggs.

Patients should choose preparations that contain vitamin E to prevent oxidation of the easily damaged oil; they should also take a little extra vitamin E to prevent oxidation within the body. To prevent stomach upset, DHA supplements should be taken with meals.

Overdosage
No information on overdosage is available.

DHEA

Why people take it
Whether or not DHEA (dehydroepiandrosterone) should be taken at all as an unregulated over-the-counter supplement is a controversial issue. There is evidence that this steroid can improve feelings of well-being and increase sexual satisfaction—but only in people whose adrenal glands are functioning poorly. There are also preliminary results indicating that it may have a beneficial effect on some people with major depression.

Much of the controversy arises because DHEA is being promoted as a cure for many other ailments and has taken on the reputation of an anti-aging remedy—kind of a modern-day fountain of youth. Advocates claim that it can encourage weight loss; boost sex drive and the immune system; enhance mood, memory, and energy; and reverse the aging process. Some proponents even suggest using it as an adjunct to conventional cancer therapy. And a number of anti-aging clinics recommend taking it as early as your 40's or 50's to fight off old age and remain biologically young. Athletes take it in large doses to enhance their performance. However, much of the research behind these claims was done on laboratory animals, and experts caution that the results of such studies cannot be translated to humans. The long-term effects of DHEA supplementation are not known and since it is a powerful hormone, it should be used with great caution and only under a doctor's supervision.

What it is; how it works

DHEA is a steroid hormone produced primarily by the adrenal glands. It is the most abundant hormone in the body, with the highest concentrations found in the brain. The only known function of DHEA is as a precursor hormone, meaning that it is a source material which the body converts into other hormones, such as estrogen and testosterone. It peaks in production by the age of 25 and gradually declines until, by age 70, levels may be more than 80 percent below their earlier highs.

Low DHEA levels have been associated with certain diseases, such as Alzheimer's, cancer, diabetes, multiple sclerosis, lupus, and other immune function disorders. For this reason, researchers have been tempted to speculate that supplementation with a synthetic form of DHEA could reverse these diseases, much like hormone replacement therapy reduces some of the symptoms of menopause by returning the hormone balance to a premenopausal state. However, it has not yet been proven that either the diseases or the aging process itself are a result of lowered levels of DHEA, and it is not yet clear whether using DHEA is helpful or, in the long run, harmful.

Despite all this, there are physicians who recommend use of this hormone to treat a variety of ailments or combat the effects of aging. Anyone who decides to try DHEA should seek out a qualified physician willing to plan and monitor their treatment.

Avoid if...

DHEA should not be used by patients who have a hormone-related cancer—or a family history of one—including breast, cervical, uterine, ovarian, and prostate cancers. The hormone should also not be given to children.

Special cautions

DHEA has been known to cause acne, facial hair growth, and deepening of the voice in some women, and there are reports of breast enlargement in men taking high doses, probably because it triggers hormone production. The hormone may also lower levels of "good" HDL cholesterol and raise levels of cancer-promoting hormones. There have been a few reports of DHEA-related hepatitis and insulin resistance.

Possible drug interactions

Natural DHEA levels may be boosted by certain drugs, including Xanax, Cardizem, testosterone, and the sports supplement androstenedione. Adding even more DHEA through supplementation increases the risk of side effects.

Certain other drugs tend to lower natural DHEA levels. Drugs in this category include Danocrine (used to treat endometriosis), corticosteroids, insulin, and morphine.

Special information about pregnancy and breastfeeding
Because of its hormonal effects, DHEA should not be used during pregnancy or while breastfeeding.

Available preparations and dosage
DHEA is available in capsule, tablet, cream, and spray form in strengths ranging from 5 milligrams to 200 milligrams. The typical daily dose is 25 to 50 milligrams.

Dosage should be set by a physician following a blood test or saliva test can tell if a true deficiency exists and how much, if any, supplemental DHEA is needed. Individuals taking DHEA will also periodically need to visit their doctor to have their blood levels monitored and the dosage adjusted accordingly.

Overdosage
No information on overdosage is available.

DL-Phenylalanine

Why people take it
An "essential" amino acid that the body can't manufacture on its own, phenylalanine is one of the raw materials for three of the nervous system's most important chemical messengers: dopamine, epinephrine, and norepinephrine. The body can also convert it to phenylethylamine, a mood-boosting substance that's said to have pain-relieving effects as well.

In light of these properties, phenylalanine has been proposed as a treatment for depression, Parkinson's disease, and chronic-pain conditions such as arthritis. Trials for arthritis have yielded conflicting results, but preliminary trials for depression have proved encouraging. Phenylalanine has also been promoted as an appetite suppressant and sexual stimulant, but its effectiveness for these purposes remains unproven.

What it is; how it works
There are two types of phenylalanine: L-phenylalanine and D-phenylalanine. The "L" variety occurs primarily in animal protein and supports production of dopamine, epinephrine, norepinephrine, and the mood elevator phenylethylamine. The "D" form of the substance is typically found in plant protein and blocks an enzyme that degrades enkephalins, a group of natural substances that the body produces to deaden pain.

Because of this action, D-phenylalanine (but not L-phenylalanine) has been proposed as a treatment for chronic pain. L-phenylalanine, on the other hand, is usually taken to relieve depression. The "L" form of the substance has also been suggested as a treatment for vitiligo, a disease characterized by abnormal white blotches of skin due to loss of pigmentation.

D-phenylalanine alone is not available as a nutritional supplement, but both forms are created during the commercial manufacturing process and are typically sold as DL-phenylalanine or DLPA. Products containing only the "L" form are also available. Phenylalanine is also an ingredient of the popular artificial sweetener aspartame.

Avoid if...

Children born without the ability to process phenylalanine can build up dangerous levels of this amino acid, leading to mental retardation, seizures, extreme hyperactivity, and psychosis. Youngsters with this condition—called phenylketonuria—must follow a special diet designed to supply no more phenylalanine than necessary, and must be monitored regularly for excess phenylalanine in the blood.

Special cautions

L-phenylalanine has also been reported to exacerbate involuntary movements (tardive dyskinesia) in schizophrenic patients. Anyone with this disorder should therefore use DL-phenylalanine with extreme caution. Caution is also warranted for people with high blood pressure or an anxiety disorder; phenylalanine tends to aggravate these conditions.

DL-phenylalanine occasionally causes mild nausea, heartburn, or headache. Because it can have significant effects on mood, it's best to use this type of phenylalanine only under a doctor's supervision.

Possible drug interactions

Phenylalanine supplements should never be combined with drugs known as MAO inhibitors, including the antidepressants Nardil and Parnate; a surge in blood pressure could result. It is also best to avoid combining phenylalanine with antipsychotic drugs, since it increases the likelihood of tardive dyskinesia.

On the other hand, taking phenylalanine with the drug Eldepryl may boost the antidepressant activity of both agents.

Special information about pregnancy and breastfeeding

Phenylalanine supplements are not recommended during pregnancy and breastfeeding.

Available preparations and dosage

DL-phenylalanine is available in capsule, tablet, and powder form. Typical dosages range from 375 milligrams to 2.25 grams daily.

Overdosage

There are no reports of overdosage.

Fish Oil

Why people take it

Fish oil is one of those nutritional megastars that holds promise for a wide variety of chronic conditions. The latest buzz focuses on its potential to alleviate symptoms of several serious psychiatric illnesses, including bipolar disorder, schizophrenia, and severe depression. Preliminary research hints that it may also be helpful for warding off Alzheimer's disease and treating attention deficit disorder. Keep in mind, however, that most of this research is still in its infancy, and more definitive answers are needed before fish oil supplements can be recommended.

While the effects of fish oil on the brain are still being investigated, more is known about its benefits for the heart. Rich in omega-3 fatty acids, fish oil seems to help protect against cardiovascular disease. Studies have found that it lowers blood pressure, keeps arteries clear following angioplasty, and reduces the risk of sudden cardiac death, death from heart attack, and stroke. If all that weren't enough, there's some evidence that fish oil could be useful for treating arthritis (particularly rheumatoid arthritis), Crohn's disease, kidney disease, and ulcerative colitis.

What it is; how it works

The two omega-3 fatty acids contained in fish oil are eicosapentaenoic acid (EPA) and docosahexaenoic acid (DHA). These acids are especially prevalent in oily cold-water fish such as cod, tuna, mackerel, herring, and salmon. Because the omega-3s come from algae that are then eaten by krill that in turn are eaten by larger fish, farm-raised fish that have been fed grain alone may contain little or none of these beneficial acids.

Researchers speculate that because Western diets have changed drastically in the last century, Americans may be deficient in omega-3 fatty acids. The brain and nervous system rely on fatty acids like EPA and DHA to regulate cell membrane function. These acids may even play a role in the proper regulation of serotonin, a chemical messenger that has gained fame for its role in depression and other mental illnesses. Indeed, depression rates have soared in recent decades, and global studies show that depression is less likely to occur in countries that consume the most fish. But while the evidence so far is tantalizing, fish oil's effectiveness against psychiatric disorders has yet to be tested in major clinical trials.

In the prevention of heart disease, omega-3s are thought to work by lowering total cholesterol and triglyceride levels, raising "good" HDL cholesterol, and thinning the blood. They lower the level of fibrinogen, the blood clotting factor, and keep blood platelets from becoming too sticky, all of which helps to prevent the buildup of artery-clogging plaque. Fish oil also tends to dilate the blood vessels, which can help to lower blood pressure in those with hypertension.

Some researchers have found that the omega-3s have anti-inflammatory properties that appear to make them helpful in the treatment of arthritis, Crohn's disease, endometriosis, lupus, and ulcerative colitis. In addition, laboratory experiments suggest that these fatty acids may have an anti-cancer effect. They are also being studied for a variety of other disorders, including eczema, psoriasis, and Raynaud's phenomenon.

Avoid if...
Because of their blood-thinning effects, fish oil supplements should be used only with great caution by patients who have a bleeding disorder such as hemophilia or a tendency to hemorrhage.

Special cautions
Although fish oil tends to have beneficial effects on "good" HDL cholesterol and total cholesterol levels, high doses sometimes cause an increase in "bad" LDL cholesterol levels. A few studies have also suggested that fish oil supplements may cause an increase in the blood sugar levels of people with diabetes. Diabetics should discuss use of these supplements with their doctor and closely monitor their blood sugar for any change.

Because fish oil supplements may slightly increase the risk of hemorrhage, patients should stop taking them before any type of surgery. Patients who have had a stroke should check with their doctor before using fish oil. It could be dangerous if the stroke involved bleeding into the brain. Give fish oil supplements to children only under a doctor's supervision.

Potential side effects of fish oil capsules include a fishy odor or taste, belching, upset stomach, nausea, diarrhea, increased bleeding (including nosebleeds), and easy bruising.

To obtain the greatest heart benefits from the fatty acids found in fish and fish oils, patients should follow a low-fat diet.

Possible drug interactions
Patients who are taking a blood-thinning drug such as aspirin or Coumadin should check with their doctor before taking fish oil supplements, which could further thin the blood. Increased bleeding could also occur if fish oil is taken with supplemental garlic or the herb ginkgo. Signs to watch for include easy bruising, nosebleeds, spitting or vomiting up blood, and blood in the stool or urine. Note, however, that these reactions are rare and may be alleviated by reducing the dose of fish oil.

Special information about pregnancy and breastfeeding

Pregnant women and nursing mothers should use fish oil capsules only under a doctor's supervision.

Some types of fish can contain high amounts of mercury, which can hurt a developing baby's brain. The Food and Drug Administration advises pregnant and breastfeeding women, and those who might become pregnant, to avoid shark, swordfish, king mackerel, and tilefish.

Available preparations and dosage

Fish oil is available in liquid, softgel, or capsule form. Most fish oil supplements range in potency from 200 to 400 milligrams of omega-3 acids. Patients should check the labels carefully, since the number of milligrams in each capsule often refers to the total weight rather than its omega-3 content. Patients should choose preparations that contain vitamin E to prevent oxidation of the easily damaged oil; they should also take a little extra vitamin E to prevent oxidation within the body.

Supplements that contain 18 percent EPA and 12 percent DHA are generally considered standard. They should be taken in divided doses, with meals, to prevent stomach upset. Patients should pay attention to expiration dates and refrigerate the package after opening. Some preparations may contain pesticides.

There is no recommended dietary allowance (RDA) for omega-3 fatty acids. When taken to prevent arterial clogging after angioplasty, doses of 4 to 5 grams per day are typical. For arthritis and high blood pressure, doses of 3 grams daily are usually recommended. A dosage of 1 gram a day has been found to have a protective effect on heart attack victims. However, the American Heart Association suggests that it may be better for patients to boost their intake by eating fish 2 or 3 times a week, rather than taking large amounts of supplements. A 7-ounce serving of salmon or bluefish provides 2.4 grams of omega-3 acids. The same serving of herring contains 3.2 grams.

Overdosage

There are no reports of serious adverse effects, even with dosages as high as 15 grams a day taken for prolonged periods of time. However, it's important for patients to make sure they are using fish oil supplements rather than fish liver oils. The latter contain large amounts of vitamins A and D, which can build up in the body until they reach toxic levels. Symptoms of vitamin A toxicity include hair loss, headache, menstrual problems, stiffness, joint pain, weakness, and dry skin. Excessive intake of vitamin D can lead to irreversible kidney and cardiovascular damage.

Gamma-Tocopherol

Why people take it

Gamma-tocopherol is a member of the vitamin E family. Although *alpha*-tocopherol is the best known form of this vitamin, there is preliminary evidence that gamma-tocopherol may be more protective against cardiovascular disease and some cancers. As a form of vitamin E, gamma-tocopherol is also thought to slow the progress of Alzheimer's disease.

What it is; how it works

Gamma-tocopherol is the most common of the tocopherols. It is found in many seeds and nuts, including soybeans, corn, and walnuts, and is the principal tocopherol in the American diet.

Like other forms of vitamin E, gamma-tocopherol is an antioxidant, scavenging the free radicals that cause cellular damage. Researchers believe that it helps to prevent fat buildup in the arteries, protects cells in the artery walls, reduces the risk of blood clots, inhibits the development of certain cancers, and stimulates the immune system.

Avoid if...

Gamma-tocopherol must be avoided by anyone with a hypersensitivity to it. There are no medical conditions that completely preclude its use.

Special cautions

Those on the blood-thinning medication warfarin should be cautious in using high doses of gamma-tocopherol (doses greater than 100 milligrams daily). Also those with vitamin K deficiencies, such as people with liver failure, should be cautious about using high doses. Gamma-tocopherol must also be used cautiously by those with bleeding ulcers and similar bleeding problems, those with a history of hemorrhagic stroke, and those with hemophilia.

To reduce the risk of bleeding problems, people preparing for surgery should stop high-dose gamma-tocopherol supplementation 1 month before the procedure.

There is one study in which high blood levels of gamma-tocopherol was associated with an increased incidence of knee osteoarthritis, especially in African-Americans.

Possible drug interactions

High doses of gamma-tocopherol may boost the effects of blood-thinning drugs, such as aspirin. Some herbs, including garlic and ginkgo, also possess blood-thinning activity and high doses of gamma-tocopherol may enhance their action as well. The following drugs may reduce the impact of gamma-tocopherol:

Cholestyramine (Questran)

Colestipol (Colestid)
Isoniazid (Rifampin)
Mineral oil
Neomycin (Neosporin)
Orlistat (Xenical)
Sucralfate (Carafate)
Alpha-tocopherol
Iron

Vitamin C and selenium may increase the effectiveness of gamma-toco-pherol.

Special information about pregnancy and breastfeeding

Since the effects of gamma-tocopherol during pregnancy have not been studied, the safest course is to forego supplementation.

Available preparations and dosage

Typical doses are about 200 milligrams daily.

Overdosage

There are no reports of gamma-tocopherol overdose.

Ginkgo

Latin name: Ginkgo biloba

Why people take it

Ginkgo is generally accepted as a remedy for minor deficits in brain function, such as those that occur with advancing age. It is used to improve concentration and combat short-term memory loss due to clogged arteries in the brain, and to treat dizziness, ringing in the ears, headache, and emotional hypersensitivity accompanied by anxiety. For people with intermittent circulation problems in the legs, it permits longer pain-free walks.

What it is; how it works

Although the ginkgo tree has been around for 200 million years, it's only during the last couple of decades that its true value has been recognized. Active compounds in ginkgo extract improve circulation, discourage clot formation, reinforce the walls of the capillaries, and protect nerve cells from harm when deprived of oxygen. These ingredients also appear to have an antioxidant effect, sparing brain tissue from the damage caused by free radicals. Because the active ingredients are limited to minute quantities in natural ginkgo leaves, only concentrated ginkgo extract is really effective.

The ginkgo tree grows over 100 feet high and can live for hundreds of years. The tree flowers for the first time when it is between 20 and 30 years old. Native to China, Japan, and Korea, it now grows worldwide, and is intensively cultivated in major plantations such as one in Sumter, South Carolina.

Avoid if...

Anyone who has been warned about the possibility of bleeding in the brain should avoid ginkgo. There have been reports of intracranial hemorrhage associated with this herb. It should also be avoided if it causes an allergic reaction.

Special cautions

Taken orally in customary doses, ginkgo is unlikely to have side effects. Spasms, cramps, and mild digestive problems are the most common reactions. On rare occasions, allergic skin problems may occur.

Possible drug interactions

Combining ginkgo with clot-busting drugs, blood-thinners, or aspirin may increase the risk of intracranial bleeding.

Special information about pregnancy and breastfeeding

There is no information available.

Available preparations and dosage

Ginkgo extract is produced in liquid, tablet, and capsule form, in strengths ranging from 30 to 500 milligrams. Tea made from ginkgo leaves, as in traditional Chinese medicine, is too weak to be effective.

A total daily intake of 120 milligrams is usually recommended, typically in three 40-milligram doses spaced throughout the day. Doses of up to 240 milligrams a day are taken by people with severe memory loss.

Strengths of commercial preparations may vary. Follow the manufacturer's labeling whenever available.

Overdosage

A massive overdose can reduce muscle tone, leading to severe weakness. If an overdose is suspected, seek medical attention immediately.

Glycine

Why people take it

In at least one carefully designed clinical trial, high-dose glycine has provided additional relief to schizophrenic patients taking antipsychotic drugs. Glycine has also been used successfully to help alleviate the symptoms of spasticity, primarily in patients with multiple sclerosis; and it has cured seizures caused by an inborn lack of the related amino acid L-serine.

Glycine is one of the many nutritional supplements adopted by body-builders to boost physical performance. Its popularity stems from its role in the formation of creatine, a key ingredient in the chemical reaction that powers muscles. Unfortunately, while there's some evidence that creatine may indeed be helpful during short bursts of physical activity, glycine alone does not seem to have the same effect. In fact, the American Dietetic Association notes that glycine and other supposedly ergogenic (energy-producing) substances may owe their standing more to psychological than to any physical effects.

Studies in laboratory animals suggest that glycine may combat certain types of cancer, including liver tumors and melanoma. Taken with other amino acids, it may also reduce the symptoms of benign prostatic hyperplasia (BPH), although the study suggesting this possibility has never been replicated.

What it is; how it works

Glycine is one of the "nonessential" amino acids that the body can produce for itself whenever they fall short in the diet. It's also available from high-protein foods such as meat, fish, beans, and dairy products.

Glycine combines with two other amino acids—arginine and methionine—to build energy-producing creatine. It also promotes the storage of blood sugar (glucose) in the form of glycogen. Together with the amino acids cysteine and glutamic acid, it produces the protective antioxidant glutathione. And on top of all these duties, it also serves as one of the nervous system's chemical regulators, inhibiting neurological responses in the spinal cord.

Glycine's beneficial effect on schizophrenia is believed to result from its ability to boost nerve impulses transmitted through N-methyl-D-aspartic acid (NMDA) receptors in the brain.

Avoid if...

Extra glycine and other amino acids increase the burden on the liver and kidneys, and should be avoided by anyone who has problems in these areas unless their doctor recommends otherwise.

Special cautions

Even when taken in megadoses, glycine rarely has unwanted side effects. Mild stomach problems are the most likely possibility.

Possible drug interactions

Theoretically glycine may add to the beneficial effects of antispastic drugs such as baclofen, diazepam (Valium), dantrolene (Dantrium), and tizanidine (Zanaflex). No other interactions are known.

Special information about pregnancy and breastfeeding

It's not known whether high levels of glycine are safe during pregnancy. As with any supplement not absolutely necessary for health, it's best to avoid glycine while pregnant or breastfeeding.

Available preparations and dosage

Glycine is available in tablet, capsule, and powder form in doses ranging from 100 to 600 milligrams. Those who use it as a performance-booster take up to 1 gram daily in divided doses. Doses for spasticity are 1 gram per day. Doses used for the management of schizophrenia have ranged from 40 to 90 grams daily.

Overdosage

There are no reports of glycine overdose.

Hops

Latin name: Humulus lupulus

Why people take it

This herb is an accepted remedy for edginess and insomnia. Effectiveness for its other uses—including stimulation of the appetite, increasing the flow of digestive juices, and treating ulcers, skin abrasions, and bladder inflammation—has never been scientifically verified.

What it is; how it works

Hops have long been associated with beer and ale, but the beverage originally called ale in English was made from fermented malt only, and contained no hops. The use of hops probably began in Holland in the early 14th century, and the resulting drink became known as "bier" or "beer." At first, there was much resistance to the use of hops, which was regarded as a "wicked weed that would spoil the taste... and endanger the people."

The plant's medicinal value lies in a set of light yellow scales adjoining the fruit. Compounds in these scales have a sedative effect. Hop tea induces calm, and pillows stuffed with hops assist sleep.

Avoid if...

No known medical conditions preclude the use of hops.

Special cautions

The fresh plant can occasionally cause a reaction. However, when taken at customary dosage levels, hops pose no problems.

Possible drug interactions

There are no known interactions.

Special information about pregnancy and breastfeeding
No harmful effects are known.

Available preparations and dosage
Hops are available in crushed and powdered form, and in commercial preparations for oral administration. A hop tea can be prepared by pouring boiling water over the ground herb and steeping for 10 to 15 minutes.

The usual single dose of Hops is 0.5 grams (about 1 heaping tea-spoonful). The strength of commercial preparations may vary, so follow the manufacturer's directions whenever available.

Store hops protected from light and moisture.

Overdosage
No information on overdosage is available.

Huperzine A

Why people take it
Huperzine A shows considerable promise as a treatment for Alzheimer's disease and age-related memory impairment. Numerous studies suggest that it may be as effective as Cognex and Aricept, two of the prescription drugs currently available for Alzheimer's.

What it is; how it works
Alzheimer's disease is marked by declining activity in certain nerve cells that respond to acetylcholine, one of the key chemical messengers in the brain. Huperzine A, like Cognex and Aricept, inhibits the breakdown of acetylcholine, thereby boosting the amount available to these cells.

Huperzine A is a plant alkaloid derived from the Chinese club moss plant, *Huperzia serrata*. In Chinese folk medicine, this herb has long been used as treatment for fever and inflammation, though there's no scientific evidence that it's effective for these problems.

Avoid if...
Huperzine A has a number of potential cardiac and neurological side effects. It should be avoided by those with seizure disorders, heartbeat irregularities, or asthma. People with irritable bowel disease, inflammatory bowel disease, and malabsorption syndromes should also refrain from using this medication.

Special cautions
Huperzine A has potent pharmacological effects and its long-term safety has not been verified. It should be used only under medical supervision and should never be given to children.

Side effects reported with huperzine A include nausea and diarrhea, sweating, blurred vision, twitching, and dizziness. Other possible effects include vomiting, cramping, asthma attacks, slow or irregular heartbeat, seizures, urinary incontinence, increased urination, and excessive salivation.

Possible drug interactions

Combining huperzine A with other medications that boost acetylcholine levels increases the likelihood of side effects. Drugs in this category include Aricept, Cognex, neostigmine, physostigmine, and pyridostigmine. Side effects are also more likely when huperzine A is taken with drugs that mimic the effects of acetylcholine, such as the bladder stimulant Urecholine.

Special information about pregnancy and breastfeeding

Safety of this medication during pregnancy has not been confirmed. It should be avoided by pregnant women and nursing mothers.

Available preparations and dosage

Huperzine A is available in natural and synthetic forms. The natural substance is three times as potent as its synthetic counterpart. Doses of natural huperzine A used in clinical trials have ranged from 60 to 200 micrograms daily.

Overdosage

There are no reports of huperzine A overdose.

Kava Kava

Latin name: Piper methysticum

Why people take it

In the past, kava kava has been taken for a host of ailments on which it has no appreciable effect, including asthma, arthritis, indigestion, cystitis, syphilis, and gonorrhea. For anxiety and insomnia, however, it is now considered a proven remedy.

What it is; how it works

One of the "new" herbs that have recently gained considerable media attention, kava kava has actually been around for centuries in the South Seas, where it's used as a ceremonial beverage. The plant's fleshy underground stem is mildly intoxicating when chewed. Prepared as a nonalcoholic drink, it is said to foster a sense of contentment and well-being, while sharpening the mind, memory, and senses.

Research shows that the active ingredients in kava kava (kava pyrones) do in fact have a calming, sedative effect. They also appear to relax the muscles, relieve spasms, and prevent convulsions. At least two scientific studies have confirmed the herb's ability to significantly reduce symptoms of anxiety. In a third study, researchers rated it as effective as prescription tranquilizers.

Avoid if...

Kava kava should not be used by women who are pregnant or nursing. It should also be avoided by anyone with a depressive disorder; it can deepen a depressed mood.

Special cautions

Patients may notice a slightly tired feeling in the mornings when first taking kava kava.

In rare cases, kava kava can cause an allergic reaction, a slight yellowing of the skin, gastrointestinal complaints, impaired or abnormal movement, loss of balance, pupil dilation, and difficulty focusing. Because of the possibility of visual disturbances, it's important to drive with caution while using this herb.

High doses of the herb have been known to trigger hepatitis, cirrhosis, and liver failure. Heavy long-term use can also cause an unusual scaly rash, and may lead to unwanted weight loss. This herb should not be taken for more than 3 months without a doctor's approval.

Possible drug interactions

Kava kava should not be combined with other substances that act on the brain, such as alcohol, barbiturates, or other mood-altering drugs. It may increase their effect. Be especially wary of taking it with the tranquilizer Xanax; the combination has caused coma.

Kava kava has an antagonistic effect on dopamine. Patients taking a levodopa-based medication for Parkinson's disease should avoid this herb.

Special information about pregnancy and breastfeeding

Remember, kava kava should be avoided during pregnancy and nursing.

Available preparations and dosage

Commercial extracts are the predominant form of kava kava. The crushed root can also be used. Daily doses delivering between 50 and 240 milligrams of the active ingredients are the customary recommendation. Commercial capsules containing between 150 and 300 milligrams of root extract may be taken twice a day. Because the potency of commercial preparations may vary, follow the manufacturer's directions whenever available. The dosage should be administered with food or liquid.

Overdosage

An overdose is usually signaled by a lack of coordination, followed by tiredness and a tendency to sleep. If an overdose is suspected, seek medical attention immediately.

Lavender

Latin name: Lavandula angustifolia

Why people take it

In Europe, lavender is considered an effective remedy for nervousness, insomnia, nervous stomach, and loss of appetite. It is also used in mineral baths to treat circulatory disorders.

Other uses remain unproven. They include migraine, cramps, asthma, and arthritis. Lavender is used in aromatherapy for sleep induction, and is added to bathwater to help treat poorly healing wounds.

What it is; how it works

Because of its wonderful fragrance, from Roman times onward lavender has always been a popular bath additive. In fact, its name derives from the Latin "lavare" meaning "to wash." Over the centuries, it has been used in a variety of forms, including oil, distilled water, and alcohol solution (tincture). One species, spike lavender, is even an effective insect repellent.

Lavender's medicinal value lies in the essential oil, customarily extracted from the flowers. Taken internally, lavender has been found to stimulate the production and flow of bile. It also has a mildly sedating effect, and gets rid of gas. Used externally, it improves circulation and brings color to the skin.

Avoid if...

No known medical conditions preclude the use of lavender.

Special cautions

Taken at customary dosage levels, lavender presents no problems, although a few people do develop a sensitivity to the oil.

Possible drug interactions

No interactions have been reported.

Special information about pregnancy and breastfeeding

No harmful effects are known.

Available preparations and dosage

Extracts, bath additives, and crushed lavender flowers are all available.

To prepare a bath additive, boil 100 grams (about one-half cup) of lavender in 2 quarts of water, then add to the tub.

The usual daily dose of lavender for internal use is:
Crushed flowers: 3 to 5 grams
Essential oil: 1 to 4 drops

Overdosage
No information on overdosage is available.

Lemon Balm

Latin name: Melissa officinalis
Other names: Balm Mint, Bee Balm, Blue Balm, Cure-all, Garden Balm, Honey Plant, Sweet Balm, Sweet Mary

Why people take it
Lemon balm is officially recognized only for its ability to calm the nerves and promote sleep. In the past it has been taken for a wide variety of problems, including bloating and gas, mood disorders, bronchial inflammation, high blood pressure, palpitations, vomiting, toothache, earache, and headache. However, its effectiveness for these purposes has never been validated by clinical trials.

Applied externally, it has also been used for arthritis, nerve pains, and stiff neck—but again without clinical validation.

What it is; how it works
Lemon balm's medicinal properties have been held in high regard for nearly two millennia. The Roman scholar Pliny believed lemon balm could prevent infection in open wounds (an action that has been clinically proven for balsamic oils in general). The noted 16th century physician Paracelsus believed lemon balm could heal even patients close to death.

Modern research on lemon balm has revealed a mild sedative effect, antibacterial and antiviral properties, and an ability to quell spasms and relieve cramps and gas. Only the plant's leaves are medicinal.

A perennial herb, lemon balm grows up to 3 feet in height. It is native to the east Mediterranean region and west Asia, but is cultivated throughout central Europe. Before flowering, it has a lemon-like taste and smell; and the fresh leaves, in addition to their medicinal applications, are commonly used in cooking.

Avoid if...
No known medical conditions preclude the use of lemon balm.

Special cautions
When taken at customary dosage levels, lemon balm poses no hazards.

Possible drug interactions
There are no known interactions.

Special information about pregnancy and breastfeeding
No harmful effects are known.

Available preparations and dosage
Lemon balm can be found in the form of dried herb, herb powder, and liquid or dry extracts, as well as various liquid and solid commercial preparations.

To make a tea, pour a cup of hot water over 1.5 to 4.5 grams (about one-quarter to 1 teaspoonful) of crushed lemon balm, steep for 10 minutes, and strain.

The usual daily dose of lemon balm is 8 to 10 grams (about 2 teaspoonfuls) Because the strength of commercial preparations may vary, follow the manufacturer's instructions whenever available.

Lemon balm can be stored in a well-sealed, non-plastic container protected from light and moisture for up to 1 year.

Overdosage
No information on overdosage is available.

L-Phenylalanine

Why people take it
An "essential" amino acid that the body can't manufacture on its own, phenylalanine is one of the raw materials for three of the nervous system's most important chemical messengers: dopamine, epinephrine, and norepinephrine. The body can also convert it to phenylethylamine, a mood-boosting substance that's said to have pain-relieving effects as well.

L-phenylalanine, the form of the substance found naturally in the diet, has shown promise as a treatment for unipolar depression. It has also proven useful in the treatment of vitiligo, a disease characterized by abnormal white blotches of skin due to loss of pigmentation. Phenylalanine has also been promoted as an appetite suppressant and sexual stimulant, but its effectiveness for these purposes remains unproven.

What it is; how it works
Researchers believe that L-phenylalanine's impact on depression stems from its role in the production of dopamine and norepinephrine, two of the chemical messengers that regulate mood. It's value in the treatment of vitiligo is thought to rest on an ability to stimulate the production of pigment-producing melanin in the affected areas of skin.

Outright deficiencies of L-phenylalanine are rare, but have been known to strike people who don't eat enough protein. (Signs of deficiency include bloodshot eyes, cataracts, and behavioral changes.) Good sources of L-phenylalanine include protein foods such as poultry, meats, fish, dairy products, soybeans, nuts, and seeds. Phenylalanine is also an ingredient of the popular artificial sweetener aspartame.

Another form of phenylalanine—D-phenylalanine—has been proposed as a treatment for chronic pain. This substance is available only in combination with L-phenylalanine, in products known as DL-phenylalanine (see separate entry).

Avoid if...

Children born without the ability to process phenylalanine can build up dangerous levels of this amino acid, leading to mental retardation, seizures, extreme hyperactivity, and psychosis. Youngsters with this condition—called phenylketonuria—must follow a special diet designed to supply no more phenylalanine than necessary, and must be monitored regularly for excess phenylalanine in the blood.

Special cautions

L-phenylalanine has also been reported to exacerbate involuntary movements (tardive dyskinesia) in schizophrenic patients. Anyone with this disorder should therefore use L-phenylalanine supplements with extreme caution. Caution is also warranted for people with high blood pressure or an anxiety disorder; phenylalanine tends to aggravate these conditions.

It's best for patients with vitiligo to use L-phenylalanine under a doctor's supervision.

Possible drug interactions

L-phenylalanine supplements should never be combined with drugs known as MAO inhibitors, including the antidepressants Nardil and Parnate; a surge in blood pressure could result. It is also best to avoid combining L-phenylalanine with antipsychotic drugs, since it increases the likelihood of tardive dyskinesia.

On the other hand, taking L-phenylalanine with the drug Eldepryl may boost the antidepressant activity of both agents.

Special information about pregnancy and breastfeeding

Phenylalanine supplements are not recommended during pregnancy and breastfeeding.

Available preparations and dosage

The estimated adult daily requirement for L-phenylalanine and the related amino acid tyrosine combined is approximately 7 milligrams per pound of body weight. Infants require almost 9 times that amount; children need 10 milligrams per pound. Most people fulfill these requirements through diet alone, but commercial L-phenylalanine supplements are available in capsule and tablet form. Typical dosages range from 500 milligrams to 1.5 grams daily. The supplements should not be taken with other amino acids or protein foods. L-phenylalanine is most effective if taken on an empty stomach prior to meals. Vitamin B_6 is said to enhance its effectiveness.

Overdosage
No overdoses have been reported

Melatonin

Why people take it
In numerous clinical studies, the hormone we call melatonin has demonstrated its value as a treatment for insomnia. For example, in one study, 14 of 18 patients taking melatonin were able to give up the sedatives they had been relying on to sleep. There is also a possibility that melatonin may relieve jet lag, though the evidence for this is mixed.

Other claims made for this hormone range from wildly exaggerated to totally baseless. Despite some hints that it may be useful for cancer and immune disorders, clinical research has yet to verify its value. Assertions that melatonin can improve the symptoms of Alzheimer's disease, lower cholesterol levels, reduce high blood pressure, prevent heart attacks, improve sexual performance, and delay the onset of aging are entirely without foundation.

What it is; how it works
Melatonin is a product of the pineal gland, where it is synthesized from the amino acid tryptophan. Under normal conditions, melatonin levels foreshadow the sleep cycle, usually increasing rapidly from the late evening until midnight, then decreasing as morning approaches. In this way, melatonin helps regulate circadian rhythm, the body's 24-hour "dark-light clock" that governs the timing of hormone production, sleep, body temperature, and more.

Not surprisingly, people with high levels of melatonin usually sleep longer and more soundly than those with a deficiency. For example, the elderly, who produce less melatonin than the young and middle-aged, are typically more susceptible to insomnia. Similarly, events that throw melatonin levels out of synch—such as a jet trip between time zones—seem to interfere with production of the hormone and thus disrupt sleep. Consumption of alcohol, tobacco, and narcotics has a similar effect.

Avoid if...
Because melatonin sometimes causes depression, those who suffer from depression should avoid it. It has been known to trigger seizures, and should not be used by anyone with epilepsy or other seizure disorders. Couples who are trying to conceive a baby should avoid this hormone. It is also not for use in children or teenagers.

Special cautions

As with other medications that cause sleepiness, melatonin should be taken only at bedtime. Patients should not drive or operate hazardous machinery after taking a dose.

Side effects are more likely with higher doses. They include stomach discomfort, morning grogginess, daytime hangover, depression, headache, lethargy, disorientation, amnesia, inhibition of fertility, increased seizures, reduced male sexual drive, low body temperature, retinal damage, and breast enlargement

Possible drug interactions

A number of drugs can reduce melatonin levels. Among them are aspirin, other nonsteroidal anti-inflammatory drugs, and beta blockers such as Inderal, Lopressor, and Tenormin. On the other hand, Luvox can increase the effect of melatonin supplements.

Use of melatonin with benzodiazepines, sedating antihistamines, sedating antidepressants and other sedating drugs may cause additive sedation and increase the likelihood of side effects. Melatonin should never be combined with Prozac.

There is a report of melatonin enhancing the activity of the tuberculosis drug isoniazid. It may also increase the anticancer effect of interleukin-2.

Special information about pregnancy and breastfeeding

Experts advise against the use of melatonin by pregnant women and nursing mothers.

Available preparations and dosage

Melatonin is available in capsules, tablets, lozenges, and liquid Those who use melatonin for sleep disturbance or jet lag should take no more than 0.3 to 3 milligrams at bedtime for short periods of time (no longer than 2 weeks). It's best to check with a doctor before taking higher doses or dosing for longer periods of time.

Overdosage

There are no reports of melatonin overdose.

Myo-Inositol

Why people take it

In a number of clinical trials, *myo*-inositol has proven to be an effective treatment for some patients with depression, panic disorder, and obsessive-compulsive disorder. It does not, however, have any beneficial effects on Alzheimer's disease, schizophrenia, or autism. And when tested for attention deficit disorder, it made the problem worse.

What it is; how it works

Myo-inositol is a small, but significant, component of cell membranes. The body manufactures it from glucose, and it's also obtained from dietary intake of foods such as dried beans, chickpeas, lentils, citrus fruit, nuts, oats, rice, and whole-grain products.

Researchers have noted a shortage of *myo*-inositol in the cerebrospinal fluid of many patients with depression. They believe its effects on depression and anxiety may stem from its ability to activate serotonin receptors in the brain. As one of the brain's chief chemical messengers, serotonin appears to play a key role in the modulation of moods—a fact that accounts for the success of such serotonin-boosting drugs as Luvox, Paxil, and Prozac. While *myo*-inositol has similar therapeutic effects, hopes that it might enhance the effect of these drugs have failed to be realized.

Avoid if...

There are no known reasons to avoid *myo*-inositol at recommended dosage levels.

Special cautions

Due to the theoretical possibility that this substance could exacerbate the manic symptoms of bipolar disorder, patients suffering from this problem should use *myo*-inositol supplements with caution and only under a doctor's supervision.

Possible drug interactions

Although it has not been observed in clinical trials, there is a theoretical possibility that high doses of *myo*-inositol may improve the action of serotonin-boosting drugs such as Celexa, Luvox, Paxil, Prozac, and Zoloft, and migraine medications such as Amerge, Axert, Imitrex, Maxalt, and Zomig. It might also add to the effects of St. John's wort.

Special information about pregnancy and breastfeeding

Because the safety of *myo*-inositol during pregnancy has not been confirmed, it should be avoided by pregnant women and nursing mothers. In very high doses, it can trigger uterine contractions.

Available preparations and dosage

The dosage that produced positive effects in clinical studies was 12 grams a day, divided into several smaller doses. Improvement, if any, can be expected in about 1 month.

Overdosage

There are no reports of *myo*-inositol overdose.

NADH

Why people take it

A chemical cousin of vitamin B_3, NADH (nicontinamide adenine dinucleotide) is naturally present in each of the body's cells, where it's needed to trigger conversion of nutrients into the cellular "fuel" adenosine triphosphate (ATP). Proponents of NADH have tested it for several serious diseases, including Parkinson's, Alzheimer's, depression, and chronic fatigue syndrome. Although results have been mixed, it seems to be helpful for many patients with Parkinson's disease. Trials for Alzheimer's disease and chronic fatigue syndrome have also been encouraging. Additionally, in one recent study NADH was found to significantly lower blood pressure and cholesterol levels.

What it is; how it works

Because of its role in the synthesis of ATP, NADH is a key factor in the body's production of energy. There's also some evidence that high levels of NADH in the brain may enhance production of such chemical messengers as dopamine, norepinephrine, and serotonin. The body produces NADH continuously, using vitamin B_3 as raw material. It's also readily available from such dietary sources as fish, poultry, beef, and products made with yeast. Deficiencies of NADH in the U.S. are almost unknown, except in rare cases of alcoholism.

Research on the use of NADH for treatment of chronic fatigue syndrome has produced encouraging—though not spectacular—results. The study included 26 patients with chronic fatigue, and found that 31 percent of those taking 10 milligrams of NADH daily had fewer symptoms. The researchers theorize that a shortage of ATP may contribute to the symptoms of chronic fatigue, and that NADH works by helping to replenish depleted cellular stores of the compound.

Because Parkinson's disease is caused by a shortage of dopamine at certain locations in the brain, researchers have speculated that NADH's dopamine-boosting effect might relieve the tremors and rigidity the disease produces. Preliminary studies seem to indicate that for many Parkinson's patients this may be true. In one uncontrolled trial of NADH in 885 people with Parkinson's disease, nearly 80 percent showed improvement.

Since NADH supports production of other chemical messengers in the brain, scientists are also eyeing it for use against Alzheimer's disease and depression. In one small trial, 17 patients suffering from Alzheimer's showed improvement after taking NADH for 8 to 12 weeks. Likewise, a 10-month trial of NADH in 205 depressed patients ended in improvement for 93 percent. But since these studies were small, uncontrolled, and conducted by advocates of NADH, experts say more rigorous testing is needed before any firm conclusions can be drawn.

Avoid if...

Given the lack of conclusive research, it would be unwise to use NADH as a replacement for more promising treatments. Although there are no known reasons to avoid the supplement, it's best used as part of an overall treatment plan. It is not recommended for children.

Special cautions

Little is known about the effects of long-term, high-dose use of NADH, but excessive use of the related compound nicotinic acid can lead to liver damage, so caution is in order.

NADH appears to have few significant side effects, but there have been isolated reports of such gastrointestinal side effects as nausea and loss of appetite.

Possible drug interactions

No drug interactions are known.

Special information about pregnancy and breastfeeding

Because of lack of long-term safety studies, NADH should be avoided by pregnant women and nursing mothers.

Available preparations and dosage

NADH is available in 2.5- and 5-milligram tablets. A typical dosage recommendation is 5 milligrams once or twice daily, with water, on an empty stomach. An injectable form is used by physicians to treat complications of alcoholism.

Overdosage

No information is available on overdosage.

Passion Flower

Latin name: Passiflora incarnata
Other names: Granadilla, Maypop, Passion Vine

Why people take it

Although proven effective only for edginess and insomnia, passion flower has also been used as a remedy for depression and nervous stomach. Applied externally, it has been used for hemorrhoids.

What it is; how it works

This perennial vine, which reaches 30 feet in length, grows naturally from the southeastern U.S. to Brazil and Argentina, and is cultivated in Europe as a garden plant. The blossoms are considered symbolic of Christ's Passion (their central corona, for instance, represents the Crown of Thorns), accounting for their name.

The above-ground parts of the plant hold its medicinal value. In animal tests, researchers found that the plant lowers blood pressure and slows the passage of food through the digestive tract.

Avoid if...
No known medical conditions preclude the use of passion flower.

Special cautions
At customary dosage levels, Passion Flower poses no risks.

Possible drug interactions
No interactions have been reported.

Special information about pregnancy and breastfeeding
No harmful effects are known.

Available preparations and dosage
Passion flower is available as an herb for tea. It is also an ingredient in certain sedative bath additives.

To make tea, pour 150 milliliters (about two-thirds of a cup) of hot water over 1 teaspoonful of passion flower, steep for 10 minutes, then strain.

To prepare an external rinse, particularly for hemorrhoids, put 20 grams (about 3 tablespoonfuls) of Passion Flower into 200 grams (about 1 cup) of simmering water, allow to cool, then strain.

The typical oral dosage is 2 to 3 cups of tea during the day and one-half hour before bedtime.

Overdosage
No information on overdosage is available.

Phosphatidylcholine

Why people take it
Two potential benefits have attracted interest in phosphatidylcholine: its impact on cholesterol levels and its effect on memory loss. In both roles, the substance gets mixed reviews.

Hopes that phosphatidylcholine might combat memory loss have been based on its ability to increase levels of acetylcholine in the brain. This important chemical messenger appears to play a role in maintaining memory, and has been found to be in short supply in Alzheimer's patients. Unfortunately an analysis of 11 carefully controlled clinical experiments with lecithin, a food supplement rich in phosphatidyl-choline, was unable to detect any significant benefit. The supplement may have very modest effects on patients with impaired thinking or dementia, but it doesn't seem to yield any major improvement.

Similarly, some experts once believed that phosphatidylcholine might relieve the symptoms of tardive dyskinesia, a severe neurological disorder that's brought on by long-term use of certain antipsychotic drugs. But when schizophrenic patients suffering from the signs and symptoms of the disorder—involuntary movements of the muscles of the face, mouth, and cheeks—were put on lecithin or related compounds, they experienced only slight improvement.

Phosphatidylcholine's performance against high cholesterol has been equally unexciting. Although it has produced moderate reductions in some studies, it has had no significant effect in a number of others.

It has been suggested that phosphatidylcholine might eventually have some therapeutic role in some cancers. Phosphatidylcholine is essential for normal liver function, and there is ample evidence that liver cancer is promoted in various animals by choline-deficient diets. In addition, phosphatidylcholine has demonstrated protective effects against a number of other liver disorders, including alcoholic fibrosis and viral hepatitis.

What it is; how it works
Phosphatidylcholine is a combination of choline, fatty acids, glycerol, and phosphorus. Its choline component serves as a raw material in the production of acetylcholine and has recently been classified as an essential nutrient by the National Academy of Sciences. (See entry on Choline.) As a source of extra choline, phosphatidylcholine is a better delivery form and is better tolerated than choline itself.

Phosphatidylcholine is one of several phosphorus-based compounds contained in lecithin, a naturally occurring substance derived from beef liver, eggs, soybeans, and peanuts. Lecithin products are generally composed of from 5 to 30 percent phosphatidylcholine. Choline constitutes about 13 percent of the total.

Avoid if...
Phosphatidylcholine is generally considered safe for everyone.

Special cautions
No major side effects need be expected. A few people suffer mild side effects such as nausea, diarrhea, and increased salivation.

Possible drug interactions
It's best to avoid choline-containing supplements if one is taking a prescription drug such as scopolamine (an antinausea medication) that works by blocking the effects of acetylcholine.

Special information about pregnancy and breastfeeding
For healthy women who eat a balanced diet, choline supplements are usually unnecessary during pregnancy and breastfeeding.

Available preparations and dosage

There are several ways to obtain supplemental phosphatidylcholine. Typical commercial lecithin supplements contain 20 to 30 percent phosphatidylcholine. Softgel capsules containing 55 to 90 percent phosphatidylcholine are available. There's also a liquid containing 3 grams of phosphatidylcholine per 5 milliliters. Typical dosages range from 3 to 9 grams of phosphatidylcholine daily, taken in several smaller doses.

Overdosage

The upper tolerable limit of choline is 3.5 grams a day. (It takes approximately 27 grams of phosphatidylcholine to supply this amount.) Dosages above this level may bring on dizziness, nausea, diarrhea, cramps, and a fishy body odor.

Phosphatidylserine

Why people take it

Phosphatidylserine (PS) is found in high concentrations in the brain. It may help to preserve, or even improve, some aspects of mental functioning in the elderly. In the largest study to date, 200 milligrams of phosphatidylserine daily made a small but significant improvement in patients with Alzheimer's disease. Other smaller studies also found phosphatidylserine to be mildly helpful. Keep in mind, however, that these studies lasted just a few months, and while phosphatidylserine may reduce symptoms in the short term, at best it probably slows the rate of deterioration rather than halting the progression altogether. Preliminary evidence also suggests that phosphatidylserine can boost the immune system, and it may blunt the effects of the stress hormone cortisol during exercise.

What it is; how it works

Phosphatidylserine belongs to a special category of fat-soluble substances called phospholipids, which are essential components of cell membranes. Brain tissues are especially rich in phosphatidylserine, but aging causes a decline in the phosphatidylserine content of cells throughout the body. Research has shown that in addition to improving neural function, phosphatidylserine may enhance energy metabolism in all cells. It also seems to boost levels of the brain chemical acetylcholine, which has been linked to improved memory function.

Some controversy exists about the source of phosphatidylserine supplements. Most research has been conducted with phosphatidylserine derived from cow brain tissue. Due to concerns about mad-cow disease, soy-based phosphatidylserine supplements have generally replaced cow-based ones. The two types are not structurally identical, however, and some researchers think these differences could be important.

Phosphatidylserine is found in only trace amounts in a typical diet. Very small amounts are present in egg yolks and soybeans.

Avoid if...
Aside from an allergy to them, there are no known reasons to avoid phosphatidylserine supplements.

Special cautions
Due to the lack of safety studies, phosphatidylserine supplements should not be given to children. Those who have a rare genetic condition known as antiphospholipid-antibody syndrome should talk to their doctor before taking phosphatidylserine.

Occasional side effects, such as nausea and indigestion, have been reported.

Possible drug interactions
There are no reported drug interactions with phosphatidylserine.

Special information about pregnancy and breastfeeding
Due to the lack of safety data, pregnant and breastfeeding women should not use phosphatidylserine.

Available preparations and dosage
Most phosphatidylserine supplements are made from soy. Due to concerns about mad-cow disease, it's best to avoid those made from cow, or "bovine," sources. PS capsules are available in strengths of 50, 100, and 500 milligrams. Typical doses are 100 milligrams three times a day.

Overdosage
There are no reports of overdosage.

Rauwolfia

Latin name: Rauwolfia serpentina

Why people take it
Rauwolfia is officially recognized in Europe as a treatment for nervousness, insomnia, and high blood pressure. In folk medicine, it has also been used for vomiting, gas, liver problems, and wounds. However, its effectiveness for such conditions remains unverified.

Indian medicine uses it as an antidote for poisonous snake bites, and as a remedy for fever, abdominal cramps, slow and painful urination, and wounds.

What it is; how it works

Reserpine, an extract of rauwolfia, combats high blood pressure, and is found in such prescription blood pressure medications as Diupres and Hydropres. Reserpine also combats irregular heartbeat and has a sedative effect.

Rauwolfia, a small shrub sporting white to pink flowers, is native to India, Indochina, Borneo, Sri Lanka, and Sumatra. Its medicinal properties lie in the dried root. The fresh root has a very bitter and unpleasant taste.

Avoid if...

Rauwolfia can trigger severe depression. No one suffering from depression should take this herb. The drug also tends to stimulate the lining of the digestive tract, so it should be avoided if an ulcer or ulcerative colitis exists. Rauwolfia should also be avoided during pregnancy and nursing.

Special cautions

Side effects can include nasal congestion, depression, fatigue, impotence, and slowed reaction time. Patients should use caution when handling machinery or driving.

Possible drug interactions

Rauwolfia must never be combined with drugs classified as monoamine oxidase inhibitors, such as the antidepressants Nardil and Parnate.

Rauwolfia enhances the sedative effect of alcohol and barbiturates; the combination should be avoided. Rauwolfia also increases the effects of antipsychotic drugs.

Taken with digitalis-based drugs such as Lanoxin, or quinidine products such as Quinaglute and Quinidex, rauwolfia can slow the heart and cause irregular beats.

The drug is also likely to interact with levodopa (Sinemet), causing twitching and other involuntary movements. Combining it with many common flu remedies and appetite suppressants can lead to a sharp rise in blood pressure.

Special information about pregnancy and breastfeeding

Rauwolfia may cause birth defects when taken during pregnancy; and it appears in breast milk. Women should avoid this drug while pregnant or breastfeeding.

Available preparations and dosage

Rauwolfia is available in ground form and as a powder for internal use.

The usual daily dose of rauwolfia is 600 milligrams. (Recommended dosage of the active ingredient reserpine is far smaller; 0.25 milligram is the daily maximum.)

Overdosage

Symptoms of overdosage include mental depression, heavy sedation, and a severe drop in blood pressure. If an overdose is suspected, seek medical attention immediately.

SAMe

Why people take it

In a series of small but promising clinical trials, this over-the-counter remedy for depression has proved itself the equal of traditional prescription drugs. Though some authorities dismiss it as a mild mood-lifter, others regard it as an important new medication, since it has not only performed as well as potent "tricyclic" antidepressants, but also starts working faster (within one or two weeks, versus three to four weeks or longer for standard drugs). Outside the U.S., it has been sold for years as a prescription antidepressant, mainly under the name AdoMet.

SAMe (S-adenosylmethionine) has been studied as an aid to the effectiveness of other antidepressants, with promising results. It also has been found to provide at least some relief from postpartum depression and depression associated with Parkinson's disease and epilepsy. In addition, it has been tested for a number of other neurological disorders, including schizophrenia, Alzheimer's disease, and dementia. Although these tests are far from conclusive, they've produced encouraging results.

SAMe is also used to treat osteoarthritis, the type of arthritis caused by wear and tear on the protective cartilage in the joints. Preliminary studies appear to confirm its ability to relieve stiffness, pain, and swelling. However, there's no evidence to support manufacturers' claims that it can renew damaged cartilage. SAMe also shows promise as a treatment for the painful muscle condition called fibromyalgia. And studies show that supplementation with SAMe can improve liver function, making it a candidate for treatment of cirrhosis, impaired bile flow, and liver damage from drugs or alcohol.

Claims that SAMe is useful in the treatment of heart disease and cancer are currently unsubstantiated, though preliminary clinical studies are underway. Assertions that SAMe fights the effects of aging also remain unproven.

What it is; how it works

The body manufactures a natural supply of SAMe from the essential amino acid methionine. In turn, SAMe plays an important role in the production of a wide variety of hormones, amino acids, antioxidants, and chemical messengers in the brain. Researchers have noted low levels of SAMe in people with depression, and have found that SAMe rises as depression improves. SAMe also helps maintain the strength and flexibility of cell walls, and participates in the production of DNA and RNA.

SAMe supplements are especially helpful in cases of liver disease, which depletes the body's natural supply. Extra vitamin B_6, B_{12}, and folic acid are usually recommended with SAMe supplementation. In fact, some products already have them added.

Avoid if...
People who have bipolar disorder should use SAMe only under a doctor's supervision; SAMe can cause episodes of mania. Those taking antidepressants should not discontinue their medication or start taking SAMe without consulting a physician. SAMe is not recommended for children.

Special cautions
Patients taking a prescription antidepressant may need to reduce their dosage gradually when attempting to replace their medication with SAMe or adding SAMe to their regimen.

Patients with high homocysteine levels (a condition associated with increased risk of heart disease) should consider adding the homocysteine-lowering supplement TMG to the regimen. Homocysteine is a byproduct of SAMe.

Unlike some prescription antidepressants, SAMe is said to have no serious side effects. However, some people suffer mild digestive upsets, anxiety, insomnia, mania, and hyperactive muscles.

There is no reason to believe that SAMe could cause cancer. But because people who already have cancer might react differently to this substance, they should check with their doctor before taking SAMe.

Possible drug interactions
SAMe may reduce the effectiveness of some medications, including the Parkinson's disease medication L-dopa.

Special information about pregnancy and breastfeeding
The safety of SAMe supplements during pregnancy has not been determined; it should be used only under a doctor's supervision. SAMe supplementation is not recommended for nursing mothers.

Available preparations and dosage
Synthetic SAMe is available in tablets and capsules, usually in strengths of 100 or 200 milligrams. For depression, some authorities recommend dosages of 400 to 1,600 milligrams daily. For arthritis, recommendations vary from 200 to 1,200 milligrams daily. For liver disease, daily dosages of 1,600 milligrams are common. The daily total is divided into smaller doses. They should be taken 1 hour before or 2 hours after meals.

Some forms of SAMe tend to degrade quickly at any temperature above freezing. Look for a temperature-stable form in a coated tablet. Store away from moisture.

Overdosage

No information on overdosage is available.

St. John's Wort

Latin name: Hypericum perforatum

Why people take it

In many—but not all—clinical trials, St. John's wort has proven to be an effective treatment for mild to moderate depressive disorders. It also has a mildly tranquilizing and sedative effect. Oily preparations of the herb are useful in the treatment of wounds, burns, blunt injuries, and inflammation of the skin.

Although its effectiveness for other ailments has not been proven, St. John's wort has also been used to treat sleep disturbances, gallbladder disorders, gastritis, bronchitis, asthma, diarrhea, bed-wetting, rheumatism, muscle pain, and gout.

What it is; how it works

St. John's wort is believed to combat depression by boosting the levels of certain chemical messengers in the brain. Like the prescription antidepressant Prozac, it seems to increase the amount of serotonin available to the nervous system. It also tends to promote higher levels of the chemical messengers norepinephrine and dopamine. In clinical trials, daily doses of 800 to 900 milligrams of St. John's wort have proven to be as effective as 20 milligrams of Prozac or 75 milligrams of the antidepressant Tofranil.

Applied to the skin, oily preparations of the herb have an antibacterial and anti-inflammatory action, though they seem to have no effect on viruses.

St. John's wort is a golden yellow perennial flower that secretes a red liquid when pinched. Cut at the start of the flowering season and processed in bunches, it must be dried quickly to preserve its oil and secretions.

This plant has been used medicinally for over 2,000 years. Ancient Greeks believed that its odor repelled evil spirits. Early Christians named the plant in honor of St. John the Baptist because they believed it released its blood-red oil on the 29th of August, the day the saint was beheaded.

Avoid if...

There are no known reasons to avoid St. John's wort at recommended dosage levels.

Special cautions

With heavy use, St. John's wort increases sensitivity to sunlight. To avoid a sunburn, patients should minimize exposure to the sun while using this medication. This herb can also cause bloating and constipation.

Possible drug interactions

Patients should avoid St. John's wort while taking a prescription MAO inhibitor such as Nardil or Parnate. At least in theory, a dangerous interaction is possible.

It's also best to avoid combining St. John's wort with serotonin-boosting drugs such as Celexa, Luvox, Paxil, Prozac, Serzone, and Zoloft. The excessive levels of serotonin that may result can trigger sweating, tremors, flushing, confusion, and agitation.

Patients taking medications for HIV, the virus that causes AIDS, should not use St. John's wort. The herb is known to interfere with at least one HIV drug—Crixivan—and may reduce the effect of others, including Agenerase, Fortovase, Invirase, Norvir, and Viracept. St. John's wort should also be avoided by people taking Neoral, a drug used to keep transplant patients from rejecting their new organs. It can inhibit the drug's life-saving effect.

Patients who use a hormonal form of contraception should remember that oral contraceptive failure has occasionally been reported in women taking St. John's wort.

Special information about pregnancy and breastfeeding

No harmful effects are known.

Available preparations and dosage

For depression, the typical dosage of standardized extract is 300 milligrams taken 3 times a day. The extract is available in tablet, capsule, and liquid form. Common brands are made by Celestial Seasonings, Centrum Herbals, Nature's Way, and Schiff. Strengths of commercial preparations may vary. Patients should follow the manufacturer's labeling whenever available.

A treatment regimen of 4 to 6 weeks is typically recommended for depression. Patients should check with their doctor if they feel no improvement. They may need a different therapy.

Overdosage

No information on overdosage is available.

Tocotrienols

Why people take it

Tocotrienols are a form of vitamin E. In general, people take them for the same reasons they take other forms of the vitamin (see separate entry), including the prevention of Alzheimer's disease, heart disease, and cancer, particularly breast cancer.

Most scientific study has focused on the alpha-tocopherol form of vitamin E because it appears to be the most active in humans. However, proponents of tocotrienols claim that they are the "missing link" in the vitamin E story; and preliminary research does indeed suggest that they may yield impressive benefits. For example, some studies suggest that tocotrienols can lower blood cholesterol levels more effectively than alpha-tocopherol can. Others hint that tocotrienols can greatly inhibit tumor formation, especially in human breast cells. Animal studies also suggest tocotrienols may be useful for healing alcohol-induced stomach lesions.

While the evidence is promising, many questions remain. There are four different types of tocotrienols, and scientists still aren't sure which ones are best, or how much should be taken. Studies also need to be done to find out the effects of taking tocotrienols and tocopherols together. (Some researchers claim that taking the two at the same time negates some of the benefits of tocotrienols.) Whatever the case, experts agree that alpha-tocopherol is still an important form of vitamin E and should not be avoided in favor of tocotrienols.

What it is; how it works

Like other forms of vitamin E, tocotrienols seem to be potent antioxidants that protect the fats in cell membranes from oxidation, or spoilage. Oxidation is thought to be a significant factor in many diseases, as well as the aging process. The antioxidant abilities of tocotrienols may explain why they are helpful for protecting the cardiovascular and nervous systems. How this form of vitamin E works to prevent cancer is still unknown.

The richest sources of tocotrienols are palm, rice bran, and coconut oils. Other plant-based oils, such as corn and canola, contain very little. Like all forms of vitamin E, tocotrienols are fat soluble.

Avoid if...

Aside from an allergy to them, there are no known reasons to avoid tocotrienol supplements.

Special cautions

Because tocotrienols could interfere with blood clot formation, patients who have bleeding problems—including those with hemophilia, peptic ulcers, vitamin K deficiency, a tendency to hemorrhage, or a history of stroke—should take care not to overdose. Likewise, patients should avoid tocotrienols about 1 month before and for 2 weeks after any surgery.

Because tocotrienol supplements are relatively new, there is little information on side effects. In general, the same precautions should be followed as those for vitamin E (see separate entry).

Possible drug interactions

Patients who are taking a blood-thinning drug such as aspirin or Coumadin should check with their doctor before taking tocotrienols, which could further thin the blood. In general, patients on blood thinners should not take more than 100 milligrams of tocotrienols per day. Likewise, tocotrienols should be used cautiously by patients taking antiplatelet drugs such as Aggrenox, Plavix, and Ticlid. In theory, increased bleeding could also occur if tocotrienols are taken with supplemental garlic or the herb ginkgo.

Patients taking cholesterol-lowering drugs such as Lescol, Pravachol, and Zocor should be aware that tocotrienols may further lower their cholesterol.

Certain drugs may decrease the absorption of tocotrienols or interfere with their use in the body. These include the cholesterol-lowering drugs Colestid and Questran, the antibiotics isoniazid and neomycin, the weight-loss drug Xenical, and the ulcer medication Carafate. Other products that may decrease absorption include mineral oil, the fat substitute olestra, and cholesterol-lowering supplements, especially the plant-based phytosterols and phytostanols.

Because of possible oxidation, tocotrienols should not be taken at the same time as iron supplements.

Special information about pregnancy and breastfeeding

Due to the lack of safety data, pregnant and breastfeeding women should use tocotrienol supplements only with their doctor's approval.

Available preparations and dosage

Most supplements contain a mixture of tocotrienols in liquid softgel form. Some manufacturers also offer "mixed" vitamin E supplements that contain the tocopherol forms as well.

Unlike the alpha-tocopherol form of vitamin E, there are no governmental recommendations for tocotrienols. Dosages used in clinical studies range from 200 to 300 milligrams per day, although some researchers believe that daily doses of 30 to 50 milligrams are sufficient for general disease prevention.

Tocotrienol supplements may be listed as "esterified," which means the formulation was chemically altered to make them more stable. Unesterified tocotrienols should not be taken with supplemental iron, since the combination could actually encourage oxidation. All tocotrienol supplements should be stored at cool temperatures in a dark, tightly closed bottle. They should be taken with fat to enhance absorption.

Overdosage

Little information is available on overdosage; so far, no serious side effects have been reported.

Valerian

Latin name: Valeriana officinalis
Other names: All-heal, Amantilla, Capon's Tail, Heliotrope, Setwall, Vandal Root

Why people take it

Valerian is an accepted remedy for insomnia, and appears to calm nervousness as well. Although its other uses have not been formally verified, valerian is also taken for mental strain, lack of concentration, excitability, hysteria, stress, headache, epilepsy, premenstrual syndrome, symptoms of pregnancy, problems of menopause, nerve pain, fainting, stomach cramps, colic, and uterine spasms.

What it is; how it works

The Ancient Greek physician Galen referred to valerian as "Phu," an expression of disgust at the plant's smell. In medieval times, it was given the name "All-heal," reflecting its many purported healing properties. It was also used as a spice and an ingredient in perfume.

The medicinal parts are the carefully dried underground stem and the dried root. Rigorous clinical trials have verified that extracts of the root do indeed have a sleep-inducing effect. Researchers believe that this action stems from the herb's tendency to boost levels of GABA (gamma-aminobutyric acid), one of the chemical messengers in the brain. Valerian also seems to relax muscles and discourage spasms.

This plant, which produces bright pink to white flowers, grows 20 to 40 inches in height. It is native to Europe and the temperate regions of Asia, and is cultivated in Europe, Japan, and the U.S.

Avoid if...

Unless a doctor approves, anyone with a large skin injury, an acute skin disorder, a severe infection, heart problems, or severe muscle tension should avoid using valerian extract or oil as a bath additive.

Special cautions

In rare instances, valerian can cause digestive problems or an allergic reaction. Long-term use can lead to headache, restlessness, sleeplessness, pupil dilation, and heart problems.

Because of valerian's sedative effect, it's best to avoid operating machinery or driving for several hours after taking the herb.

Possible drug interactions

Valerian should not be combined with other sedatives, including barbiturates such as Seconal and benzodiazepine medications such as Ativan, Halcion, Librium, Valium, and Xanax. Although there is no evidence of an interaction with alcohol, it's considered best to avoid this combination as well.

Special information about pregnancy and breastfeeding

Use of valerian during pregnancy or breastfeeding is not recommended.

Available preparations and dosage

To prepare valerian tea, combine 3 to 5 grams (about 1 teaspoonful) of crushed Valerian with 150 milliliters of hot water (about two-thirds cup), steep for 10 to 15 minutes, then strain.

To make a bath additive, combine 100 grams (about one-half cup) of crushed valerian with 2 quarts of hot water for each full bath.

`A variety of commercial preparations are available in capsule and tablet form. For relief of insomnia, typical doses of valerian extract range from 400 to 900 milligrams 30 minutes before bedtime. Because the potency of commercial tablets and capsules may vary, follow the manufacturer's directions whenever available.

For other forms of the herb, the following daily dosages are commonly recommended:

Powder: 15 grams (about 3 teaspoonfuls)
Tea: 2 to 3 cups daily, including 1 before bedtime
Alcohol solution: 1 to 3 milliliters (about one-half to one teaspoonful) 1
　　　　　　or more times per day
Alcohol solution (1:5): 15 to 20 drops in water several times daily
Pressed juice: 1 tablespoonful 3 times daily for adults; 1 teaspoonful 3
　　　　　　times daily for children

Valerian should be stored away from light. Alcohol solutions (tinctures) and extracts must be kept in tightly closed glass containers.

Overdosage

No information on overdosage is available.

Vinpocetine

Why people take it

A so-called "smart drug," vinpocetine is said to improve memory and mental function by increasing the blood supply to the brain. Advocates claim it can help healthy people, as well as those with some degree of brain impairment. It has not, however, proved capable of halting or even slowing the progress of Alzheimer's disease. Vinpocetine has also been described as a possible antioxidant, protecting cells from the damaging free radicals that can oxidize (burn) tissues throughout the body, including the brain.

Some preliminary research suggests that vinpocetine may have some protective effects in both sight and hearing. One study of patients with mild burn trauma in the eyes showed that vinpocetine enhanced healing, most likely as a result of increased blood flow to the damaged tissue. Vinpocetine has also been associated with improvements seen in retinas damaged by hepatitis B virus. Damage from acoustic trauma has been similarly been reduced by vinpocetine treatment.

Vinpocetine is sold as a drug in Germany, Japan, Mexico, and Portugal for the treatment of cerebrovascular disorders—ailments that interrupt blood circulation in the brain, starving it of oxygen. In Portugal, it's also used to treat general circulatory problems, as well as certain disorders of the eyes and ears. The drug is approved in Australia for the treatment of mental function disorders in the elderly and for other disorders of the brain. Though it has never been approved in the United States, it can be purchased here as a dietary supplement.

What it is; how it works

Like other members of the vinca alkaloid family of drugs, such as the cancer drugs vincristine, vinblastine, and vinorelbine, vinpocetine comes from the periwinkle plant. Limited research data show that vinpocetine does in fact relax the blood vessels of the brain, improve cerebral blood flow, and inhibit blood clotting to some extent. One study implies that the drug improves memory in healthy people. Studies in animals also indicate a protective effect when the brain is deprived of oxygen.

On the other hand, a number of trials have produced less encouraging results. To date, studies in people with Alzheimer's disease or stroke have been very disappointing. Trials in people with brain dysfunction due to other causes have produced mixed results, providing no clear answers for researchers. There is currently not enough evidence to determine whether vinpocetine does or does not reduce fatalities and dependence in ischemic stroke. It's evident that additional, wide-scale studies are needed before any firm conclusions can be drawn about vinpocetine's real value and most appropriate uses.

Avoid if...

Vinpocetine should not be taken if one has ever had an allergic reaction to one of the vinca-based anticancer drugs, or to vinpocetine itself.

Special cautions

It is a good idea for patients to get periodic checkups while taking vinpocetine whatever the status of their health. Blood pressure should be checked on a regular basis. A routine blood test is recommended from time to time to ensure that the liver is breaking down the drug properly. Don't forget that outside the U.S. vinpocetine is used like a potent prescription drug. A bit of extra caution is merited.

Side effects are relatively mild. People enrolled in research studies have taken up to 60 milligrams of vinpocetine per day without suffering serious adverse reactions. Some people found that their blood pressure dropped slightly, an effect that can cause dizziness. Facial flushing has also occurred among people taking vinpocetine. Other complaints reported include temporary sleep disturbances and restlessness (usually after 10 weeks of therapy), pressure headache, dry mouth, and stomach disturbances. Minor decreases in blood sugar have been noted, too, but it has not been determined whether this effect was actually caused by vinpocetine.

Possible drug interactions
Small changes in clotting time have been reported in people who combine the blood thinner warfarin with vinpocetine. While the combination does not seem to pose a great danger, more frequent monitoring of clotting time is a good idea.

Special information about pregnancy and breastfeeding
During pregnancy and breastfeeding it's best to avoid any medication that's not absolutely necessary for short-term health. Patients should forego vinpocetine throughout this period.

Available preparations and dosage
Vinpocetine is typically sold as 5-milligram tablets. Depending on the product purchased, the label may recommend anywhere from 5 to 30 milligrams daily. Do not exceed the recommended amount.

Overdosage
There are no reports of vinpocetine overdosage.

Vitamin E

Why people take it
Vitamin E has grabbed the headlines in recent years for its potential to treat—and possibly prevent—a host of devastating illnesses, including Alzheimer's disease, heart disease, peripheral nerve damage, and cancer. Researchers are particularly impressed by a study in the *New England Journal of Medicine* that showed supplemental vitamin E helped slow the progression of mild to moderate Alzheimer's disease. The results were so convincing that the American Psychiatric Association now includes the vitamin in its treatment guidelines for Alzheimer's.

The study's authors caution that one trial cannot tell the whole story, and they still don't know how vitamin E protects the brain, or whether it could stave off dementia in the first place. Also, the dose used in the study was high—2,000 International Units a day—and treatment at such high doses needs to be supervised by a doctor since, theoretically, it could cause bleeding and other problems. Even so, many researchers believe that the possible rewards of taking vitamin E seem to outweigh the risks, especially since we have so few effective treatments for Alzheimer's.

Much fanfare also surrounds the use of vitamin E for fighting heart disease and cancer. Unfortunately, for every reputable study that has found a link between vitamin E and lower rates of both diseases, another one comes along that casts doubt on the evidence. While nutritional surveys strongly suggest that vitamin E can help prevent heart disease and various cancers (including prostate, breast, and colon cancer), clinical trials of the supplement have been disappointing. It could be that some studies were too short or used a dosage that was too low. For now, the best course seems to be to get plenty of vitamin E from food and perhaps take modest amounts of supplements.

Vitamin E also gets attention for its role in strengthening the immune system and protecting the body from environmental toxins, including air pollution, tobacco smoke, and the sun's ultraviolet rays. For the same reasons, vitamin E supplements may be somewhat beneficial for treating asthma, diabetes, cataracts, and rheumatoid arthritis. It could also help relieve muscle cramps and some of the symptoms associated with premenstrual syndrome, although more research is needed. Claims that vitamin E can reverse skin aging, improve athletic abilities, and enhance fertility and sexual performance have never been substantiated.

What it is; how it works

Even though vitamin E is well known as an essential nutrient, scientists aren't sure how the body uses it. Part of the confusion stems from the vitamin's many forms. Vitamin E is actually a catchall term for a family of eight naturally occurring molecules. They are divided into two main groups, the tocopherols and the tocotrienols. The best known, and the one generally found in supplements, is alpha-tocopherol. The government bases its daily-allowance recommendation on alpha-tocopherol because, so far, it seems to be the most biologically usable form in humans. This does not, however, mean that the other forms of vitamin E are insignificant. In fact, some argue that certain tocotrienols (see separate entry) are more potent antioxidants, although the evidence is still being debated.

Scientists do know that vitamin E is a powerful antioxidant that protects the fats found in cell membranes throughout the body from oxidation, or spoilage. Oxidation is thought to play a role in numerous degenerative diseases as well as the aging process. For example, it is widely believed that the oxidation of "bad" LDL cholesterol leads to the formation of artery-clogging plaque. And oxidative stress has also been linked to many nervous system disorders because brain and nerve cells are rich in fats that are vulnerable to oxidation.

Although vitamin E's role as an antioxidant gets credit for most of its protective effects, it is not the vitamin's only beneficial property. This versatile nutrient also seems to act as a blood thinner and a cell-membrane stabilizer; and it plays an important role in the maintenance of a healthy immune system. A number of studies have shown that it can inhibit the development of certain cancers.

The richest sources of vitamin E, especially the tocopherol form, are vegetable and nut oils, including corn, sunflower, canola, soybean, and olive oils. Palm, rice bran, and coconut oils are high in the tocotrienols. Most nuts are high in vitamin E, as are fatty meats, unrefined cereal and grains, and wheat germ. Various fruits and vegetables—spinach, lettuce, onions, blackberries, apples, and pears—also contain this vitamin.

Vitamin E is fat soluble, which means that the body can store vitamin E for future use. Although high doses of fat-soluble vitamins could lead to toxic buildups in the body, vitamin E has proven safe even in much larger than standard doses.

Vitamin E deficiency is rare in humans but can occur in very premature infants. Individuals who may be deficient include those with cystic fibrosis, Crohn's disease, and certain rare genetic disorders. Vitamin E deficiency is also a concern for those who have had part of their gastrointestinal tract removed. People on a strict low-fat diet may be somewhat deficient since fatty nuts and oils are the best sources of vitamin E.

Avoid if...

Aside from an allergy to them, there are no known reasons to avoid vitamin E supplements.

Special cautions

Because vitamin E can prevent the formation of blood clots, patients who have bleeding problems—including those with hemophilia, peptic ulcers, vitamin K deficiency, a tendency to hemorrhage, or a history of stroke—should take care not to overdose. Likewise, patients should avoid vitamin E supplements about one month before and for 2 weeks after any surgery.

In general, the risk of side effects is low. Even at doses of 1,500 International Units (IU) per day, vitamin E appears to have no harmful effects. However, at doses of 2,400 IU or more bleeding problems may begin to appear. Too much vitamin E may also reduce the body's supply of vitamin A, alter the immune system, and impair sexual function.

Rare reactions to vitamin E supplements include fatigue, breast soreness, emotional disturbances, inflammation of the veins, stomach upset, altered blood fat levels, and thyroid problems.

Possible drug interactions

Patients who are taking a blood-thinning drug such as aspirin or Coumadin should check with their doctor before taking vitamin E supplements, which could further thin the blood. In general, patients taking these drugs should not exceed total daily doses of 100 milligrams of natural vitamin E or 200 milligrams of the synthetic version. Vitamin E should also be used cautiously with antiplatelet drugs such as Aggrenox, Plavix, and Ticlid. In theory, increased bleeding could also occur if vitamin E is taken with supplemental garlic or the herb ginkgo.

Certain drugs may decrease vitamin E absorption or interfere with its use in the body. These include anticonvulsants such as phenobarbital, Dilantin, and Tegretol; the cholesterol-lowering drugs Colestid and Questran; the antibiotics isoniazid and neomycin; and ulcer drugs such as Carafate. In some studies, the weight-loss drug Xenical reduced vitamin E absorption by up to 60 percent. Other products that may counter the effects of vitamin E include fiber supplements, mineral oil, the fat substitute Olestra, and cholesterol-lowering supplements, especially the plant-based phytosterols and phytostanols.

On the plus side, vitamin E may help alleviate the side effects of Cordarone, which is used to prevent abnormal heart rhythms. It may also inhibit Retrovir's harmful effects on bone marrow, and could be useful for treating the kidney damage caused by drugs used to prevent organ rejection, including the immunosuppressants Neoral and Sandimmune. Be aware, however, that in some studies vitamin E actually interfered with immunosuppressant drugs.

Because of possible oxidation, vitamin E should not be taken at the same time as iron supplements. Patients taking supplemental oils—including flaxseed, perilla, borage, blackcurrant, evening primrose, and fish oils—should take a little extra vitamin E to prevent oxidation.

The mineral selenium may boost the effectiveness of vitamin E. In addition, taking other antioxidants—such as vitamin C, glutathione, alpha-lipoic acid, and Coenzyme Q10—may help the body hold onto vitamin E.

Special information about pregnancy and breastfeeding

Pregnant women should not take more than the Recommended Dietary Allowance (RDA) of 15 milligrams (or 22 IU) of vitamin E a day. For breastfeeding women, the RDA is 19 milligrams (or 28 IU). For both cases, the RDA is measured using natural alpha-tocopherol.

Available preparations and dosage

There are several forms of vitamin E available commercially. Most consist of alpha-tocopherol in tablets, capsules, or liquid softgel form. Some manufacturers are now offering "mixed" formulations that include additional forms such as gamma-tocopherol and the tocotrienols.

Typical daily dosages for natural alpha-tocopherol range from 100 to 400 milligrams, with a recommended upper limit of 1,000 milligrams per day. The dosages for synthetic alpha-tocopherol are double that amount, since this form is not as easily stored by the body. Patients can spot the synthetic version by checking the letters listed *before* "alpha-tocopherol." The natural form lists "d," as in d-alpha-tocopherol, while the synthetic version lists "dl," as in dl-alpha-tocopherol. The RDA set by the government is much lower than the doses used in studies: 15 milligrams of natural alpha-tocopherol a day for adults.

Vitamin E is measured in milligrams or International Units (IU), with 1 milligram of alpha-tocopherol equal to approximately 1.5 IU. Therefore, to convert from milligrams to IU, multiply by 1.5. For example, the RDA for vitamin E is 15 milligrams or about 22 IU.

Vitamin E is often listed as "esterified," which means it was chemically altered to make it more stable. Unesterified vitamin E should not be taken with supplemental iron, since the combination could actually encourage oxidation. All vitamin E supplements should be stored at cool temperatures in a dark, tightly closed bottle.

Overdosage

There are no reports of overdosage with vitamin E in any form. However, extremely high doses (2,400 IU or more per day) could theoretically cause bleeding problems due to the vitamin's clot-preventing ability.

Zinc

Why people take it

Because zinc is vital for overall body function, a deficiency could lead to a host of problems. Low levels have been linked to poor brain function, delayed wound healing, a weak immune system, infertility, alcoholism, and anorexia. People who could benefit from zinc supplements include those who do not consume enough calories, vegetarians, some older infants and children with impaired growth, and people who suffer from alcoholism or digestive diseases that cause malabsorption and diarrhea. Vegetarians may need as much as 50 percent more zinc than meat eaters, since zinc is poorly absorbed from plant foods.

If taken during pregnancy, zinc may prevent certain birth defects and ensure proper fetal growth. Preliminary research suggests that zinc may be helpful for people with immune system problems such as rheumatoid arthritis and HIV. It may also slow vision loss due to macular degeneration.

Some evidence suggests that zinc may zap the common cold. In clinical trials, patients using zinc every 2 hours at the first sign of a cough or sniffle reduced their suffering by nearly 3 days. The trick is to use zinc in the form of throat lozenges or nasal spray, since these methods are thought to work by directly interfering with cold viruses in the nose and throat. Zinc capsules or tablets can also be taken to improve overall immunity, but this probably only works in people who have a zinc deficiency to begin with.

Some enthusiasts believe zinc could be beneficial for treating a wide range of other illnesses. The list includes Alzheimer's disease, attention deficit disorder, benign prostatic hyperplasia, bladder infection, cataracts, diabetes, Down's syndrome, and even baldness. While there is no doubt that a true zinc deficiency can lead to numerous problems, no credible evidence shows that zinc supplementation can benefit these conditions.

What it is; how it works

Zinc is an essential mineral that is found in almost every cell in the body. It stimulates the activity of some 100 enzymes, and plays an important role in regulating gene expression. It is needed to support normal growth and development during pregnancy, childhood, and adolescence. An adequate supply is needed for normal sperm production. Zinc is also important for maintaining a healthy immune system, healing cuts and wounds, and maintaining a normal sense of taste and smell.

How zinc works is somewhat of a mystery. Scientists do know that the mineral is needed to activate T-lymphocytes, a type of white blood cell that fights infection. Advocates suggest that it may also interfere with the replication of cold viruses. Some research suggests that zinc acts as an antioxidant and a cell-membrane stabilizer, which could explain why it's helpful for brain function.

Zinc is widely distributed in foods. Oysters are a particularly rich source, although red meat and poultry provide the majority of zinc in the American diet. Other sources include beans, nuts, certain seafood, whole grains, fortified breakfast cereals, and dairy products. Zinc absorption is greater from a diet high in animal protein than a diet rich in plant proteins, including soy. This is because plant-based compounds called phytates can decrease zinc absorption.

Even borderline zinc deficiency can have profound negative effects. General signs of zinc deficiency include growth retardation, hair loss, diarrhea, delayed sexual maturation and impotence, eye and skin lesions, and loss of appetite. There is also some evidence that weight loss, delayed healing of wounds, taste abnormalities, and mental lethargy can occur. Remember, however, that some of these symptoms can also result from a variety of medical conditions other than zinc deficiency.

Avoid if...
Aside from an allergy to the ingredients in a supplement, there are no known reasons to avoid zinc.

Special cautions
Zinc causes few problems in doses up to 30 milligrams a day. Higher doses may cause stomach problems, including pain, nausea, and vomiting. Other reactions include headache, drowsiness, and a metallic taste.

Possible drug interactions
Advise patients that zinc supplements could decrease the absorption of certain antibiotics, including penicillin, tetracycline, and quinolones such as Cipro and Floxin. The mineral could also decrease absorption of bone-building drugs such as Actonel, Fosamax, and Didronel. Likewise, these same drugs could inhibit the absorption of zinc.

Certain minerals can decrease zinc absorption, including phosphorus, calcium, and iron. Products that contain phosphates, such as the drug K-Phos and certain potassium supplements, also may decrease zinc levels. On the other hand, too much zinc can cause a copper deficiency.

Special information about pregnancy and breastfeeding
Pregnant women should not exceed the Recommended Dietary Allowance (RDA) of 11 milligrams of zinc a day. Nursing mothers can take up to 12 milligrams.

Available preparations and dosage
Zinc supplements are available in several forms as tablets, capsules, lozenges, and nasal sprays; the most common preparations use zinc gluconate and zinc picolinate. A typical dose is 15 milligrams per day, although daily RDA requirements are somewhat lower, at 8 milligrams for women and 11 milligrams for men. For colds, the usual dosage is 13 to 23 milligrams of zinc gluconate every 2 hours for a week or two (but no longer).

For best absorption, zinc should not be taken with food or beverages that contain caffeine, tea, oxalic acid (such as spinach, sweet potatoes, rhubarb, and beans), and phytic acid (unleavened bread, seeds, nuts, grains, and soy). Taking zinc supplements with foods rich in amino acids, especially meat, may enhance absorption.

Overdosage
The recommended upper limit for zinc intake by adults is 40 milligrams a day. Sustained megadoses can lead to nausea and vomiting. Intakes of more than 150 milligrams per day can cause copper deficiency, reduce "good" HDL cholesterol levels, and depress the immune system.

Prescription Drugs with Potential for Abuse

Over 500 legal prescription drug products—many of them psychotherapeutic—pose at least some danger of physical or psychological dependence leading to abuse. Such drugs are subject to the Controlled Substances Act of 1970, which assigns each drug to one of four categories of risk. Listed on the following pages are the products—both branded and generic—that fall under the Act. The meaning of their assignments is as follows:

CII = **High Potential for Abuse:** Use may lead to severe physical or psychological dependence. Prescriptions must be written or confirmed in writing. No renewals are permitted.

CIII = **Some Potential for Abuse:** Use may lead to low-to-moderate physical dependence or high psychological dependence. Prescriptions may be oral or written. Up to 5 renewals are permitted within 6 months.

CIV = **Low Potential for Abuse:** Use may lead to limited physical or psychological dependence. Prescriptions may be oral or written. Up to 5 renewals are permitted within 6 months.

CV = **Subject to State and Local Regulation:** Abuse potential is low; in some areas a prescription may not be required.

Category CII

Actiq
Adderall
Adderall XR
Alfenta
Alfentanil HCl
Alfentanil HCl Novation
Amphetamine Salt Combo
Amytal Sodium
APAP/Oxycodone
Aspirin/Oxycodone
Astramorph PF
Avinza
B & O Supprettes 15A
B & O Supprettes 16A
Belladonna/Opium
Bupivacaine/Fentanyl Citrate/Sodium
  Chloride
Bupivacaine/Hydromorphone/Sodium
  Chloride
Cocaine HCl
Codeine Phosphate
Codeine Sulfate
Concerta
Demerol Hydrochloride
Desoxyn
Dexedrine
Dexedrine Spansules
Dextroamphetamine Sulfate
Dextrose/Morphine Sulfate
Dextrostat
Dilaudid
Dilaudid-5
Dilaudid-HP
Dolophine HCl
Duragesic
Duramorph
Endocet
Endocodone
Endodan
Fentanyl Citrate
Fentanyl Citrate/Sodium Chloride
Focalin
Hydromorphone HCl
Hydromorphone HCl/Sodium
  Chloride
Infumorph
Kadian
Levo-Dromoran
Levorphanol Tartrate
Mepergan
Meperidine HCl
Meperidine HCl/Promethazine HCl
Meperidine HCl/Sodium Chloride

Meperitab
Meprozine
Metadate CD
Metadate ER
Methadone HCl
Methadone HCl Intensol
Methadose
Methylin
Methylin ER
Methylphenidate HCl
Morphine Sulfate
Morphine Sulfate/Sodium Chloride
MS Contin
MSIR
Nembutal Sodium
Numorphan HCl
Opium
Oramorph SR
Orlaam
Oxy IR
Oxycodone HCl
Oxycontin
Oxydose
Oxyfast
Percocet
Percodan
Percolone
Ritalin
Ritalin-SR
Rms
Roxanol
Roxanol 100
Roxanol-T
Roxicet
Roxicodone
Roxicodone Intensol
Roxilox
Seconal Sodium
Sublimaze
Sufenta
Sufentanil Citrate
Tuinal
Tylox

Category CIII

Ultiva
Acetaminophen/Codeine Tablets
Acetaminophen/Codeine #4
A-G Tussin
Anadrol-50
Anaplex HD
Androderm
Androgel
Android

Anexsia
APAP/Butalbital/Caffeine/Codeine
APAP/Codeine Tablets
APAP/Hydrocodone Bitartrate
Ascomp w/Codeine
Aspirin w/Codeine
Aspirin w/Codeine #3
Aspirin w/Codeine #4
Aspirin/Butalbital/Caffeine
Aspirin/Butalbital/Caffeine/Codeine
Aspirin/Carisoprodol/Codeine
Aspirin/Codeine
Atuss EX
Atuss G
Atuss HD
Atuss MS
Bancap HC
Bontril PDM
Bontril Slow-Release
Brontex Tablets
B-Tuss
Butalbital Compound
Butalbital Compound w/Codeine
Butisol Sodium
Carbinoxamine/Hydrocodone/PSE
Ceta Plus
Chlorgest HD
Codafed Expectorant
Codal-DH
Codeine Phosphate/Guaifenesin
  Tablets
Codeine/Guaifenesin
Codiclear DH
Codimal DH
Codituss DH
Codotuss
Co-Gesic
Coldcough HC
Colrex Compound
Co-Tussin
Cotuss-V
CPM/Hydrocodone/Phenylephrine
CPM/Hydrocodone/Pseudoephedrine
Crantex HC
Cytuss HC
Damason-P
Deca-Durabolin
Decotuss-HD
Delatestryl
Depo-Testadiol
Depo-Testosterone
Detussin
Didrex
Dolorex Forte

Donatussin DC
Drituss HD
Duradal HD
Duradal HD Plus
Duratuss HD
Echotuss-HC
ED-TLC
ED-Tuss HC
Efasin-HD
Efasin-HD Plus
Endagen-HD
Endal HD
Endal HD Plus
Enditussin-HD
Endotuss-HD
Enplus-HD
Entex HC
Entuss Expectorant
Exo-Tuss
Fioricet w/Codeine
Fiorinal
Fiorinal w/Codeine
First-Testosterone
Fluoxymesterone
Fortabs
Genecof-HC
Genecof-XP
GG/Hydrocodone/Pseudoephedrine
Giltuss HC
G-Tuss
Guaifenesin/Hydrocodone Bitartrate
Halotestin
H-C Tussive
H-C Tussive-D
Histex HC
Histinex HC
Histinex PV
Histussin-D
Histussin-HC
Homatrop MBR/Hydrocodone
Homatropine/Hydrocodone
Hybolin Decanoate
Hycodan
Hycomal DH
Hycomine Compound
Hycosin Expectorant
Hycotuss Expectorant
Hydone
Hydro PC
Hydro PC II
Hydrocet
Hydrocodone Compound
Hydrocodone CP
Hydrocodone GF

Hydrocodone HD
Hydrogesic
Hydromet
Hydromide
Hydron KGS
Hydropane
Hydrophene DH
Hydro-Tussin HC
Hydro-Tussin HD
Hydro-Tussin XP
Hyphed
Hyphen-HD
Iodal HD
Iotussin D
Iotussin HC
Jaycof Expectorant
Jaycof-HC
Jaycof-XP
KG-Dal HD
KG-Dal HD Plus
KG-Fed
KG-Fed Expectorant
KG-Tuss HD Expectorant
KG-Tussin
Kwelcof
Laniroif
Levall 5.0
Lorcet 10/650
Lorcet Plus
Lorcet-HD
Lortab
Lortab 10/500
Lortab 2.5/500
Lortab 5/500
Lortab 7.5/500
Lortab Asa
Marcof Expectorant
Margesic-H
Marinol
Maxidone
Maxi-Tuss HC
M-Clear
Medcodin
Medtuss HD
Melfiat
M-End
Methitest
Nalex DH
Nalex Expectorant
Nandrolone Decanoate
Norco
Notuss
Nucodine
Nucodine Expectorant

Nucofed
Nucofed Expectorant
Nucotuss Expectorant
Nudal HD
Obezine
Oxandrin
Pancof HC
Pancof XP
Panlor DC
Panlor SS
Paregoric
Pentothal
Pentothal Transfer Kit
Phenaphen w/Codeine
Phendal-HD
Phendiet
Phendiet-105
Phendimetrazine
Phendimetrazine Bitartrate
Phendimetrazine Tartrate
Phrenilin w/Caffeine/Codeine
Pneumotussin
Pneumotussin 2.5
Poly-Tussin
Poly-Tussin HD
Poly-Tussin XP
Prelu-2
Pro-Cof
Pro-Cof D
Prolex DH
Protuss
Protuss-D
P-V-Tussin
Pyregesic-C
Qrp Tussin
Quindal-HD
Quintex HC
Q-V Tussin
Soma Compound w/Codeine
S-T Forte 2
Stagesic
Stagesic-10
Status Green
Su-Tuss HD
Synalgos-DC
Teslac
Testoderm TTS
Testosterone
Testosterone Propionate
Testred
Testro AQ
Testro-L.A.
T-Gesic
Trimal DH

Tussadur-HD
Tussafed-HC
Tuss-AX
Tuss-DS
Tussend
Tussend Expectorant
Tuss-ES
Tuss-HC
Tussigon
Tussionex Pennkinetic
Tuss-PD
Tuss-S
Tylenol w/Codeine #3
Tylenol w/Codeine #4
Uni Tuss HC
Vanacet
Vanacon
Vanex-HD
Vicoclear
Vicodin
Vicodin ES
Vicodin HP
Vicodin Tuss
Vicodin Tuss Expectorant
Vicoprofen
Vi-Q-Tuss
Virilon
Vitussin Expectorant
Vortex
Winstrol
Ztuss Expectorant
Zydone

Category CIV

Acetaminophen/Pentazocine HCl
Acetaminophen/Propoxyphene HCl
Adipex-P
Alprazolam
Alprazolam Intensol
Ambien
Amidrine
Amitriptyline/Chlordiazepoxide
APAP/Dichloral/Isometheptene
APAP/Pentazocine HCl
APAP/Propoxyphene
APAP/Propoxyphene Napsylate
Aquachloral Supprettes
Aspirin/Caffeine/Propoxyphene
Ativan
Atti-Plex P Tablet #1
Brevital Sodium
Butorphanol Tartrate
Butorphanol Tartrate Novation
Chloral Hydrate

Chlordiazepoxide
Chlordiazepoxide HCl
Clonazepam
Clorazepate Dipotassium
Cylert
Dalmane
Darvocet-N 100
Darvocet-N 50
Darvon
Darvon Compound-65
Darvon-N
Diastat
Diastat Pediatric
Diastat Universal
Diazepam
Diazepam Intensol
Diethylpropion HCl
Doral
Duradrin
Epidrin
Equagesic
Estazolam
Flurazepam HCl
Flurazepam Hydrochloride
Gen-Xene
Halcion
I.D.A.
Ionamin
Iso-Acetazone
Klonopin
Librium
Limbitrol
Limbitrol DS
Lorazepam
Lorazepam Amerinet
Lorazepam Intensol
Luminal Sodium
MB-Tab
Mebaral
Meprobamate
Meridia
Micrainin
Midazolam HCl
Midazolam HCl Novation
Midrin
Migquin
Migratine
Migrazone
Miltown
Motofen
Naloxone/Pentazocine
Oxazepam
PC-Cap
Pemadd

Pemoline
Phenobarbital
Phenobarbital Sodium
Phenobarbital Sodium Solution
Phentercot
Phentermine HCl
Phentride
Placidyl
PP-Cap
Pro-Fast HS
Pro-Fast SA
Pro-Fast SR
Pronap-100
Propoxyphene Compound
Propoxyphene Compound-65
Propoxyphene HCl
Propoxyphene HCl Compound
Prosom
Provigil
Restoril
Serax
Somnote
Sonata
Stadol
Stadol NS
Talacen
Talwin Compound
Talwin Lactate
Talwin NX
Temazepam
Tenuate
Tenuate Dospan
Trancot
Tranxene SD
Tranxene T-Tab
Triazolam
Valium
Va-Zone
Versed
Xanax

Category CV

Acetaminophen/Codeine Elixir
Acetaminophen/Codeine Solution
APAP/Codeine Elixir
Atropine Sulfate/Diphenoxylate HCl
Atropine/Diphenoxylate
Biotussin AC
Biotussin DAC
Bromodiphenhydramine HCl/Codeine
Brontex Liquid
Bron-Tuss
Buprenex
Buprenorphine HCl

Capital w/Codeine
Cheracol w/Codeine
Cheratussin AC
Cheratussin DAC
Cod/Phenyl/Prometh
Codafed Pediatric Expectorant
Codeine w/Guaifenesin
Codeine/GG/Pseudoephedrine
  Expectorant
Codeine/Guaifenesin Syrup
Codeine/Promethazine
Codeine/Pseudoephedrine/Triprolidine
Codimal PH
Decohistine DH
Diabetic Tussin C Expectorant
Dihistine DH
Dihistine Expectorant
Duraganidin NR
Endal Expectorant
Gani-Tuss NR
Guaiatussin AC
Guaiatussin DAC
Guai-CO
Guaifen AC
Guaifen-C
Guaifenesin AC Expectorant
Guiatuscon A.C.
Guiatuss AC
Guiatuss DAC
Halotussin AC
Halotussin DAC
Iofen-C NF
Iophen
Iophen C-NR
KG-Fed Pediatric Expectorant
Kolephrin #1
Lomocot
Lomotil
Lonox
Mytussin AC Cough
Mytussin DAC
Novagest DH
Novagest Expectorant w/Codeine
Novahistine DH
Nucodine Pediatric
Nucofed Pediatric Expectorant
Nucotuss Pediatric Expectorant
Orgadin-Tuss
Pediacof
Phenhist Expectorant
Phenylhistine DH Expectorant
Phenylhistine Expectorant
Promethazine VC w/Codeine
Rid-A-Pain w/Codeine

Robafen AC
Robafen DAC
Robitussin-AC
Romilar AC
Ryna-C
Sudatuss-2
Sudatuss-SF
Suttar-2

Suttar-SF
Triacin C
Triacin-C
Tussi-Organidin NR
Tussi-Organidin-S NR
Tussirex
Tylenol w/Codeine
Vi-Atro

Indices

Psychotropic Drugs Indexed by Brand and Generic Name

Listed here are all psychotropic drugs profiled in the first section of the book. Generic names are shown in italics.

A

Adderall, 1
Alprazolam. See Xanax
Ambien, 4
Amitriptyline. See Elavil
Amitriptyline with Perphenazine. See Triavil
Amitriptyline with Chlordiazepoxide. See Limbitrol
Amoxapine, 8
Amphetamines. See Adderall
Anafranil, 11
Aricept, 15
Atarax, 18
Ativan, 20
Aventyl. *See* Pamelor

B

Bupropion. See Wellbutrin
BuSpar, 23
Buspirone. See BuSpar

C

Celexa, 25
Chlordiazepoxide. See Librium
Chlorpromazine. See Thorazine
Citalopram. See Celexa
Clomipramine. See Anafranil
Clonazepam. See Klonopin
Clorazepate. See Tranxene
Clozapine. See Clozaril
Clozaril, 29
Cognex, 34
Compazine, 36
Concerta. *See* Ritalin
Cylert, 41

D

Dalmane, 43
Depakote, 45
Desipramine. See Norpramin
Desoxyn, 50
Desyrel, 53
Dexedrine, 55
Dexmethylphenidate. See Focalin
Dextroamphetamine. See Dexedrine
Diazepam. See Valium

Divalproex. See Depakote
Donepezil. See Aricept
Doral, 60
Doxepin. See Sinequan

E

Effexor, 63
Elavil, 66
Eskalith, 70
Estazolam. See ProSom
Etrafon. *See* Triavil
Exelon, 74

F

Fluoxetine. See Prozac
Fluphenazine. See Prolixin
Flurazepam. See Dalmane
Fluvoxamine. See Luvox
Focalin, 76

G

Galantamine. See Reminyl
Geodon, 80

H

Halcion, 83
Haldol, 87
Haloperidol. See Haldol
Hydroxyzine. See Atarax

I

Imipramine. See Tofranil

K

Klonopin, 90

L

Librium, 94
Limbitrol, 97
Lithium. See Eskalith
Lithobid. *See* Eskalith
Lorazepam. See Ativan
Ludiomil, 100
Luvox, 104

M

Maprotiline. See Ludiomil
Mellaril, 107
Meprobamate. See Miltown

Mesoridazine. See Serentil
Metadate. *See* Ritalin
Methamphetamine. See Desoxyn
Methylin. *See* Ritalin
Methylphenidate. See Ritalin
Miltown, 111
Mirtazapine. See Remeron
Moban, 114
Molindone. See Moban

N
Nardil, 116
Navane, 120
Nefazodone. See Serzone
Nembutal, 123
Norpramin, 126
Nortriptyline. See Pamelor

O
Olanzapine. See Zyprexa
Oxazepam, 129

P
Pamelor, 132
Parnate, 135
Paroxetine. See Paxil
Paxil, 139
Pemoline. See Cylert
Pentobarbital. See Nembutal
Perphenazine. See Trilafon
Phenelzine. See Nardil
Phenergan, 143
Phenobarbital, 147
Prochlorperazine. See Compazine
Prolixin, 150
Promethazine. See Phenergan
ProSom, 154
Protriptyline. See Vivactil
Prozac, 157

Q
Quazepam. See Doral
Quetiapine. See Seroquel

R
Remeron, 161
Reminyl, 163
Restoril, 166
Risperdal, 168
Risperidone. See Risperdal

Ritalin, 172
Rivastigmine. See Exelon

S
Sarafem. *See* Prozac
Secobarbital. See Seconal
Seconal, 176
Serentil, 178
Seroquel, 181
Sertraline. See Zoloft
Serzone, 185
Sinequan, 188
Sonata, 191
Stelazine, 194
Surmontil, 197

T
Tacrine. See Cognex
Temazepam. See Restoril
Thioridazine. See Mellaril
Thiothixene. See Navane
Thorazine, 201
Tofranil, 205
Tranxene, 209
Tranylcypromine. See Parnate
Trazodone. See Desyrel
Triavil, 212
Triazolam. See Halcion
Trifluoperazine. See Stelazine
Trilafon, 216
Trimipramine. See Surmontil

V
Valium, 220
Venlafaxine. See Effexor
Vistaril. *See* Atarax
Vivactil, 223

W
Wellbutrin, 226

X
Xanax, 230

Z
Zaleplon. See Sonata
Ziprasidone. See Geodon
Zoloft, 234
Zolpidem. See Ambien
Zyprexa, 238

Psychotropic Drugs Indexed by Indication

Use this index to determine which drugs are available for a specific psychological problem. Both brand and generic names are listed; the generic names are shown in italics. Only medications profiled in the first section of the book are included.

Agitation
Amitriptyline with Perphenazine. See Triavil
Etrafon. *See* Triavil
Triavil, 212

Alcohol withdrawal
Chlordiazepoxide. See Librium
Clorazepate. See Tranxene
Diazepam. See Valium
Librium, 94
Oxazepam, 129
Tranxene, 209
Valium, 220

Alzheimer's disease
Aricept, 15
Cognex, 34
Donepezil. See Aricept
Exelon, 74
Galantamine. See Reminyl
Reminyl, 163
Rivastigmine. See Exelon
Tacrine. See Cognex

Anxiety disorders
Alprazolam. See Xanax
Amitriptyline with Chlordiazepoxide. See Limbitrol
Amitriptyline with Perphenazine. See Triavil
Atarax, 18
Ativan, 20
BuSpar, 23
Buspirone. See BuSpar
Chlordiazepoxide. See Librium
Clorazepate. See Tranxene
Compazine, 36
Diazepam. See Valium
Doxepin. See Sinequan
Effexor, 63
Etrafon. *See* Triavil
Hydroxyzine. See Atarax
Librium, 94
Limbitrol, 97
Lorazepam. See Ativan

Ludiomil, 100
Maprotiline. See Ludiomil
Meprobamate. See Miltown
Miltown, 111
Nardil, 116
Oxazepam, 129
Paroxetine. See Paxil
Paxil, 139
Phenelzine. See Nardil
Prochlorperazine. See Compazine
Sinequan, 188
Stelazine, 194
Tranxene, 209
Triavil, 212
Trifluoperazine. See Stelazine
Valium, 220
Venlafaxine. See Effexor
Vistaril. *See* Atarax
Xanax, 230

Attention Deficit Hyperactivity Disorder
Adderall, 1
Amphetamines. See Adderall
Concerta. *See* Ritalin
Cylert, 41
Desoxyn, 50
Dexedrine, 55
Dexmethylphenidate. See Focalin
Dextroamphetamine. See Dexedrine
Focalin, 76
Metadate. *See* Ritalin
Methamphetamine. See Desoxyn
Methylin. See Ritalin
Methylphenidate. See Ritalin
Pemoline. See Cylert
Ritalin, 172

Bed-wetting
Imipramine. See Tofranil
Tofranil, 205

Behavior problems in children, severe
Chlorpromazine. See Thorazine
Haldol, 87

Haloperidol. See Haldol
Thorazine, 201

Bipolar disorder
Chlorpromazine. See Thorazine
Depakote, 45
Divalproex. See Depakote
Doxepin. See Sinequan
Eskalith, 70
Lithium. See Eskalith
Lithobid. *See* Eskalith
Ludiomil, 100
Maprotiline. See Ludiomil
Olanzapine. See Zyprexa
Sinequan, 188
Thorazine, 201
Zyprexa, 238

Bulimia
Fluoxetine. See Prozac
Prozac, 157

Depression
Amitriptyline. See Elavil
Amitriptyline with Chlordiazepoxide.
   See Limbitrol
Amitriptyline with Perphenazine. See
   Triavil
Amoxapine, 8
Aventyl. See Pamelor
Bupropion. See Wellbutrin
Celexa, 25
Citalopram. See Celexa
Desipramine. See Norpramin
Desyrel, 53
Doxepin. See Sinequan
Effexor, 63
Elavil, 66
Etrafon. See Triavil
Fluoxetine. See Prozac
Imipramine. See Tofranil
Limbitrol, 97
Ludiomil, 100
Maprotiline. See Ludiomil
Mirtazapine. See Remeron
Nardil, 116
Nefazodone. See Serzone
Norpramin, 126
Nortriptyline. See Pamelor
Pamelor, 132
Parnate, 135
Paroxetine. See Paxil
Paxil, 139
Phenelzine. See Nardil
Protriptyline. See Vivactil

Prozac, 157
Remeron, 161
Sertraline. See Zoloft
Serzone, 185
Sinequan, 188
Surmontil, 197
Tofranil, 205
Tranylcypromine. See Parnate
Trazodone. See Desyrel
Triavil, 212
Trimipramine. See Surmontil
Venlafaxine. See Effexor
Vivactil, 223
Wellbutrin, 226
Zoloft, 234

Hyperactivity
See Attention Deficit Hyperactivity
   Disorder

Insomnia
Ambien, 4
Dalmane, 43
Doral, 60
Estazolam. See ProSom
Flurazepam. See Dalmane
Halcion, 83
Nembutal, 123
Pentobarbital. See Nembutal
Phenergan, 143
Phenobarbital, 147
Promethazine. See Phenergan
ProSom, 154
Quazepam. See Doral
Restoril, 166
Secobarbital. See Seconal
Seconal, 176
Sonata, 191
Temazepam. See Restoril
Triazolam. See Halcion
Zaleplon. See Sonata
Zolpidem. See Ambien

Narcolepsy
Adderall, 1
Amphetamines. See Adderall
Dexedrine, 55
Dextroamphetamine. See Dexedrine
Metadate. *See* Ritalin
Methylin. *See* Ritalin
Methylphenidate. See Ritalin
Ritalin, 172

Obsessive-compulsive disorder

Anafranil, 11
Clomipramine. See Anafranil
Fluoxetine. See Prozac
Fluvoxamine. See Luvox
Luvox, 104
Paroxetine. See Paxil
Paxil, 139
Prozac, 157
Sertraline. See Zoloft
Zoloft, 234

Panic disorder

Alprazolam. See Xanax
Clonazepam. See Klonopin
Klonopin, 90
Paroxetine. See Paxil
Paxil, 139
Sertraline. See Zoloft
Xanax, 230
Zoloft, 234

Posttraumatic stress disorder

Paroxetine. See Paxil
Paxil, 139
Sertraline. See Zoloft
Zoloft, 234

Premenstrual dysphoric disorder (PMDD)

Sarafem. *See* Prozac
Zoloft, 234

Premenstrual syndrome (PMS)

See Premenstrual dysphoric disorder

Psychotic disorders

Amitriptyline with Perphenazine. See Triavil
Chlorpromazine. See Thorazine
Clozapine. See Clozaril
Clozaril, 29
Compazine, 36
Etrafon. *See* Triavil
Fluphenazine. See Prolixin
Geodon, 80
Haldol, 87
Haloperidol. See Haldol
Mellaril, 107
Mesoridazine. See Serentil
Moban, 114
Molindone. See Moban
Navane, 120
Olanzapine. See Zyprexa
Perphenazine. See Trilafon
Prochlorperazine. See Compazine
Prolixin, 150
Quetiapine. See Seroquel
Risperdal, 168
Risperidone. See Risperdal
Serentil, 178
Seroquel, 181
Stelazine, 194
Thioridazine. See Mellaril
Thiothixene. See Navane
Thorazine, 201
Triavil, 212
Trifluoperazine. See Stelazine
Trilafon, 216
Ziprasidone. See Geodon
Zyprexa, 238

Schizophrenia

See Psychotic disorders

Sedation

See also Anxiety disorders and Insomnia
Atarax, 18
Hydroxyzine. See Atarax
Nembutal, 123
Pentobarbital. See Nembutal
Phenergan, 143
Promethazine. See Phenergan
Vistaril. *See* Atarax

Sleep attacks, recurrent

See Narcolepsy

Sleep difficulties

See Insomnia

Social anxiety disorder

Paroxetine. See Paxil
Paxil, 139

Tics

Haldol, 87
Haloperidol. See Haldol

Psychotropic Drugs Indexed by Category

This index allows you to identify all the psychotropic alternatives in a particular pharmacological category. Remember, though, that even closely related drugs may differ in their therapeutic action and adverse effects. Both brand and generic names are listed; the generic names are shown in italics. Only medications profiled in the first section of the book are included.

Antianxiety agents
Benzodiazepines and combinations
Alprazolam. See Xanax
Amitriptyline with Chlordiazepoxide. See Limbitrol
Ativan, 20
Chlordiazepoxide. See Librium
Clonazepam. See Klonopin
Clorazepate. See Tranxene
Dalmane, 43
Diazepam. See Valium
Doral, 60
Estazolam. See ProSom
Flurazepam. See Dalmane
Halcion, 83
Klonopin, 90
Librium, 94
Limbitrol, 97
Lorazepam. See Ativan
Oxazepam, 129
ProSom, 154
Quazepam. See Doral
Restoril, 166
Temazepam. See Restoril
Tranxene, 209
Triazolam. See Halcion
Valium, 220
Xanax, 230

Miscellaneous antianxiety agents
Atarax, 18
BuSpar, 23
Buspirone. See BuSpar
Doxepin. See Sinequan
Effexor, 63
Hydroxyzine. See Atarax
Meprobamate. See Miltown
Miltown, 111
Paroxetine. See Paxil
Paxil, 139
Sinequan, 188
Venlafaxine. See Effexor
Vistaril. *See* Atarax

Antidepressants
Miscellaneous antidepressants
Bupropion. See Wellbutrin
Desyrel, 53
Effexor, 63
Ludiomil, 100
Maprotiline. See Ludiomil
Mirtazapine. See Remeron
Nefazodone. See Serzone
Remeron, 161
Serzone, 185
Trazodone. See Desyrel
Venlafaxine. See Effexor
Wellbutrin, 226

Monoamine oxidase inhibitors (MAOI)
Nardil, 116
Parnate, 135
Phenelzine. See Nardil
Tranylcypromine. See Parnate

Selective serotonin reuptake inhibitors (SSRI)
Celexa, 25
Citalopram. See Celexa
Fluoxetine. See Prozac
Fluvoxamine. See Luvox
Luvox, 104
Paroxetine. See Paxil
Paxil, 139
Prozac, 157
Sertraline. See Zoloft
Zoloft, 234

Tricyclic antidepressants and combinations
Amitriptyline. See Elavil
Amitriptyline with Chlordiazepoxide. See Limbitrol
Amitriptyline with Perphenazine. See Triavil
Amoxapine, 8
Anafranil, 11
Aventyl. See Pamelor
Clomipramine. See Anafranil

Desipramine. See Norpramin
Doxepin. See Sinequan
Elavil, 66
Etrafon. *See* Triavil
Imipramine. See Tofranil
Limbitrol, 97
Norpramin, 126
Nortriptyline. See Pamelor
Pamelor, 132
Protriptyline. See Vivactil
Sinequan, 188
Surmontil, 197
Tofranil, 205
Triavil, 212
Trimipramine. See Surmontil
Vivactil, 223

Antimanic agents
Depakote, 45
Divalproex. See Depakote
Eskalith, 70
Lithium. See Eskalith
Lithobid. *See* Eskalith

Antipsychotic agents
Miscellaneous antipsychotic agents
Clozapine. See Clozaril
Clozaril, 29
Geodon, 80
Haldol, 87
Haloperidol. See Haldol
Moban, 114
Molindone. See Moban
Navane, 120
Olanzapine. See Zyprexa
Quetiapine. See Seroquel
Risperdal, 168
Risperidone. See Risperdal
Seroquel, 181
Thiothixene. See Navane
Ziprasidone. See Geodon
Zyprexa, 238

Phenothiazines and combinations
Chlorpromazine. See Thorazine
Compazine, 36
Fluphenazine. See Prolixin
Mellaril, 107
Mesoridazine. See Serentil
Perphenazine. See Trilafon
Prochlorperazine. See Compazine
Prolixin, 150
Serentil, 178

Stelazine, 194
Thioridazine. See Mellaril
Thorazine, 201
Trifluoperazine. See Stelazine
Trilafon, 216

Central nervous system stimulants
Amphetamines
Adderall, 1
Amphetamines. See Adderall
Desoxyn, 50
Dexedrine, 55
Dextroamphetamine. See Dexedrine
Methamphetamine. See Desoxyn

Miscellaneous central nervous system stimulants
Concerta. *See* Ritalin
Cylert, 41
Dexmethylphenidate. See Focalin
Focalin, 76
Metadate. *See* Ritalin
Methylin. *See* Ritalin
Methylphenidate. See Ritalin
Pemoline. See Cylert
Ritalin, 172

Cholinesterase inhibitors (Alzheimer's disease)
Aricept, 15
Cognex, 34
Donepezil. See Aricept
Exelon, 74
Galantamine. See Reminyl
Reminyl, 163
Rivastigmine. See Exelon
Tacrine. See Cognex

Sedatives and hypnotics
Barbiturates
Nembutal, 123
Pentobarbital. See Nembutal
Phenobarbital, 147
Secobarbital. See Seconal
Seconal, 176

Miscellaneous sedatives and hypnotics
Ambien, 4
Phenergan, 143
Promethazine. See Phenergan
Sonata, 191
Zaleplon. See Sonata
Zolpidem. See Ambien

Psychotropic Herbs and Supplements Indexed by Indication

This index identifies the nutritional supplements and herbs generally deemed most promising for specific mental and emotional problems. These products are profiled in Section 5. Although many of them are also used for a variety of nonpsychological ailments, only their psychotropic effects are reflected here.

Age-related memory loss
Acetylcysteine, 784
Alpha-GPC, 788
Arginine Pyroglutamate, 789
DHA, 795
DHEA, 797
Ginkgo, 805
Huperzine A, 809
Vinpocetine, 833

Alzheimer's disease
Acetyl-L-Carnitine, 786
CDP-Choline, 791
DHA, 795
Fish Oil, 801
Gamma-Tocopherol, 804
Huperzine A, 809
NADH, 819
Phosphatidylcholine, 821
Phosphatidylserine, 823
SAMe, 826
Tocotrienols, 830
Vitamin E, 835

Anxiety
St. John's Wort, 828

Attention deficit disorder
DHA, 795
Fish Oil, 801

Brain function deficit
Ginkgo, 805
Zinc, 839

Depression
5-HTP, 783
Choline, 793
DHA, 795
DL-Phenylalanine, 799
Fish Oil, 801
L-Phenylalanine, 814
Myo-Inositol, 817
NADH, 819

SAMe, 826
St. John's Wort, 828

Insomnia
Bugleweed, 790
Hops, 808
Kava Kava, 810
Lavender, 812
Lemon Balm, 813
Melatonin, 816
Passion Flower, 820
Rauwolfia, 824
Valerian, 832

Movement disorders
CDP-Choline, 791
Glycine, 806
NADH, 819
Phosphatidylcholine, 821

Nervousness
Bugleweed, 790
Hops, 808
Kava Kava, 810
Lavender, 812
Lemon Balm, 813
Passion Flower, 820
Rauwolfia, 824
Valerian, 832

Obsessive-compulsive disorder
Myo-Inositol, 817

Panic disorder
Myo-Inositol, 817

Schizophrenia
Fish Oil, 801
Glycine, 806
SAMe, 826

Stroke recovery
Alpha-GPC, 788
CDP-Choline, 791